Immunology of Agir

Ahmad Massoud   •   Nima Rezaei

Editors

Immunology of Aging

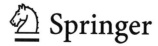 Springer

Editors

Ahmad Massoud, PharmD, MPH, PhD
Department of Immunology
School of Medicine
Tehran University of Medical Sciences
Tehran
Iran

Nima Rezaei, MD, MSc, PhD
Research Center for Immunodeficiencies
Children's Medical Center Hospital
Tehran
Iran

Department of Immunology
School of Medicine
Molecular Immunology Research Center
Tehran University of Medical Sciences
Tehran
Iran

ISBN 978-3-662-52177-9   ISBN 978-3-642-39495-9   (eBook)
DOI 10.1007/978-3-642-39495-9
Springer Heidelberg New York Dordrecht London

Springer is part of Springer Science+Business Media (www.springer.com)

Foreword

The rapidity of scientific progress over the last few years emphasizes the utility of a new collection of state-of-the-art reviews on the immunology of aging, as edited here by Drs Massoud and Rezaei. They have succeeded in putting together a remarkable set of contributions from many well-known scientists in the immunosenescence research field.

Because the number of elderly people is increasing, both in the rich world and in developing countries, aging is a huge challenge for society globally and for the science of biogerontology. Our knowledge of aging processes has exploded during this last decade, and we are starting really to understand what aging means and what causes it, even if our knowledge is still fragmentary. Nonetheless, most of this knowledge has not yet been translated meaningfully into the clinical setting. In addition to comprehensive coverage of basic research in immunity and aging, this book emphasizes the eventual clinical implications of this work.

One essential target of the complex physiological changes occurring in all organ systems with aging is the immune system. We can conceptualize this change in the immune system either as a dynamic dysregulation or an adaptation to an ever-changing universe of pathogen exposures. There is no current consensus on what the exact changes covered by the general term "immunosenescence" actually are. There is even less consensus on the causes of these changes. Also because of these controversies, it seems timely to publish a book featuring different viewpoints as represented by the many different authors. Thus, this book comprehensively treats most aspects of the immunology of aging.

The first three chapters deal with the concept of integrating age-associated changes of the immune system in the general dynamic changes of the organism, by a holistic approach. Thus, knowledge of immune system interactions (either positive or negative) with other physiological systems such as the neuroendocrine system is essential for understanding immunosenescence. Moreover, the immune system appears to be a more sensitive "marker" or "surrogate" for biological aging, being more indicative of the state of bodily functioning than chronological age. This exceptional natural aging of the immune system has been integrated and experimentally challenged in the oxy-inflamm-aging theory and the altered functions of somatic stem cells. Thereafter, Chap. 4 deals with the many different theories of aging and concludes that the inflammation theory, stated as mostly integrative of all the others, is supported by much experimental evidence, such as in the domain of oxidative stress, autophagy, and DNA repair pathways.

Because the immune system is divided into the two main arms of innate and adaptive immunity, the next four chapters deal with the innate immune system separately by describing the behavior of the individual cells which constitute it. Alterations to neutrophil, eosinophil, and basophil functions in aging are concluded to be mainly due to signaling alterations; this offers potential therapeutic targets in these cells. Another chapter discusses the essential role of dendritic cell alterations in immunosenescence. The next is devoted to changes in NK cell phenotypes and functions with aging. Their potentially important role in connection with cancer is discussed in detail. Finally, the role of the pattern recognition receptors in innate cells is reviewed from a functional and evolutionary perspective in the context of aging.

The next six chapters review changes in the adaptive immune system with age. Five of these chapters are about T-cell alterations as the most well-studied and important changes in immunosenescence, but B cells are not neglected as well. One chapter reviews the repertoire changes in T cells with aging leading to increased incidence of infections by newly encountered pathogens and an altered vaccination response. Reciprocal to this change is the increase of memory T cells, especially CD8+ T cells, induced by chronic antigenic challenges such as CMV infection. The next two chapters on T cells are dedicated to functional changes in T cells with aging and to the underlying mechanisms. The potential biomarker role of these changes for healthy aging is also mentioned. These chapters additionally describe how such alterations to T-cell function are related to many age-related diseases such as infections and cancer. T-cell aging may be considered as a hallmark of many pathological processes and changes observed with aging. The next chapter enlarges our understanding of the causes of these age-associated alterations in T cells by describing the metabolic alterations in different T-cell subsets. Finally, changes to Tregs are discussed in the next chapter in relation to aging and age-associated diseases. The last chapter in this part dealing with the adaptive immune response is devoted to B cells, changes to which are discussed in relation to the increased susceptibility to infections and decreased vaccine response in elderly subjects. Chapter 15 moves to the essential role of miRNAs in immunosenescence in relation to other genetic alterations, while the next chapter explains immunogenetics of aging. The next three chapters deal with the higher incidence of infections in elderly subjects, especially influenza infection and its prevention by vaccination. The incidence of several infections is increasing in the elderly, including sepsis due to *E. coli* or Staphylococcus infections as described in the first chapter of this section. This increased incidence of infections either at home or in hospitals is mainly due to age-associated dysregulated immune system. The next chapter specifically discusses the effects of influenza in the elderly and the possible causative immune alterations involved. Influenza is typically a disease of the elderly, and most mortality occurs in people over 60 years old. Finally, the last chapter reviews the requirement for new vaccines and new vaccine strategies in the elderly and specifically discusses recent progress in the field of influenza vaccination (such as adjuvant addition, different routes of administration, or the enhanced antigenicity of the vaccines).

The next part of the book includes three chapters dealing with an important aspect of aging and especially of immunity, specifically the effects of nutrition and diet. The first chapter in this part describes the role of body reserves and nutritional uptake as essential prerequisites for well-functioning immune responses, which do take a large amount of energy delivered by nutrients that can be deficient in most of the elderly people. The second chapter in this section describes the role and importance of a diet adequate for major nutrients, vitamins, and oligoelements as being essential for healthy aging and for a well-functioning immune system. The gut microbiota also depends on an adequate diet. Malnutrition associated with aging may largely contribute to immunosenescence. Caloric restriction and the Mediterranean diet may have some beneficial roles and are to be favored by the elderly. The last chapter discusses the specific role of Zn which intervenes in enzyme and protein functions and in genomic stability. There are several causes for decreased Zn availability in the elderly, but supplementation can yield conflicting results. Nutrigenomics and how it should be applied to the elderly need to be considered in future studies.

The next two chapters discuss the role of oxidative stress in the aging process and in immunosenescence. Oxidative stress plays an important role in cell senescence by modulating proliferative and functional capacities. There is an interplay between oxidative stress and the inflammatory process characterizing the aging immune system.

One chapter is devoted to skin aging and immunosenescence. The visible changes and the underlying molecular alterations are largely influenced by the dysregulated immune system with aging in some way specific to the skin.

The last chapter discusses the effect of physical exercise on the immune system with aging. Physical activity has many beneficial effects on the modulation of age-related diseases and even on longevity and healthy aging. Most studies are cross-sectional, but some longitudinal studies have been performed. Many immune parameters have been studied, often with disparate results. Nonetheless, it seems that exercise is able to enhance immune function in elderly subjects and possibly even postpone the occurrence of immunosenescence. Physical activity is thus beneficial for the elderly and their immune functions.

Considering the broad overview of immunosenescence and its consequences, and their potential modulation, this book should fill a gap in a timely manner. It should be on the shelves of every library as a very useful tool for researchers as well as students.

Tamas Fulop, MD, PhD
Research Center on Aging, University of Sherbrooke,
Sherbrooke, QC, Canada

Graham Pawelec, PhD
Department of Internal Medicine,
University of Tuebingen Medical School,
Tuebingen, German

Preface

Aging is defined as the accumulation of changes in a person over time. It is well established that the overall immune function declines with advancing age, a phenomenon referred to as immunosenescence. Several studies have been performed during recent decades, indicating the pathological consequences of age-related changes in the immune system, leading to a variety of manifestations such as increased susceptibility to infections and an increased tendency toward autoimmunity and immunopathology. Immune function in elderly is not deteriorating by random; rather, it appears to be under genetic control, as well as environmental factors such as diet and lifestyle. Therefore, maintaining a healthy lifestyle is an important contributing factor in supporting a more functional immune system during aging. It should be noted that average age of the world's population is increasing at an unprecedented rate. The concept that changes in the immune system may be a fundamental predisposing factor to the overall aging complications is a field of scientific inquiry and remained ambiguous in many aspects.

We are delighted to edit the book *The Immunology of Aging*, the book which is a result of extensive collaboration of more than sixty great thinkers and scholars in collaboration with a number of juniors in this field, from more than ten different countries. While we are thankful to all of them for making it possible, we would also like to acknowledge the effort of one of our medical students, Armin Hirbod-Mobarakeh, who not only contributed in drafting a chapter but also helped in technical and language edition of the whole chapters.

Whether your interests are immunological aspects of aging, age-related diseases, and longevity, this book can serve as an appropriate venue. Contributing authors in this book present a broad multidisciplinary background on the immunological facets of aging. The aim of this book is to summarize the most up-to-date information on the scientific issues in aging of the immune system research with an insight into the effect of this process on susceptibilities to diseases which are most common among elders. The retrieval strategies to slow down the decline in the immune system in the elderly are another subject detailed extensively. We hope that the book would be welcomed by the scientists and clinicians with interest in the field of aging.

Tehran, Iran   Ahmad Massoud, PharmD, MPH, PhD
Tehran, Iran   Nima Rezaei, MD, MSc, PhD

Contents

Contributors

Seyed Hossein Aalaei-andabili, MD Research Center for
Immunodeficiencies, Children's Medical Center, Tehran University of
Medical Sciences, Tehran, Iran

Giulia Accardi, MSc Department of Pathobiology and Medical and
Forensic Biotechnologies, University of Palermo, Palermo, Italy

Anshu Agrawal, PhD Division of Basic and Clinical Immunology,
University of California, Irvine, CA, USA

Ali Akbar Amirzargar, PhD Molecular Immunology Research Center,
Tehran University of Medical Sciences, Tehran, Iran

Department of Immunology, School of Medicine,
Tehran University of Medical Sciences, Tehran, Iran

Sima Balouchi Anaraki, MSc Department of Immunology,
Isfahan University of Medical Sciences, Isfahan, Iran

Fatemeh Asgari, MSc Department of Immunology, School of Medicine,
Iran University of Medical Sciences, Tehran, Iran

Carmela Rita Balistreri, PhD Department of Pathobiology and Medical
and Forensic Biotechnologies, University of Palermo, Palermo, Italy

Stuart J. Bennett, PhD Life and Health Sciences, Aston University,
Birmingham, UK

Austin B. Bigley Laboratory of Integrated Physiology, Department of
Health and Human Performance, University of Houston, Houston, TX, USA

Marcia A. Blackman, PhD Trudeau Institute, Saranac Lake, NY, USA

Diana Boraschi, PhD National Research Council, Pisa, Italy

Xavier Camous, PhD Singapore Immunology Network (SIgN),
Agency for Science Technology and Research, Singapore, Singapore

Carmen Campos, MSc Department of Immunology, IMIBIC – Reina
Sofia University Hospital – University of Cordoba, Cordoba, Spain

Giuseppina Candore, PhD Department of Pathobiology and Medical and
Forensic Biotechnologies, University of Palermo, Palermo, Italy

Calogero Caruso, MD Department of Pathobiology and Medical and Forensic Biotechnologies, University of Palermo, Palermo, Italy

Katalin Martits Chalangari, MD Monalisa Dermatology, Skin and Stem Cell Research Center, Tehran University of Medical Sciences, Tehran, Iran

Reza Chalangari, MD Monalisa Dermatology, Skin and Stem Cell Research Center, Tehran University of Medical Sciences, Tehran, Iran

Laura Costarelli, PhD Translational Centre of Research in Nutrition and Ageing, Italian National Research Centres on Ageing (INRCA), Ancona, Italy

Monica De la Fuente, PhD Department of Physiology, Faculty of Biology, Complutense University of Madrid, Madrid, Spain

Giuseppe Del Giudice, MD, PhD Research Center, Novartis Vaccines and Diagnostics, Siena, Italy

Irundika H.K. Dias, PhD Life and Health Sciences, Aston University, Birmingham, UK

Christopher R. Dunston, PhD Life and Health Sciences, Aston University, Birmingham, UK

Mohamad Bagher Eslami, PhD Immunology Division, Pathobiology Department, School of Public Health, Tehran University of Medical Sciences, Tehran, Iran

Robertina Giacconi, PhD Translational Centre of Research in Nutrition and Ageing, Italian National Research Centres on Ageing (INRCA), Ancona, Italy

Helen R. Griffiths, PhD Life and Health Sciences, Aston University, Birmingham, UK

Sudhir Gupta, MD, PhD Division of Basic and Clinical Immunology, University of California, Irvine, CA, USA

Armin Hirbod-Mobarakeh, MPH Molecular Immunology Research Center, Tehran University of Medical Sciences, Tehran, Iran

Justin W. Killick, BSc Life and Health Sciences, Aston University, Birmingham, UK

Pierre Olivier Lang, MD, MPH, PD, PhD Nescens Centre of Preventive Medicine, Clinique of Genolier, Genolier, Switzerland

Translational Medicine Research Group, School of Health, Cranfield University, Cranfield, UK

Anis Larbi, PhD Singapore Immunology Network (SIgN), Agency for Science Technology and Research, Singapore, Singapore

Emily C. LaVoy Laboratory of Integrated Physiology, Department of Health and Human Performance, University of Houston, Houston, TX, USA

Maryam Mahmoudi, MD, PhD School of Nutrition and Dietetics, Tehran University of Medical Sciences, Tehran, Iran

Marco Malavolta, PhD Translational Centre of Research in Nutrition and Ageing, Italian National Research Centres on Ageing (INRCA), Ancona, Italy

Parvin Mansouri, MD Dermatology Department, Skin and Stem Cell Research Center, Tehran University of Medical Sciences, Tehran, Iran

Ahmad Massoud, PharmD, MPH, PhD Department of Immunology, School of Medicine, Tehran University of Medical Sciences, Tehran, Iran

Amir Hossein Massoud, PhD Meakins-Christie Laboratories, McGill University, Montreal, QC, Canada

Department of Microbiology and Immunology, McGill University, Montreal, QC, Canada

Janet E. McElhaney, MD, FRCPC, FACP Vancouver Coastal Health Research Institute, University of British Columbia, Vancouver, BC, Canada

Milad Mirmoghtadaei, MBBS Department of Clinical Sciences, University of Sharjah, Sharjah, UAE

Behjat Al-Sadat Moayedi Esfahani, PharmD, SBB, MSc Department of Immunology, Isfahan University of Medical Sciences, Isfahan, Iran

Kasra Moazzami, MD, MPH Cardiovascular Research Center, Massachusetts General Hospital, Harvard Medical School, Charlestown, MA, USA

Eugenio Mocchegiani, PhD Translational Centre of Research in Nutrition and Ageing, Italian National Research Centres on Ageing (INRCA), Ancona, Italy

Sara Morgado, PhD Immunology Unit, Department of Physiology, University of Extremadura, Cáceres, Spain

Mohammad Hossein Nicknam, MD, PhD Department of Immunology, Molecular Immunology Research Center, Tehran University of Medical Sciences, Tehran, Iran

Alejandra Pera, PhD Department of Immunology, IMIBIC – Reina Sofia University Hospital – University of Cordoba, Cordoba, Spain

Rino Rappuoli, PhD Research Center, Novartis Vaccines and Diagnostics, Siena, Italy

Nima Rezaei, MD, MSc, PhD Research Center for Immunodeficiencies, Children's Medical Center, Tehran, Iran

Molecular Immunology Research Center, Tehran University of Medical Sciences, Tehran, Iran

Department of Immunology, School of Medicine, Tehran University of Medical Sciences, Tehran, Iran

Alireza Rezaiemanesh, MSc Department of Immunology, Tehran University of Medical Sciences, Tehran, Iran

Lothar Rink, PhD Institute of Immunology, Medical Faculty of the RWTH Aachen University, Aachen, Germany

Zahra Saffarian, MD Dermatology Department, Skin and Stem Cell Research Center, Tehran University of Medical Sciences, Tehran, Iran

Beatriz Sánchez-Correa, PhD Immunology Unit, Department of Physiology, University of Extremadura, Cáceres, Spain

Soledad Sánchez Mateos, PhD Immunology Unit, Department of Physiology, University of Extremadura, Cáceres, Spain

Laura Santambrogio, MD, PhD Department of Pathology, Albert Einstein College of Medicine, New York, NY, USA

Karim H. Shalaby, PhD Meakins-Christie Laboratories, Department of Physiology, Faculty of Medicine, McGill University, Montreal, QC, Canada

Meakins-Christie Laboratories, Department of Medicine, Research Institute of the McGill University Health Centre, McGill University, Montreal, QC, Canada

Mehdi Shekarabi, PhD Department of Immunology, School of Medicine, Iran University of Medical Sciences, Tehran, Iran

Richard J. Simpson, PhD Laboratory of Integrated Physiology, Department of Health and Human Performance, University of Houston, Houston, TX, USA

Rafael Solana, MD, PhD Department of Immunology, IMIBIC – Reina Sofia University Hospital – University of Cordoba, Cordoba, Spain

Guillaume Spielmann, PhD Laboratory of Integrated Physiology, Department of Health and Human Performance, University of Houston, Houston, TX, USA

Raquel Tarazona, MD, PhD Immunology Unit, Department of Physiology, University of Extremadura, Cáceres, Spain

Peter Uciechowski, PhD Institute of Immunology, Medical Faculty of the RWTH Aachen University, Aachen, Germany

Aleksandra M. Urbanska, PhD Department of Pathology, Albert Einstein College of Medicine, New York, NY, USA

Paolo Verzani Department of Pathology, Albert Einstein College of Medicine, New York, NY, USA

David L. Woodland, PhD Keystone Symposia, Silverthorne, CO, USA

Alireza Zare-Bidoki, MSc Department of Immunology, School of Medicine, Tehran University of Medical Sciences, Tehran, Iran

Valerio Zolla, PhD Department of Pathology, Albert Einstein College of Medicine, New York, NY, USA

An Introduction on the Old Age and the Aging of the Immune System

1

Mohamad Bagher Eslami

1.1 Aging and the Immune System

The period of old age is the last part of an individual's life which follows the period of middle age and terminates by death. The transition from previous periods of life into the period of old age is relatively fast in some people, while it is very slow in others. Genetics and environmental factors are the forces determining the pace of this transition.

No biomarker in blood or tissues has so far been recognized to definitely indicate the onset of the period of old age. However, telomere length has been considered a possible biomarker of aging (Sanders and Newman 2013). Telomeres are nucleotide sequences in both ends of the each chromosome which protect the chromosomes from erosion and shortening. By advancing age after each cell division, the telomeres' ends become shorter (Hohensinner et al. 2012; Goronzy et al. 2006; Sanders and Newman 2013).

The immune system is very vital for the well-being and general health of every individual by providing a state of immunity. The immune system in aged people has been the focus of several groups of researchers. Their findings indicate that the immune system is not immune from becoming ineffectual owing to advancing age (Rymkiewicz et al. 2012; Weiskopf et al. 2009). Therefore, the immune system is not a self-governing system which develops and functions independently of other systems in our bodies (Rymkiewicz et al. 2012). In general, decrease in the physiological potential of a system affects the optimum function of other systems.

B and T lymphocytes, the most vital cells of the adaptive immune system, undergo replication upon each specific immune response. Therefore, shortening of the telomeres in the activated B and T cell populations is presumably far greater than the cell population of the innate immune system such as macrophage and dendritic cells (Weng 2006; Kaszubowska 2008). Thus, if we accept the view that telomere shortening is a far more important factor than the other factors affecting the aging of systems, the adaptive immune system seems to be one of the forerunners influenced by aging, whereas the innate immune system keeps its potentials for a longer period (Kaszubowska 2008).

The immune system encompasses a large number of different cell types and molecules. The communication between different cell types in the immune system, which are often far apart, is dependent on a complex network of cytokines. The aging can affect any element of this highly complex system which in turn greatly influences all parts of the immune system (Huang et al. 2005).

M.B. Eslami, PhD
Immunology Division, Pathobiology Department,
School of Public Health, Tehran University
of Medical Sciences, Tehran, Iran
e-mail: eslamimb@tums.ac.ir

A. Massoud, N. Rezaei (eds.), *Immunology of Aging*,
DOI 10.1007/978-3-642-39495-9_1, © Springer-Verlag Berlin Heidelberg 2014

1.2   Research on Aging Immune System

There has recently been a growing body of literature on the subject of the aging of the immune system. There are now reasonable evidences indicating that a level of immunodeficiency with variable grades occurs among the elderly (Rymkiewicz et al. 2012; Larbi et al. 2008; Goronzy and Weyand 2012). However, much more research on the subject of aging of the immune system is necessary to shed light on the many untouched subjects in this field and also to clarify controversial topics (Grubeck-Loebenstein and Wick 2002; Weiskopf et al. 2009; Pahlavani 2000). The inconsistency observed between different studies on the immune system of the elderly is most probably due to the physiological differences between the groups of elderly selected as study subjects. It has been amiably showed that the interindividual differences observed in the young are even larger in the elderly individuals (Rymkiewicz et al. 2012). To reduce the differences induced by the environment and other factors among aged individuals who participate in research projects, the physiological functions of their major organs, the past and present health status, the environment where they lived, as well as their age should be all taken into consideration. Apart from this, conducting a research project on the subject of the aging of the immune system has particular limitations (Seppet et al. 2011). For example, it is not ethically feasible to take venous blood samples from a healthy aged individual on several time points.

The period of old age in some individuals could be as long as 30 years or longer. The immune system during this long period undergoes changes due to more advancing age. It is therefore very vital to acquire more knowledge about the effects of aging on this highly complex system. The well-being, health of the old people, and possible restoration of the potential of this system rely largely on the efforts of the researchers and valuable knowledge which will become available upon further research on this subject.

References

Goronzy JJ, Weyand CM (2012) Immune aging and autoimmunity. Cell Mol Life Sci 69(10):1615–1623

Goronzy JJ, Fujii H, Weyand CM (2006) Telomeres, immune aging and autoimmunity. Exp Gerontol 41(3):246–251

Grubeck-Loebenstein B, Wick G (2002) The aging of the immune system. Adv Immunol 80:243–284

Hohensinner PJ, Goronzy JJ, Weyand CM (2012) Telomere dysfunction, autoimmunity and aging. Aging Dis 2(6):524–537

Huang H, Patel DD, Manton KG (2005) The immune system in aging: roles of cytokines, T cells and NK cells. Front Biosci 10:192–215

Kaszubowska L (2008) Telomere shortening and ageing of the immune system. J Physiol Pharmacol 59(Suppl 9):169–186

Larbi A, Franceschi C, Mazzatti D, Solana R, Wikby A, Pawelec G (2008) Aging of the immune system as a prognostic factor for human longevity. Physiology (Bethesda) 23:64–74

Pahlavani MA (2000) Immune dysfunction in the elderly: the role of nutrition. Iran J Allergy Asthma Immunol 1(3):117–127

Rymkiewicz PD, Heng YX, Vasudev A, Larbi A (2012) The immune system in the aging human. Immunol Res 53(1–3):235–250

Sanders JL, Newman AB (2013) Telomere length in epidemiology: a biomarker of aging, age-related disease, both, or neither? Epidemiol Rev 35(1):112–131

Seppet E, Paasuke M, Conte M, Capri M, Franceschi C (2011) Ethical aspects of aging research. Biogerontology 12(6):491–502

Weiskopf D, Weinberger B, Grubeck-Loebenstein B (2009) The aging of the immune system. Transpl Int 22(11):1041–1050

Weng NP (2006) Aging of the immune system: how much can the adaptive immune system adapt? Immunity 24(5):495–499

The Immune System, a Marker and Modulator of the Rate of Aging

2

Monica De la Fuente

2.1 Introduction: The Process of Aging

To understand the role of the immune system in the aging process, it is necessary to remember several key concepts about this process. Aging may be defined as a progressive and general deterioration of the organism's functions that leads to a lower ability to adaptively react to changes and preserve homeostasis. Thus, elderly subjects show a lower capacity to endure extreme situations, infections, and stress in general. If the principal characteristic of a healthy organism is the maintenance of the functional balance at all levels, with aging this balance fails. This accumulation of adverse changes with the passing of time, although it should not be considered a disease, strongly increases the risk of disease and finally results in death. In fact, the difference between senescence and illness is not clearly defined (Carnes et al. 2008). As Strehler (1977) indicated, there are four rules that define aging: (a) It is universal (practically all animal species including the metazoans showing sexual reproduction suffer aging), (b) progressive (the rate of aging is similar at different ages after the adult state), (c) intrinsic (since even if animals are exposed to optimal environmental conditions throughout life, they still experience the aging process at the rate characteristic for their species), and (d) deleterious (aging is obviously detrimental to individuals since it leads to their death, although, at the species level, this detrimental character is arguable since aging is necessary for the replacement of the members of all populations).

The process of aging, which starts when the subjects achieve the adult age that allows their reproduction, finishes with their death. This period represents the mean life span or means longevity, which can be defined as the mean of the time that the subjects of a group born on the same date live. In the case of human beings, this longevity is currently very high in developed countries, where it is 75–83 years. Since we start the aging process at about 18 years of age, we spend most of our lifetime aging. Moreover, we have to consider the maximum life span or maximum longevity (the maximum time that a subject belonging to a determined species can live) and which in humans is about 122 years, whereas in mice it is 3 and in rats 4 years. If the maximum longevity is fixed in each species, and currently impossible to increase, the mean life span of individual organisms shows marked variability and can be increased by environmental factors. This allows the maintenance of good health and permits us to approach the maximum life span in a good condition. A higher mean longevity is achieved by the preservation of good health, and this depends approximately 25 % on the genes and 75 % on lifestyle and environmental factors (Kirkwood 2008) (Fig. 2.1).

M. De la Fuente, PhD
Department of Physiology, Faculty of Biology,
Complutense University of Madrid,
Madrid 28040, Spain
e-mail: mondelaf@bio.ucm.es

A. Massoud, N. Rezaei (eds.), *Immunology of Aging*,
DOI 10.1007/978-3-642-39495-9_2, © Springer-Verlag Berlin Heidelberg 2014

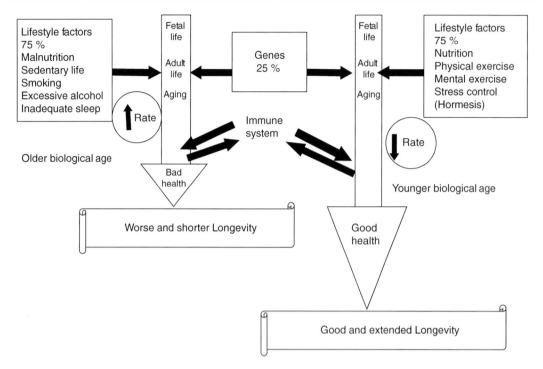

Fig. 2.1 The immune system is a good marker of the rate of aging, and it is involved in the biological age of each subjects and therefore in her/his longevity. The base of a functional longevity is the health maintenance, which depends on the genes in a proportion of 25 %, but in a proportion of 75 % it depends on the lifestyle and environmental factors. The biological age or rate of aging is the result of individual epigenetic mechanisms acting on genes since the fetal life throughout the life of the subject, and it is worth to note that they also depend on lifestyle factors. If these factors are appropriate, the rate of aging will be lower, and we will have a good and extended longevity. In addition, a poor lifestyle accelerates the pace of aging and makes it more difficult to maintain health

2.2   The Concept and Markers of Biological Age

The concept of "biological age" is justified by the fact that the aging process is very heterogeneous. Thus, it is well known that the molecular and cellular deterioration and the impairment of the physiological systems associated with aging do not occur at the same rate in all members of a population of the same chronological age. Biological age represents the rate of aging experienced by each individual and therefore his/her life expectancy, being a better predictor of longevity than chronological age (Borkan and Norris 1980). In fact, the chronological age only gives limited information on the decrease of functional capacity, longevity expectancy, and other aging characteristics (Park et al. 2009).

The problem with biological age is how to determine it. If the chronological age of a subject is easily measurable, the same is not true of biological age. Thus, a number of biochemical, physiological, and psychological parameters that change with age and that show the tendency to a premature death must be determined. Since the first publications of Benjamin (1947), followed by several relevant studies such as those by Borkan and Norris (1980), one of the most complete investigation on biological age; and by Benfante et al. (1985); Ruiz-Torres (1991); or more recently that of Nakamura and Miyao (2007) and Bulpitt et al. (2009), much research has been carried out trying to obtain the most appropriate parameters for indicating the biological age. The retrospective analysis of these studies showed that the subjects presenting certain parameters, which were "more aged" than those found in the majority of the subjects of the same chronological age, had a shorter life expectancy. These biomarkers include those related to respiratory function, systolic arterial tension, hematocrit, biochemistry markers (e.g., albumin and blood urea nitrogen), as well as reaction times determined by psychometric tests. Moreover, they proposed the characteristic that a parameter of biological age should have and suggested that the aging rate is influenced by environmental factors. In addition, since oxidation and inflammation underlies the aging process, which will be mentioned later, several inflammatory and oxidative stress markers have also been proposed recently as predictors of frailty risk (Bandeen-Roche et al. 2009) and biomarkers of aging (Pandey and Rizvy 2010). Nevertheless, in spite of all these studies attempting to extend the parameters of biological age (Bae et al. 2008), the subject is still incomplete (Bulpitt et al. 2009), and more research should be carried out.

2.3   The Immune System as a Marker of Biological Age and Predictor of Longevity

Most research on biological age did not include immune parameters. However, we have to consider that the immune system is a homeostatic system, which contributes to an appropriate functional capacity of the organism, and thus it has been proposed as one of the best markers of health (Wayne et al. 1990; De la Fuente 2004). Although these characteristics of the immune system could lead us to think of the functional capacity of this system as a possible biomarker of aging, only in recent investigations have several immune parameters been suggested as representative of the "true" biological age of a subject. A positive relation has been shown between a good function of the T cells, natural killer (NK) cells, and of phagocytic cells and longevity (Ferguson et al. 1995; Ogata et al. 1997; Guayerbas et al. 2002; Guayerbas and De la Fuente 2003). Also, the levels of immunological parameters such as excess of CD8+CD27−CD28− T cells, low T-cell

proliferative responses in vitro, and low IL-2 secretion are predictors of mortality. These together with increased IL-6 levels and a CD4:CD8 ratio <1 can define the "immune risk profile" in humans (Pawelec 2006). A number of studies carried out in our laboratory have allowed us to propose several immune parameters as being fundamental in calculating the biological age of an individual (Figs. 2.1 and 2.2). Before describing how we obtained the immune profile of biological age, we are going to briefly mention the age-related changes in the immune system or immunosenescence (which are covered in other chapters) as well as in the psychoneuroimmuno-endocrine system.

2.3.1   Age-Related Changes in the Immune System: Immunosenescence

It is known that with aging there is an increased susceptibility to infectious diseases, autoimmune processes, and cancer, which indicates the presence of a less competent immune system, exerting a great influence on the age-related morbidity and mortality (Fulop et al. 2011; Dewan et al. 2012). There are contradictory results in the investigations on immunosenescence as a consequence of many factors, which have not been taken into account (we can mention, e.g., the age, species, strain, and gender of the subjects studied as well as the locations of the immune cells used) (De la Fuente et al. 2011). Nevertheless, it is presently accepted that almost every component of the immune system undergoes striking age-associated restructuring, leading to changes that may include enhanced as well as diminished functions (De la Fuente and Miquel 2009; Arranz et al. 2010a, b, d). There is evidence of the central role played by cell-mediated immunity in immunosenescence (Lang et al. 2013). Thus, some of the key and most marked changes are a pronounced age-related decrease in T-cell functions, with a lower proliferation of lymphocytes and a decrease of several cytokines involved in this process such as interleukin 2 (IL-2) and other functions such as chemotaxis

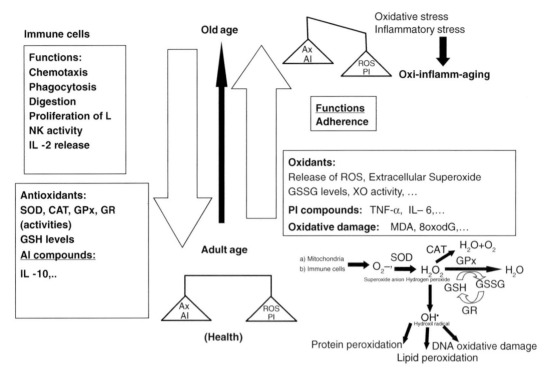

Fig. 2.2 Age-related changes in function, oxidative, and inflammatory stress parameters in immune cells. In the age-associated restructuring of the immune cells or immunosenescence, there is a decrease of several immune cell functions, but an increase in other functions. The immune cells produce in their defensive work important levels of free radicals and reactive oxygen species (*ROS*) and pro-inflammatory (*PI*) compounds, which are involved with the immune response destroying the pathogens. These oxidants and PI compounds, which in certain amounts are essential for our survival, when they are in excess, lead to oxidative and inflammatory stress and the consequent damage of cells. Therefore, the functions of our organism are based on a perfect balance between the levels of ROS and PI and those of antioxidants (*Ax*) and anti-inflammatory (*AI*) defenses. However, with aging a loss of the balance appears, with excess in the production of ROS and PI or insufficient availability of Ax and AI, which leads to an oxi-inflamm-aging. The first oxygen free radical appearing in cells is the superoxide anion (O_2^-), which produces hydrogen peroxide (H_2O_2) and hydroxyl radical ($OH^\cdot$), the most reactive free radical, which carries out the oxidation of biomolecules such as proteins, lipids, and DNA. Cells, in order to protect themselves against oxygen toxicity, have developed a variety of antioxidant mechanisms that prevent the formation of ROS or neutralize them after they are produced. Thus, superoxide dismutase (*SOD*) catalyzes the inactivation of superoxide anion, and catalase (*CAT*) inactivates hydrogen peroxide. The reduced GSH is the most important antioxidant in the organism and neutralizes peroxides using the glutathione peroxidase (*GPx*), and in this action it is transformed to oxidized glutathione (*GSSG*). The antioxidant enzyme glutathione reductase (*GR*) is used to catalyze the reduction of glutathione. Since with age there is an oxi-inflamm-aging, which is the base of the loss of health, immune cells can be involved in the rate of the aging process

(Haynes and Maue 2009; Pawelec et al. 2010; Arranz et al. 2010a, d). This age-related impairment, especially in the CD4+ T-helper (TH) cell, affects cell-mediated and humoral immunity and causes an impaired B-cell function (Frasca and Blomberg 2009). A cell type that has been relatively neglected in studies of age and immunity is the T-regulatory (Treg) subset, which seems to maintain its functional capacity and increase its number with the passing of time. This could explain the greater suppressive activity in the elderly associated with immunosenescence (Wang et al. 2010).

In cells of innate immunity, which have been less frequently studied than lymphocytes with respect to their age-related changes, the NK cells show a decrease in their antitumoral activity, although each subset may be affected differently by aging (reviewed in Shaw et al. 2010; Arranz et al. 2010a; Gayoso et al. 2011). In the phagocytic cells there are contradictory results, but in general they are less affected by the dysfunction that occurs throughout aging than lymphocytes. Nevertheless, they show a decrease in chemotaxis, ingestion, and digestion of phagocytized material (Alonso-Fernandez et al. 2010). However, adherence capacity to tissues, expression of Toll-like receptors (TLR) such as TLR-2 or TLR-4, and the pro-inflammatory cytokine production seem to increase with aging (De la Fuente and Miquel 2009; Arranz et al. 2010b, d). Although phagocytes were thought to play a less critical role in the immune dysfunction that occurs throughout aging (De la Fuente 1985), recent studies show that these cells are responsible for the susceptibility and vulnerability to infections among the aged subjects.

The network of cytokines produced in response to immune challenges has also shown changes with aging. It is important to mention the shift towards Th2 (effecting humoral antibody-mediated immunity) responses and the decrease in anti-inflammatory cytokine production (Arranz et al. 2010a, d).

Thus, currently, despite the rapidly increasing amount of data on immunosenescence in the last decades, the totality of all the changes involved in the different aspects of the immune function with age has not yet been resolved. Moreover, the specific role played by the immune system in the aging process of organisms is not wholly understood.

2.3.2 The Psychoneuro-immunoendocrine System and Its Changes with Aging

As mentioned previously, the immune system is a regulatory system, but it does not work alone. It is in constant and complex communication with the other homeostatic systems, namely, the nervous and the endocrine systems (Besedovsky and del Rey 2007, 2011). Currently, there is abundant work that confirms the bidirectional communication between these regulatory systems, which

is mediated by cytokines, hormones, and neurotransmitter through the presence of their receptors on the cells of the three systems. Therefore, any influence exerted on the immune system will have an effect on the nervous and endocrine systems and vice versa. Moreover, immune, nervous, and endocrine products coexist in lymphoid, neural, and endocrine tissues. All this shows the complexity of the regulation not only at general levels but also at local levels. Thus, presently a psychoneuroimmunoendocrine system is accepted, which allows the preservation of homeostasis and therefore of health. The scientific confirmation of the communication between these systems has permitted the understanding of why situations of depression, emotional stress, or anxiety are accompanied by a greater vulnerability to cancers, infectious, and autoimmune diseases. This agrees with the concept that the immune system is affected (Arranz et al. 2009; Salim et al. 2012). By contrast, pleasant emotions help to maintain a good immune function (Barak 2006).

With aging it is evident that not only the immune system is affected also the other regulatory systems involved in homeostasis. In the nervous system a progressive loss of its function appears, with the hippocampus being especially affected (Couillard-Depres et al. 2011). Moreover, the regulation of stress-related disorders in which the hippocampus is involved is clearly impaired with aging (Garrido 2011). Several changes accompany healthy aging in the endocrine system. These include, for example, the increase of several hormones and the decrease of others such as growth hormone/insulin-like factor-1 axis, sexual hormones, dehydroepiandrosterone, and melatonin (Makrantonaki et al. 2010). Moreover, the age-related disturbances of the hypothalamic-pituitary-adrenal (HPA) axis seem to be relevant for decreasing stress adaptability in old subjects, this being, at least in part, the cause of their health impairment (Lupien et al. 2009).

It is difficult to know if the deterioration with aging of the nervous, endocrine, and immune systems occurs simultaneously or starts in one of them (possibly the neurons are a good candidate to be the first affected), which then influences the others. Nevertheless, many age-related changes happen in the communication between the homeostatic systems (Corona et al. 2012). Thus, there are changes in the innervations of immune organs (such as the decrease of the sympathetic innervation and concentration of noradrenaline (NA) in these organs) and in the expression of receptors of neurotransmitters (as the increase of beta-receptors on the immune cells as a compensatory mechanism). Moreover, the response of immune cells in vitro to neurotransmitters changes with age (Puerto et al. 2005). This defective response of immune cells to mediators of the nervous system could contribute to the process of immunosenescence. Concretely in the case of catecholamines and their catabolites, this could explain the inadequate response to stress that occurs with aging (Bauer 2008; Gouin et al. 2008). In relation to this, the inadequate response to stress is one of the conditions leading to an acceleration of aging accompanied by the impairment of the immune system and other physiological systems. In addition, chronic stressful conditions modify immune functions and their interaction with the nervous system, causing detrimental effects on memory, neural plasticity, and neurogenesis (Yirmiya and Goshen 2011). Thus, it has been shown that mice with chronic hyperreactivity to stress and anxiety show a premature immunosenescence and are prematurely aged (Viveros et al. 2007). Recently, it was also observed that mice exposed to the stressful condition of isolation have behavioral responses that reveal an impairment of cognition, a certain degree of depression, and a more evident immunosenescence than control animals of the same age housed in groups (work in the process of publication). Likewise, human subjects suffering chronic anxiety or depression show a significant premature immunosenescence (Arranz et al. 2007, 2009; Hernanz et al. 2008).

2.3.3 Functions of the Immune System as Markers of Biological Age

The identification of parameters that measure the biological age, which is a better measurement of the rate of aging than the chronological age, is very difficult as has been mentioned previously. Since it has been demonstrated that the competence of the immune system is an excellent marker of health and several age-related changes in immune functions have been linked to longevity, we decided to investigate if some immune functions could be useful as markers of biological age and therefore as predictors of longevity (De la Fuente and Miquel 2009). Since a longitudinal study is impossible to carry out on human subjects throughout the whole aging process, we analyzed several functional parameters in leukocytes of peripheral blood in the different decades of the life of human subjects, from their 20s until their 80s. As we needed a species with a shorter life span to carry out longitudinal studies, we chose mice, which show a mean longevity of about 2 years. Although most studies on immune cells in mice involve the sacrifice of the animals (to obtain the spleen, thymus, etc.), we designed a method to extract these cells without the necessity of killing them or even using anesthesia. This consists of taking leukocytes from the peritoneum, thus allowing us to study the same functional parameters from adult age until the death of the animals.

Among all the possible functions of immune cells, we have focused on those listed in Fig. 2.2: thus, in *lymphocytes*, their ability to adhere to the vascular endothelia, migrate towards the site of antigen recognition (chemotaxis), proliferate in response to mitogens, and release cytokines such as IL-2 and in *phagocytes*, the process of adherence to tissues, chemotaxis, ingestion or phagocytosis of foreign particles, and destruction of pathogens by means of the intracellular production of free radicals such as the superoxide anion and other ROS located in the phagosome of these cells. Further, in the NK cells we have analyzed their capacity to destroy tumoral cells of the same animal species investigated.

Surprisingly our results showed that in the members of both species, similar age-related changes occur in the immune parameters studied. With aging there is a decrease of functions such as the lymphoproliferative response, the IL-2 release, the chemotaxis as well as the NK activity against tumor cells, the latex phagocytosis, and adequate levels of ROS in the phagosomes. In addition, there is an increase of other functions such as adherence of immune cells to tissue, which may prevent their arrival to the site where they have to perform their organism-protecting task (De la Fuente and Miquel 2009). There is also an increase in the release of several cytokines, especially those pro-inflammatory, which is accompanied by a decrease in others such as the anti-inflammatory cytokines (Arranz et al. 2010d).

In order to identify the above parameters as markers of biological age, it is necessary to confirm that the levels shown in particular subjects reveal their real health and senescent conditions and, consequently, their rate of aging. This has been achieved in the following two ways:

(a) Ascertaining that the individuals with those parameters showing values older than those of most subjects of the same population, sex, and chronological age die before their counterparts. This can be confirmed only in experimental animals, and we have used several murine models of premature aging, especially one of mice with poor response to stress and with anxiety, which will be covered later.

(b) Finding that the subjects reaching a very advanced age preserve these parameters at levels similar to those of adults. This can be tested on both humans (centenarians) and experimental animals, such as extremely long-lived mice. While biologically older animals showing the immune competence levels characteristic of chronologically older individuals have been found to die prematurely (Arranz et al. 2010a, d), centenarians and long-lived mice exhibit a high degree of preservation of several immune functions. This may be related to their ability to reach a very advanced age in a healthy condition (Alonso-Fernandez and De la Fuente 2011). All the above results confirm that the immune system is a good marker of biological age and a predictor of longevity.

Moreover, since the evolution of these immune functions is similar in mice and humans, it can be assumed that those humans showing immune parameters at the levels of older subjects have a higher biological age and a shorter longevity.

2.3.4 Murine Models of Premature Immunosenescence

Prematurely aging mice (PAM) in contrast to non-prematurely aging mice (NPAM) of the same population, sex, and chronological age are identified by its poor response in a simple T-maze exploration test. This provides strong support for the concept that the nervous and the immune system are closely linked. In mice showing premature aging, we have observed that the abovementioned immune functions performed at the characteristic levels of older mice. In addition to a more significant immunosenescence, the PAM showed high levels of anxiety and a brain neurochemistry similar to older animals. Nevertheless, the most convincing evidence that the abovementioned parameters are useful markers of biological age is that the PAM showed a shorter life span than their counterpart NPAM of the same age, sex, and chronological age (Viveros et al. 2007; De la Fuente 2010).

Other models of prematurely immunosenescence related with lower longevity are being carried out, such as obese animals (De la Fuente and De Castro 2012) and transgenic mice for Alzheimer's disease (Gimenez-Llort et al. 2012).

2.4 The Involvement of the Immune System in the Rate of Aging

To understand how the immune system can be involved in the rate of aging (Fig. 2.1), it is convenient to remember several concepts on aging, especially those that explain how aging occurs. Thus, herein the most relevant theories of aging will be briefly commented.

2.4.1 The How, Where, and Why of Aging: An Integrative Theory of Aging

As a consequence of the great complexity of the changes associated with aging, more than 300 theories have been proposed to explain this process (Medvedev 1990). However, presently most of these theories have been abandoned since they do not have clear research support and even the most widely accepted theories of aging offer partial explanations of the causes and effects of this process. Moreover, many of them only are based on the consequences of the aging process but do not deal with the causes of this process. For a theory to be accepted, it should be applicable to the different levels of biological organization (molecular, cellular, and physiological) in all the multicellular animals with sexual reproduction. Thus, the determinist group of theories, in which it is proposed that aging is the result of a deliberate program driven by genes, do not have this universal application. For example, Hayflick's mitotic clock theory, which was widely accepted during the last few decades of the last century, has been discarded by the author himself, mentioning in 2007 (Hayflick 2007) that "The weight of evidence indicates that genes do not drive the aging process…" and "Aging is an increase in molecular disorders. It is a stochastic process that occurs systemically after reproductive maturity in animals that reach a fixed size in adulthood." In addition, the theory of shortening telomeres (Goyns 2002), which considers aging as the cause of the shortening of telomeres (this fact occurs when the cells dividing), is also without application to those physiological systems with fundamentally only fixed postmitotic cells such as the heart and the brain and to those animals basically constitute with these postmitotic cells as is the case of Drosophila melanogaster. Thus, these determinist theories should be considered possible explanations of cell differentiation processes and replicative cellular senescence that are consequences of the aging process, but not the base of organism aging. Moreover, although a link between telomere length and longevity has been described, this seems to be explained by the levels of oxidative stress (Atzmon et al. 2010), a fact that will be commented. Another big group of theories, the "epigenetic theories," indicates that aging is the result of events that are not guided by a program but are stochastic or random events and it is not genetically programmed. In this group several theories on relevant physiological systems such as "the immune theory" and the "neuroendocrine theory" can be included. It is true that the immune system is very important for the life of animals, but it is accepted that lymphocytes, especially T cells, are the most clearly impaired with aging. However, there are many animal species without lymphocytes, and they suffer the aging process. Similar comments can be done of other theories of aging, which shows that most of these theories indicate events that are consequence of the aging process but not its cause, since they are not universal application.

Among the epigenetic theories, that of the free radical proposed by Harman (1956) probably is now the most widely accepted. This theory, which has been further developed by Haman (2006); Miquel et al. (1980) and others (Barja 2004), proposes that aging is the consequence of accumulation of damage by deleterious oxidation in biomolecules caused by the high reactivity of the free radicals produced in our cells as a result of the necessary use of oxygen (O_2). Since O_2 is mainly used in respiration to support the life-maintaining metabolic processes, the mitochondria, and more concretely their DNA (mtDNA), they are probably the first targets of this oxidation, especially in the fixed postmitotic cells that cannot fully regenerate these organelles (Miquel 1998). Moreover, it is known that the rate of mitochondrial oxygen radical generation, as well as the degree of membrane fatty acid unsaturation, and the oxidative damage to mtDNA are lower in the long-lived than in the short-lived species. Thus, the mitochondrial damage caused by free radicals results in a loss of bioenergetic competence that leads to aging and death of cells and therefore of the organism.

There is another group of theories of aging, the concepts having been published a long time ago, that attempt to explain why the aging process occurs. In this group, we can mention theories such as that proposed by Williams (1957), which suggests that aging is a consequence of characteristics selected by evolution to be of advantage to the young subjects of the species, allowing them to reach the reproductive age in the best condition (with maximal vigor) and thus preserve these species, but are a disadvantage for old subjects, not needed for species preservation. Thus, natural selection acts before the adult age (period of reproduction), and the maintenance of the species is more relevant biologically than the longevity of the individual.

Since the aging process is very complex, a theory based on only one mechanism is not able to give a satisfactory explanation for all its aspects. This justifies the proposal of a theory that integrates early concepts that offer partial explanation of the mechanism of aging with others proposed more recently. Thus, an integrated theory forms which attempts to answer the three important questions of biogerontology: the "how the aging process occurs" (oxidation), the "where" this process starts (the mitochondria from fixed differentiated cells), and the "why" the aging process is necessary (for the maintenance of an adequate number of individuals in each species) (De la Fuente and Miquel 2009).

2.4.2   The Oxidation-Inflammation Theory of Aging: Role of the Immune System in Oxi-Inflamm-Aging

Recently, a new theory of aging, the oxidation-inflammation theory, has been proposed (De la Fuente and Miquel 2009), which integrates the previously mentioned oxidation theory of aging and the idea of "inflamm-aging" suggested several years ago by Franceschi et al. (2000). The concepts that have led us to this new theory will be discussed below. As already stated, the aging process is linked to the oxidation carried out by the oxidant and reactive oxygen species (ROS), normally produced by organisms. Nevertheless, we should consider that oxygen is essential for life and that ROS, in certain amounts, are needed

for many physiological processes that are essential for our survival (Dröge 2002). In order to obtain protection against oxygen toxicity, a variety of antioxidant mechanisms that prevent the formation of ROS or neutralize them after they are produced have been developed. Thus, the functions of our organism are based on a perfect balance between the levels of ROS and those of antioxidants. It is the loss of this balance, because of an excess in the production of ROS or an insufficient availability of antioxidants, which leads to the oxidative stress than underlies ROS-related diseases and aging (Fig. 2.2).

As mentioned above, aging is accompanied by a decline of the physiological systems including the immune system, and immunosenescence occurs. Moreover, a relation between the functionality of immune cells, the health of subjects, and their longevity was observed. Given this, we asked why immunosenescence occurs. If, as it is generally accepted, the mechanisms that underlie aging must be of general application, it seems logical to accept that the cause of immunosenescence is the same as that responsible for the senescence of the other cells of the organism, namely, the oxidative disorganization linked to the unavoidable use of oxygen to support cellular functions. Further, we should remember that the immune cells need to produce free radicals and other oxidant and inflammatory compounds in order to perform their defensive functions consisting of the destruction or incapacitation of pathogens and malignant cells (Yoon et al. 2002). Nevertheless, this fact and the membrane characteristics of the immune cells make them very vulnerable to oxidative damage. Therefore, if any cell needs to maintain a balance between the production of oxidants and the antioxidant defenses in order to prevent an excess of the first and the resulting oxidative stress, this balance is even more essential to preserve the functional capacity of immune cells and, therefore, the health of the organism.

In addition, there is a close link between oxidative stress and inflammation, since uncontrolled free radical release can induce an inflammatory response, and free radicals are inflammation effectors. In fact, ROS can activate nuclear factor kappa-light-chain-enhancer of activated B cells (NFκB) inducing the production of inflammatory cytokines, and the levels of pro-inflammatory compounds (enzymes, cytokines, prostaglandins, etc.) seem to be increased with age in consistent with the proposed concept of "inflamm-aging." Based on the abovementioned points, the age-related changes in the redox and the inflammatory state of immune cells were investigated. Thus, a variety of oxidant and inflammatory compounds, and anti-inflammatory and antioxidant protectors, as well as oxidative damage to biomolecules, in immune cells (peritoneal leucocytes of mice and neutrophils and lymphocytes from human peripheral blood) were analyzed (Fig. 2.2). Our results indicate that with aging leucocytes suffer oxidative and inflammatory stress (De la Fuente et al. 2005; De la Fuente and Miquel 2009). Moreover, this also occurs in the immune cells of PAM with respect to those of NPAM (Viveros et al. 2007) as well as in the leucocytes of transgenic mice for AD with respect to the corresponding wild animals (Gimenez-Llort et al. 2012).

Therefore, with aging (chronologic or premature) the oxidant and pro-inflammatory compounds increase reaching levels higher than those of antioxidant and anti-inflammatory compounds, leading to an oxidative and inflammatory stress. Thus, oxi-inflamm-aging has been proposed as the cause of the loss of function that appears with senescence (De la Fuente and Miquel 2009).

In this context, a relationship has been found between the redox and inflammatory state of the immune cells, their functional capacity, and the life span of a subject. Thus, when an animal shows a high oxidative stress in its immune cells, these cells have an impaired function and that animal shows a decreased longevity in relation to other members of the group of the same chronological age. As examples supporting that idea and, consequently, the role of the immune system in aging, we can mention again what happens in the mouse model of premature aging, the PAM, with a shorter life span than the NPAM; they showed worse functions and a greater oxidative-inflammatory stress in their immune cells. Moreover, PAM also showed oxidative stress in

the brain, liver, heart, and kidney. The other models of premature aging previously mentioned also show this relation. Thus, in obese animals and in triple transgenic mice for Alzheimer's disease, immune cells have higher oxidative and inflammatory stress situations, worse functions than the respective controls, and the animals with these cells have a lower life span (De la Fuente and Miquel 2009; De la Fuente and De Castro 2012; Gimenez-Llort et al. 2012).

In addition, very-long-living mice and human centenarians show a redox condition in their immune cells and a functional capacity of these cells similar to that of healthy adult subjects (Arranz et al. 2010a, 2013; Alonso-Fernandez and De la Fuente 2011).

Since one of the most relevant mechanisms involved in the cellular redox state is the NFκB, which plays a key role in regulating the expression of a wide range of oxidants and inflammatory compounds, especially in the immune cells, this factor has been involved in the immunosenescence and in oxi-inflamm-aging (Salminen et al. 2008a, b). In fact, it has been observed that the NFκB activation, in resting conditions, is very high in peritoneal leucocytes from old mice but lower in extremely long-lived mice and adult animals. Moreover, only old subjects with controlled basal NFκB activation in the immune cells achieved longevity, but adults with a high basal expression of this factor died early (Arranz et al. 2010a). Thus, the level of activation of that factor in leucocytes is significantly related to the life expectancy of the subjects from which the cells were obtained. All these suggest that the immune system, if it is not well regulated and shows a high activation of factors such as the NFκB, will not be able to develop its function properly with a greater contribution to the oxi-inflamm-aging situation of the organism and consequently to the rate of aging. In conclusion, only aged individuals that maintain a good regulation of the leukocyte redox state and consequently a good function of their immune cells, with levels similar to those of healthy adults, reach very high longevity.

Thus, in the theory of oxidation-inflammation of aging, it is suggested that the immune system could play a key role not as the fundamental cause of aging but as a mechanism that modifies the rate of senescence. In this theory, it is proposed that the aging process is a chronic oxidative and inflammatory stress, which leads to damage of cell components, including proteins, lipids, and DNA, contributing to the age-related decline of all cells of organisms, but especially in those of the regulatory systems, including the immune system. Moreover, the immune system, due to its capacity of producing oxidant and inflammatory compounds in order to eliminate foreign agents, could increase the oxidative and inflammatory stress of the organism, through factors such as NFκB, if it is not well controlled. Thus, this system could be involved in the rate of aging and justifies the loss of homeostatic capacity and the consequent increase of morbidity and mortality that appears with aging (De la Fuente and Miquel 2009).

2.4.3 Can the Role of the Immune System in Aging Have a Universal Application?

The immune system is relatively well known in vertebrate animals, in which the innate and adaptive immunity collaborate to produce a very efficient immune response. However, in invertebrates this system has been less studied. Although currently it is accepted that all animals, even the plants, have some sort of immunity, the presence of lymphocytes and their specific defensive function appears only in vertebrates. For this reason "the immune theory of aging" such as originally proposed (Walford 1969) cannot be accepted since this theory suggested the impairment of the immune system as the cause of organism senescence, and this concept does not follow the principle of universality of the aging process proposed by Strehler (1977). It should be kept in mind that not all animal species have immune systems as complex as those of the mammals. Nevertheless, it seems evident, based on all the above information, that immune cells can play a fundamental role in aging.

Confirmation of this concept could be found in the fact that the immune cells produce oxidant and inflammatory compounds in high amounts with aging. However, this happens especially in the phagocytic cells, which are found, with different denominations, in all animals, including invertebrates. If during aging adaptive immunity declines, innate immunity, in several aspects, seems to be activated, inducing a prooxidative and pro-inflammatory profile. In agreement with the above, it has been observed that in the peritoneal immune cell populations of mice as in blood immune cells of human subjects, the macrophages and neutrophils, respectively, are the immune cells responsible for the generation of higher levels of oxidant compounds than those caused by lymphocytes, and these levels significantly increase with age in those phagocytic cells (De la Fuente and Miquel 2009). Thus, it is probable that these phagocytes, which already pointed out are found in all animals, can be involved in the modulation of chronic oxidative stress of senescence and, thus, in the rate of aging of the subjects of the different animal species.

2.5 Environment and Lifestyle Strategies that May Improve the Function and Redox State of the Immune System in Aging

Many strategies have been proposed to enable the maintenance of an excellent immune function with aging, resulting in a better quality of life, and consequently, greater longevity of individuals. If we agree with the oxidation-inflammation theory of aging, we should accept that the rate of aging is dependent, in part, on the degree of control of oxidation and inflammation of the immune system of each subject, which is related to its functional capacity. This theory can also be supported by research showing that this control of the immune system by lifestyle strategies results in an increased longevity (De la Fuente et al. 2011; Jenny 2012). Several of those strategies will be discussed below.

2.5.1 Nutrition

Nutrition, adequate in quality and quantity, is essential to maintain good health. Thus, a Mediterranean diet is associated with lower levels of inflammation and a decreased risk of disease compared to a Western-type diet (Pauwels 2011). Moreover, nutritional status has a relevant role in the immune system function of each subject, especially in elderly individuals (Pae et al. 2012). The results obtained from several studies in experimental animals and humans show that the impaired regulation of immune response found even in healthy elderly subjects can be attributed to deficiencies of both macronutrients and micronutrients. This fact, which is often found in older individuals because of physiological, social, and economic factors, indicates that appropriate nutrition could play a preventive role in the aging process by modulating immunosenescence. Thus, the use of "functional foods" seems to influence many cellular parameters, which can help to decrease the deleterious effect of the aging process. In this context, nutrients such as dietary fiber, omega-3 polyunsaturated fatty acids (PUFAs), probiotics, and specially antioxidant compounds are of particular interest (De la Fuente et al. 2011; Pae et al. 2012).

2.5.1.1 Antioxidants

As mentioned above, the endogenous antioxidants decrease in oxidative stress situations, such as aging, because they are spent neutralizing the excess of ROS, and this fact is very relevant in the immune cells. Since biological age and mean longevity seem to be associated with an optimal antioxidant protection, having a diet enriched with antioxidants appears adequate for maintaining an optimum redox balance and therefore protecting the organism from the impairment associated with physiological and pathological aging. Although some studies question the positive role of the ingestion of antioxidant vitamins, especially in high doses, as a consequence of a possible decrease that they may cause in the endogen antioxidant defenses, other studies show the positive role of supplementation with moderate levels of antioxidants, especially in the

immune system (De la Fuente et al. 2011; Pae et al. 2012).

There is an extensive list of antioxidant compounds with health-supporting properties. However, the effects of these antioxidants, administered by diet, on the immune functions are scarcely known for many of them. One of the most thoroughly studied antioxidants in this context is zinc (Zn). Zn is very important for optimal functioning of the immune system, especially in elderly subjects, in which a deficiency of Zn is very common (due to inadequate diet and/or intestinal malabsorption). However, higher than recommended upper limits of zinc may adversely affect immune function (Pae et al. 2012). Other antioxidants show important favorable effects on health, acting on the immune system in both laboratory animals and human subjects. This is the case of beta-carotene, coenzyme Q, alpha-tocopherol (vitamin E), ascorbic acid (vitamin C), polyphenols, as well as thiolic antioxidants such as thioproline (TP) and N-acetylcysteine (NAC), which are precursors of reduced glutathione (GSH), among others, either in isolation or in nutritional formulations containing more than one of these compounds (De la Fuente et al. 2011; Pae et al. 2012). These compounds, which have not only antioxidant but also anti-inflammatory actions, have shown immunomodulator properties since they produce an increase of the functions and antioxidant defenses that are depressed and a decrease of functions and oxidant parameters that are excessively active. Thus, they may bring each immune function and redox parameter to its optimum level. This modulating ability appears to be carried out, at least in part, through the ubiquitous intracellular factors implicated in oxidation and inflammation, such as the NFκB.

In addition, this regulatory role of the antioxidants is performed not only in the immune system but also in the other regulatory systems, including the nervous system, in which the oxidative stress also underlies its senescent impairment. Thus, the oxidative and inflammatory stress that appears to play a fundamental role in the aging of both the immune system and the nervous system could be counteracted to a certain degree by antioxidant administration. Therefore, antioxidant diet supplementation may be a useful procedure to neutralize or postpone the age-related homeostatic impairment and consequently increase life span, as has been observed in mice (De la Fuente et al. 2011). Since the effects of antioxidants on the immune system are similar in mice and humans and because these changes in mice are accompanied by an increase in longevity, it is probable that similar effects could be obtained in humans.

In summary, it seems reasonable to propose that the administration of adequate amounts of antioxidant compounds may be effective in neutralizing or slowing down the loss of homeostasis that occurs with age and consequently to slow down the aging process. Nevertheless, the effectiveness of the antioxidants depends on the administered amount of these compounds; therefore, the age-related appropriate dose, especially to improve the immune response, should be investigated further (for more details, see Chaps. 20 and 22).

2.5.1.2 Caloric Restriction (CR)

There are many studies showing that CR can slow down multiple aspects of the aging process and thus delays senescence and increases life span in a variety of animals, when these are compared to the respective controls fed ad libitum (Anderson and Weindruch 2012). Moreover, CR seems to delay the onset of numerous age-associated diseases including vascular diseases, atherosclerosis, diabetes mellitus, and autoimmune diseases and therefore decreases the death rate. Nevertheless, the universal applicability of CR as a strategy to slow down the rate of aging and extend life span is currently a highly controversial subject (Masoro 2009).

With respect to the effects of CR on immunity, several studies have reported this is a good strategy to improve immune function, protecting against infections and delaying or preventing development of cancer and metastasis. In this action, among other factors, the NFκB is involved. In aged animals CR can maintain several functional parameters of immune cells at a level typically seen in healthy adults (Messaoudi et al. 2008; Ahmed et al. 2009; Masoro 2009).

However, the delay of immunosenescence that CR produces in experimental animals needs to be verified in humans. Recent studies have even suggested that CR might compromise the host's defense against infections (Pae et al. 2012). Although it is evident that most of the effects of CR are due to the decrease in the oxidative stress produced through its action on the metabolism, the exact mechanism of the antiaging action of CR remains poorly understood (Cavallini et al. 2008) (for more details, see Chap. 20).

2.5.2 Physical Activity

Physical exercise, since its association with health is well known (Kokkinos 2012), is another of the lifestyle factors proposed to improve health and quality of life in elderly. Physical exercise modulates physiological systems such as the muscle and cardiovascular systems but also the regulatory systems such as the immune system. In fact, performance of physical exercise has been associated with lower susceptibility to infections and other pathologies related with the immune system, compared to sedentary subjects. There is a wealth of information on the effects of physical exercise on the immune function of adult experimental animals and humans. Although conflicting results have been obtained, depending on the type, intensity, and frequency of exercise, as well as the immune function studied and state of the subject, it is generally accepted that acute or strenuous physical exercise induces an impairment of immune functions, increasing the risk of infections. Moreover, moderate training exercise leads to adaptations of the immune cells with improvement of their functions (Radak et al. 2008). Nevertheless, this is not true for all cell types and in all cases. Thus, intensity training has been associated with symptoms of transient depression of many immune functions, especially those of lymphocytes, leading to increased susceptibility to infection. However, this exercise also seems to induce an overstimulation of the response of phagocytic cells. It has been suggested that this stimulation of phagocytes, which involves the activation of factors such as NFκB, might counterbalance the decreased lymphoid activity and thus help the organism to prevent infectious diseases in situations where the specific adaptive immune response seems to be depressed. In addition, moderate training exercise leads to clear benefits of the immune system with improvement of its functions, both of adaptive and innate response, and therefore, it is associated with decreased susceptibility to infection processes. Moreover, in response to repetitive or graded exercise training, a decrease in oxidative stress and a resistance to oxidative damage also appears. This seems to be due to a downregulation of the release of ROS as consequence of an adaptation of antioxidant defenses, which increases their levels and activities (Walsh et al. 2011; De la Fuente et al. 2011).

Although in old animals or elderly humans the effects of physical exercise on the immune functions have been scarcely studied, the available data show that the practice of regular and moderate exercise is an important candidate for improving the immune function throughout the aging process and in elderly subjects, delaying the onset of immunosenescence (Simpson et al. 2012). However, the conflictive results on the effect of exercise on the immune system, abovementioned, are more common in aged subjects. In this context the question is if exercise produces oxidation, how could it decrease the increased levels of ROS of immune cells from old subjects? But, it is evident that physical exercise improves immune cell functions through the recovery of the oxidant/antioxidant and inflammatory/anti-inflammatory balance of these cells and consequently decreases oxi-inflamma-aging. Since the immune system is a homeostatic system if it is well controlled and its functions take place in the physiological context, they are efficient in infections and inflammatory situations. However, a badly regulated immune response can be detrimental and cause oxidative and inflammatory diseases. Currently, the optimal level of exercise that improves, but does not impair or overstimulate, a healthy immune function is still not really known.

For the optimal use of exercise as a therapeutic strategy against aging, many aspects have to be resolved, as it was previously proposed (De la Fuente et al. 2011). For example, it should be answered when an increase in the production of ROS by immune cells, especially phagocytic cells, is positive and can enhance the microbicidal capacity and when it is negative, causing oxidative stress damage, or when an increase in inflammatory cytokine production is positive for improving the defenses of the body, or when does it become negative, causing inflammatory damage? It is possible that the levels of ROS and inflammatory compounds produced, as well as the capacity of these levels in each organism in promoting and maintaining the expression of antioxidant and anti-inflammatory defenses, could give us an answer to these questions.

In summary, before recommending physical exercise as a good therapeutic intervention in oxidative-/inflammatory-associated diseases in general and aging in particular, it is necessary to know the intensity, regularity, and duration of this exercise as well as the physiological state of each subject. Perhaps, it would be more interesting (from a physiological point of view) to think in terms of avoiding modern lifestyle-induced inactivity (sedentary), because this itself can deregulate the oxidative and inflammatory responses accelerating the aging processes. Thus, having an active life is another strategy to slow down aging (De la Fuente et al. 2011).

2.5.3 Environmental Enrichment

Environmental enrichment (EE) could be defined as an experimental approach in animal models that mimics the maintenance of an active social, mental, and physical life in humans. Thus, EE is a continuous enhancement in cognitive, sensorimotor, and physical activity, which overcomes emotional stress. In general, the positive effects of EE are manifested by many molecular, cellular, and functional modifications, which lead to an overall improvement in the physiological and physical well-being of the subjects (De la Fuente et al. 2011; Arranz et al. 2010c; De la Fuente and Arranz 2012).

The most frequently used EE protocol in rodents is housing the animals in large groups and cages with several types of objects (running wheels, tunnels, ladders, etc.) and spatial configurations, which are changed frequently. This more complex housing, with the continual introduction of new objects, induces sensory, cognitive, motor, and social stimulation. Moreover, the availability of running wheels, ropes, ladders, tunnels, or bridges allows the animal to exercise, and since EE animals are housed in relatively large cages, typically in groups of 6–12 animals, they have the opportunity for more social interaction. The beneficial effects of EE on the nervous and endocrine systems have been largely studied. Thus, EE produces improvements in learning and memory, preventing age-related cognitive impairments and reversing some of the negative consequences of neurodegenerative diseases. Moreover, it increases brain plasticity and neurogenesis, particularly at the level of the hippocampus and cerebral cortex. These effects can also be mediated, at least in part, by the effect of EE modulating the levels of hormones, such as the sexual hormones. In addition, EE can be positive in the regulation of stress-related disorders, conferring stress resistance, since it is able to protect the animal from the consequences of uncontrollable stress exposure (Schloesser et al. 2010). Nevertheless, there are few studies on the effects of EE on the immune system. We have carried out a study on mice using the type of EE mentioned above, and the results have shown an improvement in many functions of immune cells as well as a decrease in the oxidative-inflammatory stress of these cells. These positive effects were especially remarkable in old animals after a short period of EE. Moreover, when the EE starts at an adult age, a great increase in longevity occurs (Arranz et al. 2010c). A recent study showed that in triple transgenic mice for Alzheimer's disease, EE improved several immune functions in males. The results obtained also suggested that active life (by means of EE) should be maintained until the natural death of the animal in order to preserve all the positive effects that this strategy exerts on the immune system (Arranz et al. 2011).

Hydrotherapy is another strategy, which can be considered as a type of EE, for improving the neuroimmunoendocrine communication in old animals. In mice this therapy has consisted of simple baths (of 15 min/day) in normal hot tap water. After 2 and 4 weeks mice submitted to this EE showed an improvement of many behavioral parameters, which are clearly impaired with age. Moreover, this EE not only rejuvenated the nervous system of mice but also the immune system, improving all the functions of the immune cells studied, as well as their redox state (De la Fuente et al. 2011).

These results show that EE may reverse the age-related dysfunction in immunity, as well as confirm the importance of maintaining active mental and/or physical activity to improve the quality of life and even to obtain a healthy longevity.

2.5.4   Hormesis

A phenomenon called "hormesis" has been proposed as a good strategy to achieve a healthy aging (Calabrese et al. 2012). It can be defined as "a process in which exposure to a low amount of a chemical agent or environmental factors that are damaging in higher doses induces an adaptive beneficial effect on the cell or organism" (Mattson 2008). Hormesis is based on the fact that all living systems have the intrinsic ability to respond, to counteract, and to adapt to external and internal stress (Rattan 2008). In these adaptive responses to single or multiple mild stresses, after initial disruption of homeostasis, the organism responds with molecular and cellular protection and compensatory mechanisms, which provide beneficial effects activating the pathways of maintenance and repair of the biological systems. Thus, whereas excessive stress accelerates the aging process, the exposure to low doses of otherwise harmful agents, such as irradiation, food limitation, heat stress, exercise, hypoxia, and oxidant compounds, produces a variety of beneficial effects including improved health and an extended life span of organisms. These stressors which are called "hormetins" can be defined as any condition that may be potentially hormetic in physiological terms by involving one or more pathways of stress response within a cell (Rattan and Demirovic 2009).

Many of the effects of the strategies mentioned above seem to be due to their hormetic properties. Several groups of hormetins have been proposed: (1) physical hormetins, such as heat, radiation and exercise; (2) biological and nutritional hormetins, such as nutrients and infections; and (3) physiological hormetins, such as mental challenge and focused attention or mediation (Rattan and Demirovic 2009). The mentioned above strategies, such as nutrition, exercise, as well as mental and social challenges of EE, which slow down aging belong to one of these groups. Thus, the positive effects of those strategies on the immune system and on a healthy aging could be based on the capacity of these strategies to carry out hormesis mechanisms through stimulating repair systems (Gaman et al. 2011).

In spite of the recent increase in studies on hormesis, the basic nature of this phenomenon remains largely unknown (Vaiserman 2010). Nevertheless, hormetic interventions seem to be relevant strategies to improve immune function, and the functionality of the other regulatory systems, and therefore to slow down the aging process (De la Fuente et al. 2011; Calabrese et al. 2012).

2.5.4.1 Hormetic Effects of Nutrition

The mechanism of action of many antioxidant compounds in oxidative stress may not be related only to their antioxidant properties but to their hormetic activities. For example, antioxidants can activate, at a determined level, hormetic transcription factors such as NFκB and cAMP response element-binding protein (CREB), which result in the induction of genes encoding growth factors, antiapoptotic proteins, and antioxidant defenses (Mattson 2008). Moreover, several antioxidants such as polyphenols induce mitochondrial biogenesis, which is related to a more efficient energy production that contributes to a decrease in the levels of free radicals in the mitochondria and therefore to less oxidative tissue damage. Thus, many of the positive results obtained with a diet enriched with appropriated

amounts of antioxidants in the functions of the nervous, endocrine, and immune systems during aging could be attributed to the hormetic effects of these compounds. In fact, a hormetic role of dietary antioxidants with a U-shaped dose response in the redox situation of the organism has been proposed (Calabrese et al. 2010). Thus, many of the conflictive results obtained with the administration of antioxidant compounds could be due to the hormetic balance between the amount of antioxidant and the physiological state of the subject, especially at redox levels.

With respect to dietary caloric restriction (CR), this strategy represents a mild dietary stress that produces hormetic responses in the organism. For this reason, when the CR is carried out without malnutrition, it delays most age-related physiological changes and extends life span in experimental animals (Kouda and Iki 2010). CR can show its hormetic properties increasing the silent mating-type information regulation 2 homolog 1 (SIRT1) mRNA expression, SIRT1 being a key regulator of many cellular defenses that allows survival in response to stress (Kouda and Iki 2010). CR also increases the levels and functions of heat shock proteins (HSP), these chaperones enhancing the stress resistance and consequently protecting cells against otherwise lethal levels of oxidative and metabolic stress. Other cytoprotective molecules upregulated by dietary energy restriction are the antioxidant defenses, which modulate the age-related oxidative stress situation.

Many cell responses to CR are the result of the upregulation of expression of proteins involved in the regulation of mitochondrial oxidative state, which is denominated mitohormesis (Ristow and Zarse 2010; Ristow and Schmeisser 2011).

2.5.4.2 The Hormetic Effects of Physical Exercise and EE

Physical exercise is another strategy, which acts using hormetic mechanisms. Exercise performance involves the activation of NFκB signaling cascade, various stress kinases, antioxidant genes, as well as increasing levels of HSP and the expression of the mitochondrial uncoupling protein 2 (UCP2), allowing the generation of more

ATP and improving the mitochondria functions. All this provides crucial protection against oxidative stress and molecular damage in aging. Thus, exercise is a hormesis intervention, which could be a good preventive strategy in aging. It is necessary to take in account that physical exercise, even with moderate intensity, is a stress situation, and if this stress is weak, it can also generate hormetic responses. As previously mentioned, physical activity can produce a decrease in oxidative stress and a resistance to oxidative damage due to an upregulation in antioxidant enzymes. This happens especially in the skeletal muscle, which is recognized as a major source of free radical generation, but also in other tissues and cells and can be the cause of the beneficial effects on the immune function of regular and moderate physical exercise (Rattan 2008; Radak et al. 2008; De la Fuente et al. 2011).

The hormetic effect of EE is based on the fact that the continuous exposure to new objects and social interactions could be considered a mild stress condition. In fact, in experimental animals with EE, increased levels of adrenocorticotropic hormone (ACTH) and glucocorticoids along with an adrenal hypertrophy occur. This mild stress seems to be beneficial for the enriched animals to cope with other stressors (Moncek et al. 2004). The effect of EE on the hippocampus as already mentioned can explain how it may confer stress resistance, protecting the animal from the consequences of uncontrollable stress exposure. Most of the beneficial effects of hydrotherapy may also be due to thermal stress-inducing neuroendocrine reactions such as an enhancement of the HHA axis, leading to an increase of ACTH and corticosterone levels, as well as those of prolactin (PRL) and the growth hormone (GH). This therapy also induces a release of beta-endorphin that shows analgesic properties and improves the immune functions (De la Fuente et al. 2011).

2.5.4.3 Other Hormesis Interventions

Environmental toxins have also been used as possible hormetins (reviewed by Calabrese and Blain 2005). Since the response to low doses of toxins could be a good model of hormesis, we have studied the effects of an endotoxin, such as lipopolysaccharide (LPS) of *Escherichia coli*, as a hormetin, using it in very low doses during the adult life of mice to try to improve the function and redox state of the immune cells in these animals when they are old. The results showed an improvement of nervous function as well as in several functions of the immune cells and in their redox state, all the values obtained being closer to those in the adult-mature control group (De la Fuente et al. 2011).

2.6   Conclusions and Recommendations

In recent publications, much research has been proposed in order to better define immunosenescence beyond the usual relative poorer responses of old subjects compared to young subjects (Vallejo 2011). This chapter attempts to highlight the relevant involvement of the immune system in the rate of aging through its involvement in oxi-inflamm-aging, as well as the relevance of several functional parameters of immune cells as markers of biological age and, therefore, predictors of mean longevity. Although more investigations are necessary in this scientific field, and it has been questioned that if any of the markers shown in the literature are true biomarkers of aging (Vasto et al. 2010), it seems proved that maintaining an immune function in conditions similar to that of an adult can assure better health and a longer life span. In addition, having similar values in the functions of immune cells as older subjects is related to a shorter life. Thus, several lifestyle strategies such as a good nutrition, the practice of mental and physical exercise, social relationship, and overcoming emotional stress, all of which produces hormetic adaptation, could be useful, improving those immune functions, necessary for maintaining our health, and therefore increasing our mean longevity. The fact that health preservation depends on the style of life and environmental factors in about 75 % suggests all the strategies mentioned above as good candidates to achieve a long and healthy longevity, and it shows our responsibility for obtaining this state of health. Moreover, the control of the effects of these lifestyle factors on physiological systems, especially on the immune system, is very relevant, not only in the aging process but also from the fetal life of each subject (Dietert and Piepenbrink 2008).

More research is needed in order to clarify the best amount, frequency, time, moment, and organism situation for each individual with which these strategies would show higher beneficial effects. With respect to all the hormetic strategies commented, more studies are needed in order to better discriminate between their positive and possible negative effects to maintain health in the later stage of life. Nevertheless, the effectiveness of these strategies can be measured through their effects improving the immune function and thus the biological age, which allows a healthy longevity (Fig. 2.1).

Acknowledgements The author thanks Mr. D. Potter for his help with the English language revision of the manuscript and also expresses her gratitude to Dr. Ortega, Dr. Vallejo, Dr. Medina, Dr. Victor, Dr. Alvarado, Dr. Alvarez, Dr. Alonso, Dr. Arranz, Dr. Baeza, Dr, Gimenez-Llort, Ms De Castro, Ms Vida, Ms Hernandez, Ms Cruces, and Ms Maté for their invaluable help in performing several of the experiments which have allowed us to arrive at the ideas expressed in this chapter. This work was supported by grants of the MINECO (BFU2011-03336), Research Group of UCM (910379ENEROINN), and RETICEF (RD06/0013/0003) (RD12/0043/0018)(ISCIII-FEDER of the European Union).

References

Ahmed T, Das SK, Golden JK et al (2009) Caloric restriction enhances T-cell-mediated immune response in adult overweight men and women. J Gerontol A Biol Sci Med Sci 64:1107–1113

Alonso-Fernandez P, De la Fuente M (2011) Role of the immune system in aging and longevity. Curr Aging Sci 4:78–100

Alonso-Fernandez P, Maté I, De la Fuente M (2010) Neutrophils: markers of biological age and predictors of longevity. In: DeFranco JE (ed) Neutrophils: lifespan, functions and role in disease. Nova Science Publisher Inc, New York

Anderson RM, Weindruch R (2012) The caloric restriction paradigm: implications for healthy human aging. Am J Hum Biol 24:101–106

Arranz L, Guayerbas N, De la Fuente M (2007) Impairment of several immune functions in anxious women. J Psychosom Res 62:1–8

Arranz L, De Vicente A, Muñoz M et al (2009) Impairment of immune function in the social excluded homeless population. Neuroimmunomodulation 16:251–260

Arranz L, Caamaño J, Lord JM, De la Fuente M (2010a) Preserved immune functions and controlled leukocyte oxidative stress in naturally long-lived mice: possible role of nuclear factor-kappa B. J Gerontol A Biol Sci Med Sci 65A:941–950

Arranz L, De Castro NM, Baeza I et al (2010b) Differential expression of Toll-like receptor 2 and 4 on peritoneal leukocyte populations from long-lived and non-selected old female mice. Biogerontology 11:475–482

Arranz L, De Castro NM, Baeza I et al (2010c) Environmental enrichment improves age-related immune system impairment. Long-term exposure since adulthood increases life span in mice. Rejuvenation Res 13:415–428

Arranz L, Lord JM, De la Fuente M (2010d) Preserved ex vivo inflammatory status and cytokine responses in naturally long-lived mice. Age (Dordr) 32:451–466

Arranz L, De Castro NM, Baeza I (2011) Effect of environmental enrichment on the immunoendocrineageing of male and female triple-transgenic 3xTg-AD mice for Alzheimer's disease. J Alzheimers Dis 25: 727–737

Arranz L, Naudi A, De la Fuente M, Pamplona R (2013) Exceptionally old mice are highly resistant to lipoxidation-derived molecular damage. Age (Dordr) 35(3):621–635

Atzmon G, Cho M, Cawthon RM et al (2010) Evolution in health and medicine Sackler colloquium: genetic variation in human telomerase is associated with telomere length in Ashkenazi centenarians. Proc Natl Acad Sci U S A 107:1710–1717

Bae CY, Kang YG, Kim S et al (2008) Development of models for predicting biological age (BA) with physical, biochemical, and hormonal parameters. Arch Gerontol Geriat 47:253–265

Bandeen-Roche K, Walston JD, Huang Y et al (2009) Measuring systemic inflammatory regulation in older adults: evidence and utility. Rejuvenation Res 12: 403–410

Barak Y (2006) The immune system and happiness. Autoimmun Rev 5:523–527

Barja G (2004) Free radicals and aging. Trends Neurosci 27:595–600

Bauer ME (2008) Chronic stress and immunosenescence. A review. Neuroimmunomodulation 15:244–253

Benfante R, Reed R, Brody J (1985) Biological and social predictors of health in an aging cohort. J Chronic Dis 38:175–181

Benjamin H (1947) Biologic versus chronologic age. J Gerontol 2:217–227

Besedovsky HO, Del Rey A (2007) Physiology of psychoneuroimmunology: a personal view. Brain Behav Immun 21:34–44

Besedovsky HO, Del Rey A (2011) Central and peripheral cytokines mediate immune-brain connectivity. Neurochem Res 36:1–6

Borkan A, Norris AH (1980) Assessment of biological age using a profile of physical parameters. J Gerontol 35:177–184

Bulpitt CJ, Antikainen RL, Markowe HL et al (2009) Mortality according to a prior assessment of biological age. Curr Aging Sci 2:193–199

Calabrese EJ, Blain R (2005) The occurrence of hormetic dose responses in the toxicological literature, the hormesis database: an overview. Toxicol Appl Pharmacol 202:289–301

Calabrese V, Cornelius C, Trovato A, Cavallaro M, Mancuso C, Di Rienzo L, Condorelli D, De Lorenzo A, Calabrese EJ (2010) The hormetic role of dietary antioxidants in free radical-related diseases. Curr Pharm Des 16:877–883

Calabrese EJ, Iavicoli I, Calabrese V (2012) Hormesis: why it is important to biogerontologists. Biogerontology 13:215–235

Carnes BA, Staats DO, Sonntag WE (2008) Does senescence give rise to disease? Mech Ageing Dev 129:693–699

Cavallini G, Donati A, Gori Z et al (2008) Towards an understanding of the anti-aging mechanism of caloric restriction. Curr Aging Sci 1:4–9

Corona AW, Fenn AM, Godbout JP (2012) Cognitive and behavioral consequences of impaired immunoregulation in aging. J Neuroimmune Pharmacol 7:7–23

Couillard-Depres S, Iglseder B, Aigner L (2011) Neurogenesis, cellular plasticity and cognition: the impact of stem cells in the adult and aging brain. Gerontology 57:559–564

De la Fuente M (1985) Changes in the macrophage function with aging. Comp Biochem Physiol 81:935–938

De la Fuente M (2004) The immune system as a marker of health and longevity. Antiaging Med 1:31–41

De la Fuente M (2010) Murine models of premature ageing for the study of diet-induced immune changes. Improvement of leukocyte functions in two strains of old prematurely ageing mice by dietary supplementation with sulphur-containing antioxidants. Proc Nutr Soc 69:651–659

De la Fuente M, Arranz L (2012) The importance of the environment in brain aging: be happy, live longer! In: Thakur MK, Rattan SI (eds) Brain aging, therapeutic interventions. Springer, New York

De la Fuente M, De Castro NM (2012) Obesity as a model of premature immunosenescence. Curr Immunol Rev 8:63–75

De la Fuente M, Miquel J (2009) An update of the oxidation-inflammation theory of aging the involvement of the immune system in oxi-inflamm-aging. Curr Pharm Des 15:3003–3026

De la Fuente M, Hernanz A, Vallejo MC (2005) The immune system in the oxidation stress conditions of aging and hypertension favorable effects of antioxidants and physical exercise. Antioxid Redox Signal 7:1356–1366

De la Fuente M, Hernandez O, Cruces J et al (2011) Strategies to improve the functions and redox state of the immune system in aged subjects. Curr Pharm Des 17:3966–3993

Dewan SK, Zheng SB, Xia SJ (2012) Senescent remodeling of the immune system and its contribution to the predisposition of the elderly to infections. Chin Med J 125:3325–3331

Dietert RR, Piepenbrink MS (2008) The managed immune system: protecting the womb to delay the tomb. Hum Exp Toxicol 27:129–134

Dröge W (2002) Free radicals in the physiological control of cell function. Physiol Rev 82:47–95

Ferguson FG, Wikby A, Maxson P et al (1995) Immune parameters in a longitudinal study of a very old population of Swedish people: a comparison between survivors and nonsurvivors. J Gerontol A Biol Sci Med Sci 50:B378–B382

Franceschi C, Bonafe M, Valensin S et al (2000) Inflammaging. An evolutionary perspective on immunosenescence. Ann N Y Acad Sci 908:244–254

Frasca D, Blomberg BB (2009) Effects of aging on B cell function. Curr Opin Immunol 21:425–430

Fulop T, Larbi A, Kotb R et al (2011) Aging, immunity, and cancer. Discov Med 11:537–550

Gaman L, Stoian I, Atanasiu V (2011) Can ageing be slowed?: hormetic and redox perspectives. J Med Life 4:346–351

Garrido P (2011) Aging and stress: past hypothesis, present approaches and perspectives. Aging Dis 2:80–99

Gayoso I, Sanchez-Correa B, Campos C et al (2011) Immunosenescence of human natural killer cells. J Innate Immun 3:337–343

Gimenez-Llort L, Mate I, Masnassra R et al (2012) Peripheral immune system and neuroimmune communication impairment in a mouse model of Alzheimer's disease. Ann N Y Acad Sci 1262:74–84

Gouin JP, Hantsoo L, Kiecolt. Glaser JK (2008) Immune dysregulation and chronic stress among older adults: a review. Neuroimmunomodulation 15:254–262

Goyns MH (2002) Genes, telomeres and mammalian ageing. Mech Ageing Dev 123:791–799

Guayerbas N, De la Fuente M (2003) An impairment of phagocytic function is linked to a shorter life span in two strains of prematurely aging mice. Dev Comp Immunol 27:339–350

Guayerbas N, Puerto M, Víctor VM et al (2002) Leukocyte function and life span in a murine model of premature immunosenescence. Exp Gerontol 37:249–256

Haman D (2006) Free radical theory of aging: an update: increasing the functional life span. Ann N Y Acad Sci 1067:10–21

Harman D (1956) Ageing: a theory based on free radical and radiation chemistry. J Gerontol 2:298–300

Hayflick L (2007) Biological aging is no longer an unsolved problem. Ann N Y Acad Sci 1100:1–13

Haynes L, Maue AC (2009) Effects of aging on T cell function. Curr Opin Immunol 21:414–417

Hernanz A, Bayon J, Bisbal E et al (2008) Leukocyte functions are altered in patients with depressive disorder. J Neuroimmunol 197:167–168

Jenny NS (2012) Inflammation in aging: cause, effect, or both? Discov Med 13:451–460

Kirkwood TBL (2008) Gerontology: healthy old age. Nature 455:739–740

Kokkinos P (2012) Physical activity, health benefits, and mortality risk. ISRN Cardiol. doi:10.5402/2012/718789

Kouda K, Iki M (2010) Beneficial effects of mild stress (hormetic effects): dietary restriction and health. J Physiol Anthropol 29:127–132

Lang PO, Govin S, Aspinall R (2013) Reversing T cell immunosenescence: why, who and how. Age 35(3):609–620

Lupien SJ, McEwen BS, Gunnar MR (2009) Effects of stress throughout the lifespan on the brain, behaviour and cognition. Nat Rev Neurosci 10:434–445

Makrantonaki E, Schonknecht P, Hossini AM (2010) Skin and brain age together: the role of hormones in the ageing process. Exp Gerontol 45:801–813

Masoro EJ (2009) Caloric restriction induced life extension of rats and mice: a critique of proposed mechanisms. Biochim Biophys Acta 1790:1040–1048

Mattson MP (2008) Hormesis defined. Ageing Res Rev 7:1–7

Medvedev ZA (1990) An attempt at a rational classification of theories of aging. Biol Rev 65:375–398

Messaoudi I, Fischer M, Warner J et al (2008) Optimal window of caloric restriction onset limits its beneficial impact on T-cell senescence in primates. Aging Cell 7:908–919

Miquel J (1998) An update on the oxygen stress-mitochondrial mutation theory of aging: genetic and evolutionary implications. Exp Gerontol 33:113–126

Miquel J, Economos AC, Fleming J et al (1980) Mitochondrial role in cell aging. Exp Gerontol 15:575–591

Moncek F, Duncko R, Johansson BB et al (2004) Effect of environmental enrichment on stress related systems in rats. J Neuroendocrinol 16:423–431

Nakamura E, Miyao K (2007) A method for identifying biomarkers of aging and constructing and index of biological age in humans. J Gerontol A Biol Sci Med Sci 62:1096–1105

Ogata K, Yokose N, Tamura H et al (1997) Natural killer cells in the late decades of human life. Clin Immunol Immunopathol 84:269–275

Pae M, Meydani SN, Wu D (2012) The role of nutrition in enhancing immunity in aging. Aging Dis 3:91–129

Pandey KB, Rizvi SI (2010) Markers of oxidative stress in erythrocytes and plasma during aging in humans. Oxidative Med Cel Longevity 3:2–12

Park J, Cho B, Kwon H (2009) Developing a biological age assessment equation using principal component analysis and clinical biomarkers of aging in Korean men. Arch Gerontol Geriatr 49:7–12

Pauwels EK (2011) The protective effect of the Mediterranean diet: focus on cancer and cardiovascular risk. Med Princ Pract 20:103–111

Pawelec G (2006) Immunity and ageing in man. Exp Gerontol 41:1239–1242

Pawelec G, Larbi A, Derhovanesian E (2010) Senescence of the human immune system. J Comp Pathol. doi:10.1016/j.jcpa.2009.09.005

Puerto M, Guayerbas N, Alvarez P, De la Fuente M (2005) Modulation of neuropeptide Y and norepinephrine on several leucocyte functions in adult, old and very old mice. J Neuroimmunol 165:33–40

Radak Z, Chung HY, Koltai E et al (2008) Exercise, oxidative stress and hormesis. Ageing Res Rev 7:34–42

Rattan SI (2008) Hormesis in aging. Ageing Res Rev 7:63–78

Rattan SI, Demirovic D (2009) Hormesis can and does work in humans. Dose Response 8:58–63

Ristow M, Schmeisser S (2011) Extending life span by increasing oxidative stress. Free Radic Biol Med 51:327–336

Ristow M, Zarse K (2010) How increased oxidative stress promotes longevity and metabolic health: the concept of mitochondrial hormesis (mitohormesis). Exp Gerontol 45:410–418

Ruiz Torres A (1991) Basic results for assessment of human ageing. Arch Gerontol Geriatr 12:261–272

Salim S, Chugh G, Asghar M (2012) Inflammation and anxiety. Adv Protein Chem Struct Biol 88:1–25

Salminen A, Huuskonen J, Ojala J (2008a) Activation of innate immunity system during aging: NF-kB signaling is the molecular culprit of inflamm-aging. Ageing Res Rev 7:83–105

Salminen A, Kauppinen A, Suuronen T et al (2008b) SIRT 1 longevity factor suppresses NF-kappaB-driven immune responses: regulation of aging via NF-kappa B acetylation? Bioessays 30:939–942

Schloesser RJ, Lehmann M, Martinowich K et al (2010) Environmental enrichment requires adult neurogenesis to facilitate the recovery from psychosocial stress. Mol Psychiatry 15:1152–1163

Shaw AC, Joshi S, Greenwood H et al (2010) Aging of the innate immune system. Curr Opin Immunol 22:507–513

Simpson RJ, Lowder TW, Spielmann G et al (2012) Exercise and the aging immune system. Ageing Res Rev 11:404–420

Strehler BL (1977) Time, cells and aging, 2nd edn. Academic, New York

Vaiserman AM (2010) Hormesis, adaptive epigenetic reorganization, and implications for human health and longevity. Dose Response 8:16–21

Vallejo AN (2011) Is immune aging a cause of disease among the elderly, or is it a passive indicator of general decline of physiologic function? Aging Dis 2:444–448

Vasto S, Scapagnini G, Bulati M et al (2010) Biomarkers of aging. Front Biosci 2:392–402

Viveros MP, Arranz L, Hernanz A et al (2007) A model of premature ageing in mice based on altered stress-related behavioural response and immunosenescence. Neuroimmunomodulation 14:157–162

Walford L (1969) The immunologic theory of aging. Williams & Wilkins, Baltimore

Walsh NP, Gleeson M, Shepard RJ et al (2011) Positive statement. Part one: immune function and exercise. Exerc Immunol Rev 17:6–63

Wang L, Xie Y, Zhu LJ et al (2010) An association between immunosenescence and CD4(+) CD25(+) regulatory T cells: a systematic review. Biomed Environ Sci 23:327–332

Wayne SJ, Rhyne RL, Garry PJ et al (1990) Cell-mediated immunity as a predictor of morbidity and mortality in subjects over 60. J Gerontol 114:80–88

Williams GC (1957) Pleiotropy, natural selection and the evolution of senescence. Evolution 2:397–411

Yirmiya R, Goshen I (2011) Immune modulation of learning, memory, neural plasticity and neurogenesis. Brain Behav Immun 25:181–213

Yoon SO, Yun CH, Cheng AS (2002) Dose effect of oxidative stress on signal transduction in aging. Mech Ageing Dev 50:1–8

Age-Associated Alterations of Pleiotropic Stem Cell and the Therapeutic Implication of Stem Cell Therapy in Aging

Ahmad Massoud

3.1 Introduction

Aging is a complex process involving every cell and organ in the body and leads to the deterioration of many body functions over the lifespan of an individual. The reduced capacity to regenerate injured tissues or organs and an increased propensity to infections and cancers are probably the most prominent hallmarks of senescence (Hayflick 1998).

As the regenerative capabilities of a living organism is determined by the ability and potential of its stem cells to replace damaged tissue or worn-out cells, all aging phenomena, including tissue deterioration, cancer, and propensity to infections, can be interpreted as signs of aging at the level of somatic stem cells.

The research into stem cell began in 1963 when Siminovitch et al. established assays to detect hematopoietic stem cells (HSCs) (Siminovitch et al. 1963). The group has since found HSCs in the bone marrow (BM) of mice. First, their series of experiments demonstrated that cells from the BM could reconstitute hematopoiesis and hence rescue lethally irradiated animals. Second, using serial transplantations, they established the self-renewal ability of the original BM cells. When cells from splenic colonies in the first recipients of BM transplants were further transplanted into other animals that had received a lethal dose of irradiation, colonies of white and red blood corpuscles were found in the secondary recipients. On the basis of these experiments, the group defined HSCs as cells that have "the abilities of unrestricted self-renewal as well as multilineage differentiation" (Siminovitch et al. 1963). This discovery marked the beginning of modern-day stem cell research. Since then two main categories of stem cells have defined throughout different studies in both human and animals: so-called embryonic stem cells (ESCs) (Thomson et al. 1998) and somatic or tissue-specific stem cells (Gage 2000; Ho and Punzel 2003). There are differences between these cell types with respect to their regenerative capacities: ESCs have unlimited potential for growth and differentiation and have the potential to form most, if not all, cell types of the adult body over an almost unlimited period, whereas adult stem cells are committed towards specialization and have the ability to regenerate the tissue from which they are derived over the lifespan of an individual (Stojkovic et al. 2004; Bjerknes and Cheng 1999; Gage 2000; Weissman 2000b).

3.2 Evidence About the Age-Associated Stem Cell Decline

The regenerative capacity of stem cells declines with age. One of the best-studied stem cells in this respect are HSCs. HSCs differentiation is ongoing until death, as is HSCs renewal. However, there

A. Massoud, PharmD, MPH, PhD
Department of Immunology, School of Medicine,
Tehran University of Medical Sciences, Tehran, Iran
e-mail: massoud.ahmad@yahoo.com

are distinct changes as an organism ages. BM decreases in cellularity, anemias are more common, lymphopoiesis declines, and the incidence of myeloid abnormalities, such as malignancies, myelodysplastic syndromes, and myeloproliferative disorders, increases (Woolthuis et al. 2011). These changes are associated with alterations in the HSCs pool (Rossi et al. 2005; Kim et al. 2003). Hypothetically, HSCs could be affected into two ways. They can either decrease in number, or they cannot properly differentiate. Surprisingly, the number of HSCs increases with age in humans (Beerman et al. 2010; Taraldsrud et al. 2009). However, they appear to be impaired in differentiation. Specifically, the stem cells appear to be myeloid-biased and exhibit less inclination to differentiate into lymphoid lineages (Taraldsrud et al. 2009; Woolthuis et al. 2011). This would at first sight suggest and problem in differentiation. However, it has been recently shown that there is a loss of a specific HSCs subpopulation that tends to form lymphoid progeny (Challen et al. 2010; Wang et al. 2011). The other type of HSCs is mesenchymal stem cells. They are present in BM and other tissues, such as adipose. These are multipotent and can differentiate into mesodermal and nonmesodermal tissues (Deng et al. 2006; Smith et al. 2004). Studies in mice demonstrated that the number of BM mesenchymal stem cells decreases only marginally as the organism ages. However, their self-renewal ability dramatically drops. Thus, both major features of stem cells are affected by aging in this stem cell type (Chen 2004; Sun et al. 2011).

In addition, the tissue-specific stem cells involved in tissue repair are known to decline with age. This includes skin-derived precursors, which represses functionally and numerically with age (Gago et al. 2009). Another example is the age-related endothelial dysfunction (Heiss et al. 2005) which is due to decrease in bone-marrow-derived endothelial progenitor cells (EPCs), playing an important role in maintenance of endothelial function by contributing to re-endothelization and neovacularization (Asahara et al. 1997). EPCs also functionally decline with age, and this decline correlates with impairment of the endothelium (Heiss et al. 2005). A similar

situation occurs in muscles. The muscle stem cell (termed the satellite cell) is usually quiescent and mobilized when required for repair, for example, when an injury occurs. The numbers of satellite cells do not appear to change much with age (Brack and Rando 2007; Jones and Rando 2011). However, their repair, i.e., differentiation ability, is dramatically reduced (Brack et al. 2007; Conboy et al. 2003). Thus, the satellite cells are altered in at least one of the major features of stem cells.

Taken together, adult stem cells undergo age-related changes. The age-related decline is mainly functional, but in some cases, decline in stem cell numbers can be observed.

3.3   The Reciprocal Effects of Tissue and Stem Cells During Aging

Given the key role of stem cells in maintenance of many tissues, it is easy to assume that they play a central role in the aging of the tissues. This model would assume that the somatic cells can be easily replaced, and, as long as stem cells are intact, tissue aging does not occur or is reversible. However, other aspects need to be considered such as stem cell environment. In other words, the microenvironment the stem cells reside in, as well as more distant interactions, mediated by circulating proteins and growth factors might reciprocally affect each other in the process of aging. The possible role of the microenvironment has been addressed using heterochronic approaches, where young stem cells were transplanted into an old niche and vice versa. What was demonstrated is that, at least in hemopoietic stem cell case, the BM environment significantly affects stem cell aging, and a young environment can actually rejuvenate the old stem cells (Woolthuis et al. 2011; Marion and Blasco 2010). This is consistent with results from studies with induced pluripotent stem cells, which demonstrate that reprogramming of somatic cells into stem cells leads to lengthening of telomeres, and thus indicates that the rejuvenation and reversibility of the aging process is indeed possible

(Marion and Blasco 2010). Conversely, young stem cells fail to efficiently repopulate an old niche microenvironment (Mauch et al. 1982). In conclusion, stem cell aging is influenced by the aged microenvironment they are in. Thus, stem cell and organism aging is an interconnected process.

3.4 Molecular Changes Underlying the Age-Related Changes in Stem Cells

In general, mechanisms that are involved in aging of somatic cells are also involved in aging of adult stem cells. Multiple hypotheses have been proposed to address the molecular and biological age-associated changes in stem cells. These include shortening of telomeres, oxidative stress, DNA damage, epigenetic alterations of transcriptional regulation, depletion, and reduced differentiation capacity of stem cells (Goyns 2002; Li et al. 2008; Rodriguez-Rodero et al. 2010).

During DNA replication, cellular DNA has to replicate. It had been suggested first at 1970s that DNA replication may result in chromosomal shortening, due to difficulties when replicating chromosomal ends and this shortening may be related to aging (Olovnikov 1973). The chromosomal ends are protected by telomeres, which are ribonucleoprotein complexes that consist of tandem DNA repeats (TTAGGG) and several proteins, together termed shelterin (de Lange 2005). Conventional DNA polymerases cannot replicate the chromosomal ends. To prevent shortening of these ends (telomeres) with each cell cycle, cells possess the enzyme telomerase, which can add the TTAGGG repeats to the chromosomal ends. The activity of telomerase is known to decline with age (Donate and Blasco 2011). The shortening of chromosomal ends can eventually lead to the loss of telomere protection. The naked chromosomal ends then may trigger a DNA damage response, with resulting growth arrest and/or apoptosis (Vaziri and Benchimol 1996). Adult stem cells express high levels of telomerase (Zimmermann and Martens 2005). The proposed role of telomere shortening in aging is supported

by evidence from telomerase-deficient mice, which exhibit premature aging (Blasco et al. 1995; Herrera et al. 1999; Lee et al. 1998). This finding is accompanied by dramatic impairment of adult skin stem cells which can be rescued by suppression of p53, which is a key protein of cellular DNA damage response (Siegl-Cachedenier et al. 2007; Flores et al. 2005). This latter data thus support the hypothesis that naked chromosomal ends trigger DNA damage response. Consistently, p53 overexpression leads to premature aging in mice (Donate and Blasco 2011). In addition to skin stem cells, late-generation telomerase-deficient mice have also limited HSCs reserve, which is accompanied by short telomeres in this population (Donate and Blasco 2011).

The DNA damage response can be also triggered by other mechanisms than telomere shortening. The DNA damage theory of aging postulates that the main cause of the functional decline associated with aging is the accumulation of DNA damage and ensuing cellular alterations, e.g., apoptosis (Kenyon and Gerson 2007). From this point of view, telomere shortening is only a part of the picture. Cells are exposed to many types of DNA damaging agents and sources, both extrinsic and intrinsic, including reactive oxygen species (ROS). Accordingly, they possess multiple DNA repair systems, which can repair the damage. Function of many of these systems declines with age (Donate and Blasco 2011).

3.4.1 Age-Associated Epigenetic Changes

Another phenomenon associated with aging is changes in epigenetic modifications of histones and DNA and consequent dysregulation of gene expression. The epigenetic modifications that were observed during aging are related to change in histone acetylation, histone methylation, and DNA methylation. In mice, it has been observed that the level of the histone deacetylase SirT1 decreases with age (Sasaki et al. 2006). Interestingly, the well-known SirT1 activator, resveratrol, prolongs the life span of mice when added to the diet (Sasaki et al. 2006).

The second observed epigenetic change observed in senescent human stem cells is increased methylation of H4K20 (methylation of histone H4 at lysine residue 20) and decreased methylation of H3K27 (trimethylation of histone H3 at lysine residue 27) (Sarg et al. 2002). Epigenetic dysregulation of H3K9 (H3 at lysine residue 9) and H3K14 (H3 at lysine residue 14) acetylation also occurs in aging mesenchymal stem cells (Li et al. 2011).

The third aging-associated epigenetic phenomenon is a global decrease in DNA methylation (Berdyshev et al. 1967). However, there is an increase in DNA methylation at certain loci at the same time. Among these are tumor suppressor genes (Esteller 2007, 2008; Maegawa et al. 2010). DNA methylation generally suppresses expression, and therefore inactivation of tumor suppression genes may increase risk of cancer in aged individuals.

It is not yet clear if all described epigenetic changes occur in aging stem cells. However, it has been demonstrated that the levels of some DNA methyltransferases (DNMTs) control the self-renewal and differentiation of stem cells. For example, DNMT1 is essential for self-renewal of HSCs (Trowbridge et al. 2009). In summary, the presented data suggest that aging of stem cells is associated with epigenetic changes, and these changes may affect either self-renewal or differentiation of these essential cell types.

3.5 Stem Cell Exhaustion in Premature Syndromes

The hypothesis that cumulative, unrepaired DNA damage may play a role in aging is supported by some premature aging (progeria) syndromes. These include Hutchinson–Gilford (Progeria) syndrome, Werner syndrome, trichothiodystrophy, Cockayne syndrome, and ataxia telangiectasia. These are rare genetic diseases wherein symptoms resembling aging are manifested at an early age. Individuals that suffer from these syndromes have significantly shortened life span and exhibit signs on premature aging (Freitas and de Magalhaes 2011). Significantly, mutations and genes in which these mutations occur were identified for each of these syndromes. The Werner syndrome protein is a RECQ-related DNA helicase that is known to be involved in DNA repair (Lee et al. 2005). Trichothiodystrophy is caused by point mutation in the *XPD* gene, which is involved in nucleotide excision repair (NER) (Hasty et al. 2003). Similarly, Cockayne syndrome is caused by mutations in either *CSA* or *CSB* gene, both of which are required for nucleotide excision repair (Hasty et al. 2003). Finally, the gene mutated in ataxia telangiectasia is involved in double-strand break DNA repair (Rotman and Shiloh 1997). Thus, this link between DNA repair and aging strongly supports the DNA damage hypothesis of aging. Similar results were obtained with transgenic animals that carry mutations in DNA repair genes. Mutations in ligase 4, Ku80, and Ku70 genes, which are involved in double-strand DNA break (DSB) repair, lead to poor hematopoietic reconstitution due to an HSC defect in repopulation ability (Rossi et al. 2005; Nijnik et al. 2007; Qing et al. 2012). Similarly, a deficiency in another component of the DSB repair, *RAD50*, results in hematopoietic failure due to ablation of HSCs (Bender et al. 2002). In addition, mice carrying a mutation in the ataxia telangiectasia gene (*ATM*) have decreased stem cell numbers, loss of repopulation ability, and increased apoptosis of HSCs (Ito et al. 2004). These results raise a question whether this type of stem cell defects is due to a decreased DNA repair ability of HSCs. In support of this hypothesis, it has been demonstrated that antioxidants reduced the oxidative stress and maintained stem cell function in ATM-deficient mice (Ito et al. 2004). Finally, in aged humans, aged HSCs from normal individuals were shown to accumulate DNA damage, which appears to contribute to their functional decline, and exhibit increase in the numbers of H2AX foci, which are markers of double-strand DNA breaks (Rossi et al. 2007). Taken together, the presented results suggest that DNA damage may play a significant role in aging and loss of functionality of stem cells.

3.6 Stem Cell Therapy

Stem cell treatments are a type of intervention strategy that introduces new adult stem cells into damaged tissue in order to treat disease or injury. Stem cell-based therapies hold tremendous promise for the treatment of serious diseases and injuries. The ability of stem cells to self-renew and give rise to subsequent generations with variable degrees of differentiation capacities offers significant potential for generation of tissues that can potentially replace diseased and damaged areas in the body, with minimal risk of rejection and side effects (Weissman 2000a).

Medical researchers anticipate that adult and embryonic stem cells will soon be able to treat age-associated diseases, such as cancer, type 1 diabetes mellitus, Parkinson's disease, Huntington's disease, celiac disease, cardiac failure, and muscle damage and neurological disorders (Singec et al. 2007). Nevertheless, before stem cell therapies can be applied in the clinical setting, more research is necessary to understand the behavior of these cells upon transplantation as well as the mechanisms of stem cell interaction with the diseased/injured microenvironment.

It is conceivable that transplantation of appropriate cell types, either derived from embryonic or tissue-specific stem cells, is an effective method to replace cells lost due to pathology. The first demonstration that stem cells might be used for cell replacement in a solid organ, derived from work in the adult mammalian neocortex (Snyder et al. 1997). In an adult mouse model of experimentally induced apoptosis of pyramidal neurons, it was demonstrated that engrafted naïve neural stem cells (NSCs) responded to the environmental cue to differentiate specifically into that cell type and project axons to their proper target region. Outside that region, or in the neocortex of an intact adult, the same clone of NSCs yielded only glia.

Since then, many studies have documented that cell replacement is effective in generating adult tissues. However, it is important not to overgeneralize and depend on the source of transplanted cells, their cellular differentiation state, and the disease model used; grafted cells could die during cell preparation and early after implantation (Bakshi et al. 2005; Karlsson et al. 2005). Parkinson disease (PD) is a degenerative disorder of the central nervous system resulted from the death of dopamine-generating cells in the substantia nigra, a region of the midbrain; the cause of this cell death is unknown. Stem cell grafting has been utilized to treat PD in murine models. In a rat Parkinson model, it has been found that micrografting of multiple dopamine cell result in a more effective and successful stem cell transfer than single grafts (Nikkhah et al. 1994). Hence, this suggests that micrografting approach resulted in a better cell survival than did large single grafts. Defining the appropriate cell differentiation state before grafting (naïve versus predifferentiated) and improved transplantation techniques in combination with anti-apoptotic and cell-protective drugs are key areas that need to be better understood prior to clinical translation of stem cell therapy. In addition, establishing a standardized postoperative immunosuppressive regimen is critical, since insufficient immunosuppression has been suggested as a possible reason for the poor outcome in some clinical trials with patients. The continuous treatment with immunosuppressive drugs (e.g., cyclosporine alone or in combination with other drugs) over several months seems to be important in order to prevent acute and delayed immunological responses to the grafted cells (Lindvall and Bjorklund 2004).

In addition to PD, in Huntington's disease (HD) (an autosomal dominant neurodegenerative genetic disorder), transplantation of NSCs may offer a novel treatment option that may slow, halt, or even reverse the progression of this devastating illness (Peschanski et al. 2004). Experimental studies in animal models of HD have provided convincing evidence that fetal neural tissue can survive transplantation, grow, and establish functional afferent and efferent connections with the host brain. These observations correlated with an amelioration of lesion-induced behavioral deficits including abnormal locomotion, chorea, dystonia, and dementia (Peschanski et al. 2004).

Autoimmune diseases can appear in any ages, but their risk and prevalence is higher during aging. Autoimmune diseases represent a failure of normal immune regulatory processes as they are characterized by activation and expansion of immune cell subsets in response to nonpathogenic stimuli. As autoimmune diseases can be transferred, or alternatively, cured, by stem cell transplantation, a defect in the HSCs as a cause of autoimmune diseases may be postulated. The rationale for autologous hematopoietic stem cell transplantation in autoimmune diseases is the ablation of an aberrant or self-reactive immune system by chemotherapy and regeneration of a new and hopefully self-tolerant immune system from hematopoietic stem cells. Several works suggested that mesenchymal stem cells (MSCs) are defective in autoimmune diseases. These aspects are now considered the most intriguing aspect of their biology, introducing the possibility that these cells might be used as effective therapy in autoimmune diseases (Cipriani et al. 2013). Animal model of autoimmune diseases that have been shown to be effectively treated by stem cell transplantation includes multiple sclerosis, systemic sclerosis, systemic lupus erythematosus, rheumatoid arthritis, juvenile idiopathic arthritis, and idiopathic cytopenic purpura (Cipriani et al. 2013).

Cardiovascular diseases are also a group of likely age-associated disorders of the heart and blood vessels. Stem cell-based treatments are expected to have an impact on promoting cardiac myogenesis and vascularization. It is widely believed that after birth new endothelial cells are derived from resident endothelial cells during the process of angiogenesis. Multiple studies have also indicated that endothelial progenitor cells (EPCs) derived from BM contribute to postnatal vascularization (Eguchi et al. 2007). HSCs can become entrapped at the site of injury and induce neovascularization by production of growth factors. In some studies on animal models of myocardial infarction, cultured MSCs derived from BM have been shown to home in on the site of injury and to promote cardiomyocyte differentiation and vascularization (Nagaya et al. 2004), thereby resulting in a normalization of ventricular function. However, the mechanisms remain obscure. The observation that BM elements such as EPCs, HSCs, and MSCs can contribute to cardiac repair in the infarcted heart generated a therapeutic strategy for the use of adult BM cells after myocardial infarction. In clinical trials patients received mononuclear cells derived from BM by intracoronary injection exhibited improvement in cardiac function after myocardial infarction (Schachinger et al. 2004; Wollert et al. 2004). In addition to cell therapy approaches, the identification of cardiac progenitor cells (Laflamme and Murry 2005) in the adult heart opens up new therapeutic possibilities for pharmacological stimulation of the endogenous repair process in cardiac disorders. In agreement with these findings, transplantation of mobilized peripheral blood in patients with critical limb ischemia (occurs when there is a sudden lack of blood flow to a limb, such as atherosclerosis) resulted in increasing of vasculogenesis and an improvement of the symptoms (Kawamura et al. 2006).

3.7 Stem Cell-Based Gene Therapy

Depending on the specific disease, pathology can be restricted to specific sites or widely distributed. In an ideal therapeutic scenario, it would be possible to target the pathological lesions while avoiding healthy tissue. Efficient delivery of therapeutic molecules to specific regions is still a major challenge in gene therapy. Delivering therapeutic genes to specific sites via stem cells is an alternative strategy of combined gene and stem cell therapy. There are advantages for stem cell-mediated gene delivery as opposed to direct gene transfer. In recent years, some investigations have used stem cells that overexpress different neurotrophic factors, such as brain-derived neurotrophic factor (BDNF), glial cell-derived neurotrophic factor (GDNT), or neurotrophin-3 (NT3), and found that the delivery of these genetically modified stem cells to animal models of ischemic stroke is more safe and effective than delivering of naked or modifies genes (Chen et al. 2012).

NSCs also exhibit a remarkable ability to home to specific sides and are able to integrate seamlessly into the host brain while continuing to stably express a foreign transgene, it was reasoned that these cells may be ideal vehicles for the delivery of therapeutic molecules for central nervous system (CNS) disorders. In fact, inflammation and molecules released during acute or chronic injuries were found to be chemoattractants for NSCs. For instance, stromal cell-derived factor α (SDF1-α) secreted during the inflammatory response (in part by macrophages, activated microglia, reactive astrocytes, and inflamed endothelium) strongly attracts migratory human NSCs even over long distances (Imitola et al. 2004). Therefore, NSCs manipulated ex vivo (e.g., by viral transduction) and transplanted into the brain may be well suited for long-range delivery of therapeutically relevant molecules and drugs to CNS lesions. Taken together these data suggest that stem cell-based gene therapy may be a promising treatment for stroke.

3.8 Stem Cells Regenerative Medicine

Synthetic small molecules and natural products have provided useful pharmacological interventions to modulate cellular processes in stem cells. Indeed, several studies have shown that many drugs in current clinical use have the potential to modulate the function of stem cells (Kawamura et al. 2006). In addition, new chemical entities have been identified which have modulatory activity on stem cells (Ding and Schultz 2004, 2005). These chemicals might have potential for ex vivo expansion and differentiation of stem cells as well as for pharmacological intervention to stimulate self-repair processes.

Mouse embryonic stem cells are typically expanded in the presence of leukemia inhibitory factor (LIF) (Niwa et al. 1998) and bone morphogenetic protein (BMP) (Ying et al. 2003). The combination of these two factors allows these stem cells to proliferate in the absence of serum and feeder cells. LIF activates signal transducers and activators of transcription-3 (STAT-3) signaling, which promotes self-renewal and inhibits mesodermal and endodermal differentiation

(Niwa et al. 1998). BMP also inhibits mitogen-activated protein kinases signaling and neuroectodermal differentiation (Ying et al. 2003). Compared to mouse embryonic stem cells, human counterparts are more vulnerable to apoptosis upon cellular detachment and dissociation, which causes major problems for manipulations, such as subcloning, which require dissociated cultures (Watanabe et al. 2007).

Enhancing of mobilization is one of the key factors in getting stem cells, progenitor cells, macrophages, and monocytes to sites of injury, where they can induce vascularization and support regeneration. The injection of Granulocyte colony-stimulating factor (G-CSF) is one of the most common methods to mobilize HSCs for transplantation in the clinical setting (Cutler and Antin 2005). In addition, several other pharmacological agents, such as granulocyte colony-stimulating factor (G-CSF) (Yoon et al. 2007), erythropoietin (Bahlmann et al. 2004), statins (Dimmeler et al. 2001), rosiglitazone (Wang et al. 2004), estrogens (Strehlow et al. 2003), and angiotensin II receptor antagonists (Bahlmann et al. 2005), have been shown to have an effect on BM cells.

G-CSF has received attention as a possible treatment for heart failure after myocardial infarction, and it has been shown to have beneficial effects on cardiac function and cardiogenesis in animal models of myocardial infarction (Orlic et al. 2001; Minatoguchi et al. 2004). On the basis of these findings, G-CSF has been tested in patients with acute myocardial infarction (AMI) or chronic myocardial ischemia and seems to be safe and accelerating recovery. In a mouse stroke model, the combination of G-CSF and the stem cell factor (SCF) induced neurogenesis from NSCs and MSCs in the infarct area and induced functional recovery (Kawada et al. 2006). Hence, in addition to its effects on HSCs, G-CSF plays multiple roles in CNS regeneration.

The identification of regenerative pathways for pancreatic islet β cells is also an active area of research for developing regenerative treatment of diabetes type I. In this regard, three major routes for the generation of new β cells in the adult pancreas have been proposed: (1) neogenesis from ductal progenitor cells, (2) proliferation of existing β cells, and (3) transdifferentiation of pancreatic exocrine progenitor cells (Fellous et al. 2007). Glucagon-like peptide-1 (GLP-1) and its related peptide exendin-4 have been shown to prevent diabetes by enhancing β cell mass (Li et al. 2003). Therefore, in addition to cell replacement therapy using islet β cells derived from stem cells, pharmacological intervention could be an another important approach to the regenerative treatment of diabetes. However, similar to the situation in the heart, the very limited turnover capacity of these cells under normal conditions means that these studies are the subject of controversial discussion.

3.9   Concluding Remarks

In the recent year, our knowledge in the biology of stem cells and the degree to which the aging of these cells contributes to the overall aging process of human has been increased briskly. Understanding the molecular mechanisms underlies stem cell aging and utilizing technological methods for regenerating stem cells are enabling us to develop effective treatment for large spectrum of age-associated disorders. The application of human pluripotent stem cells for the treatment of a wide variety of age-associated diseases requires the development of technologies to finely regulate their growth and differentiation. In this regard, regenerative medicine, which aims to restore organ function, puts a lot of hopes into stem cell approaches. However, differences in pharmacological effects between animals and humans can be an obstacle to the selection of appropriate drug candidates for development. Techniques which allow the translation of the knowledge obtained from animal experiments to clinical application are vital for the improvement of drug development productivity and include in vitro and in vivo assay systems that mimic effects in human subjects. Although reprogramming-induced human pluripotent stem cells are not yet available, this technology would be a most efficient tool for translational medicine as well as for the generation of human cells and

tissues with specific genetic characteristics. They would provide useful tools for predicting the effects and side effects of drug candidates where these are related to genetic polymorphisms.

In summary, new stem cell findings provide new perspectives and should stimulate new research on stem cells and aging, which can potentially result in breakthrough treatments and lifespan extension.

References

Asahara T, Murohara T, Sullivan A et al (1997) Isolation of putative progenitor endothelial cells for angiogenesis. Science 275(5302):964–967

Bahlmann FH, De Groot K, Spandau JM et al (2004) Erythropoietin regulates endothelial progenitor cells. Blood 103(3):921–926

Bahlmann FH, de Groot K, Mueller O et al (2005) Stimulation of endothelial progenitor cells: a new putative therapeutic effect of angiotensin II receptor antagonists. Hypertension 45(4):526–529

Bakshi A, Keck CA, Koshkin VS et al (2005) Caspase-mediated cell death predominates following engraftment of neural progenitor cells into traumatically injured rat brain. Brain Res 1065(1–2):8–19

Beerman I, Maloney WJ, Weissmann IL et al (2010) Stem cells and the aging hematopoietic system. Curr Opin Immunol 22(4):500–506

Bender CF, Sikes ML, Sullivan R et al (2002) Cancer predisposition and hematopoietic failure in Rad50 (S/S) mice. Genes Dev 16(17):2237–2251

Berdyshev GD, Korotaev GK, Boiarskikh GV et al (1967) Nucleotide composition of DNA and RNA from somatic tissues of humpback and its changes during spawning. Biokhimiia 32(5):988–993

Bjerknes M, Cheng H (1999) Clonal analysis of mouse intestinal epithelial progenitors. Gastroenterology 116(1):7–14

Blasco MA, Funk W, Villeponteau B et al (1995) Functional characterization and developmental regulation of mouse telomerase RNA. Science 269(5228):1267–1270

Brack AS, Rando TA (2007) Intrinsic changes and extrinsic influences of myogenic stem cell function during aging. Stem Cell Rev 3(3):226–237

Brack AS, Conboy MJ, Roy S et al (2007) Increased Wnt signaling during aging alters muscle stem cell fate and increases fibrosis. Science 317(5839):807–810

Challen GA, Boles NC, Chambers SM et al (2010) Distinct hematopoietic stem cell subtypes are differentially regulated by TGF-beta1. Cell Stem Cell 6(3):265–278

Chen TL (2004) Inhibition of growth and differentiation of osteoprogenitors in mouse BM stromal cell cultures by increased donor age and glucocorticoid treatment. Bone 35(1):83–95

Chen C, Wang Y, Yang GY (2012) Stem cell-mediated gene delivering for the treatment of cerebral ischemia: progress and prospectives. Curr Drug Targets 14(1): 81–89

Cipriani P, Carubbi F, Liakouli V et al (2012) Stem cells in autoimmune diseases: implications for pathogenesis and future trends in therapy. Autoimmun Rev 12:709–716

Conboy IM, Conboy MJ, Smythe GM et al (2003) Notch-mediated restoration of regenerative potential to aged muscle. Science 302(5650):1575–1577

Cutler C, Antin JH (2005) An overview of hematopoietic stem cell transplantation. Clin Chest Med 26(4):517–527, v

de Lange T (2005) Shelterin: the protein complex that shapes and safeguards human telomeres. Genes Dev 19(18):2100–2110

Deng J, Petersen BE, Steindler DA et al (2006) Mesenchymal stem cells spontaneously express neural proteins in culture and are neurogenic after transplantation. Stem Cells 24(4):1054–1064

Dimmeler S, Aicher A, Vasa M et al (2001) HMG-CoA reductase inhibitors (statins) increase endothelial progenitor cells via the PI 3-kinase/Akt pathway. J Clin Invest 108(3):391–397

Ding S, Schultz PG (2004) A role for chemistry in stem cell biology. Nat Biotechnol 22(7):833–840

Ding S, Schultz PG (2005) Small molecules and future regenerative medicine. Curr Top Med Chem 5(4):383–395

Donate LE, Blasco MA (2011) Telomeres in cancer and ageing. Philos Trans R Soc Lond B Biol Sci 366(1561):76–84

Eguchi M, Masuda H, Asahara T (2007) Endothelial progenitor cells for postnatal vasculogenesis. Clin Exp Nephrol 11(1):18–25

Esteller M (2007) Cancer epigenomics: DNA methylomes and histone-modification maps. Nat Rev Genet 8(4):286–298

Esteller M (2008) Epigenetics in cancer. N Engl J Med 358(11):1148–1159

Fellous TG, Guppy NJ, Brittan M et al (2007) Cellular pathways to beta-cell replacement. Diabetes Metab Res Rev 23(2):87–99

Flores I, Cayuela ML, Blasco MA (2005) Effects of telomerase and telomere length on epidermal stem cell behavior. Science 309(5738):1253–1256

Freitas AA, de Magalhaes JP (2011) A review and appraisal of the DNA damage theory of ageing. Mutat Res 728(1–2):12–22

Gage FH (2000) Mammalian neural stem cells. Science 287(5457):1433–1438

Gago N, Perez-Lopez V, Sanz-Jaka JP et al (2009) Age-dependent depletion of human skin-derived progenitor cells. Stem Cells 27(5):1164–1172

Goyns MH (2002) Genes, telomeres and mammalian ageing. Mech Ageing Dev 123(7):791–799

Hasty P, Campisi J, Hoeijmakers J et al (2003) Aging and genome maintenance: lessons from the mouse? Science 299(5611):1355–1359

Hayflick L (1998) How and why we age. Exp Gerontol 33(7–8):639–653

Heiss C, Keymel S, Niesler U et al (2005) Impaired progenitor cell activity in age-related endothelial dysfunction. J Am Coll Cardiol 45(9):1441–1448

Herrera E, Samper E, Martin-Caballero J et al (1999) Disease states associated with telomerase deficiency appear earlier in mice with short telomeres. EMBO J 18(11):2950–2960

Ho AD, Punzel M (2003) Hematopoietic stem cells: can old cells learn new tricks? J Leukoc Biol 73(5):547–555

Imitola J, Raddassi K, Park KI et al (2004) Directed migration of neural stem cells to sites of CNS injury by the stromal cell-derived factor 1alpha/CXC chemokine receptor 4 pathway. Proc Natl Acad Sci U S A 101(52):18117–18122

Ito K, Hirao A, Arai F et al (2004) Regulation of oxidative stress by ATM is required for self-renewal of haematopoietic stem cells. Nature 431(7011):997–1002

Jones DL, Rando TA (2011) Emerging models and paradigms for stem cell ageing. Nat Cell Biol 13(5): 506–512

Karlsson J, Petersen A, Gido G et al (2005) Combining neuroprotective treatment of embryonic nigral donor tissue with mild hypothermia of the graft recipient. Cell Transplant 14(5):301–309

Kawada H, Takizawa S, Takanashi T et al (2006) Administration of hematopoietic cytokines in the subacute phase after cerebral infarction is effective for functional recovery facilitating proliferation of intrinsic neural stem/progenitor cells and transition of BM-derived neuronal cells. Circulation 113(5):701–710

Kawamura A, Horie T, Tsuda I et al (2006) Clinical study of therapeutic angiogenesis by autologous peripheral blood stem cell (PBSC) transplantation in 92 patients with critically ischemic limbs. J Artif Organs 9(4):226–233

Kenyon J, Gerson SL (2007) The role of DNA damage repair in aging of adult stem cells. Nucleic Acids Res 35(22):7557–7565

Kim M, Moon HB, Spangrude GJ (2003) Major age-related changes of mouse hematopoietic stem/progenitor cells. Ann N Y Acad Sci 996:195–208

Laflamme MA, Murry CE (2005) Regenerating the heart. Nat Biotechnol 23(7):845–856

Lee HW, Blasco MA, Gottlieb GJ et al (1998) Essential role of mouse telomerase in highly proliferative organs. Nature 392(6676):569–574

Lee JW, Harrigan J, Opresko PL et al (2005) Pathways and functions of the Werner syndrome protein. Mech Ageing Dev 126(1):79–86

Li Y, Hansotia T, Yusta B et al (2003) Glucagon-like peptide-1 receptor signaling modulates beta cell apoptosis. J Biol Chem 278(1):471–478

Li H, Mitchell JR, Hasty P (2008) DNA double-strand breaks: a potential causative factor for mammalian aging? Mech Ageing Dev 129(7–8):416–424

Li Z, Liu C, Xie Z et al (2011) Epigenetic dysregulation in mesenchymal stem cell aging and spontaneous differentiation. PLoS One 6(6):e20526

Lindvall O, Bjorklund A (2004) Cell therapy in Parkinson's disease. NeuroRx 1(4):382–393

Maegawa S, Hinkal G, Kim HS et al (2010) Widespread and tissue specific age-related DNA methylation changes in mice. Genome Res 20(3):332–340

Marion RM, Blasco MA (2010) Telomere rejuvenation during nuclear reprogramming. Curr Opin Genet Dev 20(2):190–196

Mauch P, Botnick LE, Hannon EC et al (1982) Decline in BM proliferative capacity as a function of age. Blood 60(1):245–252

Minatoguchi S, Takemura G, Chen XH et al (2004) Acceleration of the healing process and myocardial regeneration may be important as a mechanism of improvement of cardiac function and remodeling by postinfarction granulocyte colony-stimulating factor treatment. Circulation 109(21):2572–2580

Nagaya N, Fujii T, Iwase T et al (2004) Intravenous administration of mesenchymal stem cells improves cardiac function in rats with acute myocardial infarction through angiogenesis and myogenesis. Am J Physiol Heart Circ Physiol 287(6):H2670–H2676

Nijnik A, Woodbine L, Marchetti C et al (2007) DNA repair is limiting for haematopoietic stem cells during ageing. Nature 447(7145):686–690

Nikkhah G, Olsson M, Eberhard J et al (1994) A microtransplantation approach for cell suspension grafting in the rat Parkinson model: a detailed account of the methodology. Neuroscience 63(1):57–72

Niwa H, Burdon T, Chambers I et al (1998) Self-renewal of pluripotent embryonic stem cells is mediated via activation of STAT3. Genes Dev 12(13):2048–2060

Olovnikov AM (1973) A theory of marginotomy. The incomplete copying of template margin in enzymic synthesis of polynucleotides and biological significance of the phenomenon. J Theor Biol 41(1):181–190

Orlic D, Kajstura J, Chimenti S et al (2001) Mobilized BM cells repair the infarcted heart, improving function and survival. Proc Natl Acad Sci U S A 98(18):10344–10349

Peschanski M, Bachoud-Levi AC, Hantraye P (2004) Integrating fetal neural transplants into a therapeutic strategy: the example of Huntington's disease. Brain 127(Pt 6):1219–1228

Qing Y, Lin Y, Gerson SL (2012) An intrinsic BM hematopoietic niche occupancy defect of HSC in scid mice facilitates exogenous HSC engraftment. Blood 119(7):1768–1771

Rodriguez-Rodero S, Fernandez-Morera JL, Fernandez AF et al (2010) Epigenetic regulation of aging. Discov Med 10(52):225–233

Rossi DJ, Bryder D, Zahn JM et al (2005) Cell intrinsic alterations underlie hematopoietic stem cell aging. Proc Natl Acad Sci U S A 102(26):9194–9199

Rossi DJ, Bryder D, Seita J et al (2007) Deficiencies in DNA damage repair limit the function of haematopoietic stem cells with age. Nature 447(7145):725–729

Rotman G, Shiloh Y (1997) Ataxia-telangiectasia: is ATM a sensor of oxidative damage and stress? Bioessays 19(10):911–917

Sarg B, Koutzamani E, Helliger W et al (2002) Postsynthetic trimethylation of histone H4 at lysine 20 in mammalian tissues is associated with aging. J Biol Chem 277(42):39195–39201

Sasaki T, Maier B, Bartke A et al (2006) Progressive loss of SIRT1 with cell cycle withdrawal. Aging Cell 5(5):413–422

Schachinger V, Assmus B, Britten MB et al (2004) Transplantation of progenitor cells and regeneration enhancement in acute myocardial infarction: final one-year results of the TOPCARE-AMI Trial. J Am Coll Cardiol 44(8):1690–1699

Siegl-Cachedenier I, Flores I, Klatt P et al (2007) Telomerase reverses epidermal hair follicle stem cell defects and loss of long-term survival associated with critically short telomeres. J Cell Biol 179(2):277–290

Siminovitch L, McCulloch EA, Till JE (1963) The distribution of colony-forming cells among spleen colonies. J Cell Physiol 62:327–336

Singec I, Jandial R, Crain A et al (2007) The leading edge of stem cell therapeutics. Annu Rev Med 58:313–328

Smith JR, Pochampally R, Perry A et al (2004) Isolation of a highly clonogenic and multipotential subfraction of adult stem cells from BM stroma. Stem Cells 22(5):823–831

Snyder EY, Yoon C, Flax JD et al (1997) Multipotent neural precursors can differentiate toward replacement of neurons undergoing targeted apoptotic degeneration in adult mouse neocortex. Proc Natl Acad Sci U S A 94(21):11663–11668

Stojkovic M, Lako M, Strachan T et al (2004) Derivation, growth and applications of human embryonic stem cells. Reproduction 128(3):259–267

Strehlow K, Werner N, Berweiler J et al (2003) Estrogen increases BM-derived endothelial progenitor cell production and diminishes neointima formation. Circulation 107(24):3059–3065

Sun Y, Li W, Lu Z et al (2011) Rescuing replication and osteogenesis of aged mesenchymal stem cells by exposure to a young extracellular matrix. FASEB J 25(5):1474–1485

Taraldsrud E, Grogaard HK, Solheim S et al (2009) Age and stress related phenotypical changes in BM CD34+ cells. Scand J Clin Lab Invest 69(1):79–84

Thomson JA, Itskovitz-Eldor J, Shapiro SS et al (1998) Embryonic stem cell lines derived from human blastocysts. Science 282(5391):1145–1147

Trowbridge JJ, Snow JW, Kim J et al (2009) DNA methyltransferase 1 is essential for and uniquely regulates hematopoietic stem and progenitor cells. Cell Stem Cell 5(4):442–449

Vaziri H, Benchimol S (1996) From telomere loss to p53 induction and activation of a DNA-damage pathway at senescence: the telomere loss/DNA damage model of cell aging. Exp Gerontol 31(1–2):295–301

Wang CH, Ciliberti N, Li SH et al (2004) Rosiglitazone facilitates angiogenic progenitor cell differentiation toward endothelial lineage: a new paradigm in glitazone pleiotropy. Circulation 109(11):1392–1400

Wang J, Geiger H, Rudolph KL (2011) Immunoaging induced by hematopoietic stem cell aging. Curr Opin Immunol 23(4):532–536

Watanabe K, Ueno M, Kamiya D et al (2007) A ROCK inhibitor permits survival of dissociated human embryonic stem cells. Nat Biotechnol 25(6):681–686

Weissman IL (2000a) Stem cells: units of development, units of regeneration, and units in evolution. Cell 100(1):157–168

Weissman IL (2000b) Translating stem and progenitor cell biology to the clinic: barriers and opportunities. Science 287(5457):1442–1446

Wollert KC, Meyer GP, Lotz J et al (2004) Intracoronary autologous bone-marrow cell transfer after myocardial infarction: the BOOST randomised controlled clinical trial. Lancet 364(9429):141–148

Woolthuis CM, de Haan G, Huls G (2011) Aging of hematopoietic stem cells: intrinsic changes or microenvironmental effects? Curr Opin Immunol 23(4):512–517

Ying QL, Nichols J, Chambers I et al (2003) BMP induction of Id proteins suppresses differentiation and sustains embryonic stem cell self-renewal in collaboration with STAT3. Cell 115(3):281–292

Yoon SH, Shim YS, Park YH et al (2007) Complete spinal cord injury treatment using autologous BM cell transplantation and BM stimulation with granulocyte macrophage-colony stimulating factor: phase I/II clinical trial. Stem Cells 25(8):2066–2073

Zimmermann S, Martens UM (2005) Telomere dynamics in hematopoietic stem cells. Curr Mol Med 5(2):179–185

A Role for Epigenetic Modulation of the Innate Immune Response During Aging

4

Justin W. Killick, Stuart J. Bennett, Irundika H.K. Dias, Christopher R. Dunston, and Helen R. Griffiths

4.1 Introduction to Cellular Aging: Historical Perspective

Many theories have been suggested over the last 100 years trying to explain cellular and organismal aging. The rate of living hypothesis of Pearl in 1928 postulated that a quicker basal metabolic rate results in decreased lifespan (Pearl 1928). Denham Harman built on this notion with the free radical theory of aging which suggested that the by-products of metabolic activity such as the exposure to reactive oxygen species (ROS) OH$^\cdot$ and H_2O_2 cause damage that results in cellular aging (Harman 1956). The mutation accumulation theory of Peter Medawar in 1952 proposed that over the course of the organism's lifetime, mutations accumulate in the genome causing dysregulation of genes involved in aging and development (Medawar 1952). Others have considered aging to be a form of senescence; the process of replicative senescence was first described by Hayflick and Moorhead in 1961 as the capacity for cells to undergo a limited number of divisions, called the Hayflick limit (Hayflick and Moorhead 1961). Telomeric shortening occurs with each cell division, is accelerated under stress, and ultimately limits replicative capacity resulting in senescence.

The inflamm-aging model of cellular aging proposed by Franceschi et al. incorporates many aspects of these theories (Franceschi et al. 2007). These authors propose that the aging phenotype is the result of damage-induced inflammation that arises from a failure to adapt to stress-induced damage from ROS produced by normal cellular metabolism, exposure to ultraviolet (UV) radiation, and bacterial and viral infections. Ineffective DNA repair pathways, organelle autophagy, glutathione depletion, ineffective apoptosis, and cell clearance result in a non-resolving inflammatory response which drives aging. This is consistent with the observations of a proinflammatory state during aging.

4.2 Inflammation During Aging

The principal effectors of inflammation are cells of the innate immune system, particularly neutrophils, monocytes, and macrophages. Neutrophils from older adults have enhanced motility, but directionality of migration is poor and neutrophil-specific phagocytic activity is also decreased (Butcher et al. 2001). Such a scenario would lead to poor recruitment towards and poor clearance of damage but an accumulation of inflammatory mediators which would be secreted over a longer time. Similarly, the response to inflammatory challenge in aging mice associates with a poor acute-phase protein response from the liver in

J.W. Killick, BSc • S.J. Bennett, PhD
I.H.K. Dias, PhD • C.R. Dunston, PhD
H.R. Griffiths, PhD (✉)
Life and Health Sciences, Aston University,
Aston Triangle, Birmingham B4 7ET, UK
e-mail: h.r.griffiths@aston.ac.uk

A. Massoud, N. Rezaei (eds.), *Immunology of Aging*,
DOI 10.1007/978-3-642-39495-9_4, © Springer-Verlag Berlin Heidelberg 2014

spite of significant tissue damage (Gomez et al. 2007, 2008). Paradoxically, this associates with an enhanced inflammatory cytokine response, particularly of the acute-phase protein inducer IL-6, but this cytokine is also produced by systemic cells of the innate immune system.

It is recognized that monocyte subsets are important determinants of inflammatory persistence or resolution. Proportions and numbers of CD14⁺(high)CD16⁺ and CD14⁺(low)CD16⁺ monocytes are significantly increased, whereas proportions of CD14⁺(low)CD16⁻ monocytes are decreased in aged subjects as compared to young subjects (Nyugen et al. 2010). CD14$^{+(low)}$CD16⁺ monocytes are termed proinflammatory compared to CD14$^{(high)}$CD16⁻ monocytes based on cytokine secretion profiles, and there is a switch to proinflammatory monocytes with aging. Monocyte maturation into macrophages is vital for the innate immunity response. Macrophages produce cytokines and eicosanoids in response to exogenous and endogenous danger signals such as pathogen-derived molecules, oxidized proteins and lipids, TNF-α, and heat shock proteins (HSPs) (Vabulas et al. 2002).

We have recently reviewed the influence of aging on Toll-like receptor (TLR) expression and downstream signaling from mouse to man (Dunston and Griffiths 2010). The consensus of the literature that we reviewed is that TLRs, key receptors for innate immune signaling after gram-positive bacterial infection, are decreased on the cell surface of innate immune cells from older adults possibly due to altered trafficking. Moreover we reviewed the extent to which TLR adaptor molecules, e.g., MyD88 interleukin 1 receptor-associated kinase (IRAK)-1 and IRAK-4; tumor necrosis factor receptor-associated factor (TRAF)-6, tumor growth factor-β-activated kinase (TAK)-1, the mitogen-activated protein kinase (MAPK), and nuclear factor kappa light-chain enhancer of activated B cell (NFκB) pathways are refractory to the effect of stimulus and confirmed that there are many levels at which defective intracellular signaling can contribute to the refractory phenotype of macrophages to stimulus (Dunston and Griffiths 2010). The inability of older macrophages to mount an effective innate response to challenge poses significant health risk, notably the persistence of infection or pathogenic lipid debris and chronicity of inflammation resulting in an increased risk or morbidity and mortality as a result of infection or cardiovascular disease (Liang and Mackowiak 2007). During aging in vivo, there is a basal proinflammatory state, increased levels of circulating cytokines, and other mediators of innate immunity that are typically generated in response to lipopolysaccharide (LPS) stimulation (Lord et al. 2001).

The consequent proinflammatory environment increases the risk of disease such as rheumatoid arthritis, cardiovascular disease, and cancers which associate with a failure to resolve acute inflammatory events (Flavell et al. 2008).

4.3 Metabolism, Monocytes, and Inflammation

Metabolic state is an important contributor to monocyte function and differentiation. Early studies described that butyrate downregulates the expression of major histocompatibility complex (MHC) molecules on the cell surface that are required for antigen presentation and decreases the phagocytic capacity of treated monocytes (Millard et al. 2002). More recently, the effects of fatty acids on inflammatory responses of monocytes and macrophages have been explored and confirm that omega-3 fatty acid-treated macrophages are less inflammatory whereas saturated fatty acid (palmitate)-treated monocytes are more inflammatory (Wang et al. 2009; Gao et al. 2012). In humans, aging associates with an altered metabolic phenotype typical of insulin resistance with impaired clearance of circulating free fatty acids and glucose (Pagano et al. 1996). These studies support the hypothesis that monocyte dysfunction (proinflammatory and failure to resolve) as a result of hyperglycemia/lipidemia will be more prevalent in aging.

In further confirmation of the relationship between metabolism and inflammation, Dasu et al. described that high glucose with or without high fatty acids increased cell surface TLR-2 and

TLR-4 expression and NFκB signaling in human monocytes (Dasu et al. 2008; Dasu and Jialal 2011). High glucose or free fatty acids have also been associated with increased monocyte adhesion to human umbilical vein endothelial cells and vascular smooth muscle cells, increased rate of both monocyte migration and transendothelial migration, and impaired uptake of oxidized low-density lipoprotein (LDL) in vitro (Meng et al. 2010; Nandy et al. 2011; Gao et al. 2012).

Monocytes treated with palmitate in vitro are also resistant to insulin-stimulated glucose uptake compared to non-palmitate-treated controls, and cellular memory of this effect can be retained (Gao et al. 2009) perhaps due to epigenetic modifications. Epigenetic modifications of DNA and histone proteins have been proposed as important contributory mechanisms to the retention of metabolic memory over time. Indeed, the United Kingdom prospective diabetes study (UKPDS) and epidemiology of diabetes interventions and complications (EDIC) studies suggest that poor glycemic environment establishes a "metabolic memory" effect resulting in a poorer outcome with greater incidence of complications even after control of the glycemic environment has been established (The Diabetes Control and Complications Trial Research Group 1993; Chalmers and Cooper 2008). Assimilating these findings, it is reasonable to consider that a decline in metabolic efficiency with age drives an inflammatory phenotype which persists through epigenetic change.

4.4   A Role for Epigenetic Change in Mediating Systemic Inflammation During Aging

Epigenetic changes are believed to provide a link between the environment and nutrition to gene expression by altering the activity of some histone-modifying protein, e.g., the nicotinamide adenine dinucleotide (NAD^+)-dependent histone deacetylase enzyme silent mating type information regulation 2 homolog 1 (SIRT1) (Haigis and Sinclair 2010). As SIRT1 is an NAD^+-dependent enzyme, its activity and therefore potential for

epigenetic manipulation are dependent on energy availability within the cell.

4.4.1   Epigenetic Histone Modifications

Nucleosomes, the functional units of chromatin, are formed from genomic DNA wrapped around histone protein complexes. The posttranslational additions of methyl or acetyl groups to histone proteins are important epigenetic modifications that are implicated in gene regulation (Rice and Allis 2001).

N-terminal histone methylation is catalyzed by the histone methyl transferase (HMT) family to yield a complex series of modifications; lysine residues can be either mono-, di-, or tri-methylated and arginine residues either mono- or di-methylated, and di- or tri-methylation can be either symmetrical or asymmetrical, thereby adding further variation (Nimura et al. 2010). Although histone methylation is generally associated with gene repression, it has been shown to be capable of activating gene expression. For example, di- or tri-methylation of the histone protein H3 at lysine K4 can activate gene expression, whereas di- or tri-methylation of H3 at lysine K9 has been shown to be capable of repressing gene expression (Hou and Yu 2010).

All the HMT families use S-adenosylmethionine (SAM) as a coenzyme in the transfer of methyl groups (Varier and Timmers 2011). With the discovery of the first histone demethylase enzyme, lysine-specific histone demethylase 1 (LSD1), in 2004 by Shi et al., it became apparent that histone methylation is a dynamic process rather than a permanent one (Shi et al. 2004). Methylated histones in turn can recruit protein complexes with histone acetyl transferase (HAT) activity suggesting a mechanism by which histone methylation may influence histone acetylation (Rice and Allis 2001).

4.4.2   Histone Acetylation

N-terminal histone acetylation is mediated by HAT which requires acetyl coenzyme A (acetyl-CoA) as a source of acetyl groups (Rice and Allis 2001). The antagonistic process, deacetylation, is performed by histone deacetylases (HDAC) which remove the acetyl groups for transfer to CoA. Histone acetylation is thus a dynamic and reversible process which can affect gene expression. Histone acetylation is generally considered to result in gene activation and deacetylation to result in gene silencing (Yeung et al. 2004).

Histone acetylation results in altered gene expression; although the mechanism has not yet been fully elucidated, it is likely to be due to altered interaction between DNA and histones as acetylation neutralizes the lysine residues' positive charge weakening the interaction with the negatively charged phosphate backbone of the DNA. This relaxes the tight chromatin structure exposing the gene promoter to RNA polymerases allowing gene transcription and aiding in elongation.

4.4.3 Histone Deacetylase Enzymes and the Regulation of Histone and Protein Acetylation

Histone deacetylase enzymes like HAT enzymes are also believed to be highly conserved between mammals and yeast. At least 18 HDAC enzymes have been discovered and separated into four distinct classes based on their homology to yeast HDAC proteins. Class III HDACs contain the sirtuin family of deacetylase proteins which are NAD^+ dependent and share homology with the yeast silent information regulator 2 (Sir2) deacetylase protein (Dokmanovic et al. 2007).

The yeast Sir2 histone deacetylase protein was first discovered to have a role in regulating the aging process by Sinclair and Guarente (1997). Overexpression of Sir2 in yeast results in an approximate 30 % increase in budding yeast cellular lifespan, whereas Sir2 knockout yeast cells cause a 50 % decrease in cellular lifespan. Yeast cells subjected to reduced glucose availability (caloric restriction) also experienced increased cellular lifespan via upregulation of the Sir2 protein. Calorie restriction (CR) has also

been shown to increase lifespan in worm, fly, and mice models via invertebrate and mammalian Sir2 homologs. The mammalian homologs of yeast Sir2 belong to the sirtuin family of proteins which contains seven proteins (SIRT1–7). SIRT1 is the most closely related of the sirtuins to Sir2. SIRT1 is a NAD^+-dependent deacetylase protein which recognizes and deacetylates both histones and several other proteins and transcription factors (Haigis and Sinclair 2010).

Intracellular NAD^+ availability, increased during low nutrient availability, is rate limiting for SIRT1 activity, and deacetylation is greater during nutrient deprivation. In contrast, an increase in glycolysis arising from increased nutrient availability increases intracellular pyruvate and acetyl-CoA, a substrate necessary for acetylation. Thus increased nutrient availability results in increased acetylation frequency (Haigis and Sinclair 2010).

4.4.3.1 Acetylation, Inflammation, and Aging

SIRT1 catalyzes not only deacetylation of the histone proteins H3 and H4 at lysine residues K9 and K16, respectively, but also several proteins and transcription factors involved in metabolism and inflammation including the peroxisome proliferator gamma co-activator 1 alpha (PGC-1α) (Rodgers et al. 2005), the NFκB subunit P65 (Yeung et al. 2004), the forkhead box class O (FOXO) proteins FOXO1 and FOXO3 (Brunet et al. 2004), P53 (Vaziri et al. 2001), tyrosine-protein phosphatase non-receptor type 1 (PTP1B) (Sun et al. 2007), and the insulin receptor substrate 2 (IRS2) (Zhang 2007). SIRT1 deacetylates PGC-1a at specific lysine residues increasing PGC-1a activity. SIRT1 has also been identified as a suppressor of inflammation in several tissue types by inhibiting the NFκB pathway. Upon activation the NFκB complex translocates to the cell nucleus where it is acetylated by the protein acetylase p300 and activated causing transcription of several genes responsible for the inflammatory response such as cytokines. SIRT1 deacetylates and binds to the P65 subunit of the NFκB complex preventing acetylation and activation (Yeung et al. 2004). By acting in response to cellular nutrient availability and subsequently altering such biological processes such as inflammatory response, fatty acid and glucose metabolism, mitochondrial biogenesis, DNA repair pathways, and cellular aging, SIRT1 may form a potential link between metabolism, inflammation, and cell aging.

4.4.4 DNA Methylation

The DNA of higher organisms, especially of vertebrates, is subject to the addition of methyl groups by DNA methyltransferases (DnMT) to the 5' carbon of cytosine residues existing as part of cytosine-phosphate-guanine (CpG) dinucleotides (Illingworth and Bird 2009). DNA methylation has been shown to have a fundamental role in developmental processes such as X-chromosome inactivation and genomic imprinting (Ideraabdullah et al. 2008; Panning 2008). Addition of methyl groups is primarily carried out by proteins belonging to the DNA methyltransferase (DnMT) family and can be described as "maintenance" methylation or "de novo" methylation. Maintenance methylation is the process by which existing methylation is copied onto newly replicated DNA and is performed by the DnMT1 methyltransferase. De novo methylation is performed by the methyltransferases DnMT3a and DnMT3b and is the addition of methyl groups to previously unmodified DNA.

The sites of DNA methylation, CpG dinucleotides, are distributed throughout the genome and are generally methylated, and methylated cytosine may undergo spontaneous deamination to produce thymine. Regions of the genome containing a high concentration of CpG residues called CpG islands exist in the promoter regions of approximately 70 % of genes these regions are inherently unmethylated, although can be methylated altering gene expression (Illingworth and Bird 2009).

Methylation represses transcription after recognition of methylated CpG by specific proteins such as the protein MeCP2 which can either block the promoter region to polymerases or form a complex with histone deacetylase proteins that in turn alter chromatin conformation

restricting gene expression (Nan et al. 1997). Conversely, demethylation is likely to lead to a deregulation in gene expression.

4.4.4.1 Methylation, Inflammation, and Aging

CpG island hypermethylation has been proposed as a common mechanism in tumorigenesis and aging where aberrant hypermethylation of promoter CpG islands associates with inactivation of tumor suppressor genes. During aging, hypermethylation is reported to occur preferentially at bivalent chromatin that combine activating and repressive methylation signatures (Rakyan et al. 2010). This has led to several studies designed to characterize age-related epigenetic signatures. A recent study involved the analysis of five discrete DNA sources from dermis, epidermis, cervical smear, T cells, and monocytes, in a screen for CpG sites that are consistently and differentially methylated in aging. Koch and Wagner (2011) confirmed the presence of 19 age-predictive islands, five of which were applied to an algorithm to define age. The predictive hypermethylated genes were NPTX2, a neuronal pentraxin related to the acute-phase reactant C-reactive protein (CRP), TRIM58, GRIA2 (neuronal AMPA receptor), and KCNQ1DN which is related to Wilms' tumors. A further hypomethylated CpG site was found in the BIRC4BP gene which encodes for an antiapoptotic protein (Koch and Wagner 2011). At this time it is not clear why these combined markers are significant for aging.

A more obvious link between DNA methylation status and inflammation is from studies investigating dysregulation of tumor necrosis factor-alpha (TNF-α) expression, an important cytokine in chronic inflammation, with a decrease in TNF promoter methylation during aging (Gowers et al. 2011). This is likely to result in increased TNF-α expression however, in inflamed CKD patients global hypermethylation was associated with mortality from cardiovascular disease risk after age has been accounted for (Stenvinkel et al. 2007) suggesting a complex interaction between inflammation, age and disease on methylation status (Wilson 2008).

Age-associated inflammatory lung disease is a major cause of morbidity in the elderly. DNA methylation in nine inflammatory genes and was correlated with lung function in a cohort of 756 community-dwelling elderly men. Decreased methylation of TLR-2, CRAT, and F3 was associated with decreased lung function, whereas demethylation of IL-6 and interferon gamma (IFN-γ) was associated with better lung function possibly due to a negative feedback on the inflammatory process (Lepeule et al. 2012).

The monocyte is a good model to investigate the effect of longevity versus differentiation from a progenitor state. In a study of the maturation and differentiation of CD34[+] hematopoietic progenitor cells, methylation changes observed in older progenitor cells showed a bimodal pattern with hypomethylation of differentiation-associated genes and de novo methylation events resembling epigenetic mutations (Bocker et al. 2011). Specific targeting of epigenetic mutations may be important in regulating monocyte differentiation pathways during aging.

4.4.5 miRNA and Epigenetic Regulation

MicroRNAs (miRNA) are members of the noncoding RNA (ncRNA)—a class of nucleic acids, which regulate gene expression but do not encode any translated product. They include long ncRNA greater than 200 nucleotide bases, which may be precursors for small ncRNAs, and together are believed to regulate over 60 % of all human genes and are important in differentiation, senescence, aging, and lifespan extension (Boehm and Slack 2005, 2006; Schickel et al. 2008; Bates et al. 2009; Friedman et al. 2009). Epigenomic regulation by ncRNA is achieved by modifying chromatin structure and gene imprinting (Rinn et al. 2007; Wilkinson et al. 2007). The relevance of ncRNA for aging has been highlighted by reports of telomeric ncRNAs (TelRNAs) that regulate telomerase activity and which may play a direct role in the molecular mechanisms of aging (Azzalin et al. 2007; Schoeftner and Blasco 2008).

Since their discovery almost 20 years ago, miRNA has emerged as a critical regulator of gene expression acting at the posttranslational level to either promote degeneration or inhibit transcription of target mRNA (Lepeule et al. 2012). miRNAs with almost-perfect complementarity usually signal for mRNA cleavage, whereas miRNAs that exhibit more mismatches usually inhibit translation and/or trigger the transport of mRNA to mRNA-processing bodies where mRNA is stored or degraded (Du and Zamore 2007). The biogenesis of mature miRNAs is complex; most miRNAs are transcribed into 5′-capped poly(A)-tailed primary miRNAs (pri-miRNA) by RNAP I and after nuclear transcription fold into clusters of imperfect 3 helical-turn (33 bp) stem-and-loop structures that are recognized by DGCR8 and Drosha. These enzymes cut precursor miRNAs (pre-miRNA) to remove 22 bp from the loop and release a pre-miRNA of about 70 nucleotides (Han et al. 2006). Exportin 5 and ras-related nuclear protein (RAN) GTPase then transport pre-miRNAs into the cytoplasm for processing into double-strand intermediates by the enzyme Dicer, and the guide strand with less stable 5′ end is then incorporated into Argonaute effector complexes (Takeda et al. 2008).

The first miRNA and gene target pair to be described in any species was from *C. elegans*, *lin-4*, and the transcription factor, *lin-14*, which initially were reported to control larval development timing but later were shown to influence lifespan via the insulin/insulin-like growth factor-1 pathway (Lee et al. 1993; Boehm and Slack 2005).

4.4.5.1 miRNA, Inflammation, and Aging

Interest in the role of miRNA molecules in regulating inflammation has burgeoned in the last 5 years with the description of miR146 as an inhibitor of innate immune signaling which is turned on by NFκB and serves as a negative feedback loop to dampen down inflammatory responses (Taganov et al. 2006) and is dysregulated in aging (Jiang et al, 2012).

A role for miRNA within cells for regulating gene expression and subsequently inflammation is relatively straightforward to appreciate. However, miRNA is also found in extracellular fluids, and the roles/functions of extracellular miRNAs are poorly studied. There are several potential explanations for their presence including apoptosis, microparticle shedding, and active export with Argonaute family (Turchinovich et al. 2012). How good these molecules will prove to be as disease-specific biomarkers is therefore unknown. More interesting perhaps is the question of whether miRNA has any extracellular signaling role, and early evidence in support of this pertains to Let-7, which acts as a potent activator of TLR-7 signaling in macrophages, microglia, and neurons (Lehmann et al. 2012).

Conclusion

The aging process results from a complex interplay with genes and the environment that can precipitate uncontrolled inflammation. It is likely that epigenetic modifications may be important mediators of this relationship. A thorough understanding of the posttranscriptional and epigenetic factors involved in both normal aging and age-related disease may inform new strategies and approaches to diagnose, treat, or suppress many aspects of age-dependent frailty. The importance of the regulatory ncRNAs is only just beginning, and the potential to reverse epigenetic changes could afford significant health improvements during aging.

Acknowledgments Funding is gratefully acknowledged from the following sources BBSRC (JWK); BBSRC (SJB); Alzheimer's Research UK (IHKD); FP7 MARK-AGE (EU FP7 Large-scale integrating Project HEALTH-F4-2008-2008800 (CRD); COST CM1001 and BM1203 (HRG).

References

Azzalin CM, Reichenbach P, Khoriauli L et al (2007) Telomeric repeat-containing RNA and RNA surveillance factors at mammalian chromosome ends. Science 318:798–801

Bates DJ, Liang R, Li N et al (2009) The impact of non-coding RNA on the biochemical and molecular mechanisms of aging. Biochim Biophys Acta 1790:970–979

Bocker MT, Hellwig I, Breiling A et al (2011) Genome-wide promoter DNA methylation dynamics of human hematopoietic progenitor cells during differentiation and aging. Blood 117:e182–e189

Boehm M, Slack F (2005) Physiology: a developmental timing microRNA and its target regulate life span in C. Elegans. Science 310:1954–1957

Boehm M, Slack FJ (2006) MicroRNA control of lifespan and metabolism. Cell Cycle 5:837–840

Brunet A, Sweeney LB, Sturgill JF et al (2004) Stress-dependent regulation of FOXO transcription factors by the SIRT1 deacetylase. Science 303:2011–2015

Butcher SK, Chahal H, Nayak L et al (2001) Senescence in innate immune responses: reduced neutrophil phagocytic capacity and CD16 expression in elderly humans. J Leukoc Biol 70:881–886

Chalmers J, Cooper ME (2008) UKPDS and the legacy effect. N Engl J Med 359:1618–1620

Dasu MR, Jialal I (2011) Free fatty acids in the presence of high glucose amplify monocyte inflammation via Toll-like receptors. Am J Physiol Endocrinol Metab 300:E145–E154

Dasu MR, Devaraj S, Zhao L et al (2008) High glucose induces toll-like receptor expression in human monocytes: mechanism of activation. Diabetes 57:3090–3098

Dokmanovic M, Clarke C, Marks PA (2007) Histone deacetylase inhibitors: overview and perspectives. Mol Cancer Res 5:981–989

Du T, Zamore PD (2007) Beginning to understand microRNA function. Cell Res 17:661–663

Dunston CR, Griffiths HR (2010) The effect of ageing on macrophage Toll-like receptor-mediated responses in the fight against pathogens. Clin Exp Immunol 161:407–416

Flavell SJ, Hou TZ, Lax S et al (2008) Fibroblasts as novel therapeutic targets in chronic inflammation. Br J Pharmacol 153:S241–S246

Franceschi C, Capri M, Monti D et al (2007) Inflammaging and anti-inflammaging: a systemic perspective on aging and longevity emerged from studies in humans. Mech Ageing Dev 128:92–105

Friedman RC, Farh KKH, Burge CB et al (2009) Most mammalian mRNAs are conserved targets of microRNAs. Genome Res 19:92–105

Gao D, Bailey CJ, Griffiths HR (2009) Metabolic memory effect of the saturated fatty acid, palmitate, in monocytes. Biochem Biophys Res Commun 388:278–282

Gao D, Pararasa C, Dunston CR et al (2012) Palmitate promotes monocyte atherogenicity via de novo ceramide synthesis. Free Radic Biol Med 53:796–806

Gomez CR, Hirano S, Cutro B et al (2007) Advanced age exacerbates the pulmonary inflammatory response after lipopolysaccharide exposure. Crit Care Med 35:246–251

Gomez CR, Acuna-Castillo C, Perez C et al (2008) Diminished acute phase response and increased hepatic inflammation of aged rats in response to intraperitoneal injection of lipopolysaccharide. J Gerontol A Biol Sci Med Sci 63:1299–1306

Gowers IR, Walters K, Kiss-Toth E et al (2011) Age-related loss of CpG methylation in the tumour necrosis factor promoter. Cytokine 56:792–797

Haigis MC, Sinclair DA (2010) Mammalian sirtuins: biological insights and disease relevance. Annu Rev Pathol 5:253–295

Han J, Lee Y, Yeom KH et al (2006) Molecular basis for the recognition of primary microRNAs by the Drosha-DGCR8 complex. Cell 125:887–901

Harman D (1956) Aging: a theory based on free radical and radiation chemistry. J Gerontol 11:298–300

Hayflick L, Moorhead PS (1961) The serial cultivation of human diploid cell strains. Exp Cell Res 25:585–621

Hou H, Yu H (2010) Structural insights into histone lysine demethylation. Curr Opin Struct Biol 20:739–748

Ideraabdullah FY, Vigneau S, Bartolomei MS (2008) Genomic imprinting mechanisms in mammals. Mutat Res 647:77–85

Illingworth RS, Bird AP (2009) CpG islands–'a rough guide'. FEBS Lett 583:1713–1720

Jiang M, Xiang Y, Wang D et al (2012) Dysregulated expression of miR-146a contributes to age-related dysfunction of macrophages. Aging Cell 11(1):29–40

Koch CM, Wagner W (2011) Epigenetic-aging-signature to determine age in different tissues. Aging (Albany NY) 3(10):1018–1027

Lee RC, Feinbaum RL, Ambros V (1993) The C. elegans heterochronic gene lin-4 encodes small RNAs with antisense complementarity to lin-14. Cell 75:843–854

Lehmann SM, Kruger C, Park B et al (2012) An unconventional role for miRNA: let-7 activates Toll-like receptor 7 and causes neurodegeneration. Nat Neurosci 15:827–835

Lepeule J, Baccarelli A, Motta V et al (2012) Gene promoter methylation is associated with lung function in the elderly: the Normative Aging Study. Epigenetics 7(3):261–269

Liang SY, Mackowiak PA (2007) Infections in the elderly. Clin Geriatr Med 23:441–456

Lord JM, Butcher S, Killampali V et al (2001) Neutrophil ageing and immunesenescence. Mech Ageing Dev 122:1521–1535

Medawar PB (1952) An unsolved problem in biology. Lewis, London. Reprinted in Medawar PG (1981) The uniqueness of the individual. Dover, New York

Meng L, Park J, Cai Q et al (2010) Diabetic conditions promote binding of monocytes to vascular smooth muscle cells and their subsequent differentiation. Am J Physiol Heart Circ Physiol 298:H736–H745

Millard AL, Mertes PM, Ittelet D et al (2002) Butyrate affects differentiation, maturation and function of human monocyte-derived dendritic cells and macrophages. Clin Exp Immunol 130:245–255

Nan X, Campoy FJ, Bird A (1997) MeCP2 is a transcriptional repressor with abundant binding sites in genomic chromatin. Cell 88:471–481

Nandy D, Janardhanan R, Mukhopadhyay D et al (2011) Effect of hyperglycemia on human monocyte activation. J Investig Med 59:661–667

Nimura K, Ura K, Kaneda Y (2010) Histone methyltransferases: regulation of transcription and contribution to human disease. J Mol Med (Berl) 88:1213–1220

Nyugen J, Agrawal S, Gollapudi S et al (2010) Impaired functions of peripheral blood monocyte subpopulations in aged humans. J Clin Immunol 30:806–813

Pagano G, Marena S, Scaglione L et al (1996) Insulin resistance shows selective metabolic and hormonal targets in the elderly. Eur J Clin Invest 26:650–656

Panning B (2008) X-chromosome inactivation: the molecular basis of silencing. J Biol 7:30

Pearl R (1928) The rate of living. University of London Press, London

Rakyan VK, Down TA, Maslau S et al (2010) Human aging-associated DNA hypermethylation occurs preferentially at bivalent chromatin domains. Genome Res 20(4):434–439

Rice JC, Allis CD (2001) Histone methylation versus histone acetylation: new insights into epigenetic regulation. Curr Opin Cell Biol 13:263–273

Rinn JL, Kertesz M, Wang JK et al (2007) Functional demarcation of active and silent chromatin domains in human HOX loci by noncoding RNAs. Cell 129:1311–1323

Rodgers JT, Lerin C, Haas W et al (2005) Nutrient control of glucose homeostasis through a complex of PGC-1alpha and SIRT1. Nature 434:113–118

Schickel R, Boyerinas B, Park SM et al (2008) MicroRNAs: key players in the immune system, differentiation, tumorigenesis and cell death. Oncogene 27:5959–5974

Schoeftner S, Blasco MA (2008) Developmentally regulated transcription of mammalian telomeres by DNA-dependent RNA polymerase II. Nat Cell Biol 10:228–236

Shi Y, Lan F, Matson C et al (2004) Histone demethylation mediated by the nuclear amine oxidase homolog LSD1. Cell 119:941–953

Sinclair DA, Guarente L (1997) Extrachromosomal rDNA circles–a cause of aging in yeast. Cell 91:1033–1042

Stenvinkel P, Karimi M, Johansson S et al (2007) Impact of inflammation on epigenetic DNA methylation – a novel risk factor for cardiovascular disease? J Intern Med 261(5):488–499

Sun C, Zhang F, Ge X et al (2007) SIRT1 improves insulin sensitivity under insulin-resistant conditions by repressing PTP1B. Cell Metab 6:307–319

Taganov KD, Boldin MP, Chang K-J et al (2006) NF-κB-dependent induction of microRNA miR-146, an inhibitor targeted to signaling proteins of innate immune responses. Proc Natl Acad Sci 103:12481–12486

Takeda A, Iwasaki S, Watanabe T et al (2008) The mechanism selecting the guide strand from small RNA duplexes is different among Argonaute proteins. Plant Cell Physiol 49:493–500

The Diabetes Control and Complications Trial Research Group (1993) The effect of intensive treatment of diabetes on the development and progression of long-term complications in insulin-dependent diabetes mellitus. N Engl J Med 329:977–986

Turchinovich A, Weiz L, Burwinkel B (2012) Extracellular miRNAs: the mystery of their origin and function. Trends Biochem Sci 37:460–465

Vabulas RM, Ahmad-Nejad P, Ghose S et al (2002) HSP70 as endogenous stimulus of the toll/interleukin-1 receptor signal pathway. J Biol Chem 277:15107–15112

Varier RA, Timmers HT (2011) Histone lysine methylation and demethylation pathways in cancer. Biochim Biophys Acta 1815:75–89

Vaziri H, Dessain SK, Ng Eaton E et al (2001) hSIR2(SIRT1) functions as an NAD-dependent p53 deacetylase. Cell 107:149–159

Wang S, Wu D, Lamon-Fava S et al (2009) In vitro fatty acid enrichment of macrophages alters inflammatory response and net cholesterol accumulation. Br J Nutr 102:497–501

Wilkinson LS, Davies W, Isles AR (2007) Genomic imprinting effects on brain development and function. Nat Rev Neurosci 8:832–843

Wilson AG (2008) Epigenetic regulation of gene expression in the inflammatory response and relevance to common diseases. J Periodontol 79:1514–1519

Yeung F, Hoberg JE, Ramsey CS et al (2004) Modulation of NF-kappaB-dependent transcription and cell survival by the SIRT1 deacetylase. EMBO J 23:2369–2380

Zhang J (2007) The direct involvement of SirT1 in insulin-induced insulin receptor substrate-2 tyrosine phosphorylation. J Biol Chem 282:34356–34364

Basophil, Eosinophil, and Neutrophil Functions in the Elderly

Peter Uciechowski and Lothar Rink

5.1 Introduction

Aging is accompanied with numerous alterations in the immune system resulting in refractory responses to vaccination and a significant decrease in protective immunity (Weiskopf et al. 2009). Therefore, the elderly are more susceptible to viral and bacterial infections, chronic infectious diseases, autoimmune diseases, and neoplasia, contributing to increased morbidity and mortality (Mahbub et al. 2011). The impairment in immunity during aging is referred to as "immunosenescence." Immunosenescence is applied to describe age-associated failing systemic immunity of both innate and adaptive immunity and an imbalance between them. It is believed to contribute to the increased incidence and severity of infectious disease in old animals and people (Franceschi et al. 2007; Larbi et al. 2008; Grubeck-Loebenstein et al. 2009; Pawelec et al. 2010).

A number of proinflammatory cytokines such as interleukin (IL)-1β, IL-6, and tumor necrosis factor-α (TNFα) and acute phase proteins are detected in two- to fourfold increased levels in the serum of aged humans and mice, and there is evidence that these higher levels of inflammatory cytokines are linked to increased mortality (Swain and Nikolich-Zugich 2009). This low-grade chronic proinflammatory status is termed "inflammaging" (Franceschi et al. 2007).

To investigate immunosenescence, one has to strictly differentiate age-related changes of healthy individuals from alterations induced by medical treatment, nutrition, lifestyle, or diseases. Hence, for the study of immunosenescence, elderly donors are chosen in accordance to a protocol known as SENIEUR to distinguish healthy from frail elderly (Kita 2011; Ligthart et al. 1984).

The effects of advanced aging on T and B lymphocytes are well documented, but basophils, eosinophils, and especially neutrophils as the largest cellular part of the immune system have long been overlooked and not been studied in depth. Neutrophils are able to promote as well as to restrain inflammation, play an important role in repairing and destroying tissues, influence the adoptive system, and have the potential for pharmacological interference in preventing and treating age-related immune deficiencies (Kita 2011; Nathan 2006). Human basophil and eosinophil numbers and their function in aging are only marginally considered in aging research, often analyzed as a by-product, although manipulating their properties might be a future horizon to modify age-related burden. This article summarizes the data about age-related changes affecting these cells.

P. Uciechowski, PhD • L. Rink, PhD (✉)
Institute of Immunology,
Medical Faculty of the RWTH Aachen University,
Pauwelsstr. 30, Aachen D-52074, Germany
e-mail: lrink@ukaachen.de

A. Massoud, N. Rezaei (eds.), *Immunology of Aging*,
DOI 10.1007/978-3-642-39495-9_5, © Springer-Verlag Berlin Heidelberg 2014

5.2 Basophils

Basophils comprise only a small percentage (0.5 %) of circulating blood cells under resting conditions with a lifespan of 1–2 days, but in response to inflammatory signals, they rapidly expand in the bone marrow and migrate to the blood, spleen, lung, and liver (Min et al. 2012). They are characterized by cytoplasmic granules stained blue upon exposure to a basic dye. One major problem in studying basophils, besides their very low cell number and short lifespan, is to distinguish them from mast cells. Both cell types can be differentiated from the multipotent, lineage-restricted granulocyte–monocyte progenitor, produce similar mediators upon activation, and express the high-affinity receptor for IgE. By now, basophils can be characterized by the expression of ckit(−), FcεRI(+), CD11b(+), IL-3^{high}, and other markers. The usage of basophil-depleting monoclonal antibodies and basophil-deficient transgenic mice will hopefully lead to the further evaluation of their role in host immunity. It could be shown that basophils are a primary source of IL-4 and are involved in the differentiation from naïve CD4$^+$ T- cells into IL-4-producing Th2 effector cells (Min et al. 2012).

Basophils are also antigen-presenting cells since it was detected that they can pick up antigen–IgE complexes leading to the differentiation of antigen-specific CD4$^+$ Th2 cells (Yoshimoto et al. 2009). Regulatory factors that mediate basophil generation and functions are IL-3, immune complexes, IL-18, IL-25, IL-33, lipopolysaccharide (LPS), and complement C5a. IL-3 produced by activated parasite-specific CD4$^+$ T cells induces IL-4 expression in basophils. It also mediates the timed arrival and the number of basophils for recruitment to the infected sites. The main functions of basophils are Th2 differentiation, protective immunity against ectoparasite infection, and expulsion from the intestine (Min et al. 2012).

Denzel et al. reported a role of basophils in humoral immune responses (Denzel et al. 2008). On the other hand, basophils have been reported to play a critical role in allergic inflammation by secreting IL-4 in response to IL-3 or FcεRI cross-

linking (Denzel et al. 2008). Basophils contribute to allergic and helminth immunity; however, their exact role has not been completely understood. They are the main producers of IL-4 during primary helminth infection (van Panhuys et al. 2011). In experiments where basophils were specifically absent, it has been shown that basophils did not mediate Th2 cell priming in vivo and only interact with T cells in lung tissues. Surprisingly, deletion of IL-4 and IL-13 in T cells or basophils shows that these basophil cytokines may not be required in primary helminth immunity (Sullivan et al. 2011).

5.2.1 Basophils and Aging

Although aging research of human basophils is limited, there are contradictory reports as well (Panda et al. 2009). While the degranulation of basophils in the elderly was found to be delayed (Schwarzenbach et al. 1982), another group reported that basophils from aged subjects showed the maximum proportion of anti-IgE-induced histamine release as well as higher sensitivity to a standard concentration of anti-IgE than younger ones (Marone et al. 1986). Di Lorenzo et al. analyzed serum total IgE, serum CD23, and Th2 cytokines IL-4, IL-10, and IL-13 in samples from 37 young and 62 old individuals without finding significant differences in both groups (Di Lorenzo et al. 2003). The authors queried that the incidence of allergic diseases declines with age (Di Lorenzo et al. 2003). Song et al. reported significantly lower percentage and absolute numbers of basophils in healthy aged donors than in younger donors (Song et al. 1999).

Using two separate type 2 cytokine-dependent in vivo models, aged mice were shown to have impaired pulmonary granulomas and delayed rejection of intestinal worms. Aged mice did not develop eosinophilia and reveal decreased production of antigen-specific IgE (Smith et al. 2001). This observed impairment in type 2 responsiveness may suggest an increased incidence of various type 1 cytokine-mediated diseases but also a delayed eosinophilic and basophilic response to parasites with age. A defect in juvenile mice with

Table 5.1 Effects of aging on granulocyte cell function

Function	Basophils	Eosinophils	Neutrophils
Increased	–	–	Apoptosis (rescue)
Maintained	Number of IL-4 producing basophils (mice) IL-4 and IL-13 production under allergic conditions	Number of eosinophils (mice) Adhesion	Number of circulating neutrophils Number of precursors in bone marrow Adhesion Receptor expression (GM-CSF-R, TLR2, TLR4, TREM-1, fMLP-R) Spontaneous apoptosis
Reduced	Absolute number of basophils Delayed response to parasites (mice)	Eosinophilia in allergic airway response (rat) Delayed response to parasites (mice) Eosinophil number Degranulation (Production of ROS)	Signal transduction (calcium influx, phosphorylation of ERK, p38, Akt, PLC-γ) Pathways (JAK/STAT, ERK1/2/ MAPK) Phagocytosis Respiratory burst Degranulation (fMLP) Intracellular killing Plasma membrane fluidity Receptor recruitment to lipid rafts
Controversial	Degranulation	Chemotaxis (rat) reduced Chemotaxis (human) maintained	Chemotaxis

regard to helminth-induced innate basophil-mediated type 2 response (IL-4) is reported to be relevant to allergic conditions in contrast to older mice (Nel et al. 2011). This observation, by contrast, may support the notion that the aged have a decrease of onset of allergic symptoms and fewer allergic diseases.

Since basophils mediate CD4+ Th2 cell differentiation (Min et al. 2012) and lead to an increase in humoral immune memory responses (Denzel et al. 2008), the functions of these cells should be further examined in old individuals, particularly in regard to their newly reported abilities. Table 5.1 summarizes the age-related changes in basophils.

5.3 Eosinophils

First described in 1879 by Paul Ehrlich, eosinophils are classified as potent defenders against parasitic helminthes which are destroyed by granule proteins and superoxide radicals. Normally, eosinophils constitute about 1–6 % of blood cells. The name "eosinophil" derives from the affinity of their cytoplasmic granules for the red acid dye eosin. Eosinophils carry cytoplasmic crystalloid (also termed secretory, specific, or secondary) granules that store diverse, preformed cationic proteins (Muniz et al. 2012). They are terminally differentiated cells and their half-life in blood is almost 18 h. Most of them are located in the tissues, predominantly in the skin and mucosal surfaces of the gut, respiratory, and reproductive systems. The normal lifespan of eosinophils in healthy tissue is unknown, but they are believed to survive for several days, possibly weeks (Behm and Ovington 2000).

Eosinophils synthesize a range of Th1 cytokines [IL-12 and interferon gamma (IFN-γ)], Th2 cytokines (IL-4, IL-5, IL-9, IL-13, IL-25), proinflammatory cytokines (TNFα, IL-1β, IL-6, IL-8), suppressing cytokines (e.g., transforming growth factor-beta (TGF-β) and IL-10), chemokines, and lipid mediators such as platelet-activating factor (PAF) and leukotriene (LT)C4 (Hogan et al. 2008). Eosinophils bind IgE and can be activated by antigen–IgE complexes. By expressing CD80/86 and major histocompatibility complex (MHC)-II molecules, eosinophils can function as antigen-presenting cells (APC) as well (Behm and Ovington 2000).

Eosinophils carry pattern recognition receptors (PPR) such as toll-like receptors (TLR 1–5, 7,9) and others recognizing other pathogen-associated molecular patterns (PAMPs).

They are also included in tissue remodeling and repair by the release of TGF-β, basic fibroblast growth factors (bFGF), platelet-derived growth factor (PDGF), matrix metalloproteinases (MMPs), vascular endothelial growth factors (VEGF), and other mediators. In addition, release of secondary granule proteins, eicosanoids, leukotrienes, and ROS is probably involved in remodeling states of healthy and disease conditions (Kita 2011).

However, eosinophils are the main cellular infiltrate of the asthmatic lung and hypereosinophilia which is defined as peripheral blood eosinophil counts >1,500/μL and leads to organ damage and mortality. Additionally, by recognition of their possible deleterious role in immune hypersensitivity syndromes, including asthma, dermatitis, and rhinitis, tissue injury, tumor immunity, and allergic diseases, their status of a benign immune sentinel and effector cell began to totter (Adamko et al. 2005; Barthel et al. 2008; Hogan et al. 2008).

5.3.1 Eosinophils and Aging

Studies about age-associated changes in eosinophil numbers and functional properties are rare. Yagi et al. investigated the effect of aging on the allergic airway response in a rat model of bronchial asthma (Yagi et al. 1997). They found a significantly higher degree of specific IgE antibody in young animals and marked increase in the number of eosinophils and neutrophils in bronchoalveolar lavage fluid but no eosinophilia, like the study by Smith et al. in mice, in the aged group (Smith et al. 2001). Eosinophil chemotactic activity was only detected in the supernatant of cultured lymph node cells from young rats, while it was absent from those of aged rats. The authors suggested that aged rats have a defect in eosinophil accumulation in sites exposed to antigen, probably caused by age-modified T cells. No associations of eosinophils and basophils with

mortality, frailty, and age could be observed in women from the women's health and aging studies (Leng et al. 2005, 2009).

Di Lorenzo and colleagues investigated the course of rhinitis in a long-term follow-up study by analyzing several parameters due to age and changes in rhinitis symptom severity. They observed milder rhinitis symptoms and a decrease in allergic parameters. Interestingly, the alterations in rhinitis symptoms seemed to be associated with nasal eosinophils (Di Lorenzo et al. 2012). Others found a significant decrease in blood eosinophil and lymphocyte number with increased neutrophil and platelet counts in aged people between 79 and 87 years (Starr and Deary 2011). Eosinophils do not play a role in skin aging; at first, they are almost not present in dermis, and, secondly, their presence was independent on age (Gunin et al. 2011). Mathur et al. compared the functions of isolated blood eosinophils from a younger and an older group with asthma (Mathur et al. 2008). They could not find any differences in adhesion and chemotaxis but a significantly delayed degranulation (as measured by IL-5-induced degranulation of eosinophil-derived neurotoxin) and lower superoxide anion production in the old group (55–88 years of age) (Mathur et al. 2008). The number of eosinophils in the sputum was unchanged. Their findings regarding degranulation are comparable with those reported by Schwarzenbach et al. with basophils (Schwarzenbach et al. 1982). The authors conclude that these changes in eosinophilic function may influence the responsiveness to medications and the manifestation of asthma. These data will be important in relation to the age-associated enhancement in morbidity and mortality with allergy, asthma, autoimmune diseases, and atherosclerosis. Table 5.1 displays the age-related changes in basophils.

5.4 Neutrophils

Neutrophils are the main cellular population of the immune system in the circulation and are the first cells arriving at the site of an infection. By their ability to generate reactive oxygen and nitrogen species and by secreting a variety of proteases and antimicrobial peptides, they are able to kill and attack phagocytosed and extracellular pathogens including fungi (Mantovani et al. 2011; Panda et al. 2009; Wessels et al. 2010b). Neutrophils, as short-lived cells, have a half-life circulation time of only 6–10 h in blood (Panda et al. 2009; Schröder et al. 2006a). Therefore, a continuous production of $1–2 \times 10^{11}$ neutrophils per day is necessary for their maintenance of 60–70 % of blood leukocytes (Hellewell and Williams 1994).

Their lifespan can be prolonged in response to granulocyte-colony-stimulating factor (G-CSF), granulocyte–monocyte-colony-stimulating factor (GM-CSF), complement factors, PAF, and proinflammatory cytokines (TNFα, IL-6, IL-1β) (Gomez et al. 2008; Panda et al. 2009). Another survival factor is a hypoxic environment (Hannah et al. 1995). The prolongation of their lifespan increases neutrophil effector functions such as bactericidal ability but can also result in cumulative tissue damage via secretion of proteolytic enzymes.

To exclude further inflammatory reactions, they are eliminated by apoptosis after recognition and phagocytosis by macrophages (Panda et al. 2009; Savill et al. 1989). Because they are end-differentiated cells with few endoplasmic reticulum (Wessels et al. 2010b) and mainly phagocytic function, there are a limited number of studies investigating neutrophils. Hence, when current studies reveal that neutrophils held an armory of mediators, in part preformed in granules, and are able to de novo synthesize mediators and cytokines after stimulation (Schröder et al. 2006b; Wessels et al. 2010b), new perspectives of neutrophils as immunoregulatory cells in concert with the adaptive immune system have been formed.

Neutrophils express CD66b; CD11a, b, and c; CD18; CD14; CD15; CD16 constitutively; and MHC class II, CD64, upon stimulation (Butcher et al. 2001; Schröder et al. 2006a, b; Wessels et al. 2010b). Whether neutrophils can function as APCs or accessory cells by processing and presenting foreign antigens has been shown in some reports, but it is still not clearly determined (Fanger et al. 1997; Gosselin et al. 1993; Iking-Konert et al. 2002). Whether antigen-presenting abilities

of neutrophils change during aging process or not has not been evaluated. In this context, no data exist about the expression of MHC-I, MHC-II, or CD80/CD86 molecules on neutrophils from aged donors.

The activation of neutrophils is mediated by receptors specifically binding to PAMPs such as formyl-methionyl-leucyl-phenylalanine (fMLP), endotoxins, and other TLR ligands. Except TLR3, neutrophils express all other TLRs (Mantovani et al. 2011). Additionally, cytokines such as GM-CSF, IL-15, and IL-18 or ligands of the triggering receptor expressed on myeloid cells (TREM)-1 activate neutrophils (Ferretti et al. 2003; Fortin et al. 2007c, 2009a, b; Fulop et al. 2006; Gomez et al. 2008; Panda et al. 2009; Wessels et al. 2010b).

Conversely, activated neutrophils themselves produce cytokines and chemokines, including interferon gamma-induced protein 10 (IP-10), macrophage inflammatory protein-1α (MIP-1α), B-lymphocyte stimulator (BLyS), IL-1 receptor antagonist (IL-1RA), IL-12, IL-8, and VEGF and are substantial regulators in the induction and resolution of an immune response (Altstaedt et al. 1996; Borregaard et al. 2007; Ferretti et al. 2003; Fortin et al. 2008; Mantovani et al. 2011; Wessels et al. 2010b). On the other hand, neutrophils are described to express an array of proinflammatory cytokines such as IL-1, TNFα, IL-6, or IL-17 as well as immunoregulatory and anti-inflammatory cytokines, but some of them have only been detected via polymerase chain reaction (PCR) analysis and/or their expression is controversially discussed (Borregaard et al. 2007; Ferretti et al. 2003; Fortin et al. 2008; Mantovani et al. 2011; Wessels et al. 2010b).

During infection, the neutrophil production is upregulated leading to neutrophilia (Schröder et al. 2006b). Therefore, it is very important that the regulation of appropriate initiation but also resolution of their inflammatory responses is fine-tuned to clear infections and prevent nonspecific tissue damage, otherwise leading to chronic inflammatory disease and frailty. The finding that neutropenia due to genetic defects or chemotherapy leads to increased susceptibility to bacterial and fungal infections (Schröder and Rink 2003) points to the importance of efficient neutrophils for the immune system.

5.4.1 Neutrophils During Aging

There is strong evidence that aging exerts significant influence on all cells of the innate immune system (Agrawal and Gupta 2011; Chatta et al. 1993; De Martinis et al. 2004; Geiger and Rudolph 2009; Ginaldi et al. 1999; Gomez et al. 2008; Plackett et al. 2004; Shaw et al. 2010; Solana et al. 2006). Many studies suggest that the function of neutrophils such as phagocytic capacity, synthesis of ROS, and intracellular killing efficiency might be compromised in the elderly (Fulop et al. 2004; Di Lorenzo et al. 1999; Panda et al. 2009; Tortorella et al. 1996, 1999, 2000, 2007; Wenisch et al. 2000). This is supported by the observation that bacterial infections during aging enhance morbidity and mortality (Laupland et al. 2003) and that age is an independent risk factor for the development of chronic inflammatory diseases. For instance, impaired bactericidal activity and chemotaxis of neutrophils are very likely responsible for recurring infections of the respiratory tract and skin in aged persons (Schröder and Rink 2003; Wessels et al. 2010b).

However, many studies reported contradictory results, e.g., whether the chemotactic abilities of neutrophils are changed in the elderly population. For this purpose, there are also age-related studies in rodent animal models. But one has to keep in mind that neutrophils from aged mice did not show any functional deficiency including exocytosis, chemotaxis, respiratory burst, and phagocytosis when compared to young mice (Murciano et al. 2008).

How immunosenescence is involved into the development, progression, and treatment of cancer in elderly subjects is not clear. The low-grade inflammation in combination with resistance from apoptosis, microenvironmental imbalances, chromosomal instability, telomere shortening, and decreases of immunosurveillance may favor cancerogenesis in the elderly (Fulop et al. 2010). The role of neutrophils in defense against cancer remains unclear. The changed functions of

neutrophils may also concur to tumor progression but of lower account (Fortin et al. 2008).

As mentioned above, many conflicting data in neutrophil research of the elderly have been published by different groups. These controversial results are probably due to different neutrophil isolation techniques, purity and pre-activation of these neutrophil preparations, different methods, monocyte contaminations, and application of the SENIEUR protocol or not (Schröder et al. 2006b; Schröder and Rink 2003). Another important point is that monocytes isolated from aged donors release significantly more proinflammatory cytokines after stimulation than those of younger persons (Gabriel et al. 2002).

Although there are many studies about the changes in neutrophil function in aging, many questions remain to be answered. Which mechanisms are responsible for the delay in phosphorylation of signaling molecules, actin polymerization, second messenger generation, and changes in membrane composition and fluidity? Are experiments in mice transferable into the situation of neutrophils from the elderly in vivo?

The following sections will address, in detail, the age-associated alterations in number, function, and signal pathways of neutrophils.

5.4.2 Proliferation and Apoptosis

The total number of circulating neutrophils is constant throughout aging, and there are no alterations in the number of precursor cells in the bone marrow (Born et al. 1995; Chatta et al. 1993). Additionally, the responses to IL-3 and GM-CSF (Chatta et al. 1993; Lord et al. 2001) are sufficient enough to produce adequate neutrophil amounts during infection, while neutrophil precursor cells show a reduced proliferative response only to G-CSF (Born et al. 1995; Chatta et al. 1993).

Moreover, neutrophils have been described to be significantly increased in the aged (Cakman et al. 1997). Therefore, it is assumed that more likely functional modifications in the neutrophilic population result in observed defects of the innate immune system in the elderly. This is supported because hematopoietic stem cells from young mice proliferating and differentiating into neutrophils in an aged microenvironment showed decreased effector functions (Geiger and Rudolph 2009). Microenvironmental factors being associated with advanced age in mice may decrease neutrophil function (Mahbub et al. 2011). However, the composition of those factors may be decisive since impaired killing of *Candida albicans* (Murciano et al. 2008) has been reported, but not of other microbes such as *Streptococcus pneumoniae* (Kovacs et al. 2009).

Changes or defects in apoptosis through aging or downregulation of death receptors such as CD95 on neutrophils have not been reported in elderly donors. Contrary to that, there is consensus that rescue from apoptosis is disturbed since G-CSF, GM-CSF, IL-2, IL-6, TNFα, steroids, or LPS did not lead to an extension of lifespan of neutrophils from aged persons (Fortin et al. 2007b; Fulop et al. 1997, 1999, 2000a, b, 2004; Tortorella et al. 1998, 2006). An obvious assumption would be that the balance of pro- and anti-apoptotic molecules of the B cell leukemia (Bcl)-2 family, such as Bax, Bad, myeloid cell leukemia (Mcl)-1, or BclXL, is interrupted. This assumption is supported by the findings that the Mcl-1/Bax ratio is increased in GM-CSF-stimulated neutrophils from young donors while the ratio remains unchanged in neutrophils from aged donors (Fulop et al. 2004, 2006; Wessels et al. 2010b). Age-related failure of GM-CSF in the induction of several neutrophil functions as well as in impeding apoptosis through the inhibition of lyn, phosphoinositide-3 kinase/Akt (PI3K/Akt), extracellular signal-regulated protein kinase (ERK), and signal transducers and activator of transcription (STAT) signaling pathways is due to the increased activity of signal tyrosine phosphatase-1 (SHP-1), an inhibitor of Src family of tyrosine kinases and suppressors of cytokine signaling (SOCS) (Fortin et al. 2006, 2007b, 2009a; Tortorella et al. 2004, 2006, 2007).

There are also defects in the Janus tyrosine kinase (JAK)/STAT and mitogen-activated protein kinase (MEK)/ERK pathways regulating the expression of the Bcl-2 family members in neutrophils from the elderly (Fortin et al. 2009a). Since JAK2 is involved in the expression of anti-apoptotic

Bcl-2, a relationship between JAK2 and Mcl1 might negatively affect the rescue of neutrophils from apoptosis (Fulop et al. 2004). Fulop et al. observed a mitogen-activated protein kinase (MAPK) independent conversion from the pro-apoptotic phenotype to an anti-apoptotic phenotype in young but not aged neutrophils after GM-CSF stimulation by modification of the Bcl-2 family members Bax and Bcl-2 (Fulop et al. 2004). Together with a disturbance of caspase-3 inhibition, alterations in signaling pathways might be responsible for the damaged rescue from apoptosis.

In summary, these changes might create a pro-apoptotic milieu which causes the enhanced occurrence of infections in the elderly.

Another point is that shorter lifespan and early apoptosis are due to enhanced cell oxidative levels in neutrophils from aged donors (Tortorella et al. 1999). When superoxide dismutase (SOD) is added exogenously to cell cultures, one could detect prolonged neutrophil survival in young and aged individuals, but the addition of large amounts of SOD only caused a still increasing effect in cell cultures of young donors (Tortorella et al. 1999).

Early apoptosis and subsequently shortened lifespan will not lead to a reduction of the period of neutrophil activity alone but may also result in a higher rate of apoptotic neutrophils at the site of infection. Since this accumulation of neutrophils would not fully be cleared by macrophages, secondary necrosis followed by persistent chronic infections or frailty (Fortin et al. 2008; Leng et al. 2007; Panda et al. 2009) could be the consequence.

5.4.3 Chemotaxis

During infection, peripheral blood neutrophils follow a gradient of chemoattractants such as complement factor C5a, chemokine CXCL8 (IL-8), or bacterial peptides like formylated tripeptide fMLP. The migration to the infected tissue is mediated through binding of CD15 on neutrophils to P- and L-selectin on endothelial cells (rolling) and, secondly, via interaction of CD11a/CD18 and CD11b/CD18 on neutrophils and intercellular adhesion molecule 1 (ICAM-1) on endothelial cells (adhesion) followed by transmigration through the endothelium. Adhesion to endothelial cells, expression of adhesion molecules, and recruitment of neutrophils seem to be unaltered in aged persons (Biasi et al. 1996; Butcher et al. 2001), whereas one publication reported enhanced adhesion of fMLP/ phorbol 12-myristate 13-acetate (PMA)-stimulated neutrophils from aged donors on endothelial cells (Damtew et al. 1990).

Reduced chemotaxis of neutrophils from healthy aged donors primed with GM-CSF and fMLP is reported in a lot of in vitro studies (Alonso-Fernandez et al. 2008; Fortin et al. 2006, 2009a; Fulop et al. 2004; Niwa et al. 1989; Seres et al. 1993; Wenisch et al. 2000; Wessels et al. 2010b). A lower actin polymerization of elderly neutrophils after fMLP stimulation is discussed as one mechanism (Rao 1986; Rao et al. 1992). Changes in signaling pathways could also be involved. The consequence of chemotactic defects in neutrophils from the elderly might be an impaired infiltration of infected or injured tissues (Lord et al. 2001).

Data from in vivo studies in mice may contradict this thesis. Swift et al. reported similar numbers of neutrophils in aged and young mice in a dermal excisional injury model (Swift et al. 2001). One group found that (a) LPS-induced pulmonary inflammation was significantly increased in aged mice and associated with elevated levels of neutrophil chemokines and another (b) enhanced neutrophil infiltration after a 15 % total body surface area burn injury (Gomez et al. 2007; Nomellini et al. 2008).

In vitro studies with isolated cells or cells in culture cannot fully equate with in vivo studies, especially when human and murine approaches will be compared. Variations in analyses techniques, microenvironment, local accumulation in tissue, and time points after initiation of infection could be the reasons for observed differences in mice models and between in vivo and in vitro results. Additionally, human in vivo studies have the disadvantage that analysis take place after the progression of an infection. A further problem is that one cannot differentiate whether found discrepancies are due to differences between species. In a study comparing age-related alterations in murine and human neutrophils, a high amount of differences has been described by Kovacs et al. (Kovacs et al. 2009). This group concluded that mice models may

not be the best approach to investigate the impact of immunosenescence in neutrophils (Kovacs et al. 2009). Others stated that the existing mouse models where genes are deleted from birth are not entirely satisfactory to study immunosenescence (Swain and Nikolich-Zugich 2009).

Centenarians, in contrary, show no differences in chemotaxis (Alonso-Fernandez et al. 2008) compared to younger persons indicating that a defect in this function may contribute to the failure of a correct immune reaction in aged persons.

5.4.4 Adhesion

For diapedesis, a firm adhesion of neutrophils to endothelium is a prerequisite for the additional steps in transmigration. Most investigators found no differences in neutrophilic adhesion between young and aged individuals. There were no discrepancies in adhesion to endothelium, gelatin, plastic, or nylon (Antonaci et al. 1984; Biasi et al. 1996; Plackett et al. 2004) when cells were stimulated with calcium ionophores, PMA, zymosan, or fMLP. The expression of surface antigens such as CD11a and CD11c (Butcher et al. 2000), CD11a/ CD18, CD11b/CD18. and CD14 were reported not to be changed on neutrophils. The described slightly enhanced expression of CD11b and CD15 may contribute to increased adhesion of neutrophils from aged subjects to endothelial cell monolayers after stimulation with fMLP or PMA (Esparza et al. 1996; Wessels et al. 2010b). The correlation of enhanced adhesion and impaired chemotaxis with higher susceptibility to infections (Egger et al. 2003) is corresponding with these data. An additional surface molecule with altered expression during aging is ICAM-3 (CD50) (De Martinis et al. 2004), the ligand for LFA-1 (CD11a/CD18). Although De Martinis et al. reported a decrease of the surface density of CD50 on granulocytes of aged donors at a per cell level (De Martinis et al. 2004), the total amount of CD50+ cells was enhanced in the elderly.

The reduced Ca^{2+} mobilization from the endoplasmatic reticulum into the cytosol and vice versa after fMLP stimulation but constitutively increased cytosolic Ca^{2+} levels of unstimulated neutrophils from elderly donors (Klut et al. 2002; Lipschitz et al. 1991; Wenisch et al. 2000; Wessels et al. 2010b) are effects discussed as the outcome of the increased adhesion observed in the elderly. Additionally, this diminishes the highest possible response to fMLP stimulation in neutrophils of the aged when compared to neutrophils from young donors.

5.4.5 Phagocytosis and Respiratory Burst

Age-related impairments in the phagocytic function of neutrophils are still controversially discussed. Whereas studies report that phagocytosis is normal in the elderly (Plackett et al. 2004), others show a decreased phagocytosis of opsonized bacteria by neutrophils during aging (Alonso-Fernandez et al. 2008; Antonaci et al. 1984; Butcher et al. 2000; Esparza et al. 1996; Murciano et al. 2008; Simell et al. 2011; Tortorella et al. 2000; Wenisch et al. 2000). The percentage of neutrophils, which phagocytose more than one particle (phagocytosis efficiency), is also described to be decreased (Alonso-Fernandez et al. 2008). When decreased phagocytotic ability is reported, changes in actin polymerization (Lipschitz et al. 1991; Murciano et al. 2008; Rao 1986; Rao et al. 1992) and/or the significant age-related reduction of the Fcγ receptor (CD16), necessary for antibody dependent phagocytosis, are cited (Butcher et al. 2001).

The important killing mechanism of neutrophils is the production and release of ROS termed oxidative or respiratory burst. There are variable findings concerning changes in respiratory burst of neutrophils derived from aged individuals. In vitro studies using neutrophils from aged donors compared to young individuals found no differences in O_2^- and peroxide production after stimulation with fMLP or Gram-negative *Escherichia coli* (Butcher et al. 2000; Ito et al. 1998; Lord et al. 2001). However, more recent studies report that neither GM-CSF, LPS, TREM-1, and fMLP nor the direct injection of Gram-positive bacteria like *Staphylococcus aureus* could fully activate intracellular killing (Braga et al. 1998; Mclaughlin et al. 1986; Panda et al. 2009; Seres et al. 1993; Tortorella et al. 1999, 2000; Whitelaw et al. 1992). Stimulation with fMLP or GM-CSF led to a reduced superoxide anion production of neutrophils from aged donors after 24 h but to an increase after restimulation

(Fulop et al. 2004). Neutrophils incubated with fMLP for 48 h could be stimulated herein, resulting in the authors' suggestion that a subpopulation of "super neutrophils" may exist in the elderly (Fulop et al. 2004). Chaves and co-workers found that ROS generation by granulocytes is mediated by inositol 1,4,5-triphosphate and p38 mitogen-activated protein kinase in a cyclic AMP-dependent manner in aging (Chaves et al. 2007).

Neutrophils from young donors efficiently finalize the response to stimulation, whereas neutrophils from aged donors seem to react more heterogeneously from the aspects of intensity and duration of a response (Klut et al. 2002). These data suggest that the divergent outcomes of the studies are partly due to different time points of measurements. Since the oxidative burst is a complex reaction and can be detected by the analyses of various parameters, the difference of observations may also be a result of the usage of different analyzing methods (Wessels et al. 2010b).

Antioxidant production, e.g., glutathione, is also impaired in the elderly (Alonso-Fernandez et al. 2008; Bhushan et al. 2002; Wessels et al. 2010b), as well as the reduced ability to destroy fungi like *Candida albicans* (Murciano et al. 2008). The reasons for the alterations observed in phagocytosis and oxidative burst of the elderly are believed to be associated with changes in Ca^{2+} mobilization, membrane fluidity/composition, and modifications in signaling pathways.

Phagocytosis, respiratory burst, and, finally, killing of the invaded microorganisms are coupled mechanisms important for an efficient defense. More information about their linkage is desirable since defects of each of them or in common are correlated with age-related diseases and impaired antimicrobial functions.

5.4.6 Cytokines

As aforementioned, neutrophils store preformed molecules in their granules and are able to de novo synthesize immunoregulatory mediators and cytokines upon activation (Borregaard et al. 2007; Uciechowski and Rink 2009; Wessels et al. 2010b). Therefore, one has to leave the conception that neutrophils are only professional phagocytes or – vice versa – display the same cytokine spectrum as monocytes categorizing them as proinflammatory cells (Cassatella 1995; Lloyd and Oppenheim 1992). It is reported that neutrophils express IP-10, IL-17, IL-12, (Ferretti et al. 2003; Gomez et al. 2008) and even proinflammatory IL-1α and TNFα (Cassatella 1995; Lloyd and Oppenheim 1992; Mantovani et al. 2011), while other and own data investigating highly purified neutrophils revealed that they synthesize mainly anti-inflammatory or chemotactic molecules such as IL-8, IL-1 receptor antagonist, MIP-1α, MIP-1β, soluble TNF-R, and growth-related oncogene (GRO)-α (Altstaedt et al. 1996; von der Ohe et al. 2001; Schröder et al. 2006b; Schröder and Rink 2003; Wessels et al. 2010b).

The discrepancies and variations found in several publications may be due to low percentages of contaminating monocytes which can result in false-positive data when PCR and ELISA techniques were used (Altstaedt et al. 1996; Reato et al. 1999; Schröder et al. 2006b). Though these data have to be interpreted very carefully, particularly when cytokine data from human and murine neutrophils have not clearly been separated.

However, age-dependent alterations in cytokine production of neutrophils could not be detected; therefore, the impact of these cytokines produced by neutrophils has to be determined.

The reported amplified proinflammatory cytokine secretion by myeloid dendritic cells (DCs) and monocytes of aged donors (Agrawal et al. 2007; Rink et al. 1998) and a low-grade inflammatory situation summarizes up in the question whether cytokine production by neutrophils is also modified during aging.

Recently, it could be shown by our group that epigenetic mechanisms such as chromatin remodeling, histone methylation, and acetylation are responsible for IL-1β and TNFα expression per se and, additionally, regulate these cytokine expressions in granulocytic and monocytic differentiation (Wessels et al. 2010a). Low-grade inflammation reported for resting neutrophils of aged donors, accompanied by CD62L shedding and constitutive ROS production (Biasi et al. 1996; De Martinis et al. 2004), is initiated by

alterations in cytokine production conceivably in part due to dysregulated epigenetic mechanisms, e.g., in IL-1β and TNFα gene expression. In this context, cells cultured under long-time zinc deficiency, which is also a feature of aged persons (Biasi et al. 1996; De Martinis et al. 2004; Haase et al. 2006; Haase and Rink 2009; Rink and Kirchner 2000), undergo chromatin remodeling leading to significantly increased IL-1β, TNFα, and ROS production (Wessels et al. 2013). In addition, persistent signal transduction molecule phosphorylation (Fortin et al. 2008), altered distribution of signaling molecules in lipid rafts, and constantly elevated Ca^{2+} levels in resting neutrophils from aged donors (Fortin et al. 2006, 2007c; Fulop et al. 2004; Wessels et al. 2010b) strongly contribute to the generation of a basically proinflammatory condition in the elderly.

5.4.7 Signaling Pathways

The described alteration in neutrophilic functions of elderly persons is due to defects in signaling pathways and receptors, receptor distribution, and changes of membrane fluidity. Mainly the signaling pathways of fMLP-R, GM-CSF-R, TREM-1, and TLR4 in PMN of aged donors have been investigated (Fortin et al. 2007c; Panda et al. 2010). In contrast to age-related changes in TLR expression observed in monocytes (Shaw et al. 2011; van Duin and Shaw 2007), there was no difference in the expression of all four receptors throughout aging, indicating that the influence of aging varies from cell type to cell type.

Modified fMLP-mediated signal transduction is most probably due to the non-adequate synthesis of the second messengers diacylglycerol (DAG) and inositol triphosphate (IP_3) (Lipschitz et al. 1991) as well as Ca^{2+} mobilization (Fortin et al. 2009a). Whereas resting neutrophils of elderly persons show an enhanced level of intracellular Ca^{2+} (Mohacsi et al. 1992; Varga et al. 1988; Wenisch et al. 2000), stimulation of neutrophils leads to decreased intracellular Ca^{2+}. This in combination with altered plasma membrane composition and altered receptor and adapter protein linkage suggests that fMLP pre-activation also affects Ca^{2+} mobilization. fMLP stimulation activates the MAPKs p38 and the ERK1/2 signal pathways being involved in regulating gene transcription, chemotaxis, adhesion, and respiratory burst activity. Defects in the signal cascades of both pathways, the decrease in activation and lower phosphorylation levels of p38 and ERK1/2 after fMLP stimulation are suggested to affect chemotaxis and superoxide generation reported in PMN from aged donors (Fulop 1994; Fulop et al. 2004; Lipschitz et al. 1991).

TLRs and components of the TLR signaling pathway have also been investigated. These studies reveal that the basal expression of TLR2 and TLR4 in neutrophils from aged donors is not changed (Boehmer et al. 2004; Fulop et al. 2004b). IL-1 receptor-associated protein kinase (IRAK)-1, a key component of TLR signaling, was not found to be associated with lipid rafts after stimulation with LPS. TLR4 has to be recruited to lipid rafts in order to execute its function (Lord et al. 2001). By comparing neutrophils from young and aged subjects, TLR4 expression in unstimulated lipid rafts and non-raft fractions was increased in the elderly. LPS did not influence recruitment or redistribution of TLRs between lipid raft and non-raft fractions in the elderly. This is in contrast to findings in young mice where a significant enhancement in TLR recruitment was observed (Fulop et al. 2004). Additionally, the expression of MyD88 on neutrophils after LPS stimulation between young and old mice was unaltered with the exception that the quantity of MyD88 in the neutrophilic plasma membrane of aged subjects was significantly reduced after stimulation (Fulop et al. 2004). The latter may have an effect on the strength of the TLR4-MyD88-dependent signaling, but no direct relations between TLR-mediated signaling defects and impaired functions in neutrophils from aged donors have been reported. Surprisingly, LPS-induced chemotaxis remains unaffected.

Strikingly, the results in men and mice are varying since two studies reported that LPS-stimulated macrophages from aged mice synthesize less IL-6 and TNFα than younger ones. Furthermore, divergent results were found in mice describing a lower TLR4 mRNA level in aged macrophages, whereas others did not find

changes in TLR4 surface expression with age (Boehmer et al. 2004; Renshaw et al. 2002).

A study of 154 young and old individuals revealed an age-associated decrease in TNFα and IL-6 production in human monocytes after stimulation with a specific TLR1/2 ligand (Van Duin and Shaw 2007). The authors also found a strong correlation of impaired cytokine production with a lower surface expression of TLR1 but not TLR2 on monocytes. They also detected a reduction of TLR4 expression on monocytes of aged donors when compared to younger ones. Unfortunately, this group did not analyze neutrophils in aged donors, which, in contrast to their findings, showed an unaltered TLR4 expression (Fulop et al. 2004).

Another receptor designated triggering receptor expressed on myeloid cells (TREM)-1 is involved in phagocytosis, respiratory burst, degranulation, and survival of neutrophils after engagement by a yet unknown ligand (Fortin et al. 2007a, c). To function properly, TREM-1 has to be translocated into lipid rafts where it co-localizes with TLR4 or the NACHT-LRR (NLR) pattern recognition receptor. ERK1/2, phospholipase C-γ, Akt activation, and intracellular calcium release were detected after TREM-1 engagement. It has been described that PMN from elderly individuals displayed impaired responses concerning respiratory burst or anti-apoptotic effects after TREM-1 engagement in contrast to young donors (Fortin et al. 2007a, c). Additionally, the authors observed alterations in signal transduction following TREM-1 activation and impaired recruitment to lipid rafts of TREM-1 after stimulation in the elderly but did not found any differences in TREM-1 expression. The retention of TREM-1 in the non-raft fraction of the plasma membrane might be an explanation for the impaired TREM-1-induced functions reported for neutrophils of aged volunteers. Increased levels of soluble TREM-1 in the circulation is a sign for a divergent inflammatory state; additionally, an association with soluble TREM-1 levels in the plasma and poor outcomes for life-threatening ill patients with sepsis has been described (Routsi et al. 2008).

The disturbed interaction with the NLR receptor and TLR4, which recognizes extra- and intracellular PAMPs, abolishes the synergistic induction of cytokine and ROS production.

Reasons for the defects in translocation of TLR4 and TREM-1 could be the reduction in actin polymerization, but also the increased fluidity of the plasma membrane, which also influences the integrity of lipid rafts (Fortin et al. 2007c). It is suggested that age-associated changes in TREM-1-mediated functions may contribute to a higher incidence of sepsis in the elderly.

GM-CSF activates the JAK/STAT pathway, the Ras–Raf-1–MEK–ERK1/2 pathway, and PI-3K triggered signaling (Fortin et al. 2007b; Fortin et al. 2009a; Fulop et al. 2004; Tortorella et al. 2004, 2006). Although the GM-CSF-R expression is unchanged during aging, GM-CSF signaling is disturbed in the elderly (Fortin et al. 2009a). One mechanism of this defect is mediated by impaired phosphorylation of signaling molecules throughout the signaling cascade. Next, GM-CSF signaling may also be disturbed via delayed actions of SHP-1 (Tortorella et al. 2007), an inhibitor of Src family of tyrosine kinases. Contrary to the blocked recruitment of TLR4 and TREM-1, the action of SHP-1 is inhibited by interruption of its emigration from lipid rafts (Fortin et al. 2007c; Tortorella et al. 2007). One major consequence of the malfunction of the GM-CSF-mediated signaling in neutrophils of aged donors is impaired protection from apoptosis, in particular due to alterations in caspase-3 cleavage in combination with changes in pro- and anti-apoptotic ratios of the Bcl-2 family. Defects in GM-CSF signaling pathways during aging also influence the respiratory burst and degranulation functions of neutrophils. GM-CSF (and fMLP) is able to activate but also to prime neutrophils on a second stimulus emphasizing the relevance of the dysregulated GM-CSF signaling for the intact function of these cells.

Besides dysregulation of signaling pathways during aging, signal transduction is also dependent upon membrane fluidity. By studying the effect of altered fluidity in fMLP-induced ROS production, a correlation between increased and decreased ROS generation was detected. In contrast, protein kinase C (PKC)-mediated ROS production after PMA activation is an independent process from membrane fluidity, indicating that signaling defects are located more proximal to the receptors (Alvarez et al. 2001; Schröder and Rink 2003; Wessels et al. 2010b). There are no reports about the association of GM-CSF signaling and membrane fluidity. The disturbance in signal transduction pathways important for maintenance of apoptosis may contribute to decreased inflammatory responses during senescence.

5.5 Granulocytes in Age-Related Diseases

The roles of basophils and eosinophils in age-associated diseases have to be examined in more detail as discussed earlier. Their contribution to host immunity, allergic reactions, asthma, and autoimmune disease in aging is mostly unknown.

The relationship between age-associated changes in neutrophils and diseases is well documented (Fortin et al. 2008; Wessels et al. 2010b), but the mechanisms that induce these modifications are mainly unknown. Information about the direct contribution of neutrophils to diseases in aging is rare and much generalized. One can clearly deduce from changes in ROS production, chemotaxis, phagocytosis, signal transduction, and the lack of protection from apoptosis that the antimicrobial defense of neutrophils is attenuated in the elderly. The consequences are simply a delayed killing of bacteria, including intracellular pathogens such as *Mycobacterium tuberculosis*, parasites, and fungi. These modifications in combination with dysregulated induction of proinflammatory cytokines after septic stimuli may result in generating elderly patients at excess risk for mortality from severe sepsis and septic shock (Opal et al. 2005).

Aging is also associated with increased lung inflammation without concomitant lung disease. Bronchoalveolar lavage (BAL) fluid from donors aged 19–83 years showed an increase in BAL neutrophils and CD4+ T cells with age. Between 4 and 13 % of the population over 65 years of age has current asthma which is underdiagnosed in the elderly. In this context, increased airspace neutrophilia corresponding to increased levels of sputum neutrophil mediators including MMP-9, neutrophil elastase, and IL-8 might contribute to greater severity of asthma in the elderly (Busse and Mathur 2010).

But exposure to oxidative stress (Alonso-Fernandez et al. 2008) or epigenetic modifications (Haase et al. 2006; Issa 2003; Kim et al. 2009; Wessels et al. 2010b) and deficiency in nutrition might cause impaired phagocytosis, oxidative burst, and parasite killing (Haase and Rink 2009). Zinc deficiency, related with aging, increases susceptibility to *Salmonella enteritidis*, *M. tuberculosis*, or *Listeria monocytogenes* (Haase and Rink 2009; Prasad et al. 1993, 2007). Zinc, in addition, can influence immune cell signal transduction and is involved in cytokine gene regulation via nuclear factor kappa-light-chain-enhancer of activated B cells (NFκB), chromatin remodeling, and acetylation (Haase and Rink 2009; Wessels et al. 2010b, 2013).

Therefore, a range of age-related diseases may be originated from impaired function of neutrophils that regulate recruitment, differentiation, and activation of both innate and adaptive immune cells.

Conclusion

Granulocytes reveal age-associated modifications like all cell types of the immune system. Although no differences appear to exist in neutrophil and eosinophil number in the circulation between aged and young individuals, a delayed degranulation is observed in basophils and eosinophils, as well as a reduction of phagocytotic capacity and a delay in the production of ROS in neutrophils. If chemotaxis is also altered with aging is currently controversially discussed since a lot of contrary data exist. Other reported modifications such as decreased Ca^{2+} mobilization, receptor assembling, and impaired protection from apoptosis in concert with delayed function of neutrophils of the elderly are due to changes and defects in signal transduction pathways, protein tyrosine phosphatase activity, and membrane components and fluidity. Whereas some key molecules in these pathways have been identified, the mechanisms triggering these modifications are still uncovered. As a result, the functional consequences will be a decline in the killing of bacteria and fungi of neutrophils in the elderly. This might be the result from failures in migration to and a reduced role in inflammation accompanied by a disturbed interaction with the adaptive part of the immune system. If basophil and eosinophil functions are changed with age remained to be elucidated in future studies. Table 5.1 summarizes the age-related changes in granulocytes.

In this context, new approaches using, e.g., small interfering RNA (siRNA) knockdown assays to identify the key molecules that affect signaling or non-rodent animal models for targeting the in vivo situation may be interesting strategies to investigate granulocytes with age. In addition, the manipulation of microRNAs (Ward et al. 2011) in neutrophil senescence may also play a future role for therapeutic applications in aging.

References

Adamko DJ, Odemuyiwa SO, Vethanayagam D et al (2005) The rise of the phoenix: the expanding role of the eosinophil in health and disease. Allergy 60:13–22

Agrawal A, Gupta S (2011) Impact of aging on dendritic cell functions in humans. Ageing Res Rev 10: 336–345

Agrawal A, Agrawal S, Gupta S (2007) Dendritic cells in human aging. Exp Gerontol 42:421–426

Alonso-Fernandez P, Puerto M, Mate I et al (2008) Neutrophils of centenarians show function levels similar to those of young adults. J Am Geriatr Soc 56:2244–2251

Altstaedt J, Kirchner H, Rink L (1996) Cytokine production of neutrophils is limited to interleukin-8. Immunology 89:563–568

Alvarez E, Ruiz-Gutierrez V, Sobrino F et al (2001) Age-related changes in membrane lipid composition, fluidity and respiratory burst in rat peritoneal neutrophils. Clin Exp Immunol 124:95–102

Antonaci S, Jirillo E, Ventura MT et al (1984) Non-specific immunity in aging-deficiency of monocyte and polymorphonuclear cell-mediated functions. Mech Ageing Dev 24:367–375

Barthel SR, Johansson MW, McNamee DM et al (2008) Roles of integrin activation in eosinophil function and the eosinophilic inflammation of asthma. J Leukoc Biol 83:1–12

Behm CA, Ovington KS (2000) The role of eosinophils in parasitic helminth infections insights from genetically modified mice. Parasitol Today 16:202–209

Bhushan M, Cumberbatch M, Dearman RJ et al (2002) Tumour necrosis factor-alpha-induced migration of human Langerhans cells: the influence of ageing. Br J Dermatol 146:32–40

Biasi D, Carletto A, Dellagnola C et al (1996) Neutrophil migration, oxidative metabolism, and adhesion in elderly and young subjects. Inflammation 20:673–681

Boehmer ED, Goral J, Faunce DE et al (2004) Age-dependent decrease in toll-like receptor 4-mediated pro-inflammatory cytokine production and mitogen-activated protein kinase expression. J Leukoc Biol 75:342–349

Born J, Uthgenannt D, Dodt C et al (1995) Cytokine pro-duction and lymphocyte subpopulations in aged humans. An assessment during nocturnal sleep. Mech Ageing Dev 84:113–126

Borregaard N, Sorensen OE, Theilgaard-Wnchl K (2007) Neutrophil granules: a library of innate immunity pro-teins. Trends Immunol 28:340–345

Braga PC, Sala MT, Dal Sasso M et al (1998) Influence of age on oxidative bursts (chemiluminescence) of polymorpho-nuclear neutrophil leukocytes. Gerontology 44:192–197

Busse PJ, Mathur SK (2010) Age-related changes in immune function: effect on airway inflammation. J Allergy Clin Immunol 126:690–699

Butcher S, Chahel H, Lord JM (2000) Ageing and the neutro-phil: no appetite for killing? Immunology 100:411–416

Butcher SK, Chahal H, Nayak L et al (2001) Senescence in innate immune responses: reduced neutrophil phagocytic capacity and CD16 expression in elderly humans. J Leukoc Biol 70:881–886

Cakman I, Kirchner H, Rink L (1997) Zinc supplementa-tion reconstitutes the production of interferon-alpha by leukocytes from elderly persons. J Interferon Cytokine Res 17:469–472

Cassatella MA (1995) The production of cytokines by polymorphonuclear neutrophils. Immunol Today 16: 21–26

Chatta GS, Andrews RG, Rodger E et al (1993) Hematopoietic progenitors and aging-alterations in granulocytic precursors and responsiveness to recom-binant human G-Csf, Gm-Csf, and Il-3. J Gerontol 48: M207–M212

Chaves MM, Costa DC, Pereira CCT et al (2007) Role of inositol 1,4,5-triphosphate and p38 mitogen-activated protein kinase in reactive oxygen species generation by granulocytes in a cyclic AMP-dependent manner: an age-related phenomenon. Gerontology 53:228–233

Damtew B, Spagnuolo PJ, Goldsmith GGH et al (1990) Neutrophil adhesion in the elderly – inhibitory effects of plasma from elderly patients. Clin Immunol Immunopathol 54:247–255

De Martinis M, Modesti M, Ginaldi L (2004) Phenotypic and functional changes of circulating monocytes and polymorphonuclear leucocytes from elderly persons. Immunol Cell Biol 82:415–420

Denzel A, Maus UA, Gomez MR et al (2008) Basophils enhance immunological memory responses. Nat Immunol 9:733–742

Di Lorenzo G, Balistreri CR, Candore G et al (1999) Granulocyte and natural killer activity in the elderly. Mech Ageing Dev 108:25–38

Di Lorenzo G, Pacor ML, Pellitteri ME et al (2003) A study of age-related IgE pathophysiological changes. Mech Ageing Dev 124:445–448

Di Lorenzo G, Leto-Barone MS, La Piana S et al (2012) Clinical course of rhinitis and changes in vivo and in vitro of allergic parameters in elderly patients: a long-term follow-up study. Clin Exp Med 13(1):67–73

Egger G, Burda A, Mitterhammer H et al (2003) Impaired blood polymorphonuclear leukocyte migration and infection risk in severe trauma. J Infect 47:148–154

Esparza B, Sanchez H, Ruiz M et al (1996) Neutrophil function in elderly persons assessed by flow cytome-try. Immunol Invest 25:185–190

Fanger NA, Liu CL, Guyre PM et al (1997) Activation of human T cells by major histocompatibility complex class II expressing neutrophils: proliferation in the presence of superantigen, but not tetanus toxoid. Blood 89:4128–4135

Ferretti S, Bonneau O, Dubois GR et al (2003) IL-17, pro-duced by lymphocytes and neutrophils, is necessary for lipopolysaccharide-induced airway neutrophilia: IL-15 as a possible trigger. J Immunol 170:2106–2112

Fortin CF, Larbi A, Lesur O et al (2006) Impairment of SHIP-1 down-regulation in the lipid rafts of human neutrophils under GM-CSF stimulation contributes to their age-related, altered functions. J Leukoc Biol 79:1061–1072

Fortin CF, Lesur O, Fulop T (2007a) Effects of aging on triggering receptor expressed on myeloid cells (TREM)-1-induced PMN functions. FEBS Lett 581: 1173–1178

Fortin CF, Larbi A, Dupuis G et al (2007b) GM-CSF acti-vates the Jak/STAT pathway to rescue polymorphonu-clear neutrophils from spontaneous apoptosis in young but not elderly individuals. Biogerontology 8:173–187

Fortin CF, Lesur O, Fulop T (2007c) Effects of TREM-1 activation in human neutrophils: activation of signaling pathways, recruitment into lipid rafts and association with TLR4. Int Immunol 19:41–50

Fortin CF, McDonald PP, Lesur O et al (2008) Aging and neutrophils: there is still much to do. Rejuvenation Res 11:873–882

Fortin CF, Larbi A, Dupuis G et al (2009a) Signal trans-duction changes in fMLP, TLRs, TREM-1 and GM-CSF receptors in PMN with aging. In: Handbook on immunosenescence. Springer, Heidelberg

Fortin CF, Ear T, McDonald PP (2009b) Autocrine role of endogenous interleukin-18 on inflammatory cytokine generation by human neutrophils. FASEB J 23: 194–203

Franceschi C, Capri M, Monti D et al (2007) Inflammaging and anti-inflammaging: a systemic perspective on aging and longevity emerged from studies in humans. Mech Ageing Dev 128:92–105

Fulop T (1994) Signal-transduction changes in granulo-cytes and lymphocytes with aging. Immunol Lett 40: 259–268

Fulop T, Fouquet C, Allaire P et al (1997) Changes in apoptosis of human polymorphonuclear granulocytes with aging. Mech Ageing Dev 96:15–34

Fulop T, Goulet AC, Desgeorges S et al (1999) Changes in the apoptosis of polymorphonuclear granulocytes with aging. FASEB J 13:A519

Fulop T, Douziech N, Desgeorges S et al (2000a) Signal transduction alterations in the apoptosis of polymorphonuclear granulocytes with aging under GM-CSF stimulation. FASEB J 14:A1156

Fulop T, Douziech N, Desgeorges S et al (2000b) Apoptosis in T lymphocytes and polymorphonuclear leukocytes with aging. FASEB J 14:A194

Fulop T, Larbi A, Douziech N et al (2004) Signal transduction and functional changes in neutrophils with aging. Aging Cell 3:217–226

Fulop T, Larbi A, Douziech N et al (2006) Cytokine receptor signalling and aging. Mech Ageing Dev 127: 526–537

Fulop T, Kotb R, Fortin CF et al (2010) Potential role of immunosenescence in cancer development. Ann N Y Acad Sci 1197:158–165

Gabriel P, Cakman I, Rink L (2002) Overproduction of monokines by leukocytes after stimulation with lipopolysaccharide in the elderly. Exp Gerontol 37:235–247

Geiger H, Rudolph KL (2009) Aging in the lymphohematopoietic stem cell compartment. Trends Immunol 30:360–365

Ginaldi L, De Martinis M, D'Ostilio A et al (1999) The immune system in the elderly III. Innate immunity. Immunol Res 20:117–126

Gomez CR, Hirano S, Cutro BT et al (2007) Advanced age exacerbates the pulmonary inflammatory response after lipopolysaccharide exposure. Crit Care Med 35:246–251

Gomez CR, Nomellini V, Faunce DE et al (2008) Innate immunity and aging. Exp Gerontol 43:718–728

Gosselin EJ, Wardwell K, Rigby WFC et al (1993) Induction of Mhc class-Ii on human polymorphonuclear neutrophils by granulocyte-macrophage colony-stimulating factor, Ifn-gamma, and Il-3. J Immunol 151:1482–1490

Grubeck-Loebenstein B, Della Bella S, Iorio AM et al (2009) Immunosenescence and vaccine failure in the elderly. Aging Clin Exp Res 21:201–209

Gunin AG, Kornilova NK, Vasilieva OV et al (2011) Age-related changes in proliferation, the numbers of mast cells, eosinophils, and CD45-positive cells in human dermis. J Gerontol A Biol Sci Med Sci 66:385–392

Haase H, Rink L (2009) Functional significance of zinc-related signaling pathways in immune cells. Annu Rev Nutr 29:133–152

Haase H, Mocchegiani E, Rink L (2006) Correlation between zinc status and immune function in the elderly. Biogerontology 7:421–428

Hannah S, Mecklenburgh K, Rahman I et al (1995) Hypoxia prolongs neutrophil survival in-vitro. FEBS Lett 372:233–237

Hellewell PG, Williams TJ (1994) The neutrophil. In: The handbook of immunopharmacology: immunopharmacology of neutrophils. Academic, London

Hogan SP, Rosenberg HF, Moqbel R et al (2008) Eosinophils: biological properties and role in health and disease. Clin Exp Allergy 38:709–750

Iking-Konert C, Wagner C, Denefleh B et al (2002) Up-regulation of the dendritic cell marker CD83 on polymorphonuclear neutrophils (PMN): divergent expression in acute bacterial infections and chronic inflammatory disease. Clin Exp Immunol 130:501–508

Issa JP (2003) Age-related epigenetic changes and the immune system. Clin Immunol 109:103–108

Ito Y, Kajkenova O, Feuers RJ et al (1998) Impaired glutathione peroxidase activity accounts for the age-related accumulation of hydrogen peroxide in activated human neutrophils. J Gerontol A Biol Sci Med Sci 53: M169–M175

Kim KC, Friso S, Choi SW (2009) DNA methylation, an epigenetic mechanism connecting folate to healthy embryonic development and aging. J Nutr Biochem 20:917–926

Kita H (2011) Eosinophils: multifaceted biological properties and roles in health and disease. Immunol Rev 242:161–177

Klut ME, Ruehlmann DO, Li L et al (2002) Age-related changes in the calcium homeostasis of adherent neutrophils. Exp Gerontol 37:533–541

Kovacs EJ, Palmer JL, Fortin CF et al (2009) Aging and innate immunity in the mouse: impact of intrinsic and extrinsic factors. Trends Immunol 30:319–324

Larbi A, Franceschi C, Mazzatti D et al (2008) Aging of the immune system as a prognostic factor for human longevity. Physiology (Bethesda) 23:64–74

Laupland KB, Church DL, Mucenski M et al (2003) Population-based study of the epidemiology of and the risk factors for invasive Staphylococcus aureus infections. J Infect Dis 187:1452–1459

Leng SX, Xue QL, Huang Y et al (2005) Baseline total and specific differential white blood cell counts and 5-year all-cause mortality in community-dwelling older women. Exp Gerontol 40:982–987

Leng SX, Xue QL, Tian J et al (2007) Inflammation and frailty in older women. J Am Geriatr Soc 55:864–871

Leng SX, Xue QL, Tian J et al (2009) Associations of neutrophil and monocyte counts with frailty in community-dwelling disabled older women: results from the Women's Health and Aging Studies I. Exp Gerontol 44:511–516

Ligthart GJ, Corberand JX, Fournier C et al (1984) Admission criteria for immunogerontological studies in man – the Senieur protocol. Mech Ageing Dev 28: 47–55

Lipschitz DA, Udupa KB, Indelicato SR et al (1991) Effect of age on 2Nd messenger generation in neutrophils. Blood 78:1347–1354

Lloyd AR, Oppenheim JJ (1992) Polys lament – the neglected role of the polymorphonuclear neutrophil in the afferent limb of the immune-response. Immunol Today 13:169–172

Lord JM, Butcher S, Killampali V et al (2001) Neutrophil ageing and immunesenescence. Mech Ageing Dev 122: 1521–1535

Mahbub S, Brubaker AL, Kovacs EJ (2011) Aging of the innate immune system: an update. Curr Immunol Rev 7:104–115

Mantovani A, Cassatella MA, Costantini C et al (2011) Neutrophils in the activation and regulation of innate and adaptive immunity. Nat Rev Immunol 11:519–531

Marone G, Poto S, Dimartino L et al (1986) Human basophil releasability.1. Age-related-changes in basophil releasability. J Allergy Clin Immunol 77:377–383

Mathur SK, Schwantes EA, Jarjour NN et al (2008) Age-related changes in eosinophil function in human subjects. Chest 133:412–419

Mclaughlin B, Omalley K, Cotter TG (1986) Age-related differences in granulocyte chemotaxis and degranulation. Clin Sci 70:59–62

Min B, Brown MA, LeGros G (2012) Understanding the roles of basophils: breaking dawn. Immunology 135: 192–197

Mohacsi A, Fulop T, Kozlovszky B et al (1992) Superoxide anion production and intracellular free calcium levels in resting and stimulated polymorphonuclear leukocytes obtained from healthy and arteriosclerotic subjects of various ages. Clin Biochem 25:285–288

Muniz VS, Weller PF, Neves JS (2012) Eosinophil crystalloid granules: structure, function, and beyond. J Leukoc Biol 92:281–288

Murciano C, Yanez A, O'Connor JE et al (2008) Influence of aging on murine neutrophil and macrophage function against Candida albicans. FEMS Immunol Med Microbiol 53:214–221

Nathan C (2006) Neutrophils and immunity: challenges and opportunities. Nat Rev Immunol 6:173–182

Nel HJ, Hams E, Saunders SP et al (2011) Impaired basophil induction leads to an age-dependent innate defect in type 2 immunity during helminth infection in mice. J Immunol 186:4631–4639

Niwa Y, Kasama T, Miyachi Y et al (1989) Neutrophil chemotaxis, phagocytosis and parameters of reactive oxygen species in human aging – cross-sectional and longitudinal-studies. Life Sci 44:1655–1664

Nomellini V, Faunce DE, Gomez CR et al (2008) An age-associated increase in pulmonary inflammation after burn injury is abrogated by CXCR2 inhibition. J Leukoc Biol 83:1493–1501

Opal SM, Girard TD, Ely EW (2005) The immunopathogenesis of sepsis in elderly patients. Clin Infect Dis 41:S504–S512

Panda A, Arjona A, Sapey E et al (2009) Human innate immunosenescence: causes and consequences for immunity in old age. Trends Immunol 30:325–333

Panda A, Qian F, Mohanty S et al (2010) Age-associated decrease in TLR function in primary human dendritic cells predicts influenza vaccine response. J Immunol 184:2518–2527

Pawelec G, Larbi A, Derhovanessian E (2010) Senescence of the human immune system. J Comp Pathol 141: S39–S44

Plackett TP, Boehmer ED, Faunce DE et al (2004) Aging and innate immune cells. J Leukoc Biol 76:291–299

Prasad AS, Fitzgerald JT, Hess JW et al (1993) Zinc-deficiency in elderly patients. Nutrition 9:218–224

Prasad AS, Beck FWJ, Bao B et al (2007) Zinc supplementation decreases incidence of infections in the elderly: effect of zinc on generation of cytokines and oxidative stress. Am J Clin Nutr 85:837–844

Rao KMK (1986) Age-related decline in ligand-induced actin polymerization in human-leukocytes and platelets. J Gerontol 41:561–566

Rao KMK, Currie MS, Padmanabhan J et al (1992) Age-related alterations in actin cytoskeleton and receptor expression in human-leukocytes. J Gerontol 47:B37–B44

Reato G, Cuffini AM, Tullio V et al (1999) Co-amoxiclav affects cytokine production by human polymorphonuclear cells. J Antimicrob Chemother 43:715–718

Renshaw M, Rockwell J, Engleman C et al (2002) Cutting edge: impaired toll-like receptor expression and function in aging. J Immunol 169:4697–4701

Rink L, Kirchner H (2000) Zinc-altered immune function and cytokine production. J Nutr 130:1407S–1411S

Rink L, Cakman I, Kirchner H (1998) Altered cytokine production in the elderly. Mech Ageing Dev 102:199–209

Routsi C, Stamataki E, Nanas S et al (2008) Increased levels of serum S100B protein in critically ill patients without brain injury – Reply. Shock 30:222–223

Savill JS, Wyllie AH, Henson JE et al (1989) Macrophage phagocytosis of aging neutrophils in inflammation – programmed cell-death in the neutrophil leads to its recognition by macrophages. J Clin Invest 83:865–875

Schröder AK, Rink L (2003) Neutrophil immunity of the elderly. Mech Ageing Dev 124:419–425

Schröder AK, der Ohe M, Kolling U et al (2006a) Polymorphonuclear leucocytes selectively produce anti-inflammatory interleukin-1 receptor antagonist and chemokines, but fail to produce pro-inflammatory mediators. Immunology 119:317–327

Schröder AK, Uciechowski P, Fleischer D et al (2006b) Crosslinking of CD66b on peripheral blood neutrophils mediates the release of interleukin-8 from intracellular storage. Hum Immunol 67:676–682

Schwarzenbach HR, Nakagawa T, Conroy MC et al (1982) Skin reactivity, basophil de-granulation and Ige levels in aging. Clin Allergy 12:465–473

Seres I, Csongor J, Mohacsi A et al (1993) Age-dependent alterations of human recombinant Gm-Csf effects on human granulocytes. Mech Ageing Dev 71: 143–154

Shaw AC, Joshi S, Greenwood H et al (2010) Aging of the innate immune system. Curr Opin Immunol 22: 507–513

Shaw AC, Panda A, Joshi SR et al (2011) Dysregulation of human toll-like receptor function in aging. Ageing Res Rev 10:346–353

Simell B, Vuorela A, Ekstrom N et al (2011) Aging reduces the functionality of anti-pneumococcal antibodies and the killing of Streptococcus pneumoniae by neutrophil phagocytosis. Vaccine 29:1929–1934

Smith P, Dunne DW, Fallon PG (2001) Defective in vivo induction of functional type 2 cytokine responses in aged mice. Eur J Immunol 31:1495–1502

Solana R, Pawelec G, Tarazona R (2006) Aging and innate immunity. Immunity 24:491–494

Song C, Vandewoude M, Stevens W et al (1999) Alterations in immune functions during normal aging and Alzheimer's disease. Psychiatry Res 85:71–80

Starr JM, Deary IJ (2011) Sex differences in blood cell counts in the Lothian Birth Cohort 1921 between 79 and 87 years. Maturitas 69:373–376

Sullivan BM, Liang HE, Bando JK et al (2011) Genetic analysis of basophil function in vivo. Nat Immunol 12:527–535

Swain SL, Nikolich-Zugich J (2009) Key research opportunities in immune system aging. J Gerontol A Biol Sci Med Sci 64:183–186

Swift ME, Burns AL, Gray KL et al (2001) Age-related alterations in the inflammatory response to dermal injury. J Invest Dermatol 117:1027–1035

Tortorella C, Polignano A, Piazzolla G et al (1996) Lipopolysaccharide-, granulocyte-monocyte colony stimulating factor and pentoxifylline-mediated effects on formyl-methionyl-leucine-phenylalanine-stimulated neutrophil respiratory burst in the elderly. Microbios 85:189–198

Tortorella C, Piazzolla G, Spaccavento F et al (1998) Effects of granulocyte-macrophage colony-stimulating factor and cyclic AMP interaction on human neutrophil apoptosis. Mediators Inflamm 7:391–396

Tortorella C, Piazzolla G, Spaccavento F et al (1999) Age-related effects of oxidative metabolism and cyclic AMP signaling on neutrophil apoptosis. Mech Ageing Dev 110:195–205

Tortorella C, Piazzolla G, Spaccavento F et al (2000) Regulatory role of extracellular matrix proteins in neutrophil respiratory burst during aging. Mech Ageing Dev 119:69–82

Tortorella C, Stella I, Piazzolla G et al (2004) Role of defective ERK phosphorylation in the impaired GM-CSF-induced oxidative response of neutrophils in elderly humans. Mech Ageing Dev 125:539–546

Tortorella C, Simone O, Piazzolla G et al (2006) Role of phosphoinositide 3-kinase and extracellular signal-regulated kinase pathways in granulocyte macrophage-colony-stimulating factor failure to delay Fas-induced neutrophil apoptosis in elderly humans. J Gerontol A Biol Sci Med Sci 61:1111–1118

Tortorella C, Simone O, Piazzolla G et al (2007) Age-related impairment of GM-CSF-induced signalling in neutrophils: role of SHP-1 and SOCS proteins. Ageing Res Rev 6:81–93

Uciechowski P, Rink L (2009) Neutrophil granulocyte functions in the elderly. In: Handbook on immunosenescence. Springer, Heidelberg

Van Duin D, Shaw AC (2007) Toll-like receptors in older adults. J Am Geriatr Soc 55:1438–1444

Van Panhuys N, Prout M, Forbes E et al (2011) Basophils are the major producers of IL-4 during primary helminth infection. J Immunol 186:2719–2728

Varga Z, Kovacs EM, Paragh G et al (1988) Effect of elastin peptides and N-formyl-methionyl-leucyl phenylalanine on cytosolic free calcium in polymorphonuclear leukocytes of healthy middle-aged and elderly subjects. Clin Biochem 21:127–130

Von der Ohe M, Altstaedt J, Gross U et al (2001) Human neutrophils produce macrophage inhibitory protein-1 beta but not type 1 interferons in response to viral stimulation. J Interferon Cytokine Res 21:241–247

Ward JR, Heath PR, Catto JW et al (2011) Regulation of neutrophil senescence by MicroRNAs. PLoS One 6(1): e15810

Weiskopf D, Weinberger B, Grubeck-Loebenstein B (2009) The aging of the immune system. Transpl Int 22: 1041–1050

Wenisch C, Patruta S, Daxbock F et al (2000) Effect of age on human neutrophil function. J Leukoc Biol 67: 40–45

Wessels I, Fleischer D, Rink L et al (2010a) Changes in chromatin structure and methylation of the human interleukin-1 beta gene during monopoiesis. Immunology 130:410–417

Wessels I, Jansen J, Rink L et al (2010b) Immunosenescence of polymorphonuclear neutrophils. ScientificWorldJournal 10:145–160

Wessels I, Haase H, Engelhardt G et al (2013) Zinc deficiency induces production of the proinflammatory cytokines IL-1β and TNFα in promyeloid cells via epigenetic and redox-dependent mechanisms. J Nutr Biochem 24(1):289–297

Whitelaw DA, Rayner BL, Willcox PA (1992) Community-acquired bacteremia in the elderly – a prospective-study of 121 cases. J Am Geriatr Soc 40:996–1000

Yagi T, Sato A, Hayakawa H et al (1997) Failure of aged rats to accumulate eosinophils in allergic inflammation of the airway. J Allergy Clin Immunol 99: 38–47

Yoshimoto T, Yasuda K, Tanaka H et al (2009) Basophils contribute to T(H)2-IgE responses in vivo via IL-4 production and presentation of peptide-MHC class II complexes to CD4(+) T cells. Nat Immunol 10: 706–712

Dendritic Cells and Dysregulated Immunity in the Elderly

6

Anshu Agrawal and Sudhir Gupta

6.1 Introduction

Advancing age has a profound effect on the immune system. The capacity to mount effective immune responses against foreign antigens decreases concomitantly as the reactivity towards self increases (Liu et al. 2011). Dysregulation of the immune system at both innate and adaptive levels contributes to the change. Age-associated alterations in the adaptive immune system are more obvious with decline in naïve T cell numbers due to involution of thymus (Brunner et al. 2011). In contrast, the modifications in innate immune system cells are subtle but together cause extensive damage.

Among the innate immune cells, antigen-presenting cells (APCs) such as dendritic cells (DCs) and macrophages bridge the innate and adaptive immune systems (Steinman 2012); thus age-associated alterations in their functions also impact the functions of downstream adaptive immune cells. The activation of T and B cells, polarization of T helper (Th) cell responses, and generation of effector and memory cells are all governed by APCs particularly DCs as they are initiators of the immune response. Age-associated changes in DC function can thus significantly impact the immune status of the elderly.

A. Agrawal, PhD (✉) • S. Gupta, MD, PhD
Division of Basic and Clinical Immunology,
University of California,
Irvine, CA, USA
e-mail: aagrawal@uci.edu

6.2 Dendritic Cell Numbers and Phenotype

DCs are rare cells of the immune system which were discovered by Steinman and Cohn (Steinman et al. 1979) in 1979. DCs are derived from hematopoietic stem cells (HSCs) through gradually restricted precursors (Chopin et al. 2012). There are two major subsets of DCs – the myeloid DC (mDC) which are derived from common myeloid progenitor cells (MDP) and the plasmacytoid (PDC) which are lymphoid in origin and are morphologically similar to B plasma cells. Both subsets are widely distributed among all tissues though the myeloid DCs are more abundant than PDCs. An alternative DC developmental circuit occurring after the MDP stage involves monocytes. Under inflammatory conditions, monocytes migrate to the tissues to differentiate into monocyte-derived DCs (Liu and Nussenzweig 2010). This property of monocytes to differentiate into DCs (MDDCs) is used extensively in the laboratory to generate DCs. These MDDCs resemble mDCs in function and phenotype.

Two major populations of DCs have been identified in the blood, the myeloid or conventional DCs (cDCs, to distinguish them from other myeloid DCs present in tissues) and PDCs (Cao and Liu 2007). Extensive characterization of DCs in the circulation has been performed in aged humans. Most reports suggest that numbers and phenotype of cDC populations is not dramatically altered with age; however, various studies did observe a reduction in the number of PDCs

A. Massoud, N. Rezaei (eds.), *Immunology of Aging*,
DOI 10.1007/978-3-642-39495-9_6, © Springer-Verlag Berlin Heidelberg 2014

in circulation (Jing et al. 2009; Agrawal et al. 2007; Della Bella et al. 2007; Pietschmann et al. 2000; Uyemura et al. 2002; Panda et al. 2010; Perez-Cabezas et al. 2007; Shodell and Siegal 2002; Canaday et al. 2010; Steger et al. 1996). The expression of costimulatory (CD40, CD80, and CD86) and major histocompatibility complex (MHC) markers (HLA-DR) was also comparable between the aged and young cDC and PDC population. However, few studies also reported decreased expression of HLA-DR on cDCs (Shodell and Siegal 2002). In contrast to healthy aged population, the frail elderly populations which reside in nursing homes tended to display more differences in numbers and phenotype of DCs (Jing et al. 2009). Both the numbers and expression of DC activation markers were reduced in this subset of the elderly. In addition to cDC and PDC subsets, MDDCs have also been extensively studied in aging. The generation of MDDCs as well as the expression of DC markers is not reported to be different between aged and young subjects (Agrawal et al. 2007; Uyemura et al. 2002; Steger et al. 1996).

Studies describing DC phenotype and function in tissues from aged subjects are scarce due to the limitation in obtaining the material nevertheless there is sufficient data regarding age-associated changes in DCs in skin and oral cavity. DCs in the skin are myeloid in nature and express Langerin granules and are therefore called Langerhans cells (LCs). A reduction in the number of epidermal LCs in has been reported in elderly subjects (Bhushan et al. 2004). However, in monocytes differentiated into LCs, no significant difference was observed in the numbers or in the expression of activation markers in the aged subjects relative to young (Xu et al. 2012). Another study (Bodineau et al. 2007, 2009) examined intraepithelial LC during chronic periodontitis in elderly patients and reported a decrease in the numbers. They also observed morphological changes in LCs in that LCs from the elderly were more rounded with fewer numbers of dendrites which would affect their T cell stimulation capacity. Thus, it seems DC numbers and phenotype display more age-associated changes in tissues as compared to that in circulation in humans.

Similar to humans, DCs in tissues of mice displayed significant age-associated changes. In general, the cDC numbers in the spleen and lymph nodes were similar to young, whereas the number of cDC in the lungs increased in aged mice (Stout-Delgado et al. 2008; Tan et al. 2012). Several studies in mice have determined the age-associated modifications in DCs in the brain due to the strong correlation between neurodegeneration and immunological changes. Increased levels of CD11[+] DCs were observed (Stichel and Luebbert 2007) throughout the brains of older mice while in the young DCs were only visible in the meninges and choroid plexus. These findings were further confirmed by Kaunzner et al. (2012), who showed increased accumulation of DCs in aged brains when compared to younger control animals. Thus, it seems DC numbers can be increased or decreased with age depending on the anatomical location.

6.3 Dendritic Cells and Immunity in the Elderly

6.3.1 TLR and Cytokine Secretion

DCs are key players in generation of immunity to foreign antigens and maintain tolerance to self antigens (Steinman et al. 2000). DCs distributed throughout the body are armed with pathogen recognition receptors (PRRs) which allow them to sense and respond to threats. Engagement of PRRs leads to DC activation characterized by upregulation of several costimulatory and APC surface receptors as well as pro-inflammatory cytokine secretion. PRRs can be divided into different classes such as Toll-like receptors (TLRs), NOD-like receptors (NLRs), and C-type lectin receptors (CLRs) (Kawasaki et al. 2011; Kumar et al. 2011). TLR function, particularly in aged human MDDCs, has been reported to be largely intact at the level of both expression and function (Agrawal et al. 2007; Uyemura et al. 2002). Our own observations (Agrawal et al. 2007) suggest that inflammatory cytokine secretion particularly tumor necrosis factor-alpha (TNF-α) and interleukin (IL)-6 are increased in response to TLR4 and TLR8. In contrast to MDDCs, intracellular cytokine detection of TLR stimulated cDCs in aged blood revealed significant impairment in the production of TNF-α, IL-6, and IL-12p40 in response to nearly all TLRs (Panda et al. 2010). Other studies with blood myeloid DCs have also reported impairment in IL-12 production though these studies did not observe a reduction in TNF-α and IL-6 (Della Bella et al. 2007). Similar to MDDCs, no significant difference in baseline or inducible cytokine secretion was observed in monocyte-derived LCs from aged or young subjects. A recent study in rhesus macaques (Asquith et al. 2012) observed an increase in the frequency of myeloid DC with age but found reduced secretion of cytokines in response to TLR4, TLR2/6, and TLR7/9. Interestingly, they observed reduced expression of absent in melanoma 2 (AIM2) (Barber 2011) and retinoic acid-inducible gene I (RIG-1) (Rietdijk et al. 2008) in aged animals. Both these receptors are involved in IFN-α production.

6.3.2   Innate Interferon (IFN) Secretion

In keeping with this, the production of IFN-alpha is universally reported to be decreased in aging in response to TLR7, TLR8, or TLR9 (Canaday et al. 2010; Jing et al. 2009; Panda et al. 2010; Sridharan et al. 2011). The PDC subset in the blood is the primary IFN producer against infections. They express the intracellular TLR receptors TLR7 and TLR9 which allow sensing of ssRNA viruses such as influenza and unmethylated DNA motifs from bacteria (Gilliet et al. 2008). The production of IFN from PDCs is very rapid and the amount of IFN produced by these cells can be 100 fold more than other cells (Fitzgerald-Bocarsly 2002). Almost all studies have reported decreased type I IFN secretion by aged PDCs in response to influenza virus, TLR7 ligand Gardiquimod, and TLR9 ligand ODN which may well be responsible for the increased susceptibility of the aged to respiratory viral infections as robust IFN production by PDCs is essential to generate effective immune response against viruses. Reduced IFN secretion by PDCs in aged subjects is due to a number of reasons. Most studies observe a reduction in PDC numbers as well as reduced expression of the TLR7 and TLR9 in PDCs in the blood of aged subjects (Jing et al. 2009; Panda et al. 2009). Our own studies suggest that the defect lies in the signaling pathway downstream of TLRs (Sridharan et al. 2011). We observed impaired phosphorylation of interferon regulatory factor 7 (IRF-7), primary transcription factor required for IFN production (Honda et al. 2005). A recent study (Qian et al. 2011) reports similar deficiency in IFN production from aged PDCs in response to West Nile virus. These studies together suggest that type I IFN secretion from aged PDCs is impaired though the mechanisms may vary with the population studied.

Interestingly, this deficit in IFN production was not restricted to PDCs alone; MDDCs from aged donors also demonstrated significantly impaired IFN secretion in response to influenza virus. Here also, similar to PDCs, secretion of other cytokines was comparable to young (Prakash et al. 2012). Further investigations suggested that the defect was at the epigenetic level. Chromatin immunoprecipitation (ChIP) studies with activator histone, H3K4me3, and repressor histone, H3K9me3, antibodies revealed that the association of IFN promoter with the repressor histone is increased in aged DCs at the basal level which reduces the association of the promoter with activation histone on activation with influenza. Similar reduction in type I IFN secretion in by MDDCs from aged donors was also observed in response to West Nile virus (Qian et al. 2011). Their observations suggested that DCs from older donors had diminished late-phase responses, such as induction of the transcription factors signal transducers and activators of transcription 1 (STAT1) and IRF-7, and lower expression of IRF-1, suggesting defective positive-feedback regulation of type I IFN expression. Altogether, DCs (both PDCs and MDDCs) from aged donors show selective defect in IFN secretion in response to viruses while the secretion of other pro-inflammatory cytokines is largely intact.

In addition to type I IFNs, PDCs also produce type III IFNs – IL28/IL29 or IFN-lambda (Ank et al. 2006, 2008; Yin et al. 2012). These are more recently discovered innate IFNs which have been reported to play a major role in protection against viral infections of the mucosa particularly of the respiratory tract (Mordstein et al. 2010b). In support of this, *IL28R* knockout mice were reported to be more susceptible to several pneumotropic viruses than *IFNAR1-knockout* mice (Mordstein et al. 2010a). This is because their induction in DCs utilizes the same pathways as type I IFN however; their mode of action is restricted as the receptor for type III IFN is expressed mainly on epithelial cells of the mucosa (Ank et al. 2006). Thus, IFN-III seems to selectively contribute to innate immunity at mucosal surfaces, which are the most frequent entry sites of viruses. Our group has observed reduced type III IFN secretion from both PDCs and MDDCs from aged in response to influenza virus (Sridharan et al. 2011; Prakash et al. 2012). Reduced IFN-III is also observed in asthmatic individuals (Edwards and Johnston 2011). Thus, impaired secretion of IFN-III by aged DCs could be a major factor in the susceptibility of the elderly to not only respiratory viral infections but also other respiratory disorders such asthma and COPD. Given the selective nature of IFN deficiency observed in aged donors, supplementation of IFN particularly of the type III subtype during viral infections may help reduce the incidence and severity of respiratory viral infections in the elderly provided the response to IFN is not compromised.

6.3.3 Inflammasome

Most studies in the elderly are focused on TLRs and there is a scarcity of information on the functions of other PRRs, which are emerging as major players in the immune response. A recent mouse study with influenza infection demonstrates that activation of NOD receptor NLRP3 is impaired in aged mice resulting in reduced IL-1β production (Stout-Delgado et al. 2012). There is reduced expression of ASC, NLRP3, and caspase-1 but increased expression of pro-IL-1β, pro-IL-18, and pro-IL-33 in DCs from aged mice as compared to DCs from young mice. The authors also showed that treatment of mice with nigericin reduced the influenza infection in mice by enhancing the IL-1β production. In another study, the authors have demonstrated that increased generation of danger signals in the thymus activates the caspase-1 via NLRP3 inflammasome resulting in thymic atrophy (Youm et al. 2012). Inhibition of inflammasome activity restored the thymic epithelium and T cell repertoire. One other study has examined the activity of inflammasomes in nonimmune cells. In this study (Mawhinney et al. 2011), the activation of NLRP1 was reported to be enhanced in hippocampus of aged rats resulting in increased secretion of IL-1β and IL-18 which contributed to cognitive decline in the elderly. A recent microarray study (Cribbs et al. 2012) of aged human brain tissue also observed signatures reminiscent of activation of microglia and perivascular macrophages in the aging brain. Almost all innate immune response genes such as TLR signaling, complement components, as well as inflammasome signaling were upregulated in aged brain. These studies suggest that activity of NOD-like receptors may be increased or decreased with age and vary with different receptors and anatomical location.

6.4 Phagocytosis and Migration

Sensing of pathogens by DC leads to antigen uptake by phagocytosis and activation of DCs which upregulates chemokine receptor type 7 (CCR7) receptor on DCs allowing their migration to draining lymph nodes to prime T cells. Our studies indicate that MDDCs from aged are impaired in phosphorylation of AKT, a kinase in the PI3kinase signaling pathway which controls cytoskeletal proteins (Agrawal et al. 2007). This impairment leads to reduced phagocytic uptake of antigens by DCs as well as reduced migration in response to macrophage inflammatory protein-3 (MIP3-β). Similar impairment in migratory capacity of epidermal LCs to TNF-α has also been reported in the elderly (Cumberbatch et al. 2003).

However, differentiated monocyte (Ogden et al. 2011) showed migration equivalent to young in response to the chemokine ligand chemokine (C-C motif) ligand 19 (CCL19). A decrease in the capacity of migration of adoptively transferred aged DCs is also observed in aged mice. Reduced CCR7 signaling as well as reduced response to CCL21 was considered to be the primary culprit (Grolleau-Julius et al. 2008). A recent study (Zhao et al. 2011) also observed impaired migration of lung DCs to draining lymph nodes in aged mice in an influenza infection model. They attributed it to increased expression of prostaglandin D2 (PGD2) in mouse lungs. In summary advancing age seems to slow down aged DCs.

6.5 T Cell Priming

Once DCs migrate to lymph nodes they activate CD4+ Th cell, CD8+ T cytotoxic and B cell antibody responses. Almost all studies in humans studying DC-T interaction have been performed using MDDCs. Most studies did not observe a significant difference in the capacity of aged MDDCs to induce T cell proliferation compared to young DCs (Steger et al. 1997; Agrawal et al. 2009, 2012b). This was true for MDDCs and PDCs. However, we did observe (Agrawal et al. 2012b) increased basal level of proliferation and IFN-γ secretion by young CD4+ T cells when cultured with aged MDDCs as compared to young which may be a consequence of increased basal level of DC activation in the elderly. Culture of unstimulated PDCs with CD8+ T cells also resulted in higher basal level of IFN-γ secretion and granzyme and perforin induction (Sridharan et al. 2011). However, influenza-stimulated PDCs from aged subjects were deficient in inducing granzyme and perforin in CD8+ T cells of young subjects due to the reduced secretion of IFN-I and IFN-III by aged PDCs.

DCs also dictate the polarization of Th cells (Manicassamy and Pulendran 2009a). The cytokines secreted by DCs direct the differentiation of Th cells towards Th1/Th2/Th17/Treg/Tfh cells. Evidence suggests that Th1 response is predominant in healthy old subjects which changes to Th2 in the frail elderly probably due to increase in histamine which enhances Th2 polarization (Rafi et al. 2003). Treatment with antihistamine reduced Th2 responses and improved immune function in the frail elderly. Most studies with MDDC-T interaction do not report any change in Th cell cytokine secretion in aged donors. We have observed an increase in basal level of IFN-γ secretion from young Th cells when cultured with aged DC. This increase was more prominent in aged DC-aged T coculture (Agrawal et al. 2012b). We also observed increased differentiation of aged CD4 T cells of aged towards IL-21 secreting T follicular helper (Tfh) cells (Agrawal et al. 2012b). IL-21 affects almost all immune cells of the body and increased secretion of IL-21 is associated with autoimmune diseases (Shekhar and Yang 2012). IL-21 enhances IL-17 production and also increases the differentiation of B cells towards antibody secreting plasma cells thus IL-21 enhances autoantibody production in autoimmune and inflammatory diseases (Sarra et al. 2011). Increased levels of autoantibodies are common in aged individuals (Howard et al. 2006). Furthermore, IL-21 enhances the formation of IL-10 secreting B regulatory cells which suppress immune responses (Yoshizaki et al. 2012). IL-21 also enhances the cytotoxicity of CD8+ T cells and natural killer (NK) cells which may account for increased granzyme and perforin observed in aged CD8+ T cells in the absence of infection. Increased IL-21 was found to enhance the susceptibility of mouse to pneumovirus infection (Spolski et al. 2012). IL-21 also promotes allergic inflammation (Spolski and Leonard 2008). Therefore, increased IL-21 in aging may be detrimental for generating efficient immune responses against infections and enhance the susceptibility of the elderly to respiratory diseases.

6.6 Dendritic Cell and Tolerance

6.6.1 Peripheral Tolerance

DCs are unique among the APCs due to their constitutive low level expression of MHC and costimulatory molecules. This low level expression of MHC allows DCs to sample and present endogenous antigens to T cells and induces the formation of T regulatory (Treg) cells. DCs are therefore crucial for maintenance of tolerance (peripheral and mucosal) in the body (Hu and Wan 2011). Impaired capacity of DCs to maintain tolerance is one of the primary mechanisms of induction of autoimmunity (Agrawal et al. 2012a). Increased response of DCs to self antigens induces the secretion of pro-inflammatory cytokines and decreases the formation of Treg cells. Most studies in aging have not focused on the tolerizing function of DCs. Our own group determined the response of aged MDDCs to self-antigen, human DNA and demonstrated that aged MDDCs secrete significantly higher level of IFN-α and IL-6 compared to young MDDCs (Agrawal et al. 2009). The capacity of aged MDDCs to prime T cells was also enhanced. Increased response to self antigens would enhance chronic inflammation as DCs are constantly sampling self antigens from the surrounding milieu. Investigations into the signaling mechanisms suggest that DCs from aged display increased basal level of activation as evidenced by increased phosphorylation of the p65 subunit of nuclear factor kappa-light-chain-enhancer of activated B cells (NF-κB) in aged MDDCs. Increased basal level activation of DCs may induce secretion of pro-inflammatory cytokines and other inflammatory mediators from aged DCs. This was confirmed by study of Panda et al. (2010) where they observed increased secretion of TNF and IL-6 from cDCs from aged donors in the absence of stimulation. Our unpublished observations from gene expression analysis using microarrays suggest a pro-inflammatory signature in aged MDDCs.

6.6.2 Mucosal Tolerance

Besides maintaining peripheral tolerance, DCs play a major role in mediating tolerance at mucosal surfaces. The airways and the mucosa are continuously exposed to millions of harmless pathogens, toxins, etc. DCs are present just below the mucosal epithelium and can sense these stimuli via extension of their dendrites as well as via activation of epithelial cells (Allam et al. 2011; Lambrecht and Hammad 2012). The mucosal environment is rich in immunosuppressive cytokines such as transforming growth factor beta (TGF-β) and vitamin A metabolite, retinoic acid (RA), which prevent activation of DCs to these stimuli and results in the generation of Treg cells (Manicassamy and Pulendran 2009b; Feng et al. 2010). Majority of the DCs in the mucosa are myeloid in origin though it has recently been shown DCs in the mucosa can be divided into two subsets: one expressing the CD103$^+$ which are immunosuppressive and induces Tregs and the other CD103 subset which react to pathogens and activate T cells (Haniffa et al. 2012; Ivanov et al. 2012; Nakano et al. 2012; Leepiyasakulchai et al. 2012). Increased activation of DCs from aged donors may disturb the mucosal equilibrium as they may react to harmless antigens to induce chronic inflammation which would result in airway hyperresponsiveness and increase the susceptibility of the elderly to mucosal infections.

Conclusion

In summary, DC function changes significantly with age. Certain responses such as the production of innate IFNs in response to viruses decrease while the basal levels of pro-inflammatory cytokines increase. Reduced IFN secretion impairs the ability of the aged subjects to fight viral infections particularly of the respiratory mucosa, while enhanced basal level of inflammation causes erosion of tolerance both at the peripheral level and in the mucosa. Increased IL-21 secretion further impairs the capacity of the elderly to fight infections. Thus, DCs from aged subjects display defects at multiple levels and therapeutic measures targeting DCs may restore the immune functions in the elderly.

References

Agrawal A, Agrawal S, Cao JN et al (2007) Altered innate immune functioning of dendritic cells in elderly humans: a role of phosphoinositide 3-kinase-signaling pathway. J Immunol 178(11):6912–6922

Agrawal A, Tay J, Ton S et al (2009) Increased reactivity of dendritic cells from aged subjects to self-antigen, the human DNA. J Immunol 182(2):1138–1145

Agrawal A, Sridharan A, Prakash S et al (2012a) Dendritic cells and aging: consequences for autoimmunity. Expert Rev Clin Immunol 8(1):73–80

Agrawal A, Su H, Chen J et al (2012b) Increased IL-21 secretion by aged CD4+T cells is associated with prolonged STAT-4 activation and CMV seropositivity. Aging (Albany NY) 4(9):648–659

Allam JP, Duan Y, Winter J et al (2011) Tolerogenic T cells, Th1/Th17 cytokines and TLR2/TLR4 expressing dendritic cells predominate the microenvironment within distinct oral mucosal sites. Allergy 66(4):532–539

Ank N, West H, Bartholdy C et al (2006) Lambda interferon (IFN-lambda), a type III IFN, is induced by viruses and IFNs and displays potent antiviral activity against select virus infections in vivo. J Virol 80(9):4501–4509

Ank N, Iversen MB, Bartholdy C et al (2008) An important role for type III interferon (IFN-lambda/IL-28) in TLR-induced antiviral activity. J Immunol 180(4):2474–2485

Asquith M, Haberthur K, Brown M et al (2012) Age-dependent changes in innate immune phenotype and function in rhesus macaques (macaca mulatta). Pathobiol Aging Age Relat Dis. doi:10.3402/pba.v2i0.18052

Barber GN (2011) Cytoplasmic DNA innate immune pathways. Immunol Rev 243(1):99–108

Bhushan M, Cumberbatch M, Dearman RJ et al (2004) Exogenous interleukin-1beta restores impaired Langerhans cell migration in aged skin. Br J Dermatol 150(6):1217–1218

Bodineau A, Coulomb B, Folliguet M et al (2007) Do Langerhans cells behave similarly in elderly and younger patients with chronic periodontitis? Arch Oral Biol 52(2):189–194

Bodineau A, Coulomb B, Tedesco AC et al (2009) Increase of gingival matured dendritic cells number in elderly patients with chronic periodontitis. Arch Oral Biol 54(1):12–16

Brunner S, Herndler-Brandstetter D, Weinberger B et al (2011) Persistent viral infections and immune aging. Ageing Res Rev 10(3):362–369

Canaday DH, Amponsah NA, Jones L et al (2010) Influenza-induced production of interferon-alpha is defective in geriatric individuals. J Clin Immunol 30(3):373–383

Cao W, Liu YJ (2007) Innate immune functions of plasmacytoid dendritic cells. Curr Opin Immunol 19(1):24–30

Chopin M, Allan RS, Belz GT (2012) Transcriptional regulation of dendritic cell diversity. Front Immunol 3:26

Cribbs DH, Berchtold NC, Perreau V et al (2012) Extensive innate immune gene activation accompanies brain aging, increasing vulnerability to cognitive decline and neurodegeneration: a microarray study. J Neuroinflammation 9:179

Cumberbatch M, Bhushan M, Dearman RJ et al (2003) IL-1beta-induced Langerhans' cell migration and TNF-alpha production in human skin: regulation by lactoferrin. Clin Exp Immunol 132(2):352–359

Della Bella S, Bierti L, Presicce P et al (2007) Peripheral blood dendritic cells and monocytes are differently regulated in the elderly. Clin Immunol 122(2):220–228

Edwards MR, Johnston SL (2011) Interferon-lambda as a new approach for treatment of allergic asthma? EMBO Mol Med 3(6):306–308

Feng T, Cong Y, Qin H et al (2010) Generation of mucosal dendritic cells from bone marrow reveals a critical role of retinoic acid. J Immunol 185(10):5915–5925

Fitzgerald-Bocarsly P (2002) Natural interferon-alpha producing cells: the plasmacytoid dendritic cells. Biotechniques 22(Suppl. 16):24–29

Gilliet M, Cao W, Liu YJ (2008) Plasmacytoid dendritic cells: sensing nucleic acids in viral infection and autoimmune diseases. Nat Rev Immunol 8(8):594–606

Grolleau-Julius A, Harning EK, Abernathy LM et al (2008) Impaired dendritic cell function in aging leads to defective antitumor immunity. Cancer Res 68(15):6341–6349

Haniffa M, Shin A, Bigley V et al (2012) Human tissues contain CD141hi cross-presenting dendritic cells with functional homology to mouse CD103+ nonlymphoid dendritic cells. Immunity 37(1):60–73

Honda K, Yanai H, Negishi H et al (2005) IRF-7 is the master regulator of type-I interferon-dependent immune responses. Nature 434(7034):772–777

Howard WA, Gibson KL, Dunn-Walters DK (2006) Antibody quality in old age. Rejuvenation Res 9(1):117–125

Hu J, Wan Y (2011) Tolerogenic dendritic cells and their potential applications. Immunology 132(3):307–314

Ivanov S, Fontaine J, Paget C et al (2012) Key role for respiratory CD103(+) dendritic cells, IFN-gamma, and IL-17 in protection against Streptococcus pneumoniae infection in response to alpha-galactosylceramide. J Infect Dis 206(5):723–734

Jing Y, Shaheen E, Drake RR et al (2009) Aging is associated with a numerical and functional decline in plasmacytoid dendritic cells, whereas myeloid dendritic cells are relatively unaltered in human peripheral blood. Hum Immunol 70(10):777–784

Kaunzner UW, Miller MM, Gottfried-Blackmore A et al (2012) Accumulation of resident and peripheral dendritic cells in the aging CNS. Neurobiol Aging 33(4):681–693 e681

Kawasaki T, Kawai T, Akira S (2011) Recognition of nucleic acids by pattern-recognition receptors and its relevance in autoimmunity. Immunol Rev 243(1):61–73

Kumar H, Kawai T, Akira S (2011) Pathogen recognition by the innate immune system. Int Rev Immunol 30(1):16–34

Lambrecht BN, Hammad H (2012) Lung dendritic cells in respiratory viral infection and asthma: from protection to immunopathology. Annu Rev Immunol 30:243–270

Leepiyasakulchai C, Ignatowicz L, Pawlowski A et al (2012) Failure to recruit anti-inflammatory CD103+ dendritic cells and a diminished CD4+ Foxp3+ regulatory T cell pool in mice that display excessive lung inflammation and increased susceptibility to Mycobacterium tuberculosis. Infect Immun 80(3):1128–1139

Liu K, Nussenzweig MC (2010) Origin and development of dendritic cells. Immunol Rev 234(1):45–54

Liu WM, van der Zeijst BA, Boog CJ et al (2011) Aging and impaired immunity to influenza viruses: implications for vaccine development. Hum Vaccin 7(Suppl):94–98

Manicassamy S, Pulendran B (2009a) Modulation of adaptive immunity with Toll-like receptors. Semin Immunol 21(4):185–193

Manicassamy S, Pulendran B (2009b) Retinoic acid-dependent regulation of immune responses by dendritic cells and macrophages. Semin Immunol 21(1):22–27

Mawhinney LJ, de Rivero Vaccari JP, Dale GA et al (2011) Heightened inflammasome activation is linked to age-related cognitive impairment in Fischer 344 rats. BMC Neurosci 12:123

Mordstein M, Michiels T, Staeheli P (2010a) What have we learned from the IL28 receptor knockout mouse? J Interferon Cytokine Res 30(8):579–584

Mordstein M, Neugebauer E, Ditt V et al (2010b) Lambda interferon renders epithelial cells of the respiratory and gastrointestinal tracts resistant to viral infections. J Virol 84(11):5670–5677

Nakano H, Free ME, Whitehead GS et al (2012) Pulmonary CD103(+) dendritic cells prime Th2 responses to inhaled allergens. Mucosal Immunol 5(1):53–65

Ogden S, Dearman RJ, Kimber I et al (2011) The effect of ageing on phenotype and function of monocyte-derived Langerhans cells. Br J Dermatol 165(1):184–188

Panda A, Arjona A, Sapey E et al (2009) Human innate immunosenescence: causes and consequences for immunity in old age. Trends Immunol 30(7):325–333

Panda A, Qian F, Mohanty S et al (2010) Age-associated decrease in TLR function in primary human dendritic cells predicts influenza vaccine response. J Immunol 184(5):2518–2527

Perez-Cabezas B, Naranjo-Gomez M, Fernandez MA et al (2007) Reduced numbers of plasmacytoid dendritic cells in aged blood donors. Exp Gerontol 42(10):1033–1038

Pietschmann P, Hahn P, Kudlacek S et al (2000) Surface markers and transendothelial migration of dendritic cells from elderly subjects. Exp Gerontol 35(2):213–224

Prakash S, Agrawal S, Cao JN et al (2012) Impaired secretion of interferons by dendritic cells from aged subjects to influenza: role of histone modifications. Age (Dordr). doi:10.1007/s11357-012-9477-8

Qian F, Wang X, Zhang L et al (2011) Impaired interferon signaling in dendritic cells from older donors infected in vitro with West Nile virus. J Infect Dis 203(10):1415–1424

Rafi A, Castle SC, Uyemura K et al (2003) Immune dysfunction in the elderly and its reversal by antihistamines. Biomed Pharmacother 57(5–6):246–250

Rietdijk ST, Burwell T, Bertin J et al (2008) Sensing intracellular pathogens-NOD-like receptors. Curr Opin Pharmacol 8(3):261–266

Sarra M, Franze E, Pallone F et al (2011) Targeting interleukin-21 in inflammatory diseases. Expert Opin Ther Targets 15(6):695–702

Shekhar S, Yang X (2012) The darker side of follicular helper T cells: from autoimmunity to immunodeficiency. Cell Mol Immunol 9(5):380–385

Shodell M, Siegal FP (2002) Circulating, interferon-producing plasmacytoid dendritic cells decline during human ageing. Scand J Immunol 56(5):518–521

Spolski R, Leonard WJ (2008) The Yin and Yang of interleukin-21 in allergy, autoimmunity and cancer. Curr Opin Immunol 20(3):295–301

Spolski R, Wang L, Wan CK et al (2012) IL-21 promotes the pathologic immune response to pneumovirus infection. J Immunol 188(4):1924–1932

Sridharan A, Esposo M, Kaushal K et al (2011) Age-associated impaired plasmacytoid dendritic cell functions lead to decreased CD4 and CD8 T cell immunity. Age (Dordr) 33(3):363–376

Steger MM, Maczek C, Grubeck-Loebenstein B (1996) Morphologically and functionally intact dendritic cells can be derived from the peripheral blood of aged individuals. Clin Exp Immunol 105(3):544–550

Steger MM, Maczek C, Grubeck-Loebenstein B (1997) Peripheral blood dendritic cells reinduce proliferation in in vitro aged T cell populations. Mech Ageing Dev 93(1–3):125–130

Steinman RM (2012) Decisions about dendritic cells: past, present, and future. Annu Rev Immunol 30:1–22

Steinman RM, Kaplan G, Witmer MD et al (1979) Identification of a novel cell type in peripheral lymphoid organs of mice. V. Purification of spleen dendritic cells, new surface markers, and maintenance in vitro. J Exp Med 149(1):1–16

Steinman RM, Turley S, Mellman I et al (2000) The induction of tolerance by dendritic cells that have captured apoptotic cells. J Exp Med 191(3):411–416

Stichel CC, Luebbert H (2007) Inflammatory processes in the aging mouse brain: participation of dendritic cells and T-cells. Neurobiol Aging 28(10):1507–1521

Stout-Delgado HW, Yang X, Walker WE et al (2008) Aging impairs IFN regulatory factor 7 up-regulation in plasmacytoid dendritic cells during TLR9 activation. J Immunol 181(10):6747–6756

Stout-Delgado HW, Vaughan SE, Shirali AC et al (2012) Impaired NLRP3 inflammasome function in elderly mice during influenza infection is rescued by treatment with nigericin. J Immunol 188(6):2815–2824

Tan SY, Cavanagh LL, d'Advigor W et al (2012) Phenotype and functions of conventional dendritic cells are not compromised in aged mice. Immunol Cell Biol 90(7):722–732

Uyemura K, Castle SC, Makinodan T (2002) The frail elderly: role of dendritic cells in the susceptibility of infection. Mech Ageing Dev 123(8):955–962

Xu YP, Qi RQ, Chen W et al (2012) Aging affects epidermal Langerhans cell development and function and alters their miRNA gene expression profile. Aging (Albany NY) 4(11):742–754

Yin Z, Dai J, Deng J, Sheikh F et al (2012) Type III IFNs are produced by and stimulate human plasmacytoid dendritic cells. J Immunol 189(6):2735–2745

Yoshizaki A, Miyagaki T, DiLillo DJ et al (2012) Regulatory B cells control T-cell autoimmunity through IL-21-dependent cognate interactions. Nature 491(7423):264–268

Youm YH, Kanneganti TD, Vandanmagsar B et al (2012) The Nlrp3 inflammasome promotes age-related thymic demise and immunosenescence. Cell Rep 1(1):56–68

Zhao J, Legge K, Perlman S (2011) Age-related increases in PGD(2) expression impair respiratory DC migration, resulting in diminished T cell responses upon respiratory virus infection in mice. J Clin Invest 121(12):4921–4930

Natural Killer Cell Immunosenescence and Cancer in the Elderly

7

Beatriz Sánchez-Correa, Carmen Campos,
Alejandra Pera, Soledad Sánchez Mateos,
Sara Morgado, Raquel Tarazona, and Rafael Solana

7.1 Introduction

The population of the world is aging, and since cancer predominantly affects older people, the increase in the numbers of elderly individuals will lead to more incidence of cancer (Ferlay et al. 2010). The overall incidence of cancer and cancer-related mortality increase with age (Agostara et al. 2008; Mazzola et al. 2012). In animals, the genetic background seems to influence age-related cancer incidence that usually are specie and strain specific. In humans, more than 80 % of malignancies are diagnosed after age 50 (Anisimov 2003). Several causes may explain the higher incidence of cancer in the elderly. The development of tumors is a multistage process that usually occurs over the course of many years, acting a large number of factors to disturb normal cell growth. Moreover, an increased susceptibility of aged cells to carcinogens has also been described. It has been also suggested that the age-associated deterioration of the

immune system can also be an additional cause for the high incidence of cancer in the elderly. Immunosenescence can make elderly individuals less able to mount an effective immune response after challenges with tumors (Derhovanessian et al. 2008; Pawelec and Solana 2008).

Cancer immunosurveillance refers to the capacity of the immune system to identify and destroy tumor cells. Both innate and adaptive immune responses have been involved in cancer elimination, and consequently, alterations of one or more components of the immune system will affect this process (Derhovanessian et al. 2008; Fulop et al. 2010a; Malaguarnera et al. 2010; Pawelec et al. 2010). It is generally accepted that cancer cells of different origins are immunogenic and that the immune system can target these antigens to destroy cancer cells. Supporting evidences of this hypothesis mainly come from the analysis of the phenotype of the cancer cells obtained ex vivo that, in many instances, reflects alterations compatible with an immunoediting process associated with the escape of immune recognition and lysis (Schreiber et al. 2011; Vesely et al. 2011). Thus, a decreased immunosurveillance against cancer could also contribute to the increased incidence of cancer in the elderly (Derhovanessian et al. 2008; Fulop et al. 2010a).

Immunosenescence, the age-related decline in the immune function, renders older individuals more susceptible to infectious diseases and tumors (Fulop et al. 2010b; Pawelec and Solana 1997). It involves both innate and adaptive

B. Sánchez-Correa, PhD • S. Sánchez Mateos, PhD
S. Morgado, PhD • R. Tarazona, MD, PhD (✉)
Immunology Unit, Department of Physiology,
University of Extremadura, Cáceres, Spain
e-mail: rtarazon@unex.es

C. Campos, MSc • A. Pera, PhD
R. Solana, MD, PhD
Department of Immunology, IMIBIC – Reina Sofia
University Hospital – University of Cordoba,
Cordoba, Spain
e-mail: rsolana@uco.es

A. Massoud, N. Rezaei (eds.), *Immunology of Aging*,
DOI 10.1007/978-3-642-39495-9_7, © Springer-Verlag Berlin Heidelberg 2014

immunity (DelaRosa et al. 2006; Pawelec et al. 1997, 1998b; Solana et al. 2006; Tarazona et al. 2000). Age-related changes in the adaptive immune system have been extensively studied. Immunosenescence of T cells is characterized by loss of naïve T cells and a shift towards memory phenotype T cells, especially increasing highly differentiated effector-memory CD8 T cells and a decline in T cell repertoire diversity (Koch et al. 2006; Pawelec et al. 1998a). Significant alterations on B cell numbers and function and a decreased diversity of the B cell repertoire have also been described (Siegrist and Aspinall 2009). In addition, immunosenescence is also accompanied by changes in the cells of innate immunity including alteration of natural killer (NK) cells and by increased systemic inflammation believed to contribute to the development and/or exacerbation of several age-related diseases (De et al. 2005; Larbi et al. 2008; Solana et al. 2006; Vasto et al. 2007; Wagner et al. 2004; Wikby et al. 2006).

7.2 NK Cells

NK cells are lymphocytes involved in the early defense against tumors and virus-infected cells. NK cells are part of the innate immunity arsenal and are able to lyse tumor and virus-infected cells without the requirement of prior sensitization. NK cells were originally defined as large lymphocytes which respond spontaneously to abnormal cells using their germline-encoded receptors and require no prior exposure to antigen in contrast to cytotoxic CD8$^+$ T lymphocytes. Human NK cells are defined by the expression of CD56$^+$ and/or CD16$^+$ and lack of expression of CD3$^+$. Two phenotypic and functionally distinct NK cell subsets, CD56^{dim} and CD56^{bright}, can be defined according to the level of expression of CD56$^+$. CD56^{dim} NK cells represent mature cells with high cytolytic capacity and the CD56^{bright} cells are immature cells with high cytokine production (Freud and Caligiuri 2006). A third subpopulation of CD56$^-$ NK cells expressing CD16$^+$ that is expanded in some chronic viral infections has also been defined (Solana et al. 2006, 2012; Tarazona et al. 2002).

NK cells express a wide array of germline-encoded inhibitory and activating NK cell receptors that are capable of recognizing major histocompatibility complex (MHC) class I and class I-like molecules, as well as other ligands frequently overexpressed on virus-infected or tumor transformed cells (Bryceson et al. 2011; Vivier et al. 2008). There are two main types of inhibitory receptors with different specificities for different alleles of MHC class I molecules: killer immunoglobulin-like receptors (KIRs) that belong to the Ig superfamily and are specific for determinants shared by groups of human leukocyte antigen (HLA)-A, HLA-B, or HLA-C allotypes and the heterodimeric receptors CD94/NKG2A related to C-type lectins that recognizes HLA-E, an HLA class Ib molecule (Thielens et al. 2012; Zamai et al. 2007). NK cytotoxicity is not due to the simple absence of MHC class I molecules but also requires the triggering of NK activating receptors. One of these receptors is the NK cell marker CD16$^+$, the low-affinity IgG Fc receptor (FcγRIII-A). Its cross-linking by antibody-coated target cells triggers the so-called antibody-dependent cell cytotoxicity (ADCC). Other NK activating receptors have been characterized, NKG2D, CD94/NKG2C, CD244, the natural cytotoxicity receptors (NCRs: NKp30, NKp44, and NKp46), and NKp80 (Pegram et al. 2011; Thielens et al. 2012). Among these NK cell-activating receptors, the role of NKp30 and NKp46 that are expressed constitutively and NKp44 expressed after NK cell activation, the C-type lectin-like receptor NKG2D, and the DNAX accessory molecule-1 (DNAM-1) in the killing of a different types of tumor target cell has been highlighted (Levy et al. 2011; Morgado et al. 2011; Sanchez-Correa et al. 2011). NK cell function is regulated by the tune balance between signals transmitted through activating and inhibitory receptors. NK cell-mediated killing of target cells requires not only triggering of activating NK receptors but also the lack of inhibitory signals initiated by the interaction of NK inhibitory receptors with MHC class I molecules on target cells. Total or partial loss of MHC-I expression, a frequent event in tumor cells, sensitizes them to NK cell-mediated cytotoxicity (Bernal et al. 2012; Garrido et al. 2010; Mendez et al. 2009).

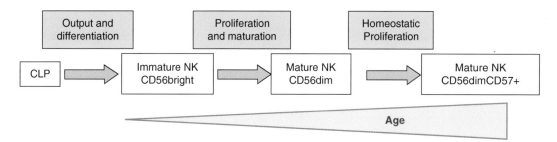

Fig. 7.1 Redistribution of NK cell subsets in healthy aging. Decreased proportion of CD56[bright] and increase of CD56[dim] CD57+ NK cells during aging

Target cell recognition by NK cells also induces the production of different cytokines and chemokines that directly participate in the elimination of pathogens or activate other cellular components of immunity. Thus, NK cells also play a crucial role in promoting the activation of dendritic cells (DCs) and vice versa. In this bidirectional crosstalk, NK cells induce the maturation of DCs and increase their capacity to produce proinflammatory cytokines and to stimulate T cell responses. This effect is dependent on activating receptors as NKp30 and cytokines as tumor necrosis factor (TNF)-α and interferon (IFN)-γ (Wehner et al. 2011). Recently, it has been shown that NK cells also interact with macrophages and that this crosstalk exerts important role in anti-infection and antitumor responses (Bellora et al. 2010; Zhou et al. 2012).

7.3 NK Cells in the Elderly

Several alterations have been described in human NK cell function with advancing aging, therefore contributing to immunosenescence (Camous et al. 2012; Solana et al. 2006, 2012). Although the NK cell frequency and absolute numbers tend to increase in healthy aging, a redistribution of NK cell subsets is also found in the elderly (Fig. 7.1). A shrinkage of the subset of immature CD56[bright] NK cells and an increase of the mature CD56[dim] NK cells are also observed, indicating that the increased frequency of NK cells is due to the expansion of the more mature NK cell subset (Borrego et al. 1999; Chidrawar et al. 2006; Gayoso et al. 2011;

Le Garff-Tavernier et al. 2010). In addition, the expression of CD57 (HNK-1epitope, sialyl-Lewis X) on CD56[dim] NK cells from elderly individuals is increased (Borrego et al. 1999). It has been shown that CD57+CD56[dim] cells are highly differentiated NK cells with poor response to cytokines and decreased proliferative response but higher cytotoxic capacity than their CD57− counterpart (Bjorkstrom et al. 2010; Lopez-Verges et al. 2010).

Healthy elderly and centenarians, in particular those with criteria of healthy status, have an overall increase of NK cell number and well-preserved cytotoxicity whereas the decrease in NK cell activity is associated to increased incidence of infectious and inflammatory diseases and to increased mortality risk in the first 2 years of follow-up compared to those with high NK cell numbers (Ogata et al. 2001; Remarque and Pawelec 1998; Solana and Mariani 2000; Tarazona et al. 2009).

The decreased proportion of immature CD56[bright] NK cells is likely associated to the lower production rates of NK cells in healthy elderly subjects compared to young healthy individuals (Zhang et al. 2007). An age-associated loss of telomeres on NK cells together with a reduction of telomerase activity has been shown, in particular in the oldest individuals and in those with increased NK cell numbers (Mariani et al. 2003a, b). Taken together, these results support the hypothesis that the preservation of NK cell numbers in healthy aging depends on the accumulation of terminally differentiated CD56[dim]CD57+ long-lived NK cells (Gayoso et al. 2011; Le Garff-Tavernier et al. 2010).

Whereas the overall NK cell cytotoxicity is maintained in healthy elderly, the analysis of cytotoxicity per NK cell shows a decreased lysis of the NK cell-susceptible K562 target cell, suggesting that the maintenance of overall NK cell cytotoxicity in healthy elderly individuals is associated with an increased number of NK cells (Gayoso et al. 2011; Le Garff-Tavernier et al. 2010; Solana and Mariani 2000). Neither CD16+- (FcγRIII-A) nor CD16−-dependent NK cell activation is affected by aging, indicating NK activation and cytotoxic granule release remain intact in the elderly (Bruunsgaard et al. 2001; Gayoso et al. 2011; Le Garff-Tavernier et al. 2010; Lutz et al. 2005; Solana et al. 2006; Solana and Mariani 2000). Scarce and conflicting data exists regarding the effects of aging on the expression and function of other NK receptors. Discordant results have been published in relation with the expression of HLA-specific KIR. KIR and CD94 expression was either not significantly affected in NK cells from elderly compared to young donors (Le Garff-Tavernier et al. 2010; Mariani et al. 1994) or increased (Lutz et al. 2005). A decrease of NKG2A (Lutz et al. 2005), CD94 (Hayhoe et al. 2010, Lutz et al. 2005), and the inhibitory receptor KLRG-1 was observed on NK cells from elderly donors (Hayhoe et al. 2010). These discordances may probably be due to the criteria used for selection of the individuals, healthy versus frail elderly, and the broad age ranges considered in the different studies (Gayoso et al. 2011). The expression or the functionality of some activating NK cell receptors is defective in the elderly. A decreased expression of the activating receptors NKp30 and DNAM-1 has been shown in NK cells from elderly donors (Sanchez-Correa et al. 2012; Tarazona et al. 2009). Elderly individuals show a decrease in the expression of activating receptors whereas the expression of KIR is increased only in the CD56bright subset (Almeida-Oliveira et al. 2011). The expression of NKG2D is not affected by age (Gayoso et al. 2009).

In addition to their cytotoxic functions against infected and tumor cells, NK cells also secrete cytokines upon activation. It has been reported that in the elderly the secretion of IFN-γ by interleukin (IL)-2-stimulated NK cells either shows an early decrease which can be overcome by prolonging the incubation time (Murasko and Jiang 2005) or is maintained (Le Garff-Tavernier et al. 2010) with an increased production of IFN-γ by CD56bright cells (Hayhoe et al. 2010). The production of chemokines in response to IL-2 or IL-12 is decreased in NK cells from elderly individuals (Mariani et al. 2002). Considering that CD56dim NK cells can produce high amounts of IFN-γ and whereas chemokines are mainly produced by CD56bright NK cells, these alterations can be explained the decrease of this subset in the elderly. Due to the co-stimulatory role of chemokines on NK responses, the decreased production of chemokines can be involved in the defective functional activity of NK cells in elderly. As a consequence, the defective production of cytokines and chemokines may also compromise NK cell-driven adaptive immune responses in the elderly (Panda et al. 2009).

NK cell activation by cytokines results in proliferation and enhanced cytotoxicity. IL-2-induced NK cell proliferation is decreased in old donors (Borrego et al. 1999), whereas the enhancement of the cytotoxic activity in response to IL-2, IL-12 or IFN-α, and IFN-γ is well preserved in the healthy elderly (Kutza and Murasko 1994, 1996; Le Garff-Tavernier et al. 2010; Murasko and Jiang 2005).

In addition, aging is characterized by a pro-inflammatory status called "inflamm-aging" with an increase in the level of several cytokines (e.g., IL-6, IL-1β, TNFα) and chemokines (e.g., IL-8, regulated upon activation normal T cell expressed and presumably secreted (RANTES), MIPα) (Franceschi et al. 2000). It has been suggested that inflamm-aging is involved in the pathogenesis of inflammatory diseases including cancer (Lustgarten 2009; Myers et al. 2011). The alterations in cytokine production in the elderly can also play a role in the age-associated alterations observed in NK cells in the elderly.

These studies support the significance of age-associated changes in NK cell function and NK receptor expression in the increased susceptibility of elderly subjects to infectious, inflammatory, and neoplastic diseases.

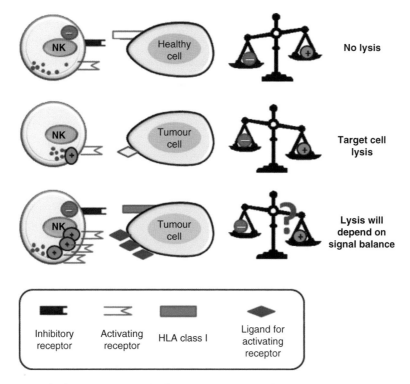

Fig. 7.2 NK cell activation depends on the balance between inhibitory and activating signals transmitted through surface receptors. NK cells are inhibited by crosslinking of inhibitory receptors that recognize MHC class I molecules, and thus, healthy cells expressing normal levels of MHC class I are generally protected from NK cell-mediated lysis. However, malignant cells may express reduced levels of MHC class I molecules or have lost the expression of one or more MHC class I alleles, and thus, provided that they also express appropriate ligands for activating receptors, they become vulnerable to NK cell attack. The lysis of tumor cells expressing both MHC class I molecules and ligands for activating receptors depends on the tune balance of signals transmitted through inhibitory and activating NK cell receptors

7.4   NK Cells in Cancer

As stated before, NK cells have the capacity of recognizing tumor cells that have lost the expression of MHC class I molecules ("missing self" hypothesis), an escape mechanism used frequently by tumors cells to avoid CD8$^+$ T cell recognition (Levy et al. 2011; Stojanovic and Cerwenka 2011). Activation of NK cells is the result of a balance between inhibitory and activating signals (Fig. 7.2). In the absence of inhibitory signals, NK cell cytotoxicity depends on the signals transmitted by a set of triggering receptors. Different activating receptors have been described that participate in NK cell-mediated killing of tumor targets. The role of NKp30, NKp46, NKG2D, and DNAM-1 in the interaction of NK cells with

tumor cells from different lineages has been highlighted. Since the threshold of activating signals required to overcome the inhibitory signals is usually high, the collaboration of several activating receptors in the destruction of tumor cells occurs frequently (Casado et al. 2009; Morgado et al. 2011; Morisaki et al. 2012; Pegram et al. 2011; Sanchez-Correa et al. 2011; Solana et al. 2007).

NK cells play an important role in the immune response against hematological malignancies as demonstrated by the low relapse in allogenic stem cell transplantation when there is KIR-ligand mismatch between the donor and the recipient. Thus, NK cells in the haploidentical hematopoietic stem cell transplantation setting are very effective in eradicating residual blasts (Farnault et al. 2012; Verheyden and Demanet 2008). In non-Hodgkin lymphoma, NK cell count after autologous peripheral blood hemato-poietic stem cell transplantation is a prognostic factor for overall survival and progression-free survival (Porrata et al. 2008).

The role of NK cells in the defense against solid tumors is highlighted by different studies showing a role in the protection against metastasis. In pancreatic cancer it has been observed a small number of tumor-infiltrating NK cells (Ademmer et al. 1998). It was showed that apoptotic pancreatic tumor cells are very good activators of NK and T cells and immunotherapeutic strategies directed to the local administration of autologous NK cells may be relevant for clinical outcome (Schnurr et al. 2002). In stomach cancer, NK activity could be a good marker for tumor volume and dissemination and patient survival (Ishigami et al. 2000a, b; Takeuchi et al. 2001). In lung cancer, tumor-infiltrating NK cells are mainly CD56[bright] noncytotoxic NK cells (Carrega et al. 2008). Intratumoral NK cells display phenotypic alterations such as reduced NK cell receptor expression that lead to an impaired degranulation and secretion of cytokines, like IFN-γ. Because of these defects, NK cells are not correlated to the clinical outcome of these patients, supporting the existence of tumor escape mechanism to avoid NK cell cytotoxicity (Platonova et al. 2011). Tumor-infiltrating NK cells are very rare in colorectal carcinoma, but NK activity could be used as a marker of colorectal progression (Halama et al. 2011). Thus, a reduction of NK cell activity was related to colon cancer metastasis (Nüssler et al. 2007).

Several NKG2D ligands (NKG2DL) have been identified in humans and mice that exhibit different affinities for NKG2D. NKG2DL are homologous to MHC class I molecules and they exhibit considerable allelic variation. In humans, NKG2DL include MHC class I chain-related proteins (MIC) A and B and up to six different proteins called UL16-binding proteins (ULBPs). NKG2D ligands are likely regulated differently by diverse stress pathways; thus, the same receptor can stimulate a response in different situations as viral infection or tumor transformation. It has been proposed that the existence of multiple NKG2DL may also difficult pathogen (or tumor cell) evasion from NKG2D-mediated immune response (Pegram et al. 2011; Raulet et al. 2013).

Ligands for DNAM-1 (DNAM-1L) include nectin-2/CD112 and PVR/CD155 belonging to the nectin/nectin-like family of adhesion molecules. DNAM-1 ligands are broadly distributed on hematopoietic, epithelial, and endothelial cells as well as on tumors from different origins (Casado et al. 2009; Fuchs and Colonna 2006; Pende et al. 2005; Sanchez-Correa et al. 2011). Interestingly, TIGIT, an inhibitory receptor expressed on activated lymphocytes including NK cells, also binds to CD112 and CD155 and to CD113 (PVRL3, nectin-3) and may play a role in tumor escape from NK cells (Chan et al. 2012).

By analyzing a large panel of melanoma cell lines, it has been shown that melanoma cells frequently express ligands for NKG2D and DNAM-1 activating NK receptors. NK cell-mediated recognition and killing of melanoma cells depend on multiple receptor-ligand interactions (Casado et al. 2009; Morgado et al. 2011; Solana et al. 2007). However, melanoma cells have developed several mechanisms to escape NK recognition and killing, including the shedding of NKG2DL and the induction of the NKG2D downregulation (Paschen et al. 2009; Schwinn et al. 2009). We have previously analyzed the expression of ligands for NK cell-activating receptors on acute myeloid leukemia (AML) blasts, showing that 85 % of patients expressed ligands for DNAM-1 and about 55 % expressed MICA/B, a ligand for NKG2D (Sanchez-Correa et al. 2011, 2012).

Different reports have demonstrated that patients with cancer of different origins have low NK cell cytotoxicity although the bases of this alteration remain unclear (Levy et al. 2011; Stojanovic and Cerwenka 2011; Verheyden and Demanet 2008). It has been shown that the expression of activating receptors such as NCR and DNAM-1 is reduced in NK cells from cancer patients (Carlsten et al. 2009; Farnault et al. 2012; Fauriat et al. 2007; Markel et al. 2009; Sanchez-Correa et al. 2011, 2012). Altered NK cell subset distribution has been observed in metastatic melanoma showing an expansion of CD16⁻ NK cells that was associated with elevated plasma levels of transforming growth factor-beta (TGF-β) (Holtan et al. 2011).

Diminished expression of NCRs (Fauriat et al. 2007; Sanchez-Correa et al. 2011, 2012) and DNAM-1 (Sanchez-Correa et al. 2012) on NK cells from myeloid leukemia patients has been correlated with the expression of their ligands on leukemic blasts. In ovarian carcinoma, reduced expression of DNAM-1 on NK cells was correlated with low cytotoxicity and was induced by chronic ligand exposure (Carlsten et al. 2009). Decreased expression of NKG2D (Konjevic et al. 2009) and NKp30 (Markel et al. 2009) has been found on NK cells from metastatic melanoma patients that correlated with a lower NK cell cytotoxicity against melanoma.

Shedding of ligands for activating receptors are escape mechanisms used frequently by tumor cells to evade immune recognition. The presence of soluble NKG2D ligands in serum from cancer patients has been related with an impaired NKG2D-mediated cytotoxicity (Fernandez-Messina et al. 2012; Hilpert et al. 2012; Salih et al. 2008). Tumor-derived exosomes which have been viewed as a source of tumor antigens that can be used to induce antitumor immune responses can also negatively regulate NK cells (Whiteside 2013; Yang and Robbins 2011). Shedding of NKG2DL has been correlated with poor prognosis in human melanoma and prostate cancer, supporting previous evidences that tumor cells also evolve to escape from NK cells (Vivier et al. 2011).

The frequent expression of ligands for NKG2D and DNAM-1 on tumor cells and the possibility of modulating ligand expression by cytokines and chemotherapeutic agents may open new avenues for immunotherapy in cancer patients (Krieg and Ullrich 2013; Morisaki et al. 2012). A better understanding of the mechanisms involved in NK recognition and lysis of tumor cells of different origins may explain why some tumors are resistant to NK cell lysis even when tumors express low levels of MHC class I molecules.

7.5 NK Cells in Elderly Patients with Cancer and Cancer-Induced NK Cell Immunosenescence

The incidence of cancer increases with age, but not all types of cancers. The epidemiological studies indicate that the most frequent tumors in patients over 65 years are represented by lung, colon, rectum, prostate, and bladder in men and breast, lung, colon-rectum, bladder, pancreas, and non-Hodgkin lymphoma in women (Malaguarnera et al. 2010). Chronic lymphoid and acute myeloid leukemia also have higher prevalence in patients over age 65 (Gribben 2011; Jabbour et al. 2006). The accumulation of DNA damage constitutes one of the main characteristics during aging, and consequently the accumulation of senescent cell in tissue could promote cancer initiation (Falandry et al. 2013). However, the contribution of immunosenescence to the high prevalence of cancer in the elderly remains elusive. Interestingly a decrease in cancer incidence in centenarians has been observed (Anisimov 2003). Data analysis has demonstrated that cancer in the very elderly is uncommon, the number of metastases is less, and cancer-related mortality is also decreased after age 90, suggesting that cancer in centenarians is a more silent disease, of slower growth and of less-threatening potential (Pavlidis et al. 2012).

As indicated above, it has been suggested that age-associated alterations of the immune system may also contribute to the development of cancer in the elderly. Immunosenescence affects principally the T cell compartment (Appay et al. 2010; Ferrando-Martinez et al. 2011; Pawelec et al. 2002; Tarazona et al. 2000) but also has an effect on NK cells (Gayoso et al. 2011; Sanchez-Correa et al. 2012). Altered NK-DC crosstalk may disrupt their ability to induce DC maturation and to cooperate in the initiation of the adaptive immune response against tumors or virus-infected cells (Gayoso et al. 2009; Tarazona et al. 2009; Wehner et al. 2011). Several studies support the notion that NK cells play a role in tumor immunosurveillance (Fuchs and Colonna 2006; Morgado et al. 2011; Stojanovic and Cerwenka 2011; Zamai et al. 2007).

The presence of NK cells in colorectal carcinoma tissue has been negatively correlated with the age of the patients probably due to an age-related decrease in adherence molecule expression (Papanikolaou et al. 2004).

We have previously analyzed NK cells from elderly patients with AML and compared with healthy elderly individuals. The expression of the activating receptor NKp46 was found diminished in elderly AML patients in comparison to healthy elderly individuals (Sanchez-Correa et al. 2011, 2012). Interestingly, NKp46 expression on NK cells has also been associated to patient survival in AML (Fauriat et al. 2007) and Sanchez-Correa et al. (2013). The expression of NKp30 and DNAM-1 was low in the elderly compared to young healthy donors and no significant differences were found between healthy elderly and elderly AML patients (Sanchez-Correa et al. 2011, 2012). Neither the expression of the DNAM-1 ligands on AML blasts (Sanchez-Correa et al. 2012) nor the expression of NKG2D ligands were associated with patient age (Sanchez-Correa et al. 2013).

Tumor progression is associated with immunosuppression. It has been reported that the number of regulatory T cells (Tregs) increases with age (Gregg et al. 2005). It is discussed that the accumulation of Tregs in the old may inhibit or prevent the activation of immune responses against cancer (Lustgarten 2009; Myers et al. 2011). Regarding NK cells, a bidirectional interaction between these cells and Tregs has been described. Tregs can suppress NK cell function although the molecular mechanism by which Treg cells perform its regulatory/suppressor function on NK cells has not been fully characterized (Zimmer et al. 2008).

Several biomarkers of human immunosenescence identified in elderly individuals have been also observed in cancer patients due to chronic activation of the immune system by tumor antigens. Thus, alterations at the CD8$^+$ T cell compartment observed in the elderly without cancer can also be found in younger individuals with cancer (Hirokawa et al. 2009) and recently, it has been observed that the altered phenotype of NK cells in young and middle-age acute myeloid leukemia patients resembles in some aspects the NK cell phenotype of elderly individuals (Sanchez-Correa et al. 2011, 2012).

The age-associated alterations observed on cytokine production, inflamm-aging, can also play a role in cancer pathogenesis (Lustgarten 2009; Myers et al. 2011). Recently, we have described an altered cytokine profile in AML patients. Our results showed that patient survival was inversely correlated with IL-6 and directly correlated with IL-10 levels. IL-8 levels were higher in AML patients over 65 years compared with younger patients (Sanchez-Correa et al. 2013).

Altogether, evidences support that tumor-induced alterations of activating NK cell receptors have an effect on immunosurveillance and may promote tumor progression. However, the identification of the factors involved in the decreased expression of these activating receptors in elderly individuals remains elusive.

7.6   Concluding Remarks

NK cells are known to be involved in the recognition and lysis of tumor cells. The results reviewed here indicate that aging may affect not only NK cell cytotoxicity but also NK cell response to cytokines and in sum provokes a detriment in NK cell capacity to kill target cells and to synthesize cytokines and chemokines (Solana et al. 2006). Age-related changes on NK cell function can also contribute to the dysregulation of other cells of the adaptive and innate immune system since NK cells may interact with monocytes promoting inflammation and also induce the maturation of DCs (Tarazona et al. 2009; Wehner et al. 2011).

The analysis of NK cells in elderly individuals with cancer and the possibility to enhance NK cell function by the modulation of activating receptor expression on NK cells or their ligands on tumors may open new therapeutic strategies. In addition, clinical trials testing novel methods to enhance NK cytotoxicity against cancer will favor the development of NK cell-based immunotherapy to fight cancer (Lee and Gasser 2010).

Further studies are required to analyze NK cell immunosenescence in healthy elderly individuals compared with the frail elderly, who have a higher morbidity and mortality risk and represent the majority of elderly individuals.

Acknowledgments We apologize to our colleagues whose work was not cited due to space limitations. This work was supported by grants PS09/00723 (to R.S.) from Spanish Ministry of Health and SAF2009-09711 from the Ministry of Science and Innovation of Spain and PRI09A029 (to RT) and grants to INPATT research group from Junta de Extremadura (GRU10104) and from University of Extremadura, cofinanced by European Regional Development Fund (FEDER).

References

Ademmer K, Ebert M, Muller-Ostermeyer F et al (1998) Effector T lymphocyte subsets in human pancreatic cancer: detection of CD8 + CD18+ cells and CD8 + CD103+ cells by multi-epitope imaging. Clin Exp Immunol 112:21–26

Agostara B, Carruba G, Usset A (2008) The management of cancer in the elderly: targeted therapies in oncology. Immun Ageing 5:16

Almeida-Oliveira A, Smith-Carvalho M, Porto LC et al (2011) Age-related changes in natural killer cell receptors from childhood through old age. Hum Immunol 72:319–329

Anisimov VN (2003) The relationship between aging and carcinogenesis: a critical appraisal. Crit Rev Oncol Hematol 45:277–304

Appay V, Sauce D, Prelog M (2010) The role of the thymus in immunosenescence: lessons from the study of thymectomized individuals. Aging (Albany NY) 2:78–81

Bellora F, Castriconi R, Dondero A et al (2010) The interaction of human natural killer cells with either unpolarized or polarized macrophages results in different functional outcomes. Proc Natl Acad Sci U S A 107:21659–21664

Bernal M, Ruiz-Cabello F, Concha A et al (2012) Implication of the beta2-microglobulin gene in the generation of tumor escape phenotypes. Cancer Immunol Immunother 61:1359–1371

Bjorkstrom NK, Riese P, Heuts F et al (2010) Expression patterns of NKG2A, KIR, and CD57 define a process of CD56dim NK cell differentiation uncoupled from NK cell education. Blood 116:3853–3864

Borrego F, Alonso MC, Galiani MD et al (1999) NK phenotypic markers and IL2 response in NK cells from elderly people. Exp Gerontol 34:253–265

Bruunsgaard H, Pedersen AN, Schroll M et al (2001) Decreased natural killer cell activity is associated with atherosclerosis in elderly humans. Exp Gerontol 37:127–136

Bryceson YT, Chiang SC, Darmanin S et al (2011) Molecular mechanisms of natural killer cell activation. J Innate Immun 3:216–226

Camous X, Pera A, Solana R et al (2012) NK cells in healthy aging and age-associated diseases. J Biomed Biotechnol 195956

Carlsten M, Norell H, Bryceson YT et al (2009) Primary human tumor cells expressing CD155 impair tumor targeting by down-regulating DNAM-1 on NK cells. J Immunol 183:4921–4930

Carrega P, Morandi B, Costa R et al (2008) Natural killer cells infiltrating human nonsmall-cell lung cancer are enriched in CD56 bright CD16(−) cells and display an impaired capability to kill tumor cells. Cancer 112:863–875

Casado JG, Pawelec G, Morgado S et al (2009) Expression of adhesion molecules and ligands for activating and costimulatory receptors involved in cell-mediated cytotoxicity in a large panel of human melanoma cell lines. Cancer Immunol Immunother 58:1517–1526

Chan CJ, Andrews DM, Smyth MJ (2012) Receptors that interact with nectin and nectin-like proteins in the immunosurveillance and immunotherapy of cancer. Curr Opin Immunol 24:246–251

Chidrawar SM, Khan N, Chan YL et al (2006) Ageing is associated with a decline in peripheral blood CD56bright NK cells. Immun Ageing 3:10

De MM, Franceschi C, Monti D et al (2005) Inflammageing and lifelong antigenic load as major determinants of ageing rate and longevity. FEBS Lett 579:2035–2039

DelaRosa O, Pawelec G, Peralbo E et al (2006) Immunological biomarkers of ageing in man: changes in both innate and adaptive immunity are associated with health and longevity. Biogerontology 7:471–481

Derhovanessian E, Solana R, Larbi A et al (2008) Immunity, ageing and cancer. Immun Ageing 5:11

Falandry C, Gilson E, Rudolph KL (2013) Are aging biomarkers clinically relevant in oncogeriatrics? Crit Rev Oncol Hematol 85:257–265

Farnault L, Sanchez C, Baier C et al (2012) Hematological malignancies escape from NK cell innate immune surveillance: mechanisms and therapeutic implications. Clin Dev Immunol 2012:421702

Fauriat C, Just-Landi S, Mallet F et al (2007) Deficient expression of NCR in NK cells from acute myeloid leukemia: evolution during leukemia treatment and impact of leukemia cells in NCRdull phenotype induction. Blood 109:323–330

Ferlay J, Shin HR, Bray F et al (2010) Estimates of worldwide burden of cancer in 2008: GLOBOCAN 2008. Int J Cancer 127:2893–2917

Fernandez-Messina L, Reyburn HT, Vales-Gomez M (2012) Human NKG2D-ligands: cell biology strategies to ensure immune recognition. Front Immunol 3:299

Ferrando-Martinez S, Ruiz-Mateos E, Hernandez A et al (2011) Age-related deregulation of naive T cell homeostasis in elderly humans. Age (Dordr) 33:197–207

Franceschi C, Bonafe M, Valensin S et al (2000) Inflamm-aging. An evolutionary perspective on immunosenescence. Ann N Y Acad Sci 908:244–254

Freud AG, Caligiuri MA (2006) Human natural killer cell development. Immunol Rev 214:56–72

Fuchs A, Colonna M (2006) The role of NK cell recognition of nectin and nectin-like proteins in tumor immunosurveillance. Semin Cancer Biol 16:359–366

Fulop T, Kotb R, Fortin CF et al (2010a) Potential role of immunosenescence in cancer development. Ann N Y Acad Sci 1197:158–165

Fulop T, Larbi A, Witkowski JM et al (2010b) Aging, frailty and age-related diseases. Biogerontology 11: 547–563

Garrido F, Cabrera T, Aptsiauri N (2010) "Hard" and "soft" lesions underlying the HLA class I alterations in cancer cells: implications for immunotherapy. Int J Cancer 127:249–256

Gayoso I, Peralbo E, Sanchez-Correa B et al (2009) Phenotypic analysis of human NK cells in healthy elderly. Medimond s.r.l, Bologna, pp 105–109

Gayoso I, Sanchez-Correa B, Campos C et al (2011) Immunosenescence of human natural killer cells. J Innate Immun 3:337–343

Gregg R, Smith CM, Clark FJ et al (2005) The number of human peripheral blood CD4+ CD25high regulatory T cells increases with age. Clin Exp Immunol 140: 540–546

Gribben JG (2011) Are prognostic factors in CLL overrated? Oncology (Williston Park) 25:703–706

Halama N, Braun M, Kahlert C et al (2011) Natural killer cells are scarce in colorectal carcinoma tissue despite high levels of chemokines and cytokines. Clin Cancer Res 17:678–689

Hayhoe RP, Henson SM, Akbar AN et al (2010) Variation of human natural killer cell phenotypes with age: identification of a unique KLRG1-negative subset. Hum Immunol 71:676–681

Hilpert J, Grosse-Hovest L, Grunebach F et al (2012) Comprehensive analysis of NKG2D ligand expression and release in leukemia: implications for NKG2D-mediated NK cell responses. J Immunol 189: 1360–1371

Hirokawa K, Utsuyama M, Ishikawa T et al (2009) Decline of T cell-related immune functions in cancer patients and an attempt to restore them through infusion of activated autologous T cells. Mech Ageing Dev 130:86–91

Holtan SG, Creedon DJ, Thompson MA et al (2011) Expansion of CD16-negative natural killer cells in the peripheral blood of patients with metastatic melanoma. Clin Dev Immunol 2011:316314

Ishigami S, Natsugoe S, Tokuda K et al (2000a) Clinical impact of intratumoral natural killer cell and dendritic cell infiltration in gastric cancer. Cancer Lett 159:103–108

Ishigami S, Natsugoe S, Tokuda K et al (2000b) Prognostic value of intratumoral natural killer cells in gastric carcinoma. Cancer 88(3):577–583

Jabbour EJ, Estey E, Kantarjian HM (2006) Adult acute myeloid leukemia. Mayo Clin Proc 81:247–260

Koch S, Solana R, Dela RO et al (2006) Human cytomegalovirus infection and T cell immunosenescence: a mini review. Mech Ageing Dev 127:538–543

Konjevic G, Mirjacic MK, Jurisic V et al (2009) Biomarkers of suppressed natural killer (NK) cell function in metastatic melanoma: decreased NKG2D and increased CD158a receptors on CD3-CD16+ NK cells. Biomarkers 14:258–270

Krieg S, Ullrich E (2013) Novel immune modulators used in hematology: impact on NK cells. Front Immunol 3:388

Kutza J, Murasko DM (1994) Effects of aging on natural killer cell activity and activation by interleukin-2 and IFN-alpha. Cell Immunol 155:195–204

Kutza J, Murasko DM (1996) Age-associated decline in IL-2 and IL-12 induction of LAK cell activity of human PBMC samples. Mech Ageing Dev 90: 209–222

Larbi A, Franceschi C, Mazzatti D et al (2008) Aging of the immune system as a prognostic factor for human longevity. Physiology (Bethesda) 23:64–74

Le Garff-Tavernier M, Beziat V, Decocq J et al (2010) Human NK cells display major phenotypic and functional changes over the life span. Aging Cell 9: 527–535

Lee SK, Gasser S (2010) The role of natural killer cells in cancer therapy. Front Biosci (Elite Ed) 2:380–391

Levy EM, Roberti MP, Mordoh J (2011) Natural killer cells in human cancer: from biological functions to clinical applications. J Biomed Biotechnol 2011: 676198

Lopez-Verges S, Milush JM, Pandey S et al (2010) CD57 defines a functionally distinct population of mature NK cells in the human CD56dimCD16+ NK cell subset. Blood 116:3865–3874

Lustgarten J (2009) Cancer, aging and immunotherapy: lessons learned from animal models. Cancer Immunol Immunother 58:1979–1989

Lutz CT, Moore MB, Bradley S et al (2005) Reciprocal age related change in natural killer cell receptors for MHC class I. Mech Ageing Dev 126:722–731

Malaguarnera L, Cristaldi E, Malaguarnera M (2010) The role of immunity in elderly cancer. Crit Rev Oncol Hematol 74:40–60

Mariani E, Monaco MC, Cattini L et al (1994) Distribution and lytic activity of NK cell subsets in the elderly. Mech Ageing Dev 76:177–187

Mariani E, Meneghetti A, Neri S et al (2002) Chemokine production by natural killer cells from nonagenarians. Eur J Immunol 32:1524–1529

Mariani E, Meneghetti A, Formentini I et al (2003a) Telomere length and telomerase activity: effect of aging on human NK cells. Mech Ageing Dev 124: 403–408

Mariani E, Meneghetti A, Formentini I et al (2003b) Different rates of telomere shortening and telomerase activity reduction in CD8 T and CD16 NK lymphocytes with ageing. Exp Gerontol 38:653–659

Markel G, Seidman R, Besser MJ et al (2009) Natural killer lysis receptor (NKLR)/NKLR-ligand matching as a novel approach for enhancing anti-tumor activity of allogeneic NK cells. PLoS One 4:e5597

Mazzola P, Radhi S, Mirandola L et al (2012) Aging, cancer, and cancer vaccines. Immun Ageing 9:4–9

Mendez R, Aptsiauri N, Del CA et al (2009) HLA and melanoma: multiple alterations in HLA class I and II expression in human melanoma cell lines from ESTDAB cell bank. Cancer Immunol Immunother 58:1507–1515

Morgado S, Sanchez-Correa B, Casado JG et al (2011) NK cell recognition and killing of melanoma cells is controlled by multiple activating receptor-ligand interactions. J Innate Immun 3:365–373

Morisaki T, Onishi H, Katano M (2012) Cancer immunotherapy using NKG2D and DNAM-1 systems. Anticancer Res 32:2241–2247

Murasko DM, Jiang J (2005) Response of aged mice to primary virus infections. Immunol Rev 205:285–296

Myers CE, Mirza NN, Lustgarten J (2011) Immunity, cancer and aging: lessons from mouse models. Ageing Dis 2:512–523

Nüssler NC, Stange BJ, Petzold M et al (2007) Reduced NK-cell activity in patients with metastatic colon cancer. Exp Clin Sci 6:1–9

Ogata K, An E, Shioi Y et al (2001) Association between natural killer cell activity and infection in immunologically normal elderly people. Clin Exp Immunol 124:392–397

Panda A, Arjona A, Sapey E et al (2009) Human innate immunosenescence: causes and consequences for immunity in old age. Trends Immunol 30:325–333

Papanikolaou IS, Lazaris AC, Apostolopoulos P et al (2004) Tissue detection of natural killer cells in colorectal adenocarcinoma. BMC Gastroenterol 4:20

Paschen A, Sucker A, Hill B et al (2009) Differential clinical significance of individual NKG2D ligands in melanoma: soluble ULBP2 as an indicator of poor prognosis superior to S100B. Clin Cancer Res 15:5208–5215

Pavlidis N, Stanta G, Audisio RA (2012) Cancer prevalence and mortality in centenarians: a systematic review. Crit Rev Oncol Hematol 83:145–152

Pawelec G, Solana R (1997) Immunosenescence. Immunol Today 18:514–516

Pawelec G, Solana R (2008) Are cancer and ageing different sides of the same coin? Conference on Cancer and Ageing. EMBO Rep 9:234–238

Pawelec G, Adibzadeh M, Solana R et al (1997) The T cell in the ageing individual. Mech Ageing Dev 93:35–45

Pawelec G, Remarque E, Barnett Y et al (1998a) T cells and aging. Front Biosci 3:d59–d99

Pawelec G, Solana R, Remarque E et al (1998b) Impact of aging on innate immunity. J Leukoc Biol 64:703–712

Pawelec G, Barnett Y, Forsey R et al (2002) T cells and aging, January 2002 update. Front Biosci 7:d1056–d1183

Pawelec G, Derhovanessian E, Larbi A (2010) Immunosenescence and cancer. Crit Rev Oncol Hematol 75:165–172

Pegram HJ, Andrews DM, Smyth MJ et al (2011) Activating and inhibitory receptors of natural killer cells. Immunol Cell Biol 89:216–224

Pende D, Bottino C, Castriconi R et al (2005) PVR (CD155) and Nectin-2 (CD112) as ligands of the human DNAM-1 (CD226) activating receptor: involvement in tumor cell lysis. Mol Immunol 42:463–469

Platonova S, Cherfils-Vicini J, Damotte D et al (2011) Profound coordinated alterations of intratumoral NK cell phenotype and function in lung carcinoma. Cancer Res 71:5412–5422

Porrata LF, Inwards DJ, Ansell SM et al (2008) Early lymphocyte recovery predicts superior survival after autologous stem cell transplantation in non-Hodgkin lymphoma: a prospective study. Biol Blood Marrow Transplant 14:807–816

Raulet DH, Gasser S, Gowen BG et al (2013) Regulation of ligands for the NKG2D activating receptor. Annu Rev Immunol 31:413–441

Remarque E, Pawelec G (1998) T cell immunosenescence and its clinical relevance in man. Rev Clin Gerontol 8:5–14

Salih HR, Holdenrieder S, Steinle A (2008) Soluble NKG2D ligands: prevalence, release, and functional impact. Front Biosci 13:3448–3456

Sanchez-Correa B, Morgado S, Gayoso I et al (2011) Human NK cells in acute myeloid leukaemia patients: analysis of NK cell-activating receptors and their ligands. Cancer Immunol Immunother 60:1195–1205

Sanchez-Correa B, Gayoso I, Bergua JM et al (2012) Decreased expression of DNAM-1 on NK cells from acute myeloid leukemia patients. Immunol Cell Biol 90:109–115

Sanchez-Correa B, Bergua JM, Campos C et al (2013) Cytokine profiles in acute myeloid leukemia patients at diagnosis: survival is inversely correlated with IL-6 and directly correlated with IL-10 levels. Cytokine 61(3):885–891

Schnurr M, Scholz C, Rothenfusser S et al (2002) Apoptotic pancreatic tumor cells are superior to cell lysates in promoting cross-priming of cytotoxic T cells and activate NK and gammadelta T cells. Cancer Res 62:2347–2352

Schreiber RD, Old LJ, Smyth MJ (2011) Cancer immunoediting: integrating immunity's roles in cancer suppression and promotion. Science 331:1565–1570

Schwinn N, Vokhminova D, Sucker A et al (2009) Interferon-gamma down-regulates NKG2D ligand expression and impairs the NKG2D-mediated cytolysis of MHC class I-deficient melanoma by natural killer cells. Int J Cancer 124:1594–1604

Siegrist CA, Aspinall R (2009) B-cell responses to vaccination at the extremes of age. Nat Rev Immunol 9:185–194

Solana R, Mariani E (2000) NK and NK/T cells in human senescence. Vaccine 18:1613–1620

Solana R, Pawelec G, Tarazona R (2006) Aging and innate immunity. Immunity 24:491–494

Solana R, Casado JG, Delgado E et al (2007) Lymphocyte activation in response to melanoma: interaction of NK-associated receptors and their ligands. Cancer Immunol Immunother 56:101–109

Solana R, Tarazona R, Gayoso I et al (2012) Innate immunosenescence: effect of aging on cells and receptors of
the innate immune system in humans. Semin Immunol
24:331–341

Stojanovic A, Cerwenka A (2011) Natural killer cells and
solid tumors. J Innate Immun 3:355–364

Takeuchi H, Maehara Y, Tokunaga E et al (2001)
Prognostic significance of natural killer cell activity in
patients with gastric carcinoma: a multivariate analysis. Am J Gastroenterol 96:574–578

Tarazona R, DelaRosa O, Alonso C et al (2000) Increased
expression of NK cell markers on T lymphocytes in
aging and chronic activation of the immune system
reflects the accumulation of effector/senescent T cells.
Mech Ageing Dev 121:77–88

Tarazona R, Casado JG, DelaRosa O et al (2002) Selective
depletion of CD56(dim) NK cell subsets and maintenance of CD56(bright) NK cells in treatment-naive
HIV-1-seropositive individuals. J Clin Immunol 22:
176–183

Tarazona R, Gayoso I, Alonso C et al (2009) NK cells in
human ageing. In: Fulop T, Franceschi C, Hirokawa
K, Pawelec G (eds) Handbook on Immunosenescence.
Springer, New York, pp 533–546

Thielens A, Vivier E, Romagne F (2012) NK cell MHC
class I specific receptors (KIR): from biology to clinical intervention. Curr Opin Immunol 24:239–245

Vasto S, Candore G, Balistreri CR et al (2007)
Inflammatory networks in ageing, age-related diseases
and longevity. Mech Ageing Dev 128:83–91

Verheyden S, Demanet C (2008) NK cell receptors and
their ligands in leukemia. Leukemia 22:249–257

Vesely MD, Kershaw MH, Schreiber RD et al (2011)
Natural innate and adaptive immunity to cancer. Annu
Rev Immunol 29:235–271

Vivier E, Tomasello E, Baratin M et al (2008) Functions
of natural killer cells. Nat Immunol 9:503–510

Vivier E, Raulet DH, Moretta A et al (2011) Innate or
adaptive immunity? The example of natural killer
cells. Science 331:44–49

Wagner WM, Ouyang Q, Sekeri-Pataryas K et al (2004)
Basic biology and clinical impact of immunosenescence. Biogerontology 5:63–66

Wehner R, Dietze K, Bachmann M et al (2011) The bidirectional crosstalk between human dendritic cells and
natural killer cells. J Innate Immun 3:258–263

Whiteside TL (2013) Immune modulation of T-cell and
NK (natural killer) cell activities by TEXs (tumour-
derived exosomes). Biochem Soc Trans 41:245–251

Wikby A, Nilsson BO, Forsey R et al (2006) The immune
risk phenotype is associated with IL-6 in the terminal
decline stage: findings from the Swedish NONA
immune longitudinal study of very late life functioning. Mech Ageing Dev 127:695–704

Yang C, Robbins PD (2011) The roles of tumor-derived
exosomes in cancer pathogenesis. Clin Dev Immunol
2011:842849

Zamai L, Ponti C, Mirandola P et al (2007) NK cells and
cancer. J Immunol 178:4011–4016

Zhang Y, Wallace DL, de Lara CM et al (2007) In vivo
kinetics of human natural killer cells: the effects of
ageing and acute and chronic viral infection.
Immunology 121:258–265

Zhou Z, Zhang C, Zhang J et al (2012) Macrophages help
NK cells to attack tumor cells by stimulatory NKG2D
ligand but protect themselves from NK killing by
inhibitory ligand Qa-1. PLoS One 7:e36928

Zimmer J, Andres E, Hentges F (2008) NK cells and Treg
cells: a fascinating dance cheek to cheek. Eur
J Immunol 38:2942–2945

Pattern Recognition Receptors and Aging

Karim H. Shalaby

8.1 Introduction

About two decades ago, Charles Janeway Jr. proposed the existence of pathogen-sensing receptors through which the innate immune system instructs the initiation of adaptive immune responses to antigens of foreign microbial origin (Janeway 1989). Specifically, he postulated that these innate "pattern recognition receptors" (PRRs) are germline-encoded and recognize conserved microbial structural or biosynthetic products, known as pathogen-associated molecular patterns (PAMPs), in contrast to the receptors associated with adaptive immunity (T cell receptors and B cell immunoglobulins), which are generated *de novo* by random gene rearrangement, recognize unique antigen-specific epitopes, and are clonally distributed (reviewed in Janeway and Medzhitov (2002), Medzhitov (2009), and O'Neill et al. (2013)). Importantly, he hypothesized that activated PRRs would be capable of stimulating pro-inflammatory pathways, such as nuclear factor κB (NFκB) signaling, and costimulatory molecule expression in antigen-presenting

cells such as dendritic cells and macrophages, thus permitting the immune system to distinguish infectious nonself from noninfectious self-antigens under normal physiological conditions. Janeway's theory also provided an explanation for the well-established immunostimulatory and adjuvant effects of certain microbial molecules, such as lipopolysaccharide (LPS), and led to the discovery of the toll-like receptors (TLRs), the most extensively studied family of PRRs (O'Neill et al. 2013). To date, 12 murine and 10 human functional TLRs have been identified that recognize a variety of bacterial, viral, fungal, and protozoal ligands, including DNA, RNA, carbohydrates, lipopeptides, and glycolipids (Iwasaki and Medzhitov 2010; Kawai and Akira 2011). The resulting activation of TLRs can promote the production of pro-inflammatory cytokines, chemokines, type I interferons (IFNs), costimulatory and adhesion molecules, major histocompatibility complex (MHC) expression, and antibody production to ensure the stimulation of rapid and robust immune responses against pathogenic environmental signals (Iwasaki and Medzhitov 2010; Janeway and Medzhitov 2002). However, PRRs play an even more expansive role in regulating immunity in that their activation can additionally be triggered by nonpathogenic organisms, including commensals, as well as endogenous ligands or damage-associated molecular patterns (DAMPs) that are exposed in the context of cellular stress, tissue injury, or autoimmunity such as host DNA, the intracellular high-mobility group box protein 1, heat shock

K.H. Shalaby, PhD
Meakins-Christie Laboratories,
Department of Medicine,
Research Institute of the McGill University
Health Centre, McGill University,
Montreal, QC H2X 2P2, Canada

Meakins-Christie Laboratories,
Department of Physiology, Faculty of Medicine,
McGill University, Montreal, QC H2X 2P2, Canada
e-mail: karim.shalaby@mail.mcgill.ca

A. Massoud, N. Rezaei (eds.), *Immunology of Aging*,
DOI 10.1007/978-3-642-39495-9_8, © Springer-Verlag Berlin Heidelberg 2014

...nd the extracellular matrix components, onan, biglycan, and versican (Iwasaki and edzhitov 2010; Medzhitov 2009). Thus, TLR signaling occurs constitutively under normal physiological conditions and is further induced by foreign or endogenous ligands within pathophysiological contexts.

Other families of PRRs have also been identified (reviewed in Iwasaki and Medzhitov (2010) and Medzhitov (2009)); the cell-surface C-type lectin receptors (CLRs or dectins) participate particularly in antifungal immunity (Hardison and Brown 2012). The cytosolic family of nucleotide-binding oligomerization domain and leucine-rich repeat-containing receptors (NLRs) detects bacterial and viral components, and some members of this family form multiprotein complexes, inflammasomes, which activate IL-1β production in response to pathogens, noninfectious stimuli, and DAMPs that compromise cellular membrane integrity (Elinav et al. 2011a; Ting et al. 2008). More recently, numerous nucleic acid-detecting receptors have been discovered which participate in antiviral and bacterial immunity, including the intracellular RNA-sensing helicases (the retinoic acid-inducible gene I (RIG-I)-like receptors (RLRs)) and DNA-sensing PRRs (Absent in Melanoma-2 (AIM2) and interferon-inducible protein 16 (IFI16), which constitute the AIM2-like receptors (ALRs)), as well as the cytosolic DNA-dependent activator of interferon regulatory factor 3 (DAI), RNA polymerase III (Pol III), and aspartate-glutamate-any amino acid-aspartate/histidine box helicases, which activate the core signaling molecule "stimulator of type I interferon genes" (STING) (reviewed in Atianand and Fitzgerald (2013), Dixit and Kagan (2013), and Rathinam and Fitzgerald (2011)). The pentraxins (C-reactive protein, serum amyloid protein, and pentraxin 3), as well as the lectin families of ficolins and collectins (including mannan-binding lectin and surfactant proteins A and D), are secreted, extracellular PRRs that activate the complement system and opsonize pathogens for phagocytosis, accounting for most of the remaining pathogen-sensing capabilities of the mammalian host (Iwasaki and Medzhitov 2010). Thus, PRRs can occur on the cell surface and in intracellular com-

partments or can be secreted into the bloodstream and tissue fluids, and their localization is an important determinant of the ligands that they detect and the ensuing signaling pathways that are activated (Blasius and Beutler 2010; Kagan and Iwasaki 2012). Most, if not all, PRRs that activate the transcription factors NFκB, interferon regulatory factors (IRFs), or nuclear factor of activated T cells (NFAT) are sufficient to induce T and B cell responses, whereas the secreted PRRs and some phagocytic PRRs (scavenger receptors) are not (Iwasaki and Medzhitov 2010). Research in the domain of PRRs is flourishing and for many of the newly discovered families is still in its infancy. However, numerous PRRs and their associated signaling molecules have already been implicated in various inflammatory and autoimmune conditions, as well as hereditary immunodeficiencies (Atianand and Fitzgerald 2013; Casanova et al. 2011; Netea et al. 2012). PRRs have additionally been established to play a crucial role in the immunostimulatory effects of vaccine adjuvants to native antigens lacking intrinsic immunogenic activity (Eisenbarth et al. 2008; Palm and Medzhitov 2009; Pasare and Medzhitov 2005). The subsequent sections will address the impact of immunosenescence on PRR expression and function and its consequences upon immune regulation in the context of healthy aging, pathophysiology of diseases associated with aging, and responsiveness of an aging immune system to vaccination.

8.2 PRR Expression and Function from Birth to Old Age

8.2.1 Ontogeny of TLR Responses in Infancy

TLRs are selectively expressed on numerous cell types, including the innate immune cells (monocytes, macrophages, dendritic cells, granulocytes, and natural killer cells) as well as T and B cells. Beyond the immune system, specific TLRs are also expressed by epithelial and endothelial cells, fibroblasts, smooth muscle, osteoblasts and osteoclasts, neurons, neuron progenitor cells, microglia, and astrocytes, among other cells. The expression and function of TLRs in these various cells is gradually being elucidated. Interestingly, newborns demonstrate heightened susceptibility to infection and diminished responsiveness to vaccines compared to older children and adults, similarly to the elderly (Kollmann et al. 2012; Levy 2005). Newborns (defined as those less than 28 days of age) demonstrate Th2-biased immunity and have generally been reported to display attenuated responsiveness to TLR stimulation compared to adults in studies that have assayed whole cord blood versus peripheral blood mononuclear cell (PBMC) responses or cord blood-derived monocyte versus PBMC-derived monocyte responses (Kollmann et al. 2012; Levy 2005, 2007). Various reports have collectively evaluated neonatal responses to agonists of TLR1-9. A number of studies have shown that the production of pro-inflammatory and/or Th1-polarizing cytokines, such as TNF-α, IL-12 and IFN-γ, by neonatal monocytes is diminished in response to the TLR4 ligand, LPS, as well as di- and tri-acylated bacterial lipoproteins that are recognized by TLR2/6 or TLR2/1 heterodimers, respectively (Belderbos et al. 2009; Goriely et al. 2001; Levy et al. 2004). Type I IFN production by neonatal plasmacytoid dendritic cells in response to TLR7/8 and TLR9 agonists has also been shown to be diminished (Corbett et al. 2010; Gold et al. 2006) and is associated with posttranscriptional downregulation of the TLR9/IRF-7 signaling pathway (Charrier et al. 2012). However, other TLR-induced cytokine responses, such as IL-1β, IL-6, IL-23, and the anti-inflammatory IL-10, remain equivalent to or even greater than responses of adult mononuclear cells, indicating that the impairment in TLR responses may be specific to certain mediators and, therefore, distinct TLR signaling pathways (Burl et al. 2011; Kollmann et al. 2012; Yerkovich et al. 2007). In one study, blood TNF-α and IL-12 responses to LPS, as well as induction of costimulatory molecules on DCs, were reported to reach adult levels within 1 year of birth, whereas type I IFN production in response to the TLR9 ligand, CpG-containing oligodeoxynucleotides (CpG DNA), remained low (Nguyen et al. 2010). However,

apart from TLR-induced IFN-γ production which appears to gradually increase from birth to adulthood, the reported acquisition of adult-like cytokine responses to TLR stimulation has been variable, with one study indicating that even at 12 years of age, IL-12 production still remains lower compared to adults (Upham et al. 2002). Some studies have reported augmented induction of IL-10 from neonatal mononuclear cells stimulated with TLR4, TLR7/8, or TLR9 agonists and a decline in IL-10 induction through infancy and childhood (Belderbos et al. 2009; Corbett et al. 2010; Upham et al. 2002). In contrast, TLR-mediated cytokine responses in Gambian and Papua New Guinean infants showed stable or increasing IL-10 production during infancy (Burl et al. 2011; Lisciandro et al. 2012), indicating that geographical diversity is also likely to affect innate immune responses to TLR ligands. Interestingly, LPS-induced IL-12p40, IL-6, and IL-23 production which is thought to support Th17 immunity was found to peak at birth and declined throughout the first year of infancy, while BCG immunization at birth has also been shown to promote stronger Th17 responses compared to vaccination at 4 months of age (Burl et al. 2010, 2011). Furthermore, differential LPS-induced upregulation of various transcription factors, cytokines, and chemokines in neonatal versus adult mononuclear cells has been documented (Jiang et al. 2004).

The altered TLR stimulatory capacity in neonatal blood cells may be related to cell-intrinsic as well as extrinsic environmental factors. Though basal expression of various TLRs and the membrane-bound TLR4 coreceptor CD14 on neonatal monocytes has been reported to be equivalent to that of adults (Dasari et al. 2011; Levy 2005), TLR4 expression actually increased more substantially in neonatal monocytes in response to LPS than in infant or adult monocytes (Levy et al. 2009; Yerkovich et al. 2007). Neonatal neutrophils also expressed normal TLR4 levels but lower levels of the primary TLR signaling adaptor, MyD88, and displayed reduced p38 MAPK activation (Al-Hertani et al. 2007). Soluble factors in neonatal plasma, including vitamin D, have been shown to affect TLR-induced antimicrobial peptide gene expression and cytokine responses (Levy et al. 2004; Walker et al. 2011). Levels of soluble CD14 and bactericidal/permeability-increasing protein, which affect the delivery of LPS to the TLR4 receptor complex, are different in neonatal compared to adult plasma (Levy 2005). Also, cyclic adenosine monophosphate (cAMP) synthesis, induced by adenosine and prostaglandins in neonatal plasma, inhibits TLR-induced TNF-α and IL-12 production while preserving or enhancing Th2-polarizing IL-6 and IL-10 production (Levy et al. 2006; Levy 2007). Maternal influences such as atopic status and breast-feeding additionally affect TLR expression and function in the newborn (LeBouder et al. 2006; Liu et al. 2011).

Collectively, the evidence indicates that the ontogeny of the immune response to TLR stimulation is variable and is ligand-, cell-, as well as cytokine-specific. It is also dependent upon external environmental influences and does not appear to progress linearly from birth to adulthood, but is rather likely to be governed by age-specific regulatory mechanisms, such as the expression of plasma-modulating factors (Kollmann et al. 2012). The functional immaturity of TLR responses in neonates may be associated with their enhanced susceptibility to infectious agents and dampened reactivity to vaccination, whereas aberrant TLR responsiveness has also been associated with neonatal preterm birth and sepsis (Kollmann et al. 2012; Sadeghi et al. 2007). Other PRR families are also critical to neonatal immunity. The mannan-binding lectin is implicated in neonatal sepsis, and the collectins (surfactant proteins) play a central role in neonatal lung development and disease (Bersani et al. 2012; Cedzynski et al. 2012; Schlapbach et al. 2010). In contrast to TLR responses, NLR and inflammasome responses to alum, the most widely used commercial vaccine adjuvant, were shown to peak immediately after birth and decline thereafter, suggesting differential regulation of distinct PRR families and innate immune functions through infancy (Lisciandro et al. 2012).

8.2.2 Disequilibrium of PRR Responses in the Aged

Similar to infants, there is evidence that TLR function is altered in monocytes and macrophages of aged adults. However, with regard to LPS-mediated cytokine responses, the evidence is conflicting, with some studies indicating increased LPS-induced cytokine secretion and others showing unchanged or decreased secretion (reviewed in Panda et al. (2009) and Van and Shaw (2007)). The divergent results may be related to differences in experimental protocols, such as cell enrichment, the origin and dose of the LPS preparations, cytokine assays (ELISA or flow cytometry), as well as sample size and enrolment criteria for subjects. For example, use of the highly selective SENIEUR protocol, which excludes participants taking prescribed medications or showing abnormalities in serum, urine, and blood count or a history of malignancy, while on the one hand permitting standardization of studies of human aging, may also be restricting such studies to a subset of uncommonly healthy, successfully aged individuals. The application of statistical models that adjust for potential confounding covariates such as age, gender, ethnicity, medication use, and comorbidities may uncover useful information with respect to TLR-induced cytokine responses in aging humans; one study that employed less stringent enrolment criteria and multivariable mixed statistical analysis reported that whereas peripheral blood monocyte responses to TLR2/6, TLR4, and TLR5 ligands were similar in aged compared to young adults, aged individuals demonstrated lower TNF-α, IL-6, and IL-8 production in response to TLR1/2 ligands, even after adjustment for covariates, which was associated specifically with lower surface expression of TLR1 (Van et al. 2007b). IL-6 synthesis in response to a TLR7/8 ligand was also diminished in monocytes from older adults (Van et al. 2007b). A more recent study which evaluated responses to a TLR1/2 ligand in subpopulations of monocytes, stratified on the basis of their expression of CD14 and CD16, confirmed the impaired TNF-α and IL-6 production as well as reduced TLR1 expression among multiple monocyte subsets in aged subjects and particularly those expressing CD16 (Nyugen et al. 2010). In contrast to the study by Van Duin et al. (2007b), elevated TLR5 expression and MAPK signaling resulting in higher IL-8 production from monocytes of older adults and diminished NFκB activation and TNF-α production were recently demonstrated (Qian et al. 2012). Therefore, cytokine responses of peripheral blood monocytes to TLR1/2 ligand, as well as TLR1 expression, have been reproducibly shown to be impaired in aged individuals, whereas cytokine responses to TLR4 and TLR5 stimulation are inconclusive. However, analysis of TLR-induced upregulation of CD80 and CD86 costimulatory molecules on monocytes revealed an age-associated defect that was significant for all tested TLR agonists, including ligands of TLR1/2, TLR2/6, TLR4, TLR5, and TLR7/8, supporting that aging (and potentially even that which is considered "normal" or healthy) is associated with diminished TLR responsiveness in these cells (Van et al. 2007a).

Studies comparing dendritic cells (DCs) from young and old adults have also indicated age-associated differences in TLR function. Due to the limited abundance of DCs in peripheral blood, a number of studies have examined DCs that are derived *in vitro* from monocytes using a concoction of growth factors and cytokines (monocyte-derived DCs or MDDCs). Agrawal et al. observed elevated cytokine production by MDDCs from older individuals in response to LPS, single-stranded RNA (TLR7/8 ligand), and self-DNA (TLR9 ligand) but simultaneously reported defective phagocytic and migratory function of these cells (Agrawal et al. 2007). In contrast, MDDCs and peripheral blood plasmacytoid DCs (pDCs) from older donors produced significantly lower levels of type I IFNs when infected with West Nile virus (TLR3 stimulation) (Kong et al. 2008; Shaw et al. 2011). pDCs are copious producers of type I IFNs and therefore play an important role in antiviral immunity (Diebold et al. 2004). Myeloid DCs (mDCs) are crucial for promotion of Th1 or Th2 immune

responses and express a diverse repertoire of TLRs (GeurtsvanKessel and Lambrecht 2008). Primary mDCs isolated from older individuals displayed reduced IL-12 production upon TLR4 stimulation (Della et al. 2007) but no difference in response to TLR3 activation (Jing et al. 2009). In the latter study, primary pDCs from older individuals had decreased influenza-virus (TLR7 and TLR9)-induced IFN-α production. The relative proportion of pDCs expressing TLRs 7 and 9 was also found to be reduced in aged individuals, whereas no difference in TLR2- or TLR4-expressing mDCs was observed. An age-associated decline in TLR7- and TLR9-induced IFN-α production by pDCs was confirmed more recently in a larger study, which also revealed a broad defect in TNF-α, IL-6, and IL-12p40 production by mDCs in response to most TLR ligands that were tested (TLR1/2, TLR2/6, TLR3, TLR4, TLR5, and TLR8). These age-related defects remained significant when the subjects were reevaluated nearly 2 years later (Panda et al. 2010). Age-associated reductions in mRNA and/or protein expression of specific TLRs has also been noted in mDCs and pDCs, suggesting that both transcriptional and posttranscriptional regulatory processes may underlie the TLR dysfunction observed with aging. Overall, the aforementioned studies support that aging results in diminished responsiveness of human DCs to TLR ligands. Curiously, basal intracellular cytokine production in the absence of TLR stimulation was in contrast found to be elevated in mDCs and pDCs of older compared to young adults (Panda et al. 2010; Shaw et al. 2011), perhaps suggesting that other PRR families or innate immune mechanisms may become hyperactive with aging or that regulatory mechanisms in DCs may become compromised. Several neutrophil functions have also been shown to be reduced with aging, such as chemotaxis, phagocytosis, and respiratory burst in response to a range of ligands including LPS (Solana et al. 2012). Although TLR expression in neutrophils is thought to be unaffected, aging may be associated with dysregulated trafficking of signaling molecules to cell membrane microdomains called lipid rafts, which facilitate the aggregation of TLR receptors and their downstream adaptor molecules during activation and signaling (Fortin et al. 2007a, b; Fulop et al. 2004). Other families of receptors expressed on neutrophils also appear to be implicated in the age-associated functional deficiencies of these cells (Solana et al. 2012).

That TLR responsiveness declines with aging is also supported by data from animal studies, although many dendritic cell and neutrophil functions do not appear to be affected as markedly in aged, but otherwise healthy, rodents as compared to their human counterparts. Neutrophils isolated from aged mice were reported to be functionally intact but became impaired only *in vivo* and upon exposure to an additional environmental stress, such as dietary deficiency or infection, emphasizing that the age-associated impairment of cell function is caused by not only cell-intrinsic but also extrinsic microenvironmental factors (Kovacs et al. 2009). In accordance with human studies, pDCs from aged mice were found to produce less type I IFN in response to synthetic or viral TLR9 ligand, as well as TLR7 ligand (Kovacs et al. 2009). However, TLR function in response to TLR2/6, TLR3, TLR4, TLR5, or TLR9 ligands was reportedly preserved in aged murine mDCs (Tesar et al. 2006). Gene expression analysis of splenic macrophages revealed lower expression of all tested TLRs (TLRs 1–9) in aged compared to young mice (Renshaw et al. 2002). Functional deficiency of aged macrophages in response to numerous TLR ligands as well as lower surface expression of TLR4 protein was also reported. However, these age-associated effects have not been consistently confirmed in other studies (Boehmer et al. 2004, 2005; Tesar et al. 2006).

The data discussed thus far from both human and rodent studies collectively support that TLR responsiveness declines with aging and may be a strong contributing factor to the age-associated increase in susceptibility to infectious disease and reduction of immunostimulatory capacity of vaccines. However, the role of TLRs in aging is complicated by the widely recognized observation that aging is paradoxically associated with chronic, low-grade inflammation characterized by elevated levels of circulating IL-6, TNF-α, and the pentraxin, C-reactive protein (sometimes also IFN-γ, IL-12, IP-10, and CXCL9) (Franceschi et al. 2007; Kollmann et al. 2012). It has therefore been hypothesized that constitutive TLR function in the elderly may be elevated, thus causing this phenomenon of "inflammageing," which may be particularly pertinent in the context of noninfectious age-associated diseases as will be discussed in the ensuing sections. Furthermore, this pro-inflammatory environment may precipitate the apparent age-associated refractory or hyporesponsive TLR activation by infectious stimuli (Kollmann et al. 2012). Increased NFκB (and mitogen-activated protein kinase (MAPK)) activity is also a prominent feature of inflammageing (Chung et al. 2009), having been consistently documented in older adults; however, definitive evidence demonstrating augmented basal activity of TLRs in relation to these processes is scarce. Nevertheless, there are a number of plausible mechanisms implicating TLRs in inflammageing. Although the expression and functional relevance of other PRR families in relation to aging has not been studied as extensively, there is increasing evidence to suggest a role for NLRs, RLRs, and inflammasome activation in inflammageing, as well as the pentraxins, C-reactive protein (CRP) and serum amyloid A. Circulating CRP levels have been shown to correlate with numerous age-associated diseases, including metabolic syndrome, cardiovascular disease, and osteoporosis, but are curiously found at even higher levels in centenarians than in old adults (Arai et al. 2001; Chung et al. 2009). Increased serum levels of serum amyloid A also correlate with the risk of cardiovascular disease (Johnson et al. 2004). Furthermore, this molecule was shown to trigger NLRP3 inflammasome activation via TLRs 2 and 4 in human and murine macrophages, thus implying that coordinated cross talk between multiple PRR families may underlie age-related inflammation (Niemi et al. 2011). Moreover, aberrant inflammasome activation has in recent years emerged as a leitmotif in inflammageing and age-related inflammatory disorders, though in certain contexts of aging, inflammasome and other PRR responses actually may be protective (see Sect.

8.4.4 and 8.4.6). Before elaborating upon the roles of PRRs in specific age-associated immune disorders, the ensuing section addresses the preeminent hypotheses regarding the mechanisms underlying altered PRR function in aging.

8.3 Mechanisms of TLR Hyporesponsiveness and PRR Disequilibrium in Aging

8.3.1 TLR Hyporesponsiveness

Reduced age-associated expression in human or murine cells of most TLRs (except TLR5 which may be expressed at higher levels) has been documented in a number of studies, as mentioned. However, the extent to which the altered expression contributes to the reduced functionality of TLRs with aging is unclear. Microarray gene expression analysis of macrophages isolated from older mice has also revealed altered expression of several downstream signaling molecules, including decreased expression of the primary TLR adaptor molecule myeloid differentiating factor 88 (MyD88) and TNF receptor-associated factor 6 (TRAF-6), as well as elevated expression of the adaptor Toll/IL-1R-associated protein (TIRAP) and TLR-inhibitory molecule IL-1R-associated kinase-M (IRAK-M) (Chelvarajan et al. 2006). MyD88 and TIRAP work in tandem to direct signaling downstream of all TLRs, with the exception of TLR3, promoting the phosphorylation of IRAK molecules and TRAF-6 which results in the activation of NFκB, MAPKs, and IRFs and, eventually, production of pro-inflammatory mediators. Numerous endogenous inhibitors within the TLR signaling network have been identified, although apart from IRAK-M, it is unclear how these molecules are affected in the context of aging. Elevated expression of IRAK-M and reduced expression of MyD88 and TRAF-6 might, nevertheless, contribute to the age-associated hyporesponsiveness of TLRs. Macrophages of aged mice have also been found to express lower levels of CD14 (Chelvarajan et al. 2005), a coreceptor

for LPS which facilitates signaling through the MyD88 pathway and particularly the other major TLR signaling pathway governed by the "TIR domain-containing adaptor-inducing IFN-β" (TRIF) which leads to the production of antiviral type I IFNs (Jiang et al. 2005; Wright et al. 1990; Zanoni et al. 2011). Systems genetics approaches are additionally being employed to delineate TLR signal transduction networks relevant to aging (Diego et al. 2012), whereas functional studies have thus far described lower NFκB and p38 MAPK signaling via TLR4 in macrophages (Boehmer et al. 2004; Boehmer et al. 2005), as well as diminished induction of type I IFNs in DCs of older donors due to reduced activity of signal transducer and activator of transcription (STAT) 1, IRF-1, and IRF-7 (Qian et al. 2011; Stout-Delgado et al. 2008). Although TLR1 surface expression was determined to be lower in macrophages of aged individuals, intracellular TLR1 expression was equivalent to that of the young, suggesting that impaired regulation of TLR trafficking to the cell surface may be another mechanism leading to reduced TLR responsiveness (Nyugen et al. 2010; Van et al. 2007b). Dysregulated recruitment of TLRs and their signaling molecules into membrane lipid rafts has also been postulated as a common mechanism to explain the broad decline in responsiveness of numerous TLRs with aging (Fortin et al. 2006, 2007a, b).

TLR-induced responses may also be downregulated by cross talk with other age-related pathological mechanisms that are not intrinsically part of the TLR signaling pathway. For example, increased expression and activity of Axl, a receptor tyrosine kinase, and broad inhibitor of various TLR responses is also believed to negatively regulate TLR signaling in DCs and further impair antiviral immunity in aging (Lemke and Rothlin 2008). Finally, oxidative stress and redox imbalance caused by weakening antioxidant defense mechanisms is a hallmark of aging that may have substantial implications upon TLR signaling (Peters et al. 2009). Reactive oxygen and nitrogen species (ROS and RNS) can react with and modify several cellular components including nucleic acids, proteins, and lipids. The resulting oxidation products, such as oxidized membrane phospholipids, have been shown to interact with multiple PRR pathways, including the TLRs, inflammasomes, C-reactive protein, and scavenger receptors (Weismann and Binder 2012). For example, 4-hydroxynonenal, an end product of membrane lipid peroxidation, can inhibit TLR4 receptor dimerization and signaling (Kim et al. 2009b) but is also capable of activating the NLRP3 inflammasome (Kauppinen et al. 2012). Oxidized phospholipids have been reported to inhibit TLR2, 3, 4, and 9 signaling (Kim et al. 2013; Weismann and Binder 2012). Moreover, reduction of the augmented oxidative stress levels observed in pDCs of aged mice can alleviate the impaired upregulation of IRF7 and induction of IFN-α in response to TLR9 activation (Stout-Delgado et al. 2008), additionally demonstrating the potential of oxidative stress to negatively regulate TLR responses. A recent study reported that the reduced type I IFN production by MDDCs of aged subjects in response to influenza virus infection was associated with altered chromatin structure and histone interactions with the IFN promoter (Prakash et al. 2012), supporting that various mechanisms may contribute to the hyporesponsiveness of TLRs in the elderly (Peters et al. 2009; Stout-Delgado et al. 2009).

8.3.2 PRR Disequilibrium in Inflammageing

Inflammageing refers to the heightened pro-inflammatory status associated with aging (Franceschi et al. 2007). In contrast to the generally diminished TLR function described thus far in innate immune cells, TLRs may also contribute to the pathophysiology of inflammageing given the additional evidence demonstrating hyperresponsiveness of certain TLRs in specific contexts. For example, Agrawal et al. reported augmented TLR4-, 7-, or 9-induced cytokine and costimulatory responses in MDDCs from aged subjects (Agrawal et al. 2007, 2009). The augmented TLR4 or TLR7 responsiveness was suggested to be due to decreased activation of the PI3K pathway, possibly caused by enhanced expression of

the phosphatase and tensin homolog (PTEN), a negative regulator of PI3K signaling which is now also known to promote pro- rather than anti-inflammatory TLR responses (Agrawal et al. 2007; Siegemund and Sauer 2012). The increased TLR9 activity occurred in response to self-DNA and was associated with augmented basal activation of NFκB and p38 MAPK in DCs (Agrawal et al. 2009). Elevated TLR5 mRNA and protein expression in monocytes of aged subjects, as well as augmented TLR5-induced cytokine production, has also been demonstrated and associated particularly with augmented p38 MAPK and ERK activity in these cells rather than NFκB activation (Qian et al. 2012). Furthermore, whereas resting macrophages from aged individuals were found to express lower basal levels of TLR3, activation of this TLR was enhanced and prolonged following West Nile virus infection (Kong et al. 2008). This was due to impaired downregulation of TLR3 resulting from increased STAT1 activity in the elderly. Thus, hyperresponsiveness of TLR3 was implicated in the over-exuberant inflammatory response and therefore potentially in the increased morbidity and mortality of aged individuals to this virus.

Interestingly, whereas splenic and peritoneal macrophages from aged mice produce lower amounts of pro-inflammatory mediators in response to LPS treatment *ex vivo* than those of young mice, the same mediators are augmented in aged mice following *in vivo* exposure to LPS or other bacterial products (Kovacs et al. 2009). This indicates that TLR4 activation on additional cell types, such as adipocytes or endothelial and epithelial cells, may perhaps be an important source of these cytokines in the context of aging. Indeed, epithelial cells in particular are receiving greater recognition for their substantial role in the initiation of PRR-mediated pro-inflammatory responses (Lambrecht and Hammad 2012). Alternatively, the presence of various microenvironmental stimuli *in vivo*, such as reactive oxygen species, hormones, cytokines, chemokines, adrenergic and cholinergic agonists, fatty acids, and immunoglobulins, may additionally contribute to the elevated inflammatory status associated with aging and TLR hyperresponsiveness that is evident in certain instances (Kovacs et al. 2009). Also, epigenetic and transcriptional mechanisms have been suggested to enhance TLR-induced cellular expression of specific cytokines, such as IL-23, which can contribute to age-related autoimmune disease (rheumatoid arthritis) (El et al. 2009).

A growing repertoire of endogenous PRR ligands or DAMPs has also been linked to age-associated immunopathology, such as mitochondrial DNA, saturated fatty acids, and phospholipid peroxidation products which can activate both cellular and soluble PRRs including TLRs, scavenger receptors, C-reactive protein, and inflammasomes (Salminen et al. 2012; Weismann and Binder 2012; West et al. 2010). Despite having the potential to inhibit TLR signaling, oxidative stress is perhaps predominantly considered to be a significant amplifier of TLR responses. For instance, oxidants can trigger TLR2 and TLR8 signaling, while oxidized phospholipids have also been documented to promote TLR2 and 4 activation (Kadl et al. 2011; Paul-Clark et al. 2009; Yanagisawa et al. 2009). Moreover, increases in cellular oxidative stress and nuclear translocation of antioxidant enzymes, such as thioredoxin, are believed to contribute to the age-related upregulation of the redox-sensitive transcription factors, NFκB and AP-1, which are central to TLR signaling (Chung et al. 2009). Heme oxygenase I, a major antioxidant gene, has also been demonstrated to be necessary for the activation of IRF3 and the expression of its primary target genes following TLR3 or TLR4 stimulation, as well as viral infection, while ROS production correlates with the increased ERK, JNK, and p38 MAPK activation associated with the aging process (Chung et al. 2009; Koliaraki and Kollias 2011; Tzima et al. 2009). Furthermore, mouse macrophages lacking a master transcription factor that regulates antioxidant genes, Nrf2, therefore having impaired antioxidant defense, were reported to exhibit augmented LPS-induced NADPH oxidase activity and ROS production, which enhanced TLR4 signaling via both the MyD88 and TRIF signaling pathways (Kong et al. 2010). Finally, ROS accumulation from damaged mitochondria can amplify RLR and inflammasome activation, as will be discussed in the ensuing sections (Tal et al. 2009; Zhou et al. 2011). Therefore, there is considerable evidence to support that a redox imbalance associated with aging has significant and broad effects upon PRR signaling pathways and amplification of inflammatory mediators.

Although reduced TLR function has generally been described in mDCs and pDCs of older adults, the elevated basal production of intracellular cytokines in these cells in the absence of TLR stimulation suggests that alternative mechanisms are also at play in inflammageing. Recent evidence supports that TLRs are not the only family of PRRs with relevance to inflammageing. In this regard, another important feature of age-associated immunopathology in innate immune cells is a decline in phagocytosis and autophagy, the process of sequestration of intracellular organelles within double-membrane vacuoles called "autophagosomes" and their eventual delivery to lysosomes for degradation (Kollmann et al. 2012). The persistence of damaged or senescent cells or intracellular components (resulting from deficient phagocytosis or autophagy, respectively) may thus augment inflammation by eliciting sustained PRR activation. Such defects may occur and may exacerbate inflammation in concert with the described redox imbalance associated with aging given that oxidized phospholipids have been shown to inhibit phagocytosis in macrophages, while this in turn, as well as impaired autophagy, can augment cellular oxidative stress (Knapp et al. 2007; Lee et al. 2012). In addition to providing homeostatic controlled clearance of toxic macromolecular aggregates and defunct cellular organelles, such as mitochondria, the major functions of autophagy include restoration of nutrient supply during cell starvation and clearance of cytosol-invading microbes (xenophagy) in cooperation with innate and adaptive immunity (Deretic 2012; Into et al. 2012). Whereas starvation-induced autophagy degrades cellular components nonspecifically via digestion of bulk cytoplasm, certain stressful stimuli induce "selective autophagy" in which specific cell constituents or intracellular microbes are targeted by autophagy-related ubiquitin-binding proteins, also referred to as autophagic receptors, such as sequestosome 1/p62-like receptors (SLRs), which in and of themselves have been proposed to be a class of PRRs (Deretic 2012; Into et al. 2012; Johansen and Lamark 2011). SLRs possess numerous protein interaction domains through which they can interact with microbial components and endogenous signaling molecules to expand pro-inflammatory immune responses but are normally consumed when autophagy proceeds efficiently. It is now known that canonical autophagy-related proteins and SLRs interact with numerous "conventional" PRR signaling pathways and vice versa, including TLRs (TLR2, 4, and 7), NLRs (Nod1/2, NLRC4, NLRP3, and NLRP4), RLRs, and inflammasomes. Endogenous alarmins or DAMPs such as IL-1β, high-mobility group box 1 (HMGB1), and ATP also stimulate autophagy (Bortoluci and Medzhitov 2010; Deretic 2012; Into et al. 2012). Several TLRs, such as TLRs 2, 4, and 7, rely upon autophagic clearance of specific intracellular microbes. For example, TLR7 engagement induces autophagy which is necessary for elimination of bacillus Calmette-Guerin, as well as recognition of RNA viruses by TLR7 in autolysosomes (Delgado and Deretic 2009; Into et al. 2012). However, autophagy also plays an important role in restraining TLR- and PRR-mediated inflammatory responses, as well as cross talk between PRR pathways (Deretic 2012; Into et al. 2012). This is primarily achieved by efficient sequestration and clearance of intracellular pathogens, autophagic receptors, as well as cellular material, such as mitochondrial DNA, that could otherwise, in the case of inefficient autophagy, provoke persistent innate immune activation. For instance, disruption of autophagy causes accumulation of physiologically abnormal mitochondria which, under normal circumstances, are continuously removed by a form of housekeeping autophagy (mitophagy) (Into et al. 2012; Lee et al. 2012). When this basal autophagy is defective, leaky mitochondria provide an ongoing source of ROS which can amplify RLR signaling as well as NLRP3 (or NALP3) inflammasome activation in macrophages (Nakahira et al. 2011; Tal et al. 2009; Zhou et al. 2011). The result-

ing damage releases mitochondrial DNA which further augments NLRP3 inflammasome activation (Nakahira et al. 2011; Shimada et al. 2012). Mitochondrial DNA that has escaped autophagy can also activate TLR9, promoting autoimmune and cardiovascular disease (Oka et al. 2012) (Therefore, defects in DNA clearance and/or repair mechanisms may also be substantial in relation to age-associated inflammation and vice versa (Nijnik et al. 2007)). Autophagic proteins also negatively regulate RLR signaling by directly binding RLRs and their adaptor proteins (Jounai et al. 2007). Autophagy additionally appears to serve the housekeeping function of tempering inflammation by eliminating components of the RLR pathway, such as the adaptor "IFN-β promoter stimulator 1" (Tal et al. 2009), as well as activated AIM2 and NLRP3 inflammasomes (Shi et al. 2012), and therefore could perhaps be involved in the increased RLR and inflammasome activation that has been documented in several age-associated diseases, such as Alzheimer's (Halle et al. 2008; Heneka et al. 2013). Although other NLRs, such as NOD1/2, are known to induce autophagy, while NLRC4 and NLRP4 negatively regulate autophagy, further studies will be necessary to determine whether these processes are reciprocally regulated (Deretic 2012). Also, the functional consequences of the interaction of NLRP1, NLRP3, and NLRP10 with autophagy-related proteins are unknown. Moreover, TLR4 engagement by LPS in the context of defective autophagy augments mitochondrial ROS production, NLRP3 inflammasome activation, and subsequent IL-1β and IL-18 secretion (Juliana et al. 2012; Nakahira et al. 2011; Saitoh et al. 2008; West et al. 2011), indicating that autophagy additionally constrains TLR-induced inflammation and cross talk with inflammasomes. In summary, the clearance of mitochondria seems to be at least one chief mechanism by which autophagy maintains innate immune homeostasis.

Furthermore, several autophagic receptors are also known to interact with and negatively regulate TLR signaling (Into et al. 2012; Saitoh et al. 2008). For example, following TLR4 signaling via MyD88 and TRIF, the resulting activation of TRAF6 and TRAF3 mediates the recruitment and activation of various SLRs which in turn promote clearance of cytosolic bacteria via selective xenophagy but also accumulate signaling proteins, including MyD88, TRIF, and TRAF6, in cytosolic aggregates for degradation via a category of selective autophagy known as aggrephagy (Into et al. 2012). TLR4-mediated activation of p38 MAPK and JNK was thus attenuated, while other SLRs have also been shown to suppress TLR3/4-induced NFκB and IRF3 activation, as well as TRIF or TRAF3-dependent type I IFN production. Thus, age-associated deficiency in autophagy may very well contribute to the pathophysiology of inflammageing, potentially by facilitating dysregulation of TLR and other PRR pathways. However, it remains to be established how pervasive impaired phagocytosis/autophagy is among elderly individuals, what the precise mechanistic consequences are of such a defect upon specific PRR pathways, and whether defective autophagy may be the cause or result of dysregulated PRR activity in the context of inflammageing. The following section summarizes our current knowledge regarding PRRs that have been implicated in specific age-related immune disorders.

8.4   Age-Related Diseases

8.4.1   Declining Immunity: Susceptibility to Infection

Reduced PRR activity in innate immune cells is possibly a major factor in the increased susceptibility and/or morbidity of elderly individuals to specific infections, such as tuberculosis, bacterial pneumonia, listeria, Candida albicans, herpes, and influenza (reviewed in Kollmann et al. (2012)). In particular, reduced TLR1 expression in monocytes and TLR7/9 activity in pDCs have been shown to be important in some of these contexts (Canaday et al. 2010; Van et al. 2007b), while reduced expression in the lungs of TLRs 1, 2, and 4 was associated with impaired immunity against pneumonia in aged mice (Hinojosa et al. 2009). Also, impaired NLRP3 inflammasome activation was recently discovered in DCs of

aged mice infected with influenza virus, causing increased morbidity and mortality (Stout-Delgado et al. 2012). In contrast, excessive activation of certain PRRs can also modulate immune responses to infection in the aged; sustained upregulation of TLR3 in macrophages in response to West Nile virus (WNV) was shown to cause excessive inflammation and, thus, increased severity and mortality in the elderly (Kong et al. 2008). The dysregulation of TLR3 was apparently the indirect result of impaired signaling downstream of the CLR, dendritic cell-specific intercellular adhesion molecule 3 grabbing nonintegrin (DC-SIGN) which binds a WNV envelope protein in the initial stages of infection. Thus, age-dependent impairment in CLR function was determined to amplify TLR3 activation in macrophages in response to WNV. Moreover, immunosenescence of adaptive immune responses may perhaps also be influenced by dysfunction or dysregulation of PRRs. B cells, for example, express various TLRs, the ligands of which can directly modulate B cell functions, while CD4+ or CD8+ T cell responses are primarily influenced by antigen-presenting cell activation via numerous PRRs and inflammasomes (Dostert et al. 2013; Manicassamy and Pulendran 2009; Pasare and Medzhitov 2005). Age-associated defects in CD4+ T cell functions, such as chemotaxis, priming by DCs, and transition to a T follicular helper cell phenotype, are not only caused by cell-intrinsic defects but are also the result of the aged microenvironment (Lefebvre et al. 2012; Schindowski et al. 2002). Thus, altered PRR function might additionally contribute to age-associated deficiencies in germinal center formation, memory B cell generation and survival, immunoglobulin production, and changes in the quality and quantity of CD4+, CD8+, and regulatory T cell responses (Arnold et al. 2011; Frasca and Blomberg 2011; Raynor et al. 2012; Sridharan et al. 2011). However, a recent study reported that a specific subset of B cell receptor-refractory but TLR-responsive B cells preferentially expands with aging, suggesting that TLR responses are intact in aged B cells (Hao et al. 2011). Notably, NLRP3 inflammasome activation has recently been shown to promote age-dependent thymic demise and T cell senescence, which might occur as a result of accumulation of by-products of thymic fatty acids and lipids acting as DAMPs (Dixit 2012; Youm et al. 2012). Deletion of the NLRP3 inflammasome also accelerated T cell reconstitution in hematopoietic stem cell transplants (Youm et al. 2012). Finally, chronic exposure to endogenous or pathogen-derived TLR ligands such as in the context of persistent low-grade infection has also been suggested to contribute to aspects of hematopoietic stem cell senescence (Esplin et al. 2011).

8.4.2 Metabolic Syndrome

The term "metabolic syndrome" encompasses the immunologically and clinically associated disorders of obesity, type 2 diabetes, and cardiovascular disease (Hotamisligil 2006; Mokdad et al. 2003). Obesity is characterized by increased storage of fatty acids in an expanded adipose tissue and chronic low-grade inflammation even in the absence of overt infection or autoimmunity (De Nardo and Latz 2011; Konner and Bruning 2011). Obesity predisposes individuals to chronic metabolic diseases, namely, type 2 diabetes mellitus and atherosclerosis (Hotamisligil 2006; Mokdad et al. 2003). High-fat diet and resulting obesity-associated inflammation cause resistance, not only in peripheral tissues but also in the central nervous system (CNS), to the peptide hormones insulin and leptin which regulate metabolism and energy homeostasis (Sandoval et al. 2008). This effect is even more pronounced when food intake contains high levels of carbohydrates (Dasu and Jialal 2011; Ferreira et al. 2011). Obesity-associated inflammation is caused by adipose tissue-infiltrating inflammatory macrophages as well as adipocytes, which themselves are a significant source of pro-inflammatory mediators or "adipokines", such as TNF-α and IL-6 (Weisberg et al. 2003). Adipose tissue, apart from its classical role as an energy storage depot, has thus increasingly been recognized as a dynamic endocrine organ whose secretion of metabolic and pro-inflammatory factors varies according to the degree of adiposity

(Chung et al. 2009; Konner and Bruning 2011). Perhaps not surprisingly, age-related accumulation of visceral adipose tissue is directly associated with systemic inflammation in the elderly, and adipokines are believed to contribute significantly to inflammageing (Chung et al. 2009; Xu et al. 2003). Moreover, caloric restriction and exercise are currently the two most effective antiageing regimens known to man, and their anti-inflammatory effects are widely documented (Chung et al. 2009; Salminen et al. 2012). Leptin is the major adipocyte-derived hormone controlling energy homeostasis by promoting energy expenditure, by inhibiting food (or energy) intake, and by regulating glucose metabolism and peripheral insulin sensitivity (Frederich et al. 1995; Mistry et al. 1997). The vast majority of obese individuals, as well as obese mice fed a high-fat diet, present with increased circulating leptin concentrations indicative of neuronal leptin resistance (Friedman 2009). Insulin regulates glucose and fat metabolism by reducing blood glucose levels, food intake, and body weight via its actions on peripheral tissues and the brain (Obici et al. 2002; Plum et al. 2006). Insulin resistance peripherally and in the CNS is another hallmark of obesity (Konner and Bruning 2011). Insulin resistance is driven by activation of JNK, NFκB, and protein kinase C inflammatory pathways in metabolically active sites in response to various obesity-related stress signals such as cytokines and metabolic or cellular disturbances (increased circulating fatty acid levels, hyperglycemia, endoplasmic reticulum stress, as well as NADPH oxidase- and mitochondria-derived ROS) (Dasu et al. 2012; Konner and Bruning 2011; Nguyen et al. 2007). Various PRRs are activated in these contexts and are recognized to contribute to the pathophysiology of obesity and its related disorders. For instance, circulating CRP levels in humans have been reported to correlate with increased adiposity and leptin resistance, suggesting that the pentraxin, CRP, is associated with metabolic syndrome (Bruunsgaard et al. 1999; Chen et al. 2006c).

Though recent studies indicate that numerous TLRs have the capacity to stimulate inflammatory mediator production and induce insulin resistance in adipocytes (Franchini et al. 2010;

Kopp et al. 2010, 2009; Schaeffler et al. 2009), the most extensively studied PRRs described to play a prominent role in insulin and leptin resistance are the TLRs 2 and 4. Increased expression and activity of these TLRs in monocytes and adipose tissues have been demonstrated in obese and type 2 diabetic patients, as well as in murine models of these diseases (Bes-Houtmann et al. 2007; Creely et al. 2007; Dasu et al. 2010; Jialal et al. 2012; Roncon-Albuquerque et al. 2008; Song et al. 2006). Obese individuals and those with type 2 diabetes also display significantly elevated TLR4 gene and protein expression in their muscle which correlates with the severity of insulin resistance (Reyna et al. 2008). Studies have shown that saturated fatty acids, the circulating levels of which are increased in obesity, are capable of stimulating TLR2 and 4 activation in macrophages and adipocytes, whereas unsaturated fatty acids are not (Lee et al. 2001; Shi et al. 2006; Tripathy et al. 2003). Also, the induction of inflammation in these cells is TLR4 dependent. Furthermore, the stimulatory capacity of saturated fatty acids and consequential insulin resistance in skeletal muscle is chain length dependent; the longer-chain fatty acids, palmitate and stearate, were shown to trigger inflammation and insulin resistance, whereas the short-chain fatty acid laurate was unable to activate TLR4 or induce insulin resistance (Hommelberg et al. 2009). Mice with either targeted disruption or naturally occurring mutation in TLR4 are protected from the development of obesity and insulin resistance, although TLR4 deficiency appears to selectively protect against obesity and insulin resistance caused by a diet rich in saturated fats but not by an isocaloric diet high in unsaturated fats (Davis et al. 2008; Poggi et al. 2007; Shi et al. 2006; Tsukumo et al. 2007). More recently, hematopoietic cell-specific deletion of TLR4 was shown to ameliorate high-fat-diet-induced hepatic and adipose tissue insulin resistance (Saberi et al. 2009).

The aforementioned findings support that TLR4 activation by specific saturated fatty acids, such as palmitate, plays a substantial role in mediating obesity-associated insulin resistance elicited by high-fat diet. However, numerous studies have shown that TLR2 deficiency or pharmacological inhibition also improves insulin sensitivity in the muscle, liver, and adipose tissues of mice fed a high-fat diet and, furthermore, prevents pancreatic islet β cell death and palmitate-induced insulin resistance, implying redundancy between TLR2 and TLR4 in mediating fatty acid-induced insulin resistance (Caricilli et al. 2008; Davis et al. 2011; Ehses et al. 2010; Himes and Smith 2010; Kuo et al. 2011; Senn 2006). Furthermore, both TLRs 2 and 4 have been shown to mediate high-fat-diet-induced vascular inflammation and impaired responsiveness of vascular endothelial cells to insulin, thus providing a potential link to the cardiovascular complications associated with obesity and diabetes (Jang et al. 2013; Kim et al. 2007a). However, the capacity of saturated fatty acids to directly stimulate TLRs 2 and 4 was also challenged in one study which raised the possibility of LPS and lipopeptide contamination of fatty acid preparations (Erridge and Samani 2009). Thus, alternative mechanisms or endogenous ligands are additionally likely to contribute to the activation of TLR4 by high-fat foods. For instance, saturated fatty acids may be capable of activating TLR-dependent signaling via intermediate molecules produced during metabolic processing, such as the sphingolipid ceramide, a specific product of long-chain saturated fatty acid metabolism which has been shown to activate TLR4 (Fischer et al. 2007). Metabolic processing of fatty acids to ceramide has also been shown to activate TLR4-independent inflammatory events that will be described shortly (Schwartz et al. 2010).

The receptor for advanced glycation end products (RAGE) is a nonclassical PRR which interacts with numerous endogenous ligands and can subsequently activate NFκB, PI3K, and MAPKs (Kierdorf and Fritz 2013). The high-mobility group box protein 1 (HMGB1) and heat shock protein 60 are additional TLR2, TLR4, and/or RAGE-activating DAMPs which are increased in the plasma of obese individuals and have been reported to function as mediators of adipose tissue inflammation and insulin resistance (Dasu et al. 2010; Marker et al. 2012; Nogueira-Machado et al. 2011). Moreover, a high blood glucose level (or hyperglycemia) increases the expression of TLRs 2 and 4 in human monocytes (an effect that is amplified in the presence of fatty acids), as well as RAGE, and thus could potentially enhance the sensitivity of obese and diabetic patients to endogenous ligands of these receptors (Dasu et al. 2008; Dasu and Jialal 2011; Yao and Brownlee 2010). TLR2 also appears to contribute to autoimmune diabetes by sensing DAMPs released from injured or dying pancreatic islet β cells (Kim et al. 2007b). Finally, there is a growing literature indicating that the gut microbiota also plays a key role in metabolism and energy storage by activating TLR2- and TLR4-dependent signaling (Cani and Delzenne 2009; Caricilli et al. 2011; Turnbaugh et al. 2006). Interestingly, high-fat diet increases the proportion of LPS-containing microbes in the gut as well as plasma LPS levels, and the resulting metabolic endotoxemia triggers TLR4-dependent inflammation, weight gain, and diabetes (Cani et al. 2007, 2008; Kim et al. 2012). Although TLR2-deficient mice are protected from diet-induced obesity and insulin resistance under germ-free conditions, it was recently reported that conventional, non-germ-free housing caused these mice to develop a phenotype resembling metabolic syndrome, characterized by changes in gut microbiota, increased serum LPS concentrations, glucose intolerance, obesity, and TLR4-dependent insulin resistance (Caricilli et al. 2011). These effects were reproducible in wild-type animals following transplantation of microbiota. Furthermore, recent studies have shown that such features may be prevented by antibiotic treatment of high-fat-diet-fed mice (Caricilli et al. 2011; Carvalho et al. 2012). Exercise training in rodents also reduces circulating LPS levels, adipose tissue inflammation, and TLR4 activation while improving glucose and insulin tolerance (Kawanishi et al. 2010; Oliveira et al. 2011). These findings indicate an additional layer of complexity in the role of TLRs in metabolic syndrome.

The specific signaling pathways and effector molecules downstream of TLR activation which promote or counteract the development of obesity-associated disorders are still in the process of being resolved. Despite the abundant evidence supporting the prominent role of TLR2 and TLR4 signaling in obesity and insulin resistance, a study examining the consequences of MyD88 deficiency in high-fat-diet-induced disease curiously reported an exacerbation of circulating insulin, leptin, and cholesterol levels, as well as liver dysfunction in MyD88 knockout compared to wild-type mice, which was not related to TNF-α (Hosoi et al. 2010). MyD88 signaling was therefore concluded to prevent the development of diabetes caused by high-fat diet. Meanwhile, CNS-restricted deletion of MyD88 protected mice from weight gain, leptin resistance, and impaired peripheral glucose metabolism induced by either high-fat diet or intracerebroventricular injection of palmitate (Kleinridders et al. 2009). These results indicate that MyD88 signaling in the CNS is important in diet-induced leptin and insulin resistance and suggest that the activation of these innate immune pathways in different tissues could have variable consequences upon the pathophysiology of obesity and diabetes. Global CD14 deficiency also attenuates cardiovascular and metabolic complications in a murine model of diet-induced obesity (Roncon-Albuquerque et al. 2008), while TRIF deficiency can affect glucose metabolism and insulin production in mice after fasting, without causing insulin resistance (Hutton et al. 2010). Therefore, there is abundant evidence indicating the regulatory role of TLR signaling in glucose and fatty acid metabolism. TNF-α is likely to be an important effector molecule downstream of TLR activation given its increased expression in both adipose and muscle tissues of obese individuals and established role in promoting insulin resistance in rodent models of obesity (Hardy et al. 2013; Konner and Bruning 2011; Uysal et al. 1997). In contrast, certain mediators such as IL-6 and IL-18 may actually have protective effects against obesity and insulin resistance (Konner and Bruning 2011).

Recent studies have also revealed NLRP3 inflammasome activation as a key mechanism in obesity and insulin resistance (Stienstra et al. 2011; Vandanmagsar et al. 2011; Wen et al. 2012). One seminal study demonstrated that caloric restriction and exercise-mediated weight loss in obese individuals with type 2 diabetes was associated with a reduction in adipose tissue expression of Nlrp3, as well as with decreased inflammation and improved insulin sensitivity (Vandanmagsar et al. 2011). Ablation of Nlrp3 in mice also prevented obesity-induced inflammasome activation, effector T cell accumulation in adipose tissues and augmented insulin signaling. A comparison of abdominal adipose tissue from obese men with impaired glucose tolerance with lean normal glucose tolerant age-matched controls confirmed that the former group exhibited signs of enhanced NLRP3 inflammasome activation and augmented T helper 1 and T helper 17 immune responses (Goossens et al. 2012). Another study reported that inflammasome deficiency in mice attenuated features of high-fat-diet-induced obesity and insulin resistance, such as hepatic triglyceride content, adipocyte size, and macrophage infiltration of adipose tissues, while also affecting plasma concentrations of insulin and the energy-regulating hormones leptin and resistin (Stienstra et al. 2011). Therefore, these findings suggest that inflammasome activation not only regulates the inflammatory profile associated with obesity but also controls energy expenditure and adipogenic gene expression during chronic overfeeding, similar to what has been described for the TLRs. Inflammasome deficiency in mice or caspase 1 inhibitor treatment of obese mice has also been shown to enhance metabolic activity and insulin sensitivity of adipocytes (Stienstra et al. 2010).

NLRP3 inflammasome activation in adipose tissues of mice can occur as a result of increases in intracellular ceramide, further supporting its role as a potential obesity-associated DAMP (De Nardo and Latz 2011). Palmitate also induces NLRP3 inflammasome activation in hematopoietic cells and production of IL-1β in adipose tissues, which is known to play a major role in insulin resistance (Wen et al. 2011). Interestingly, as in the case of TLR4, inflammasome activation and insulin resistance occurred only in response to this saturated fatty acid and not the unsaturated fatty acid oleate. Inflammasome activation by palmitate was mediated by a mechanism involving mitochondrial ROS production and

inhibition of autophagy which consequently impaired insulin signaling in several target tissues (Wen et al. 2011). Moreover, the activation of the NLRP3 inflammasome in dendritic cells and adipocytes of mice by dietary saturated fatty acids depended on priming via TLR4 of the dendritic cells (Reynolds et al. 2012). These findings further highlight the significance of saturated fatty acid metabolism to the manifestation of insulin resistance, which occurs not only as a result of TLR activation but also the activation of the NLRP3 inflammasome. Another signature feature of obesity-induced insulin resistance is the accumulation of pancreatic islet amyloid polypeptide which, when taken up by DCs and macrophages, has also been shown to stimulate activation of the NLRP3 inflammasome and IL-1β production in the pancreas (Masters et al. 2010). Accordingly, chronic obesity-induced pancreatic damage is also attenuated in inflammasome-deficient mice (Youm et al. 2011). The polypeptide-induced inflammasome activation is also apparently primed by TLR4 signaling triggered by modified low-density lipoprotein, the concentration of which is characteristically elevated in obesity, type 2 diabetes, and cardiovascular disease (Masters et al. 2010). Taken together, these findings indicate the contribution of multiple obesity-associated DAMPs in the development of type 2 diabetes and support that inhibitors of TLRs, NLRP3, and perhaps other inflammasomes could be useful therapeutic agents in the treatment of obesity and type 2 diabetes. To date, no therapeutics directly targeting TLRs or the NLRP3 inflammasome have been tested in this context, while therapies that neutralize the major downstream product of inflammasome activation, IL-1β, such as the recombinant human IL-1 receptor antagonist, anakinra, or monoclonal anti-IL-1β antibody, have thus far yielded mixed results (reviewed in De Nardo and Latz (2011)). Recent studies in mice, however, indicate that deficiency in the inflammasome component caspase 1 dramatically reduces high-fat-diet-induced weight gain and increases insulin sensitivity (Kotas et al. 2013; van Diepen et al. 2013). This is a result of increased triglyceride clearance and possibly reduced intestinal triglyceride absorption and hepatic triglyceride secretion into the blood in the absence of caspase 1. Interestingly, caspase 1-mediated triglyceride clearance was independent of IL-1 family cytokine signaling, indicating that inflammasomes may potentially influence lipid metabolism and insulin sensitivity via IL-1β- and IL-18-dependent as well as independent mechanisms (Kotas et al. 2013). As mentioned, the non-inflammasome cytokine TNF-α also contributes to impaired glucose homeostasis and insulin resistance in patients with type 2 diabetes, perhaps necessitating the development of combined therapies that target multiple cytokines or PRR pathways simultaneously (Wen et al. 2012). Finally, metabolic syndrome is a common malady in aging, perhaps by default, due to the chronicity of the processes leading to the disorder. But despite the similarities between obesity-associated inflammation and age-related inflammageing, much work remains to clarify whether the mechanisms driving inflammation in obesity and type 2 diabetes are equivalent to those underlying the inflammageing process.

8.4.3   Cardiovascular Disease

Atherosclerosis is the leading cause of cardiovascular disease. TLRs are differentially regulated by several cardiovascular risk factors, such as hypercholesterolemia, hyperlipidemia, and hyperglycemia (Moghimpour Bijani et al. 2012). A peripheral blood gene expression profile indicating elevated TLR and IL-1R signaling was suggested to be a strong indicator of atherosclerotic burden, and importantly, even in women who were at lower risk based on predictive clinical factors (Huang et al. 2011). Obesity was also shown to be a significant risk factor for enhanced peripheral blood responses to bacterial TLR2 and 4 ligands in patients suffering from established atherosclerotic disease (Scholtes et al. 2011). TLR4 expression has been found to be upregulated in atherosclerotic tissues, and various pro-inflammatory mediators produced by TLR4 activation, such as IL-6 and TNF-α, exert atherogenic effects (Katsargyris et al. 2011; Michelsen et al. 2004; Spirig et al. 2012). Bacterial ligands

of TLR2 and TLR4 accelerate atherosclerosis, but various endogenous DAMPs which contribute to atherogenesis and cardiovascular disease have also been identified (reviewed in De Nardo and Latz (2011), Moghimpour Bijani et al. (2012)). For instance, oxidized low-density lipoprotein and phospholipids can function as endogenous TLR ligands to promote cytoskeletal changes, pro-inflammatory cytokine secretion, and ROS production in macrophages and endothelial cells and, thus, contribute to the chronic inflammation in atherosclerotic lesions (Miller et al. 2011; Moghimpour Bijani et al. 2012). The atherogenic effects of modified low-density lipoproteins have been attributed to both TLR4-MyD88-dependent and MyD88-independent signaling, as well as TLR2 activation (Miller et al. 2012, 2011); mice deficient in either TLR4, TLR6, MyD88, CD14, or IRAK-4 exhibit reduced atherosclerotic burden (Erridge 2009; Michelsen et al. 2004; Spirig et al. 2012). The activation of these pathways can additionally prime NLRP3 inflammasome activation (De Nardo and Latz 2011). Furthermore, oxidized low-density lipoprotein can also activate the NLRP3 inflammasome through ROS production and by facilitating the formation of inflammasome-activating cholesterol crystals (Duewell et al. 2010; Rajamaki et al. 2010). Other TLR2- and/or TLR4-activating DAMPs that are abundant in atherosclerotic plaques include the high-mobility group box protein 1, the heat shock proteins 60 and 70, fibrinogen, tenascin C, and the extracellular matrix components hyaluronan and versican (reviewed in Moghimpour Bijani et al. (2012)).

Cardiovascular disease is influenced by both genetic and environmental factors, and common single-nucleotide polymorphisms (SNPs) in the CD14 and TLR4 genes have been shown to modify the risk of myocardial infarction, one of the major complications in cardiovascular disease. The CD14/-260 gene variant may be associated with augmented systemic levels of IL-6 and TNF-α and higher risk of myocardial infarction (Giacconi et al. 2007), although this finding has not been replicated in all studies (Longobardo et al. 2003; Zee et al. 2001). There are also discordant results regarding the role of the TLR4/-299 gene variant upon the risk of myocardial infarction; although some studies indicate a potential for the TLR4/-299 SNP to modify the effect of specific environmental factors such as pharmacological treatments or smoking, resulting in increased risk of myocardial infarction (Edfeldt et al. 2004; Holloway et al. 2005; Olivieri et al. 2006), most studies have reported no association (Dzumhur et al. 2012; Nebel et al. 2007; Zee et al. 2005). Interestingly, a single study found this loss-of-function mutation to occur at a significantly lower frequency in individuals affected by myocardial infarction and at a higher frequency in centenarians, suggesting that a genetic predisposition to developing weaker inflammatory responses via TLR4 may be protective against cardiovascular disease (Balistreri et al. 2004). Therefore, while enhancing risk of infections in the elderly, this polymorphism was proposed to decrease atherogenesis and perhaps confer longevity to individuals living in an environment with lower microbial burden and advanced control of severe infections. However, two subsequent studies were unable to confirm an association of the TLR4/-299 SNP with longevity and/or acute myocardial infarction, whereas a SNP in the TLR2 gene was found to be expressed less frequently in afflicted subjects, suggesting a protective role for this SNP (Dzumhur et al. 2012; Nebel et al. 2007). Another group failed to detect an association between TLR2 gene variants and acute myocardial infarction (Balistreri et al. 2008a), implying that the influence of gene polymorphisms may depend on the specific mutation and gene-environment interactions. TLR4 deficiency has also been shown to reduce tissue damage in a mouse model of myocardial infarction (Zhao et al. 2009). A protective effect has similarly been observed in mice deficient in TLR2 (Favre et al. 2007), although, in contrast, TLR2 ligands have also been reported to induce cardioprotection (Ha et al. 2010). Furthermore, TLR4 may partially contribute to lipid accumulation in cardiac muscle and reduced cardiac function in the nonobese diabetic mouse model of type 1 diabetes (Dong et al. 2012). Finally, blockade of TLR2 or TLR4 by antagonists has shown benefit in murine models of ischemia/reperfusion injury (reviewed in Spirig et al.

(2012)), and TLR4 antagonism reduced disease parameters in spontaneously hypertensive rats (Bomfim et al. 2012). These findings support a role for TLRs 2 and 4 in the inflammatory events associated with both the development of heart disease (e.g. atherosclerosis) as well as actual injury of the heart (e.g. myocardial infarction).

Growing evidence indicates an additional role for other TLRs and PRRs in cardiovascular disease. TLR3-, TLR4-, or TLR9-mediated signaling can contribute to excessive lipid accumulation in macrophages resulting in foam cell formation, a major hallmark of atherosclerosis (Moghimpour Bijani et al. 2012; Spirig et al. 2012). Mitochondrial DNA that escapes from autophagy was shown to elicit TLR9-mediated inflammatory responses in cardiomyocytes causing myocarditis and dilated cardiomyopathy, also supporting that declining autophagy and resultant mitochondrial DNA release may contribute to the chronic inflammation leading to age-related heart disease (Oka et al. 2012). Meanwhile, ablation of TLR3 or TLR7 function has recently been shown to accelerate the onset of atherosclerosis in hypercholesterolemic mice, suggesting a protective role for these TLRs in vascular health (Cole et al. 2011; Salagianni et al. 2012). The receptor for advanced glycation end products (RAGE) may also contribute to atherogenesis and arterial aging (Lin et al. 2009).

Moreover, there is increasing evidence implicating inflammasome activation in the development of heart disease. Although vascular tissues and the heart were found to express fewer members of the NLR family compared to tissues associated with immunity, inflammasome and NLR upregulation is inducible in these tissues (Yin et al. 2009). The atherogenic role of IL-1β and IL-18 is well established; however, there are conflicting reports regarding the contribution of NLRP3 inflammasome activation to the pathogenesis of atherosclerosis in different murine models (Duewell et al. 2010; Garg 2011; Menu et al. 2011). Nevertheless, recent studies indicate that genetic ablation of NLRP3 or an important signaling molecule in inflammasomes, the apoptosis-associated speck-like protein containing a caspase recruitment domain (ASC), markedly diminished myocardial ischemia/reperfusion injury in mice (Kawaguchi et al. 2011; Sandanger et al. 2013). Inflammasome activation particularly in cardiac fibroblasts rather than cardiomyocytes appeared to be an important mediator of injury in these studies. However, inflammasome formation also occurred in cardiomyocytes in a murine model of acute myocardial infarction in which it was shown to contribute to the loss of the myocardium and cardiac remodeling (Mezzaroma et al. 2011). ROS production and ATP release from apoptotic cells were suggested to play an important role as DAMPs in these experimental models of sterile inflammation, while uric acid and calcium pyrophosphate crystals could also constitute relevant endogenous danger signals (Garg 2011). Elevated blood cholesterol and high-cholesterol diet are intimately linked to atherosclerosis (De Nardo and Latz 2011). Recent studies have additionally identified cholesterol crystals, which are found to accumulate in atherosclerotic lesions, as NLRP3 inflammasome-activating atherogenic DAMPs (Duewell et al. 2010; Rajamaki et al. 2010). It has also been suggested that cholesterol-induced membrane microvesicles could function as carriers of certain DAMPs which may contribute to age-related cardiovascular disease (Liu et al. 2012). Bacterial PAMPs could perhaps also activate the inflammasome to cause heart disease, such as in the context of periodontitis which is a significant risk factor for atherosclerosis (Garg 2011; Roth et al. 2007). Finally, a synthetic derivative of a bacterial ligand of the NOD1 (or NLRC1) receptor was also demonstrated to promote cardiac dysfunction, fibrosis, and cardiomyocyte apoptosis in mice, common features associated with heart failure (Fernandez-Velasco et al. 2012).

8.4.4 Cancer

Cancer is commonly viewed as a process that originates from cell-autonomous defects, but which evolves as a result of complex microenvironmental factors (Zitvogel et al. 2012). Specifically, cancer cells engage in stimulatory and inhibitory interactions with stromal constituents and can escape from or suppress immunosurveillance mechanisms. A link between a chronic inflammatory microenvironment and carcinogenesis has been established since the nineteenth century; in 1858, Rudolf Virchow noticed that cancer often developed at sites of chronic inflammation (Basith et al. 2012). However, the capacity of innate immunity to fight cancer has also been appreciated for quite some time, since the 1890s, when surgical oncologist William Coley observed spontaneous tumor regressions in some patients who had contracted bacterial infections and demonstrated that repeated administration of crude microbial extracts (known as "Coley's toxin") could promote an antitumor response against different types of cancer (Coley 1894) (TLR ligands were later discovered to account for this antitumor effect (Garay et al. 2007)). It has therefore been postulated that carcinogenesis and tumor progression are either stimulated or restrained by inflammatory or immune processes, respectively. Thus, PRRs, such as TLRs and inflammasomes, have the potential to influence the formation, progression, and, conversely, the treatment of cancer given their contribution to tissue homeostasis and immunity (reviewed in Basith et al. (2012), Zitvogel et al. (2012)).

Numerous forms of cancer have been etiologically linked to local chronic inflammatory processes in which the activation of inflammasomes, as well as various other PRRs, may be implicated. A few examples include the association of inflammatory bowel disease with colorectal cancer, chronic *Helicobacter pylori* infections with gastric cancer, chronic bronchitis with lung cancer, chronic pancreatitis with pancreatic cancer, and papillomavirus infection with cervical cancer (Balkwill and Coussens 2004; Balkwill and Mantovani 2001). A role for augmented IL-1β activity has been described in various experimental models of carcinogenesis, including stomach, breast, and skin cancer (reviewed in Zitvogel et al. (2012)). Tumor-derived IL-1β and IL-18 production can render the tumor stroma carcinogenic by stimulating the production of trophic factors, such as IL-6, and growth factors. This is one mechanism by which the tumor microenvironment provides support to malignant cells. IL-1β and fibroblast growth factor, another mediator whose secretion requires inflammasome-dependent proteolysis, may also play a major role in promoting angiogenesis, tumor growth, and metastasis (Voronov et al. 2003; Zitvogel et al. 2012). Furthermore, NLRP3 inflammasome activation and IL-1β activity have been shown to promote the accumulation of tumor-associated myeloid-derived suppressor cells which can dampen anti-tumor immunity and thereby suppress tumor immunosurveillance (Bunt et al. 2006, 2007; Song et al. 2005; Tu et al. 2008; van Deventer et al. 2010). Notably, dendritic cell-based vaccination against experimental melanoma was more efficient in Nlrp3 knockout compared to wild-type mice (van Deventer et al. 2010). Activation of the NLRP3 inflammasome may also suppress natural killer cell-mediated antitumor responses (Chow et al. 2012). NLR members such as NLRP3 and NLRP6 and the adaptor ASC have certainly been shown to affect the gut microflora and transmission of colitogenic microbiota (Elinav et al. 2011b); however, there are conflicting reports regarding the role of inflammasomes and NLRs in colitis and colitis-associated cancer; the absence of NLRP3 and caspase 1 has been shown to attenuate experimental colitis in mice (Bauer et al. 2010; Siegmund et al. 2001), whereas others have demonstrated enhanced susceptibility to experimental colitis and tumorigenesis in mice lacking NLRP3, NLRP6, NLRP12, ASC, or caspase 1 compared to their wild-type counterparts (Allen et al. 2010; Chen et al. 2011; Dupaul-Chicoine et al. 2010; Normand et al. 2011; Zaki et al. 2010a, 2011). Furthermore, bone marrow reconstitution experiments revealed that NLRP3 expression in hematopoietic cells was oncosuppressive, whereas its expression in intestinal epithelial or stromal cells did not exert similar function (Allen et al. 2010). NLRP3 and NLRP6 have, however, been shown to be important in maintaining epithelial membrane integrity and homeostasis, thus protecting against colitis and associated tumorigenesis (Normand et al. 2011; Zaki et al. 2010a), a phenomenon in which the inflammasome substrate IL-18 may play a major role (Zaki et al. 2010b; Zitvogel et al. 2012).

A major cell-autonomous hallmark of cancer is that tumor cells escape from or are resistant to programmed cell death, such as that mediated by apoptosis or programmed necrosis (Zitvogel et al. 2012). Classical inflammasomes involving the adaptor ASC and either NLRs (most commonly NLRP3) or the cytoplasmic DNA receptor AIM2 can also induce a form of cell death referred to as "pyroptosis" which is characterized by activation of caspase 1 and secretion of IL-1β and IL-18, hence precipitating local inflammation, unlike classical apoptosis (Fernandes-Alnemri et al. 2009; Hornung et al. 2009; Rathinam et al. 2010). Pyroptosis may also be induced by an ASC-independent, NLRC4-dependent pathway (Miao et al. 2010). Though primarily described to play a role in killing bacterially infected macrophages, pyroptosis has been postulated to potentially contribute to cell-autonomous tumor suppression, a mechanism which may be compromised in specific forms of cancer. This is supported by the observed down-regulation of caspase 1 in human prostate cancers (Winter et al. 2001), as well as animal studies indicating resistance to apoptosis and enhanced proliferation of colon epithelial cells from caspase 1- or Nlrc4-deficient mice compared to their wild-type counterparts (Hu et al. 2010). There are also reports that Nlrp3 or Nlrc4 knockout mice are more susceptible to colitis-associated experimental colon cancer (Allen et al. 2010; Hu et al. 2010).

The transformation of normal melanocytes to malignant melanoma cells results from an accumulation of genetic alterations, most frequently in chromosomes 1, 6, and 9. Interestingly, the introduction of a normal copy of human chromosome 6 suppressed the tumorigenicity or metastasis of melanoma cell lines and permitted the identification of novel genes that were differentially expressed in association with chromosome 6-mediated suppression (DeYoung et al. 1997; Ray et al. 1996). An overexpressed gene located on chromosome 1 whose expression was found to coincide with tumor regression was thus isolated and cloned (DeYoung et al. 1997). The gene, which shared homology with the gene for interferon-inducible protein

16 (IFI16), was named "Absent in Melanoma 2" (AIM2). A subsequent study determined that the overexpression of AIM2 retarded the proliferation of murine fibroblasts, thus confirming the growth-inhibitory effects of this protein (Choubey et al. 2000). AIM2 has since been shown to suppress human breast cancer cell proliferation *in vitro* and mammary tumor growth in a murine model (Chen et al. 2006a). A high frequency of frameshift mutations in the AIM2 gene, as well as promoter hypermethylation, have been detected in colorectal tumors, indicating that inactivation of AIM2 by genetic and epigenetic mechanisms is frequent in colorectal cancers (Woerner et al. 2007). AIM2 and IFI16 have only very recently been recognized to function as intracellular DNA-sensing PRRs that are important in immunity against cytosolic bacteria and DNA viruses and which induce inflammasome formation and type I IFN production, respectively (Fernandes-Alnemri et al. 2009; Hornung et al. 2009; Rathinam et al. 2010; Unterholzner et al. 2010). It is noteworthy that an estimated 15 % of all human cancers worldwide may be attributed to viruses, particularly DNA viruses (Liao 2006). Additionally, a number of human and viral proteins with oncogenic potential such as the antiapoptotic proteins, Bcl-2 and Bcl-x_L, or the Kaposi sarcoma virus protein Orf63 are known to interact with members of the NLR family (NLRP1 and NLRP3) (reviewed in Zitvogel et al. (2012)), while IFI16 interacts with and is upregulated by the tumor suppressor p53 (Johnstone et al. 2000; Song et al. 2008). IFI16 expression is higher in old compared to young human fibroblasts (as is AIM2 expression), is induced by DNA-damaging agents or oxidative stress, augments p53 transcriptional activity, and is associated with cellular senescence-mediated cell growth arrest (Duan et al. 2011b; Gugliesi et al. 2005; Song et al. 2008, 2010; Xin et al. 2003, 2004). Furthermore, IFI16 was shown to constitutively bind to the BRCA1 breast cancer tumor suppressor, and its subcellular localization depended on BRCA1 (Aglipay et al. 2003). These proteins were crucial to the p53-mediated apoptosis caused by damaged DNA. Immunocytochemical and histological analyses of breast cancer cell lines and specimens revealed that IFI16 levels are frequently attenuated, supporting the notion that loss of IFI16 expression is associated with tumor development (Aglipay et al. 2003; Choubey et al. 2008). Lastly, in human prostate cancer cell lines, IFI16 protein expression was also lower than normal, or undetectable, and its overexpression inhibited cell growth (Xin et al. 2003). The loss of IFI16 expression in malignant prostate epithelial cells could be attributed to histone deacetylase-dependent transcriptional silencing of the IFI16 gene (Alimirah et al. 2007), suggesting that epigenetic regulation of IFI16 may contribute to the development of prostate cancer and may additionally influence the variable constitutive and IFN-inducible expression of IFI16 among different individuals (Choubey et al. 2008). In conclusion, both AIM2 and IFI16 possess oncosuppressive activity. Additionally, IFI16 augments autophagy and cell death triggered by glucose restriction, suggesting that reduction or loss of IFI16 expression may provide a survival advantage for cancer cells in microenvironments with low glucose levels (Duan et al. 2011a). Oxidative DNA damage which is a key factor in cellular senescence can also activate the AIM2-like receptors (ALRs). However, enhanced expression of both AIM2 and IFI16 was detected in oral squamous cell tumors, which augmented tumorigenesis in the p53-deficient cells (Kondo et al. 2012). Interestingly, in the presence of wild-type p53, co-expression of the receptors had the opposite effect and suppressed cell growth. Recent studies also indicate that IFI16 can itself interact with ASC and pro-caspase 1, forming a functional inflammasome in response to certain viruses, including the Kaposi sarcoma-associated herpesvirus, a DNA virus etiologically linked to Kaposi sarcoma, an angioproliferative tumor of the skin (Johnson et al. 2013; Kerur et al. 2011). However, IFI16 has also been reported to suppress AIM2 or NLRP3 inflammasome-induced caspase 1 activation and thus can antagonize IL-1β production (Veeranki et al. 2011). The regulatory cross talk between these ALRs and their significance in tumor development continues to be investigated.

Beyond AIM2 and IFI16, it remains to be examined whether deficient activation of inflammasomes or DNA-sensing PRRs and whether loss-of-function mutations or epigenetic silencing of their components may contribute to oncogenesis, such as through defective pyroptosis or apoptosis. Notably, that many tumors constitutively produce IL-1β indicates that defective inflammasome activation in cancer cells is unlikely to be a general mechanism of oncogenesis (Zitvogel et al. 2012). Collectively, the contribution of inflammasomes to pro-carcinogenic "sterile" inflammation, production of trophic factors, and promotion of angiogenesis and metastasis versus anticarcinogenic immunity, pyroptotic cell death, and tissue homeostasis remains to be reconciled, and the specific conditions for each of these processes require delineation. As alluded to previously, there is mounting evidence that inflammasome activation and particularly IL-1β are essential in stimulating adaptive immune responses that are important in antitumorigenic immunosurveillance (Zitvogel et al. 2012). Anticancer chemotherapeutics tend to be particularly efficient when they succeed in killing cancer cells through immunogenic cell death, wherein dying cells release tumor antigens which elicit a cytotoxic T cell response that can control the residual disease (Zitvogel et al. 2010, 2011). For instance, ATP release from dying cells constitutes one such immunogenic signal that can trigger the P2RX7 purinergic receptor on dendritic cells causing activation of the NLRP3 inflammasome and generation of IL-1β (Iyer et al. 2009; Martins et al. 2009). This in turn elicits the recruitment and activation of γδ T cells and CD8+ αβ T cells which can attack and eradicate therapy-resistant cancer cells (Ma et al. 2011; Michaud et al. 2011; Sutton et al. 2009). *In vitro* and animal studies indicate that this T cell-mediated anticancer immunity may be very important in enhancing the efficiency of chemotherapy (reviewed in Zitvogel et al. (2012)). Deficiency in P2RX7, NLRP3 inflammasome components (NLRP3, ASC, or caspase 1), or IL-1R renders unresponsiveness in mice to chemotherapy with immunogenic cell death inducers, such as anthracyclines (Ghiringhelli et al. 2009; Zitvogel et al. 2012).

A few studies in humans also support a role for ATP in colorectal cancer as well as metastatic melanoma and breast cancer, while a loss-of-function mutation in P2RX7 that negatively affects IL-1β and IL-18 production by monocytes was associated with reduced efficacy of anthracycline-based adjuvant chemotherapy of human breast cancer (Kunzli et al. 2011; Sluyter et al. 2004a, b; Stagg and Smyth 2010). Finally, a recent study reported increased expression of the NLRP3, AIM2, and RIG-I inflammasomes in Epstein-Barr virus (EBV)-associated nasopharyngeal carcinoma, wherein expression levels correlated with patient survival (Chen et al. 2012). In tumor cells, AIM2 and RIG-I were required for IL-1β induction by EBV genomic DNA and EBV-encoded small RNAs, respectively, while NLRP3 was activated by extracellular ATP and ROS. Irradiation and chemotherapy were shown to further augment NLRP3 and AIM2 activation, while tumor inflammasome-derived IL-1β inhibited tumor growth, enhanced survival in mice, and promoted the infiltration of neutrophils. Lastly, tumor-associated neutrophilia significantly correlated with enhanced survival in cancer patients (Chen et al. 2012). These findings strongly support the therapeutic benefit of ATP-dependent, P2RX7-mediated activation of the NLRP3 inflammasome, as well as nucleic acid-induced inflammasome activation.

Conversely, various inhibitors of IL-1β and its receptor, including ones that have been approved by the US Food and Drug Administration for the treatment of several autoinflammatory diseases, are currently in preclinical and clinical trials to determine their efficacy in the prophylaxis or treatment of inflammation-related cancers (reviewed in Zitvogel et al. (2012)). Small compounds that specifically target the inflammasome, as well as caspase 1 inhibitors, are also in development. Therapeutic efficacy of the recombinant IL-1R antagonist, anakinra, has been correlated with reduced circulating levels of C-reactive protein and IL-6 (Lust et al. 2009). The use of IL-1β inhibitors has also been suggested to perhaps be effective in reducing toxicity or side effects associated with NLRP3 inflammasome activation by specific chemotherapeutics (Zitvogel et al. 2012). Thus, although such inhibitors may interfere with the induction of anticarcinogenic adaptive immune responses by immunogenic cell death inducers, they are still regarded as promising candidates for the inhibition of tumor growth and metastasis. In summary, inflammasomes and their products have pleiotropic and contrasting effects upon oncogenesis in that they contribute to tissue homeostasis, cell-autonomous death of malignant cells, and anticancer immunosurveillance but also stimulate autocrine or paracrine processes that favor carcinogenic inflammation, tumor growth, metastasis, and angiogenesis. Therefore, cancer therapies that aim to inhibit inflammasome activation appear promising but require careful refinement. Moreover, it is unknown whether inflammasome inhibition would abolish the efficacy of established anticancer immunotherapies that employ adjuvants, such as the TLR7 ligand imiquimod and bacterial BCG, or dendritic cell vaccines. Inflammasome inhibitors would thus be contraindicated during chemotherapy or immunotherapy which relies upon activation of anticancer immune responses via inflammasome activation. The epidemiological association between metabolic syndrome, its inflammatory complications that are characterized by augmented activation of the inflammasome, and greater incidence of tumors also supports the notion that inflammasome inhibition could be a viable therapeutic option in these various diseases (Zitvogel et al. 2012).

Like the inflammasomes, TLRs also appear to have a dual role in cancer development. In addition to their primary function of protecting tissues against pathogens, TLRs are important in tissue homeostasis due to their role in regulating injury, repair, apoptosis, and regeneration occurring in response to infectious or noninfectious tissue damage (Ioannou and Voulgarelis 2010). Uncontrolled TLR signaling can provide a microenvironment that supports tumor cell proliferation and immune evasion, whereas impaired TLR function or hyporesponsiveness, such as that associated with aging, could potentially increase susceptibility to and persistence of infection, hence sustaining inflammation which is favorable

to oncogenesis (Basith et al. 2012). Conversely, appropriate TLR activation can augment the anticancer immune response, thereby inhibiting tumor progression. TLRs may therefore participate in the development of inflammation-associated cancers or could alternatively be harnessed in cancer therapy. In contrast to the generally reduced expression of the DNA-sensing ALRs, mostly elevated expression of numerous TLRs has been noted in various tumors and cancer cell lines (reviewed in Basith et al. (2012)). The effect of TLR stimulation varies according to the expression of the receptors as well as the specific type of tumor but generally promotes tumorigenesis by establishing an inflammatory tumor microenvironment that facilitates cell survival and migration, while also suppressing immunosurveillance (Huang et al. 2005; Pikarsky et al. 2004; Vaknin et al. 2008). Activation of the transcription factors, NFκB and Akt, appears to be crucial in this effect, as well as in chemotherapy resistance (Clark et al. 2002; Doan et al. 2009; Pikarsky et al. 2004; Xu et al. 2010). NFκB activation generates pro-inflammatory mediators, antiapoptotic proteins, and pro-angiogenic and remodeling factors, thus promoting resistance in preneoplastic and malignant cells to apoptosis-based tumor surveillance and enhancing tumor invasiveness (Karin 2006) (although in some models, its inhibition can also promote tumorigenesis (Pikarsky and Ben-Neriah 2006)). TLR2, for instance, is highly expressed in human hepatocellular carcinoma (Huang et al. 2012b), breast cancer (Xie et al. 2009) and ovarian cancer cell lines (Zhou et al. 2009), laryngeal (Szczepanski et al. 2007) and intestinal cancer specimens (Pimentel-Nunes et al. 2011), as well as malignant keratinocytes from oral squamous cell carcinoma (Ng et al. 2011). Functional TLR3 expression has also been reported in numerous human cancers, including neuroblastoma, breast adenocarcinoma, and cervical, ovarian, hepatocellular, thyroid, nasopharyngeal, laryngeal, and lung carcinoma (reviewed in Basith et al. (2012)). TLR4 is overexpressed in various forms of cancer and in cancer cell lines, as well (reviewed in Basith et al. (2012)), and is associated with augmented cell survival and invasiveness, suppression of immunosurveillance, and resistance to apoptosis and chemotherapy (He et al. 2007; Huang et al. 2005; Kelly et al. 2006; Killeen et al. 2009; Sun et al. 2012; Szczepanski et al. 2009). Altered expression of TLRs 5, 7, and 9 has also been demonstrated in numerous cancers (reviewed in Basith et al. (2012)). TLR9 expression, for example, is altered in tumor specimens of patients with prostate, breast, brain, or lung cancer, among other cancers, as well as in cancer cell lines (Droemann et al. 2005; Ilvesaro et al. 2007; Ren et al. 2009).

A number of SNPs in TLR genes have been reported to influence susceptibility to cancer or identified as potential candidates in further studies that examine the association of TLR SNPs with cancer risk (reviewed in Kutikhin (2011a, b)). Different SNPs within the TLR1-TLR6-TLR10 gene cluster have opposing effects on the risk of non-Hodgkin's lymphoma (Purdue et al. 2009), and TLR10 gene polymorphisms may also affect the risk of meningioma and breast cancer (Barnholtz-Sloan et al. 2010; Rajaraman et al. 2010). TLR2 gene variants have been associated with increased risk of mucosa-associated lymphoid tissue (MALT) lymphoma (Nieters et al. 2006), follicular lymphoma (Purdue et al. 2009), and gallbladder (Srivastava et al. 2010), cervical (Pandey et al. 2009), gastric (de Oliveira and Silva 2012; Tahara et al. 2007), and colorectal cancers (Boraska Jelavic et al. 2006). TLR4 gene SNPs have also been linked to numerous forms of cancer (reviewed in Kutikhin (2011b)), and some of these associations were confirmed in a recent meta-analysis (Zhang et al. 2013). Whereas TLR9 gene variants may increase the risk of Hodgkin's lymphoma (Mollaki et al. 2009), a TLR7 gene polymorphism was associated with a lower risk of this malignancy (Monroy et al. 2011). Apart from these polymorphisms, the majority of studies have reported no association of TLR gene SNPs with various cancers (reviewed in Kutikhin (2011a)). This is also the case among studies which have screened for polymorphisms of genes encoding proteins that are part of TLR signaling networks (Kutikhin 2011a). However, interferon regulatory factor 3; TNF receptor-associated factors 1, 3,

and 5; and IRAK3 (or IRAK-M) gene polymorphisms have been detected to significantly affect cancer risk (Cerhan et al. 2007; Du et al. 2011; Lee et al. 2009; Rajaraman et al. 2009; Wang et al. 2009b, c; Zhang et al. 2004), although further studies will be necessary to corroborate these findings, particularly in larger studies as well as to determine the penetrance of such gene variants. Individual TLR polymorphisms may influence cancer development to only a modest degree, and future studies may need to examine the role of gene-gene and gene-environment interactions in modifying the effect of TLR SNPs in cancer. Although there is evidence to support that many of the loss-of-function polymorphisms in TLR genes or their signaling components may be linked to cancer by virtue of impaired protective immunity against oncogenic pathogens, such as *Helicobacter pylori*, human papillomavirus, or Epstein-Barr virus, further studies will be necessary to confirm this hypothesis (Kutikhin and Yuzhalin 2012b).

TLR activation in tumors or cancer cell lines typically promotes cell proliferation, production of trophic factors—such as pro-inflammatory cytokines (IL-6, IL-8, and IL-12)—growth factors (TGF-β and vascular endothelial growth factor), and remodeling factors (matrix metalloproteinase (MMP) 9), and, thus, tumor invasiveness and metastasis (Goto et al. 2008; Huang et al. 2005, 2012b; Jego et al. 2006; Szczepanski et al. 2009; Xie et al. 2009). For example, TLR4 or TLR9 ligands increase the proliferation of primary and immortalized prostate epithelial cells (Kundu et al. 2008), and a recent study reported that higher expression of TLRs 3, 4, and 9 in prostate carcinomas conferred an increased susceptibility to biochemical recurrence of the cancer (Gonzalez-Reyes et al. 2011). TLR4-MyD88-dependent signaling was important in ovarian cancer progression and chemoresistance (Szajnik et al. 2009). MyD88, the adaptor molecule through which almost every TLR signals (with the exception of TLR3), as well as the structurally related IL-1, IL-18, and IL-33 cytokine receptors, was also shown to be necessary for chronic colitis and either spontaneous or carcinogen-induced intestinal tumorigenesis in mice (Hoebe et al. 2003; Rakoff-Nahoum and Medzhitov 2007; Tomita et al. 2008). Expression of TLR7 and 8, which recognize single-stranded RNA, was detected in tumor cells in human lung cancer *in situ*, as well as in human lung tumor cell lines in which TLR7/8 stimulation favored tumor development and chemoresistance (Cherfils-Vicini et al. 2010). TLR7 or 9 activation in myeloma cells induces tumor growth and prevents chemotherapy-induced apoptosis (Jego et al. 2006). Furthermore, gradually increasing expression of TLR5 and TLR9 was shown to contribute to cervical carcinogenesis and cell invasiveness (Kim et al. 2008; Lee et al. 2007), while TLR9 overexpression in breast, ovarian, prostate, and lung cancers and stimulation by hypomethylated CpG DNA also augments the migratory capacity and invasiveness of the malignant cells (Berger et al. 2010; Droemann et al. 2005; Ilvesaro et al. 2007; Merrell et al. 2006; Ren et al. 2009). In addition to the factors mentioned earlier, NFκB-regulated antiapoptotic proteins, Bcl-2 and Bcl-x_L, as well as the cellular and X-linked inhibitors of apoptosis proteins, cIAP1, cIAP2, and XIAP, also contribute to TLR ligand-induced resistance of cancer cells to apoptosis and chemotherapy (Cherfils-Vicini et al. 2010; Kelly et al. 2006; Luo et al. 2004). Increased expression or shedding of matrix metalloproteinases (MMP2 and MMP13), cell adhesion molecules (β1 integrin), and chemokine receptors (CXCR7) enhances tumor cell adhesion, invasiveness, and metastasis in response to TLR activation (Harmey et al. 2002; Hsu et al. 2011; Ilvesaro et al. 2008; Ilvesaro et al. 2007; Merrell et al. 2006; Wang et al. 2003, 2012; Xu et al. 2011). Finally, several studies have shown that TLR deficiency in animals or loss of function in tumor cells prevents tumor development. Knockdown or neutralization of TLRs, such as TLR2, TLR4, TLR5, or TLR9, has been shown in several instances to inhibit the survival, growth, and metastasis of various cancers and the associated oncogenic, metastatogenic, and angiogenic mediators (Fukata et al. 2007; Hua et al. 2009; Huang et al. 2012b; Ilvesaro et al. 2008; Park et al. 2011; Xie et al. 2009; Yang et al. 2010). Altogether, there is considerable evidence to support the oncogenic effect of tumor-intrinsic TLR expression.

Furthermore, adoptive transfer of tumor cell lines has also revealed a contribution, or in some cases requirement, of recipient TLR signaling for tumor growth which is enhanced by either exogenously administered or tumor-derived TLR ligands, indicating that TLR activation beyond that which is tumor-intrinsic can additionally contribute to tumorigenesis (Kim et al. 2009a; Luo et al. 2004). For instance, TLR4 signaling in recipient mice was necessary for LPS-stimulated tumor growth in a murine model of cancer metastasis (Luo et al. 2004). The proposed mechanism for this involves the host hematopoietic cell-dependent (or tumor-extrinsic) increase in the circulating levels of TNF-α which then elicits the upregulation of NFκB-dependent antiapoptotic proteins in the tumor cells, such as Bcl-x_L, cIAP1, and cIAP2. Interestingly, tumor-specific ablation of NFκB signaling yielded LPS-induced tumor regression rather than growth (Luo et al. 2004). Furthermore, bone marrow expression of TLR2 in mice receiving lung cancer cells was necessary for the activation of macrophages and myeloid suppressor cells producing TNF-α which specifically amplified tumor metastasis but not tumor growth (Kim et al. 2009a). These studies, as well as others, additionally indicate that the tumorigenic effects of TLR ligands may be due to actions on both tumor cells and accessory or immune cells, such as stromal cells or myeloid suppressor cells, in the tumor microenvironment (Kim et al. 2009a, 2008; Lee et al. 2007). Such mechanisms might also explain the association of systemic low-grade inflammation, or "inflammageing," with the development of cancer. Remarkably, similar effects have also been observed in the context of immunotherapy, wherein TLR9 expression was necessary in either the tumor or the host for effective combination chemotherapy with CpG DNA (Li et al. 2007a).

Hepatocarcinoma is a particularly interesting type of cancer given how many different PRR pathways have been shown to influence its development. Hepatitis C virus (HCV) is an RNA virus which causes chronic infection that can often lead to liver cancer. This virus is capable of evading the RNA-sensing RIG-I receptor-induced immunity (Liu and Gale 2010), whose role in carcinogenesis will be discussed shortly, but can also activate TLR3- and TLR7-dependent signaling which can influence hepatocarcinoma (Gondois-Rey et al. 2009; Imran et al. 2012; Li et al. 2012a; Tanaka et al. 2010; Wang et al. 2009a). Interestingly, TLR2/1 and TLR2/6 heterodimers are activated by HCV-associated proteins (Chang et al. 2007), and recent studies indicate a role for overexpression of TLR2 and TLR4 (Soares et al. 2012) or SNPs of the TLR2 gene in modulating susceptibility to HCV-associated hepatocarcinoma (Junjie et al. 2012; Nischalke et al. 2012). Furthermore, TLR2 was essential in tumor growth accelerated by direct contact of a murine hepatocarcinoma cell line with *Listeria monocytogenes* bacteria or interaction of *Helicobacter pylori* with tumor cells from gastric carcinoma patients (Huang et al. 2007). *Helicobacter pylori*-induced gastritis and gastric carcinogenesis were also associated with higher TLR2 expression and lower expression of TLR inhibitors (Pimentel-Nunes et al. 2013). Peptidoglycan from *Staphylococcus aureus* bacteria also enhances invasiveness of breast cancer cells TLR2-dependently (Xie et al. 2010). Lastly, hepatitis B virus (HBV) is a DNA virus (also epidemiologically associated with hepatocellular carcinoma) whose CpG DNA-mediated activation of TLR9 is important in the virus-induced carcinogenesis of human normal liver cells (Liu et al. 2009). These findings provide further compelling evidence of the PRR-mediated oncogenic properties of infectious agents.

Moreover, numerous studies have established the importance of various TLRs and other PRR families in immune defense against oncogenic pathogens, although no direct link to cancer was necessarily shown (Kutikhin and Yuzhalin 2012b). TLR4, for instance, mediates innate immunity to Kaposi sarcoma-associated herpesvirus (Lagos et al. 2008). Furthermore, it is possible that chronic TLR activation resulting from persistent infection or release of TLR ligands from cancer cells, in addition to contributing to the production of trophic or immunosuppressive cytokines in the tumor microenvironment as mentioned earlier,

could compromise the function of immune cells that are important in tumor immunosurveillance. For example, activation of TLRs (e.g., TLRs 2, 3, and 7) by HCV-associated proteins induces tolerance in human APCs and PBMCs to further stimulation by exogenous ligands of various TLRs and impairs subsequent CD4 T cell immunity (Chung et al. 2010, 2011; Dolganiuc et al. 2006; Gondois-Rey et al. 2009; Qian et al. 2013; Wang et al. 2013a), thus potentially contributing to the persistence of infection as well as suppression of antitumor immunity. Chronic HBV infection also impairs TLR7 and 9 expression and function in PBMCs, including plasmacytoid dendritic cells and B cells, of patients with HBV-associated chronic hepatitis and hepatocellular carcinoma (Vincent et al. 2011; Xu et al. 2012). Whether the virus-induced TLR hyporesponsiveness in PBMCs is comparable to that which has been described in the context of aging is intriguing. Importantly, these observations indicate that oncogenic, immune evasive pathogens may impair TLR function and, furthermore, imply that loss of PRR function, for instance due to gene polymorphisms or age-related immunosenescence, could further enhance susceptibility to oncogenic infectious agents. Therefore, it remains unclear whether oncogenic pathogens take advantage of augmented or attenuated TLR expression and function to promote cancer development. It appears that augmented TLR activation in the tumor microenvironment but reduced TLR function in immune cells would manifest the optimal environment for carcinogenesis.

Moreover, in addition to the described tumor-specific overexpression of TLRs 2 and 4 in HCV-induced hepatocarcinoma and TLR hyporesponsiveness in immune cells, recent studies have shown that TLR2 or 4 deficiency in murine models of genotoxic carcinogen-induced liver cancer augmented susceptibility to hepatocarcinogenesis due to the loss of proteins that are important in DNA repair, as well as due to autophagic dysfunction (Lin et al. 2012, 2013a; Wang et al. 2013b, c). Thus, TLRs 2 and 4 have been shown to maintain DNA repair mechanisms and efficient autophagic control of oxidative stress by regulating the expression of

DNA repair proteins which ensure cancer cell apoptosis. As such, in preventing the dysfunction of autophagy and DNA repair processes by supporting cellular senescence and autophagic flux, TLRs 2 and 4 would additionally be expected to negatively regulate the ensuing pro-inflammatory cascades such as activation of inflammasomes in response to cellular stress or various DNA-sensing PRRs such as TLR9. That TLRs influence DNA repair mechanisms implies that PRRs could potentially play an even more substantive role than was previously appreciated in cellular senescence and homeostasis. Moreover, these studies further support the importance of TLRs 2 and 4 in liver cancer and suggest that their role may differ depending on whether the cancer is virally or chemically induced. Recently, there has also been progress in our understanding of microRNA (miRNA) regulation by TLRs which may be relevant to carcinogenesis. TLR9-enhanced human lung cancer progression *in vitro* or *in vivo* in mice was mediated by miRNA-574-5p-dependent inhibition of the cell cycle transcription factor "checkpoint suppressor 1" (Li et al. 2012b). Expression levels of these molecules in cancer patients were also congruent with such a mechanism. Conversely, TLR9-dependent inhibition of miRNA-7 in human lung cancer cells augments activity of the pro-survival PI3K/Akt pathway (Xu et al. 2013). There is emerging evidence of inhibition of TLR signaling components in infected cells by viral miRNAs, such as that of the Kaposi sarcoma-associated herpesvirus (Abend et al. 2012), although the direct significance of this in relation to carcinogenesis remains to be clarified. To date, one of the most striking findings in this area is the reported activation of murine TLR7 and human TLR8 by tumor-secreted miRNAs which trigger a TLR-mediated pro-metastatic inflammatory response (Fabbri et al. 2012). MiRNAs have been detected in the blood of cancer patients and can serve as circulating biomarkers of cancer (Gibbings et al. 2009; Lawrie et al. 2008; Mitchell et al. 2008). They can be secreted in exosomes from one cell to another and may therefore function as key regulators of the tumor microenvironment by acting as paracrine agonists of TLRs (Valadi

et al. 2007). MiRNAs could potentially also enhance the inflammatory microenvironment of cancer cells by regulating signaling components of the TLR-NFκB pathway (Chen et al. 2008). Therefore, miRNAs could also be an important effector of "inflammageing." Whether this might additionally be a key mechanism in the suppression of antitumor immunity remains to be determined. Interestingly, *in vivo* infusion of miRNAs in murine peripheral blood was actually found to protect against cancer development through the TLR1-NFκB-dependent activation of natural killer cells (He et al. 2013).

An increasing array of endogenous TLR ligands that may be pertinent to oncogenesis and cancer metastasis is being identified. Such ligands could potentially originate from tumor cells themselves, as previously alluded to, and facilitate tumor progression or may be released as DAMPs or alarmins by cells surrounding the tumor microenvironment to alert the host immune system. The extracellular matrix proteoglycan, versican, is upregulated in many human tumors including lung tumors and was identified in lung cancer cell cultures as a factor activating the TLR2/6 heterodimer to induce myeloid cell production of TNF-α. This was specifically crucial to metastasis rather than growth of tumors *in vivo* (Kim et al. 2009a). Other matrix components that activate TLRs 2 and 4, namely, biglycan and hyaluronan, have also been implicated in metastasis (Lokeshwar et al. 2005; Schaefer et al. 2005; Scheibner et al. 2006). More recently, an end product of lipid oxidation, a carboxyalkylpyrrole, was discovered as an endogenous TLR2 ligand which was elevated in tissues of aged mice and promoted angiogenesis in highly vascularized tumors of murine and human melanoma (West et al. 2010). This TLR2 ligand is thus also a potential link between senescence-associated oxidative stress and carcinogenesis. Stimulation of a human lung cancer cell line with TLR9 agonist CpG DNA also dose-dependently increased the expression of the high-mobility group box 1 (HMGB1), a protein involved in an array of biological processes, including gene transcription, DNA repair, cell differentiation, development, and extracellular signaling (Wang et al. 2012). Blockade of HMGB1 abrogated the CpG-enhanced tumor progression. The tumorigenic effects of HMGB1, including MMP2 and 9 upregulation, were also dependent on the TLR4 and RAGE receptors, as well as MyD88. Therefore, there is considerable evidence indicating that endogenous PRR agonists, especially TLR ligands, can contribute particularly to cancer metastasis. Perhaps microbial TLR ligands play an important role in the initial stages of carcinogenesis by causing inflammation which promotes tumor growth, invasiveness, and tissue injury, thereby releasing endogenous TLR ligands as DAMPs which facilitate further tumor progression and metastasis.

In the 1890s, William Coley reported the successful use of bacterial toxins in cancer treatment (Coley 1894). LPS, or the "hemorrhage-producing fraction" of Coley's toxin, was subsequently shown in 1943 to account for its antitumor effects (Garay et al. 2007). Since then, various bacterial components, such as endotoxins/exotoxins, lipoteichoic acid, and DNA, have been recognized to possess potent antitumor activities, in some instances promoting complete tumor regression (Ishii et al. 2003). In recent years, a number of studies have also described antitumorigenic effects of TLR signaling (reviewed in Basith et al. (2012)). Moreover, despite the extensive literature discussed thus far indicating an oncogenic potential of TLR signaling, virtually all existing TLR-targeting immunotherapeutics that are currently in clinical trials for cancer treatment consist of TLR agonists. This is due to the capacity of TLRs to stimulate (i) direct tumoricidal effects and (ii) innate inflammatory responses that kill cancer cells, e.g., natural killer cells and neutrophils, or (iii) to serve as adjuvants enhancing tumor antigen-specific immune responses, e.g. T helper 1 cells as well as cytotoxic $CD8^+$ $\alpha\beta$ T cells and $\gamma\delta$ T cells (Brignole et al. 2010; Chew et al. 2012; De Cesare et al. 2008; Huang et al. 2012a; Ishii et al. 2003; Ren et al. 2008; Salaun et al. 2006; Simons et al. 2008; Wang et al. 2006a, b). Animal studies using mice genetically deficient in TLRs have demonstrated protective effects of TLRs 2 and 4 against tumor development; TLR2 knockout mice developed significantly greater numbers and larger tumors than wild-type mice in a model of colitis-associated colorectal cancer (Lowe et al. 2010), while TLR4 deficiency exacerbated inflammation-mediated lung cancer elicited by chemical carcinogenesis (Bauer et al. 2005). Stimulation of human primary cancer cells or cell lines with poly(I:C), a synthetic double-stranded RNA which can trigger TLR3, RNA-activated protein kinase, as well as RLR activation, induces apoptosis and direct killing of tumor and ancillary cells, such as vascular endothelial cells in the tumor microenvironment (Matijevic et al. 2009; Nomi et al. 2010; Salaun et al. 2006). Therefore, TLR3 has also been suggested to have a dual effect upon cancer cells (Matijevic and Pavelic 2011). Poly(I:C)- or imiquimod (TLR7/8-ligand)-treated cancer cells enhance the cytotoxic activity of co-cultured human $\gamma\delta$ T cells (Shojaei et al. 2009), further indicating that tumor-intrinsic TLR activation may also carry antitumorigenic potential, in addition to the oncogenic activity described earlier. The most extensively studied TLR ligand in cancer therapy is the TLR9 agonist CpG oligodeoxynucleotide (ODN), whose antitumor potential has been evaluated in breast cancer, colorectal cancer, lung cancer, melanoma, as well as leukemias and lymphomas (reviewed in Basith et al. (2012) and Krieg (2008)). TLR9 activation can also directly induce apoptosis of cancer cells and enhances antitumor immunity by augmenting dendritic cell and B cell responses (Brignole et al. 2010; De Cesare et al. 2008; Wang et al. 2006a).

Numerous TLR agonists are under development as immunotherapeutic agents, and a substantial number have successfully advanced through preclinical trials, including TLR2, 3, 4, 5, 7, 8, and 9 ligands (summarized in Basith et al. (2012)). Although results from clinical trials have generally been less promising, some TLR agonists have been approved for treatment by the US Food and Drug Administration, such as the *Mycobacterium bovis* BCG vaccine possessing TLR2/4 (and some TLR9) agonist activity, which has been approved for the treatment of bladder cancer (Morales et al. 1976; Simons et al. 2008). Also, monophosphoryl lipid A, a TLR4 agonist with potent immunostimulatory capacity and reduced toxicity compared to the diphosphorylated lipid A-carrying LPS, has been approved as a vaccine adjuvant for cervical cancer, specifically that which is caused by human papillomavirus types 16 and 18 (D'Souza et al. 2007; Rietschel et al. 1987). Imiquimod, the TLR7 agonist belonging to the small-molecule imidazoquinoline family, is the first topical TLR therapeutic approved for the treatment of basal skin tumors (Schon and Schon 2008). TLR7 agonists are believed to act by inducing immunogenic cell death, type I IFN production, and Th1 immune responses (Schon and Schon 2008; Spaner et al. 2010). BCG and imiquimod have also been approved as monotherapies, as opposed to the combination of TLR agonists with chemotherapeutic agents. The TLR9 agonist CpG ODNs, in particular, have shown considerable promise as vaccine adjuvants and monotherapies or combination therapies in early trials (reviewed in Basith et al. (2012)). However, recent clinical trials of TLR agonists have been disappointing, the latest being the phase II failure of Idera Pharmaceutical's immunostimulatory oligodeoxynucleotide-2055 in head and neck cancer (Guha 2012). Other high-profile failures include Pfizer's ODN-based CpG-7909 which was ineffective in combination with chemotherapy in phase III trials in non-small cell lung cancer (Guha 2012). Although experts in the field are lacking optimism that TLR agonists will prove successful as monotherapies, the belief remains that TLRs would be promising as vaccine adjuvants or when combined with immunogenic cell death-inducing agents (Guha 2012). Indeed most TLR agonists currently in clinical trials are formulated in such a manner, although in many of the failed trials the TLR agonists had been combined with chemotherapy or a targeted anticancer agent. Moreover, there is uncertainty regarding the choice and dosage of TLR agonists and which specific tumor antigens, chemotherapies, or anticancer drugs to combine them with for the generation of maximal antitumor immune responses while limiting toxicity.

There are also those who have questioned whether the rapidly growing metastatic tumors in which most novel anticancer drugs are initially investigated are an appropriate setting for testing TLR agonists, given that such cancers are likely to involve multiple immune evasive mechanisms and TLR immunotherapeutics have thus far been unsuccessful in the treatment of metastatic malignancies (Guha 2012). That TLR agonists have been found to sometimes drive tumorigenesis in preclinical models is also a potentially confounding issue, although such effects have not been observed directly in the clinic. Furthermore, the differential expression and function of certain TLRs in humans and mice may also be a factor in the failure of certain TLR agonists to treat human cancer. This might be overcome using ligands that target TLRs which are more highly expressed in humans or which induce more potent immune responses in human cells, such as agonists of TLR3 or TLR8, which may be capable of inducing greater T cell responses than TLR7 or 9 agonists (Gorden et al. 2006; Guha 2012). Simultaneous targeting of different TLRs or TLRs and other PRRs, such as the CLR dectin receptors or the NLR NAIP5 (neuronal apoptosis inhibitor protein 5), is being tested in order to determine whether the combined activation of multiple TLR or PRR signaling pathways could boost anticancer immunity (Dzopalic et al. 2012; Garaude and Blander 2012). Finally, tumor-derived immunosuppressive mechanisms are a major hurdle for TLR agonists to overcome, and it is possible that TLR ligands may thus need to be combined with agents that counteract such factors. However, TLRs themselves also stimulate negative feedback mechanisms to prevent uncontrolled inflammation. One example is the anti-inflammatory IL-10 cytokine production elicited by imiquimod, the blockade of which enhanced the efficacy of this TLR ligand (Lu et al. 2010). Similarly, administration of a PI3K inhibitor suppressed the IL-10 and TGF-β activity induced by the TLR5 ligand flagellin in preclinical trials (Marshall et al. 2012), while the inhibitory costimulatory molecule CTLA-4 is also being examined as a viable target for overcoming tumor-mediated immunosuppression (Egen et al. 2002; Leach et al. 1996; Sotomayor et al. 1999; Wolchok et al. 2013). Moreover, though TLR ligands augment anticancer immune responses in part by relieving regulatory T cell suppressive activity in the tumor microenvironment (Peng et al. 2005; Sharma et al. 2010; Zhang et al. 2011), repeated administration of various TLR agonists can promote counterproductive myeloid suppressor cell-mediated inhibition of natural killer and T cell responses (Cohen et al. 2012; Dang et al. 2012; Vaknin et al. 2008). Therefore, although TLR agonists may acutely enhance anticancer immunity, their long-term use is undetermined. Moreover, the challenge posed by the therapeutic antagonism of immunoregulatory processes is the risk of excessive immune reactions. Given the dual nature of TLRs in cancer, a major outstanding question is distinguishing the difference between the inflammation that drives tumorigenesis and the inflammation that drives tumor regression, particularly as it pertains to specific TLR signaling pathways (Basith et al. 2012).

Finally, studies have shown that additional PRR families, namely, the CLRs and RLRs, are also likely to play a role in tumorigenesis. Certain CLRs and RLRs are known to recognize PAMPs of oncogenic infectious agents (Kutikhin and Yuzhalin 2012a). Moreover, there is some, albeit very limited and preliminary, evidence supporting the hypothesis that inherited genetic variants of these receptors may be associated with increased cancer risk, keeping in mind that this area of oncogenomics is still in its nascency (Kutikhin and Yuzhalin 2012a, b; Lu et al. 2013; Moumad et al. 2013). The CLRs are a family of transmembrane carbohydrate-binding receptors that recognize pathogens as well as endogenous glycoproteins (Garcia-Vallejo and van Kooyk 2009; Geijtenbeek and Gringhuis 2009). A number of studies have demonstrated that at least some CLRs elicit anti-inflammatory or immunosuppressive responses, supporting the possibility that pathogens may exploit this property to overcome innate immune defenses and survive within the host and, furthermore, that tumors may release endogenous ligands of CLRs which facilitate immunosuppression (Allavena et al. 2010; Geijtenbeek and Gringhuis 2009). Tumor-associated macrophages isolated from human ovarian carcinoma or cell lines were shown to express a number of CLRs, the most abundant of which is the mannose receptor.

Engagement and activation of this receptor by tumor-derived mucins (which are known to be heavily glycosylated) modulated the phenotype of tumor-associated macrophages towards an immune-suppressive profile (Allavena et al. 2010). Mannose receptor activation by tumor-released mannose residue-containing glycolipids has also been shown to induce the polarization of immune-suppressive tumor-associated macrophages (Dangaj et al. 2011). Recent studies have shown that RLR signaling and IFN-β mediate protection against experimental colitis and colitis-associated cancer and contribute to gastrointestinal homeostasis (Gonzalez-Navajas et al. 2012; Li et al. 2011; Wang et al. 2007). Furthermore, the endoribonuclease RNAse-L is a type I IFN-regulated enzyme that produces RNA agonists of RLRs and functions in antiviral, antibacterial, and antiproliferative activities (Malathi et al. 2007). A newly published study demonstrated that RNAse-L deficiency exacerbates experimental colitis and colitis-associated cancer and that the RNAse-L-mediated production of IFN-β in response to bacterial RNA may be an important protective mechanism against gastrointestinal inflammatory disease and malignancy (Long et al. 2013). These findings indicate a protective role of RLR signaling in cancer. Furthermore, RIG-I expression is elevated in head and neck squamous cell carcinoma, and it was recently reported that RIG-I activation by low-dose viral dsRNA augmented tumor cell proliferation, invasion, and metastasis, whereas a high dose of this RIG-I ligand triggered cell apoptosis (Hu et al. 2013). This indicates an agonist dose-dependent bimodal effect of RLR signaling in cancer with higher levels of activation promoting antitumorigenic activity. Another study assessing the contribution of the TLR3/TRIF or the RLR, MDA5/MAVS, pathways in antitumor immunity elicited by RNA adjuvants determined that systemic activation of the MAVS pathway was required for robust cytokine and type I IFN production, whereas TRIF signaling is important for the maturation of dendritic cells and subsequent effector responses, including natural killer cell and cytotoxic T lymphocyte responses (Seya et al. 2013). The authors concluded, however, that TLR3-targeting RNA duplexes were effective in cancer immunotherapy, even in the absence of RLR signaling. Interestingly, a novel therapeutic approach to cancer, termed "virotherapy," utilizes the capacity of naturally occurring and engineered oncolytic viruses to selectively infect and cause cytotoxicity to tumor cells without affecting healthy cells (Patel and Kratzke 2013; Russell et al. 2012). However, the tumor selectivity and efficacy of such viruses, like the Newcastle disease virus, depend on a reduced antiviral IFN-α response in tumor cells and, effectively, reduced expression of RLRs (specifically RIG-I) (Biswas et al. 2012; Elankumaran et al. 2010; Fournier et al. 2012b). In contrast, the Newcastle disease virus is a potent inducer of IFN-β and pro-inflammatory cytokines in dendritic cells and Tregs and is therefore believed to mediate antitumor immunity not only via its oncolytic activity but also by promoting effector T cell responses and additionally blunting Treg activity (Fournier et al. 2012a). Both of the latter effects appear to rely on RLR signaling in these immune cells, given that RLRs are important for the production of the mentioned virus-induced mediators in dendritic cells and that RLR activation in Tregs inhibits the suppressive function of these cells (Anz et al. 2010; Fournier et al. 2012a). In summary, these findings suggest that reduced expression of RLRs in tumor cells facilitates infection and oncolytic activity of this virus, whereas enhanced RLR activation in immune cells would ensure maximal antitumorigenic immunity by promoting effector cell responses and simultaneously counteracting tumor-mediated immunosuppression. Time will tell whether the great potential of RLR modulation in cancer immunotherapy can be realized.

8.4.5 Cognition and Neurodegenerative Disease

TLR expression has been recognized among cells in the brain and central nervous system that contribute to immune homeostasis, namely, microglia and astrocytes, but also among oligodendrocytes, neurons, and neural stem/progenitor cells (NPCs)

(reviewed in Okun et al. (2011)). It has also become evident that TLRs influence the differentiation and proliferation of NPCs and neurons in early stages of human development, in the adult brain, and perhaps during the course of aging. Therefore, TLRs additionally affect neurogenesis and plasticity of the central nervous system. In some cases the cells of the central nervous system, such as microglia, express and signal via the same TLR4 co-receptors (CD14 and MD2) and adaptor molecules (MyD88 and TRIF) as those that are utilized by conventional immune cells. However, other cell types can exhibit more selective signaling via the MyD88- or TRIF-dependent pathways depending on the TLR ligand (e.g. astrocytes) or express an unusual assortment of TLR adaptor proteins, such as MD-1 instead of MD-2, and are not known to signal via either the MyD88 or TRIF proteins (as in the case of neurons) (Bsibsi et al. (2006), Gorina et al. (2011) and reviewed in Okun et al. (2011)). Interestingly, neurons also do not translocate NFκB to the nucleus, transcribe IFN-β, or activate AP-1 in response to TLR3, TLR4, or TLR8 activation (Tang et al. 2007). Therefore, the signaling mechanisms ensuing from TLR activation in neurons remain elusive. However, in NPCs, TLR4 activation can induce both MyD88- and TRIF-dependent signaling, though the downstream effectors are mostly undefined. TLRs 2, 3, and 4 have been shown to differentially affect NPC differentiation and/or proliferation and depending on the stage of embryonic, neonatal, or adult development. This has been demonstrated by TLR or TIR adaptor protein deficiency, by pharmacological inhibition, or by activation of TLRs using PAMPs, thus demonstrating that TLRs can modulate NPC proliferation even in the absence of exogenous stimuli, suggesting the existence of endogenous ligands (Martino and Pluchino 2007; Okun et al. 2011; Zhang and Schluesener 2006). TLR3, 4, or MyD88 signaling suppresses NPC proliferation, whereas TLR2 alters NPC differentiation by preferentially promoting the differentiation of neurons rather than astrocytes (reviewed in Martino and Pluchino (2007) and Okun et al. (2011)). TLR4 has the opposite effect on neuronal differentiation. Similar modulatory effects of these TLRs upon neurogenesis in the adult mammalian brain have also been noted (Rolls et al. 2007). TLR3 and 8 stimulation have additionally been shown to affect neurite growth and therefore the development of neuronal circuits (Okun et al. 2011). Furthermore, cells of the central nervous system, particularly microglia, can be activated via TLRs that facilitate the clearance of bacterial and viral infections of the CNS or by specific systemic infections, suggesting that certain PAMPs may be able to cross the blood–brain barrier to promote neurodegenerative disease (Arroyo et al. 2013; Combrinck et al. 2002; Cunningham et al. 2005; Field et al. 2010; Okun et al. 2011). TLRs 2 and 4 are important in the immune response against cerebral meningitis, while TLRs 2, 3, and 9 protect against herpes simplex viral encephalitis. TLR3 and MyD88 also protect against West Nile virus infection of the brain (reviewed in Okun et al. (2011)).

The involvement of TLRs in neurogenesis, neurite outgrowth, and neuronal survival suggests that they may also influence cognitive function in health and disease (Okun et al. 2011; Rolls et al. 2007). TLR3 deficiency in mice enhances various memory functions, and ligands of TLRs 3, 4, and 9 have also been shown to affect cognitive performance, though it is not clear whether these phenomena are related to developmental effects, neurotoxicity, or effects on synaptic plasticity (Okun et al. 2010; Palin et al. 2009; Sloane et al. 2010; Tanaka et al. 2006; Tauber et al. 2009; Watson et al. 2010). Increased expression and production of various innate immune genes and pro-inflammatory mediators and declining levels of anti-inflammatory molecules have been described during "normal" or physiological aging of the brain (Cribbs et al. 2012; Godbout and Johnson 2004; Ye and Johnson 2001). The expression of numerous TLR genes is also altered in this context, suggesting that TLRs may be involved in both healthy and pathological aging of the brain (Letiembre et al. 2007, 2009). Alzheimer's disease, the most common age-related neurodegenerative disease, is characterized by the accumulation of extracellular fibrillar amyloid β peptide deposits or "senile plaques" on neurons as well as intracellular tau protein

"tangles" within brain regions that are crucial for learning and memory (Mattson 2004; Weiner and Frenkel 2006). Increased expression in the brain, and particularly within amyloid plaques, of TLRs 2 and 7 or TLRs 2 and 4 has been described in murine models or human Alzheimer's disease, respectively (Bsibsi et al. 2002; Frank et al. 2009; Letiembre et al. 2007; Walter et al. 2007). TLR activation in microglia may play a significant role in the clearance of amyloid β from the brain (Reed-Geaghan et al. 2009). *In vitro*, agonists of TLRs 2, 4, or 9 were shown to be capable of promoting such function in microglia (Iribarren et al. 2005; Tahara et al. 2006), while *in vivo* administration of TLR2/4 or 9 ligands also reduces amyloid β accumulation and ameliorates cognitive function in mice (Chen et al. 2006b; Frenkel et al. 2005, 2008; Herber et al. 2007; Iribarren et al. 2005; Lifshitz et al. 2012; Tahara et al. 2006). Furthermore, TLRs 2 and 4 might be required for the activation of microglia by amyloid β itself and amyloid plaques *in vivo*; TLR4 deficiency in mice attenuates the activation of microglia and monocytes by amyloid β, resultant production of pro-inflammatory mediators, and causes a decline in cognitive function (Reed-Geaghan et al. 2009; Song et al. 2011; Walter et al. 2007). Thus, TLR4 was shown not to be necessary for the initiation of β-amyloidosis, but rather contributed to the clearance of amyloid β deposits and preservation of cognitive functions (Song et al. 2011). A recent gene association study also suggests that a loss-of-function SNP in the TLR4 gene is associated with increased susceptibility to late-onset Alzheimer's disease in a Han Chinese population (Wang et al. 2011). In contrast, earlier studies linked the loss-of-function TLR4/-299 SNP with reduced risk of developing late-onset Alzheimer's in Italians (Balistreri et al. 2008b; Minoretti et al. 2006), suggesting that TLR4 activation might sustain the damaging inflammatory environment that is conducive to the disease (in t' Veld et al. 2001; Stewart et al. 1997). Thus, although microglial activation by TLRs (particularly TLRs 2, 4, and 9) may be important in the clearance of protein deposits, it may also mediate damage to the central nervous system (Hoffmann et al. 2007;

Lehnardt et al. 2002, 2003; Li et al. 2007b). Active immunization with amyloid β peptide which is used in immunotherapy to reduce plaque formation in the CNS of Alzheimer's patients but can also promote serious meningoencephalitis was shown to reduce murine cognitive function in a TLR2/4-dependent manner (Vollmar et al. 2010). Furthermore, deletion of the CD14 gene attenuated experimental Alzheimer's disease, namely, amyloid β deposition, plaque burden, and microglial cell numbers (Reed-Geaghan et al. 2010). TLR activation in other cell types, such as in neurons, can also promote neuronal damage and degeneration. Indeed, TLR4 expression in neurons was shown to be important in their response to amyloid β and the resulting neuronal damage (Tan et al. 2008; Tang et al. 2008). TLR2- and, in particular, TLR4-deficient mice are also protected from cerebral ischemic injury or "stroke" (reviewed in Okun et al. (2009)). Furthermore, in multiple sclerosis, the most common demyelinating disease which is characterized by damage to myelinated axons in the brain and spinal cord, TLR2 and TLR8 activation may promote the progression of the disease (reviewed in Okun et al. (2011)). Interestingly, whereas MyD88-dependent signaling is crucial to the development of experimental autoimmune encephalitis (EAE), a rodent model of multiple sclerosis, TLRs 3 and 4 may have a protective role (Marta et al. 2008; Tanaka et al. 2008; Touil et al. 2006). TLR expression is markedly augmented in MS lesions, as well as in the brains of animals suffering from EAE. There is also limited evidence to support that TLR2 and 4 may be important in promoting neuronal repair following injury, specifically remyelination, perhaps via their action on oligodendrocytes (Kigerl et al. 2007). Finally, it is possible that alteration of the physicochemical structure of membrane lipid raft microdomains, or "premature lipid raft aging," described in Alzheimer's patients and in murine models could be a contributing factor to the dysregulation of TLR function in this disease (Chadwick et al. 2010; Fabelo et al. 2012; Martin et al. 2010). In summary, TLRs can influence the development and function of various cells of the CNS in health and disease and have also been shown to mediate the responsiveness of numerous cells to amyloid β. However, both pathophysiological and protective roles have been attributed to TLR function in the context of age-related or autoimmune brain disease, and further studies will be necessary to clarify the contribution of individual TLRs, their signaling pathways and downstream effector molecules, as well as the identity of the ligands that are responsible for their activation.

Recent studies have indicated a potentially crucial role for NLRP3 inflammasome activation in the pathogenesis of Alzheimer's disease. First, Halle et al. demonstrated that fibrillar amyloid β elicits cleavage of caspase 1 and production of IL-1β in microglia and macrophages which is dependent on the NLRP3 inflammasome. Also, microglial accumulation and activation was found to be lower in the brains of ASC- and caspase 1-deficient mice injected with amyloid β (Halle et al. 2008). Furthermore, increased expression of active caspase 1 was demonstrated in the brains of humans with mild cognitive impairment, as well as Alzheimer's disease (Heneka et al. 2013). Mice carrying mutations associated with familial Alzheimer's disease but deficient in either NLRP3 or caspase 1 exhibited reduced activation of IL-1β and deposition of amyloid β in the brain as well as enhanced cognitive function. NLRP3 inflammasome deficiency also altered the microglial phenotype and enhanced the clearance of amyloid β, altogether suggesting that inhibition of the NLRP3 inflammasome may represent a new therapeutic avenue for the treatment of Alzheimer's disease (Heneka et al. 2013). Lysosomal "destabilization" or permeabilization appears to be a key mechanism in the activation of the NLRP3 inflammasome, which could occur upon phagocytosis of amyloid fibrils by microglia (Willingham and Ting 2008). Intralysosomal amyloid β content in neurons is also substantially increased in Alzheimer's disease, to which impaired amyloid β secretion and oxidative stress-triggered autophagy are thought to contribute (Zheng et al. 2009, 2011, 2012). The resultant lysosomal permeabilization leads to neuronal death, though it remains to be investigated whether this is necessarily associated with activation of the NLRP3 inflammasome. On the other hand, there are indications that autophagic capacity is compromised in certain neurodegenerative diseases, such as Alzheimer's, though the consequences of this are yet to be determined (Martinez-Vicente and Cuervo 2007; Nixon and Yang 2011). Using mice deficient in Nlrp3 or other components of the inflammasome (caspase 1 or IL-18), NLRP3 inflammasome activation was also found to be an important contributor to CNS inflammation, neuronal demyelination, and oligodendrocyte loss in experimental autoimmune encephalitis (Gris et al. 2010; Jha et al. 2010). Finally, age-related cognitive decline in rats was correlated with heightened hippocampal NLRP1 inflammasome activation (Mawhinney et al. 2011), while inhibition of the NLRP1 inflammasome was also shown to be protective in the context of traumatic brain injury (de Rivero Vaccari et al. 2009). Amyloid β oligomers can potentially activate the NLRP1 inflammasome (Salminen et al. 2008), and multiple single-nucleotide variations in the NLRP1 gene were recently associated with Alzheimer's disease (Pontillo et al. 2012). The possible role of other NLR members and PRR families in age-related neurodegeneration remains to be explored.

8.4.6 Macular Degeneration and Retinopathy

Age-related macular degeneration (AMD) is one of the leading causes of blindness in the elderly. A hallmark of early stage AMD is the accumulation of extracellular lipid deposits at the retina, called "drusen," and chronic inflammation (Chen and Smith 2012; Hageman et al. 2001; Mullins et al. 2000). These deposits gradually separate the retinal pigment epithelium from the underlying choroidal vascular bed which provides oxygen and nutrients to photoreceptors. Disruption of the epithelial-choroid interface by drusen results in degeneration of photoreceptors and what is known as "dry" or non-neovascular AMD which is characterized by atrophy of the retinal pigment epithelium. Neovascularization in the form of abnormal leaky blood vessels arising from the

choroid and growing through the disrupted epithelium causes rapid and substantial vision loss, referred to as "wet" AMD (Chen and Smith 2012; Rosenbaum 2012). Innate immune mechanisms are commonly believed to play a major role in AMD, and the relevant PRRs are beginning to be elucidated. For example, advanced glycation end products (AGEs) and their receptors (RAGEs) are found at high levels within drusen deposits and have been postulated to contribute to the abundant oxidative stress, apoptosis, and lipofuscin accumulation that occurs in AMD (Glenn et al. 2009; Yamada et al. 2006). Stimulation of retinal pigment epithelial cells by AGEs induces the expression of numerous pro-inflammatory mediators which could contribute to the pathogenesis of AMD (Lin et al. 2013b). Interestingly, two recent studies implicated the NLRP3 inflammasome in macular degeneration. One study described the activation of the inflammasome by drusen isolates from the eyes of AMD donors or known drusen components, the complement factor C1q, and the protein carboxyethylpyrrole, a lipid oxidation product (Doyle et al. 2012). Another group corroborated the activation of the NLRP3 inflammasome in patients with AMD but used an RNA motif known as an *Alu* repeat which may also be relevant to the pathogenesis of AMD to activate the inflammasome in murine and tissue culture studies (Tarallo et al. 2012). The former study suggested that NLRP3 inflammasome activation in myeloid cells inhibits choroidal neovascularization and thus protects against "wet" AMD, whereas the latter one suggested that activation of this inflammasome in the retinal pigment epithelium causes its atrophy and thus promotes "dry" AMD. The two studies also arrived at opposite conclusions regarding the role of inflammasome-produced IL-18 in AMD. The study by Doyle et al. suggests that innate immunity in the form of NLRP3 inflammasome activation may be beneficial in preventing the progression of dry to wet AMD (Doyle et al. 2012). However, taken together, the two studies present challenges to therapies that aim to target the NLRP3 inflammasome. Stimulation of a retinal pigment epithelial cell line with the lipid peroxidation product, 4-HNE, also triggers NLRP3 inflammasome activation, further supporting that oxidative stress and its associated endogenous danger signals contribute to AMD pathology by promoting epithelial lysosomal destabilization and resultant inflammasome-mediated pyroptosis (Kauppinen et al. 2012; Tseng et al. 2013).

8.5   Vaccination of the Elderly

TLR dysfunction has been shown to impede immune responses of aged subjects to vaccines (Kollmann et al. 2012; Van and Shaw 2007). Reduced cytokine production in response to TLR1/2, TLR2/6, TLR3, TLR5, or TLR8 ligands in mDCs, as well as TLR7 or TLR9 ligands in pDCs, was associated with diminished antibody responses to a trivalent influenza vaccine in old compared to young adults (Panda et al. 2010), as was TLR-induced B7 costimulatory molecule expression in human monocytes (Van et al. 2007a). These studies therefore suggested that TLR function in antigen-presenting cells is predictive of influenza vaccine responses in the elderly. On the other hand, higher IL-10 production in response to LPS, possibly indicative of skewed TLR4 signaling, was associated with a reduced antibody response to an influenza vaccine (Corsini et al. 2006). It is not clear whether TLR dysfunction is also relevant to the suboptimal efficacy of pneumococcal polysaccharide vaccines in older individuals (Van and Shaw 2007). Therefore, it may be necessary to specially tailor vaccines for the elderly population such that they target individual PRRs whose function is intact or even augmented in aging, or activate multiple PRR families in concert, to enable enhanced immunostimulatory capacity in this poorly responsive demographic. For example, elevated TLR5 expression and responsiveness in the elderly has been proposed as a potential avenue for enhancing immune responses in older individuals, and the inclusion of TLR5 ligand, flagellin, in influenza vaccines has indeed shown early promise (Huleatt et al. 2008; Qian et al. 2012; Skountzou et al. 2010). A recent study also indicated that adjuvants targeting TLR3

(poly(I:C)) or the NLRP3 inflammasome (alum) could enhance the efficacy of an influenza vaccine in aged mice (Schneider-Ohrum et al. 2011). Poly(I:C) was also shown to enhance T cell helper activity, thereby augmenting B cell differentiation and expansion and immunoglobulin affinity maturation (Maue et al. 2009). Another study demonstrated that various TLR ligands (TLR1/2, TLR3, or TLR9) were capable of activating DCs such that certain age-associated defects in CD4+ T cell responses could be ameliorated (Jones et al. 2010). TLR9 agonists have also been shown to be effective as adjuvants in restoring adaptive immune responses in the elderly (Sen et al. 2006; Sharma et al. 2008). Finally, it is not clear whether age-associated aberrations in other PRR families may also influence vaccine responses in the elderly.

Conclusions

The influence of immunosenescence on innate immune responses and particularly the function of PRRs deserves greater attention given its potential to substantially impact the health of a growing population of aging individuals and, consequently, the health policies directed towards this demographic. The expression and function of various TLRs and the adaptor molecules that transduce their signals is known to decrease in the aging population and is perhaps directly associated with reduced responsiveness of the immune system to vaccination and increased susceptibility to infectious disease, as well as the emergence of other health disorders in the elderly. Amplification of constitutive PRR signaling by infectious or noninfectious agents may be a major contributing factor towards the elevated basal inflammatory status or "inflammageing" that is associated with aging and various age-related disorders such as cancer and cardiovascular disease, whereas age-associated dysfunction of processes associated with cellular homeostasis such as autophagy and DNA repair may also contribute to persistent PRR activation, such as in the case of neurodegenerative disease. Moreover, chronic inflammation and PRR activation may actually be the driving force behind impaired responsiveness of inflammatory cells, such as monocytes and dendritic cells, from aged individuals to certain types of PRR ligands, such as TLR agonists. It remains to be confirmed, however, whether the age-associated decline in TLR function in PBMCs is the cause or result of inflammageing due to the activation of compensatory innate immune mechanisms or dampening of TLR signaling, respectively. Defining the role of PRR families other than the TLRs in immunosenescence may help to reconcile these observations and advance the selection and design of appropriate therapeutic countermeasures to overcome the age-associated dampening or dysregulation of PRR responses. In this regard, the past few years have seen an emergence in data suggesting that inflammasome activation may be a central component underlying age-associated systemic inflammation and disease pathogenesis, upon which numerous PRR pathways, including those of the TLRs, NLRs, and ALRs appear to converge. The NLRP3 inflammasome, in particular, could perhaps be the most promising target of novel therapeutics aimed at resolving age-associated diseases. It is also very likely that with time, the recently discovered RNA- and DNA-sensing PRRs will be found to play a prominent role in age-related diseases in addition to the TLRs and NLRs. The study of PRRs in age-related diseases will continue to broaden our understanding of their diverse functions that extend beyond immunity and encompass the regulation of cellular senescence and tissue homeostasis. A vast number of endogenous ligands of PRRs have also been discovered and many more are likely to follow. The priority of future research endeavors is likely to be the delineation of the specific mechanisms and pathways leading to the dysregulation of PRR responses in the elderly, the endogenous or exogenous ligands that engage the implicated PRR pathways in the context of each disease, the discrete signaling events that are triggered, and the selection of appropriate therapeutic options. Nevertheless, PRRs serve the fundamental purpose of maintaining immunity and health by recognizing microbial components, and a major challenge facing the scientific community is to determine the specificity and degree of inhibition or stimulation of various PRRs that effectively ameliorates age-associated disease without jeopardizing immune defenses or conversely triggering excessive inflammatory reactions.

References

Abend JR, Ramalingam D, Kieffer-Kwon P, Uldrick TS, Yarchoan R, Ziegelbauer JM (2012) Kaposi's sarcoma-associated herpesvirus microRNAs target IRAK1 and MYD88, two components of the toll-like receptor/interleukin-1R signaling cascade, to reduce inflammatory-cytokine expression. J Virol 86(21):11663–11674

Aglipay JA, Lee SW, Okada S, Fujiuchi N, Ohtsuka T, Kwak JC, Wang Y, Johnstone RW, Deng C, Qin J, Ouchi T (2003) A member of the Pyrin family, IFI16, is a novel BRCA1-associated protein involved in the p53-mediated apoptosis pathway. Oncogene 22(55):8931–8938

Agrawal A, Agrawal S, Cao JN, Su H, Osann K, Gupta S (2007) Altered innate immune functioning of dendritic cells in elderly humans: a role of phosphoinositide 3-kinase-signaling pathway. J Immunol 178(11):6912–6922

Agrawal A, Tay J, Ton S, Agrawal S, Gupta S (2009) Increased reactivity of dendritic cells from aged subjects to self-antigen, the human DNA. J Immunol 182(2):1138–1145

Al-Hertani W, Yan SR, Byers DM, Bortolussi R (2007) Human newborn polymorphonuclear neutrophils exhibit decreased levels of MyD88 and attenuated p38 phosphorylation in response to lipopolysaccharide. Clin Invest Med 30(2):E44–E53

Alimirah F, Chen J, Davis FJ, Choubey D (2007) IFI16 in human prostate cancer. Mol Cancer Res 5(3):251–259

Allavena P, Chieppa M, Bianchi G, Solinas G, Fabbri M, Laskarin G, Mantovani A (2010) Engagement of the mannose receptor by tumoral mucins activates an immune suppressive phenotype in human tumor-associated macrophages. Clin Dev Immunol 2010:547179

Allen IC, TeKippe EM, Woodford RM, Uronis JM, Holl EK, Rogers AB, Herfarth HH, Jobin C, Ting JP (2010) The NLRP3 inflammasome functions as a negative regulator of tumorigenesis during colitis-associated cancer. J Exp Med 207(5):1045–1056

Anz D, Koelzer VH, Moder S, Thaler R, Schwerd T, Lahl K, Sparwasser T, Besch R, Poeck H, Hornung V, Hartmann G, Rothenfusser S, Bourquin C, Endres S (2010) Immunostimulatory RNA blocks suppression by regulatory T cells. J Immunol 184(2):939–946

Arai Y, Hirose N, Nakazawa S, Yamamura K, Shimizu K, Takayama M, Ebihara Y, Osono Y, Homma S (2001) Lipoprotein metabolism in Japanese centenarians: effects of apolipoprotein E polymorphism and nutritional status. J Am Geriatr Soc 49(11):1434–1441

Arnold CR, Wolf J, Brunner S, Herndler-Brandstetter D, Grubeck-Loebenstein B (2011) Gain and loss of T cell subsets in old age–age-related reshaping of the T cell repertoire. J Clin Immunol 31(2):137–146

Arroyo DS, Soria JA, Gaviglio EA, Garcia-Keller C, Cancela LM, Rodriguez-Galan MC, Wang JM, Iribarren P (2013) Toll-like receptor 2 ligands promote microglial cell death by inducing autophagy. FASEB J 27(1):299–312

Atianand MK, Fitzgerald KA (2013) Molecular basis of DNA recognition in the immune system. J Immunol 190(5):1911–1918

Balistreri CR, Candore G, Colonna-Romano G, Lio D, Caruso M, Hoffmann E, Franceschi C, Caruso C (2004) Role of toll-like receptor 4 in acute myocardial infarction and longevity. JAMA 292(19):2339–2340

Balistreri CR, Candore G, Mirabile M, Lio D, Caimi G, Incalcaterra E, Caruso M, Hoffmann E, Caruso C (2008a) TLR2 and age-related diseases: potential effects of Arg753Gln and Arg677Trp polymorphisms in acute myocardial infarction. Rejuvenation Res 11(2):293–296

Balistreri CR, Grimaldi MP, Chiappelli M, Licastro F, Castiglia L, Listi F, Vasto S, Lio D, Caruso C, Candore G (2008b) Association between the polymorphisms of TLR4 and CD14 genes and Alzheimer's disease. Curr Pharm Des 14(26):2672–2677

Balkwill F, Coussens LM (2004) Cancer: an inflammatory link. Nature 431(7007):405–406

Balkwill F, Mantovani A (2001) Inflammation and cancer: back to Virchow? Lancet 357(9255):539–545

Barnholtz-Sloan JS, Shetty PB, Guan X, Nyante SJ, Luo J, Brennan DJ, Millikan RC (2010) FGFR2 and other loci identified in genome-wide association studies are associated with breast cancer in African-American and younger women. Carcinogenesis 31(8):1417–1423

Basith S, Manavalan B, Yoo TH, Kim SG, Choi S (2012) Roles of toll-like receptors in cancer: a double-edged sword for defense and offense. Arch Pharm Res 35(8):1297–1316

Bauer AK, Dixon D, DeGraff LM, Cho HY, Walker CR, Malkinson AM, Kleeberger SR (2005) Toll-like receptor 4 in butylated hydroxytoluene-induced mouse pulmonary inflammation and tumorigenesis. J Natl Cancer Inst 97(23):1778–1781

Bauer C, Duewell P, Mayer C, Lehr HA, Fitzgerald KA, Dauer M, Tschopp J, Endres S, Latz E, Schnurr M (2010) Colitis induced in mice with dextran sulfate sodium (DSS) is mediated by the NLRP3 inflammasome. Gut 59(9):1192–1199

Belderbos ME, van Bleek GM, Levy O, Blanken MO, Houben ML, Schuijff L, Kimpen JL, Bont L (2009) Skewed pattern of toll-like receptor 4-mediated cytokine production in human neonatal blood: low LPS-induced IL-12p70 and high IL-10 persist throughout the first month of life. Clin Immunol 133(2):228–237

Berger R, Fiegl H, Goebel G, Obexer P, Ausserlechner M, Doppler W, Hauser-Kronberger C, Reitsamer R, Egle D, Reimer D, Muller-Holzner E, Jones A, Widschwendter M (2010) Toll-like receptor 9 expression in breast and ovarian cancer is associated with poorly differentiated tumors. Cancer Sci 101(4):1059–1066

Bersani I, Speer CP, Kunzmann S (2012) Surfactant proteins A and D in pulmonary diseases of preterm infants. Expert Rev Anti Infect Ther 10(5):573–584

Bes-Houtmann S, Roche R, Hoareau L, Gonthier MP, Festy F, Caillens H, Gasque P, Lefebvre d'Hellencourt C, Cesari M (2007) Presence of functional TLR2 and TLR4 on human adipocytes. Histochem Cell Biol 127(2):131–137

Biswas M, Kumar SR, Allen A, Yong W, Nimmanapalli R, Samal SK, Elankumaran S (2012) Cell-type-specific innate immune response to oncolytic Newcastle disease virus. Viral Immunol 25(4):268–276

Blasius AL, Beutler B (2010) Intracellular toll-like receptors. Immunity 32(3):305–315

Boehmer ED, Goral J, Faunce DE, Kovacs EJ (2004) Age-dependent decrease in toll-like receptor 4-mediated proinflammatory cytokine production and mitogen-activated protein kinase expression. J Leukoc Biol 75(2):342–349

Boehmer ED, Meehan MJ, Cutro BT, Kovacs EJ (2005) Aging negatively skews macrophage. Mech Ageing Dev 126(12):1305–1313

Bomfim GF, Dos Santos RA, Oliveira MA, Giachini FR, Akamine EH, Tostes RC, Fortes ZB, Webb RC, Carvalho MH (2012) Toll-like receptor 4 contributes to blood pressure regulation and vascular contraction in spontaneously hypertensive rats. Clin Sci 122(11):535–543

Boraska Jelavic T, Barisic M, Drmic Hofman I, Boraska V, Vrdoljak E, Peruzovic M, Hozo I, Puljiz Z, Terzic J (2006) Microsatellite GT polymorphism in the toll-like receptor 2 is associated with colorectal cancer. Clin Genet 70(2):156–160

Bortoluci KR, Medzhitov R (2010) Control of infection by pyroptosis and autophagy: role of TLR and NLR. Cell Mol Life Sci 67(10):1643–1651

Brignole C, Marimpietri D, Di Paolo D, Perri P, Morandi F, Pastorino F, Zorzoli A, Pagnan G, Loi M, Caffa I, Erminio G, Haupt R, Gambini C, Pistoia V, Ponzoni M (2010) Therapeutic targeting of TLR9 inhibits cell growth and induces apoptosis in neuroblastoma. Cancer Res 70(23):9816–9826

Bruunsgaard H, Andersen-Ranberg K, Jeune B, Pedersen AN, Skinhoj P, Pedersen BK (1999) A high plasma concentration of TNF-alpha is associated with dementia in centenarians. J Gerontol A Biol Sci Med Sci 54(7):M357–M364

Bsibsi M, Ravid R, Gveric D, van Noort JM (2002) Broad expression of toll-like receptors in the human central nervous system. J Neuropathol Exp Neurol 61(11):1013–1021

Bsibsi M, Persoon-Deen C, Verwer RW, Meeuwsen S, Ravid R, Van Noort JM (2006) Toll-like receptor 3 on adult human astrocytes triggers production of neuroprotective mediators. Glia 53(7):688–695

Bunt SK, Sinha P, Clements VK, Leips J, Ostrand-Rosenberg S (2006) Inflammation induces myeloid-derived suppressor cells that facilitate tumor progression. J Immunol 176(1):284–290

Bunt SK, Yang L, Sinha P, Clements VK, Leips J, Ostrand-Rosenberg S (2007) Reduced inflammation in the tumor microenvironment delays the accumulation of myeloid-derived suppressor cells and limits tumor progression. Cancer Res 67(20):10019–10026

Burl S, Adetifa UJ, Cox M, Touray E, Ota MO, Marchant A, Whittle H, McShane H, Rowland-Jones SL, Flanagan KL (2010) Delaying bacillus Calmette-Guerin vaccination from birth to 4 1/2 months of age reduces postvaccination Th1 and IL-17 responses but leads to comparable mycobacterial responses at 9 months of age. J Immunol 185(4):2620–2628

Burl S, Townend J, Njie-Jobe J, Cox M, Adetifa UJ, Touray E, Philbin VJ, Mancuso C, Kampmann B, Whittle H, Jaye A, Flanagan KL, Levy O (2011) Age-dependent maturation of toll-like receptor-mediated cytokine responses in Gambian infants. PLoS One 6(4):e18185

Canaday DH, Amponsah NA, Jones L, Tisch DJ, Hornick TR, Ramachandra L (2010) Influenza-induced production of interferon-alpha is defective in geriatric individuals. J Clin Immunol 30(3):373–383

Cani PD, Delzenne NM (2009) Interplay between obesity and associated metabolic disorders: new insights into the gut microbiota. Curr Opin Pharmacol 9(6):737–743

Cani PD, Amar J, Iglesias MA, Poggi M, Knauf C, Bastelica D, Neyrinck AM, Fava F, Tuohy KM, Chabo C, Waget A, Delmee E, Cousin B, Sulpice T, Chamontin B, Ferrieres J, Tanti JF, Gibson GR, Casteilla L, Delzenne NM, Alessi MC, Burcelin R (2007) Metabolic endotoxemia initiates obesity and insulin resistance. Diabetes 56(7):1761–1772

Cani PD, Bibiloni R, Knauf C, Waget A, Neyrinck AM, Delzenne NM, Burcelin R (2008) Changes in gut microbiota control metabolic endotoxemia-induced inflammation in high-fat diet-induced obesity and diabetes in mice. Diabetes 57(6):1470–1481

Caricilli AM, Nascimento PH, Pauli JR, Tsukumo DM, Velloso LA, Carvalheira JB, Saad MJ (2008) Inhibition of toll-like receptor 2 expression improves insulin sensitivity and signaling in muscle and white adipose tissue of mice fed a high-fat diet. J Endocrinol 199(3):399–406

Caricilli AM, Picardi PK, de Abreu LL, Ueno M, Prada PO, Ropelle ER, Hirabara SM, Castoldi A, Vieira P, Camara NO, Curi R, Carvalheira JB, Saad MJ (2011) Gut microbiota is a key modulator of insulin resistance in TLR 2 knockout mice. PLoS Biol 9(12):e1001212

Carvalho BM, Guadagnini D, Tsukumo DM, Schenka AA, Latuf-Filho P, Vassallo J, Dias JC, Kubota LT, Carvalheira JB, Saad MJ (2012) Modulation of gut microbiota by antibiotics improves insulin signalling in high-fat fed mice. Diabetologia 55(10):2823–2834

Casanova JL, Abel L, Quintana-Murci L (2011) Human TLRs and IL-1Rs in host defense: natural insights from evolutionary, epidemiological, and clinical genetics. Annu Rev Immunol 29:447–491

Cedzynski M, Swierzko AS, Kilpatrick DC (2012) Factors of the lectin pathway of complement activation and their clinical associations in neonates. J Biomed Biotechnol 2012:363246

Cerhan JR, Ansell SM, Fredericksen ZS, Kay NE, Liebow M, Call TG, Dogan A, Cunningham JM, Wang AH, Liu-Mares W, Macon WR, Jelinek D, Witzig TE, Habermann TM, Slager SL (2007) Genetic variation in 1253 immune and inflammation genes and risk of non-Hodgkin lymphoma. Blood 110(13):4455–4463

Chadwick W, Brenneman R, Martin B, Maudsley S (2010) Complex and multidimensional lipid raft alterations in a murine model of Alzheimer's disease. Int J Alzheimer's Dis 2010:604792

Chang S, Dolganiuc A, Szabo G (2007) Toll-like receptors 1 and 6 are involved in TLR2-mediated macrophage activation by hepatitis C virus core and NS3 proteins. J Leukoc Biol 82(3):479–487

Charrier E, Cordeiro P, Cordeau M, Dardari R, Michaud A, Harnois M, Merindol N, Herblot S, Duval M (2012) Post-transcriptional down-regulation of toll-like receptor signaling pathway in umbilical cord blood plasmacytoid dendritic cells. Cell Immunol 276(1–2):114–121

Chelvarajan RL, Collins SM, Van Willigen JM, Bondada S (2005) The unresponsiveness of aged mice to polysaccharide antigens is a result of a defect in macrophage function. J Leukoc Biol 77(4):503–512

Chelvarajan RL, Liu Y, Popa D, Getchell ML, Getchell TV, Stromberg AJ, Bondada S (2006) Molecular basis of age-associated cytokine dysregulation in LPS-stimulated macrophages. J Leukoc Biol 79(6):1314–1327

Chen J, Smith LE (2012) Protective inflammasome activation in AMD. Nat Med 18(5):658–660

Chen IF, Ou-Yang F, Hung JY, Liu JC, Wang H, Wang SC, Hou MF, Hortobagyi GN, Hung MC (2006a) AIM2 suppresses human breast cancer cell proliferation in vitro and mammary tumor growth in a mouse model. Mol Cancer Ther 5(1):1–7

Chen K, Iribarren P, Hu J, Chen J, Gong W, Cho EH, Lockett S, Dunlop NM, Wang JM (2006b) Activation of toll-like receptor 2 on microglia promotes cell uptake of Alzheimer disease-associated amyloid beta peptide. J Biol Chem 281(6):3651–3659

Chen K, Li F, Li J, Cai H, Strom S, Bisello A, Kelley DE, Friedman-Einat M, Skibinski GA, McCrory MA, Szalai AJ, Zhao AZ (2006c) Induction of leptin resistance through direct interaction of C-reactive protein with leptin. Nat Med 12(4):425–432

Chen R, Alvero AB, Silasi DA, Kelly MG, Fest S, Visintin I, Leiser A, Schwartz PE, Rutherford T, Mor G (2008) Regulation of IKKbeta by miR-199a affects NF-kappaB activity in ovarian cancer cells. Oncogene 27(34):4712–4723

Chen GY, Liu M, Wang F, Bertin J, Nunez G (2011) A functional role for Nlrp6 in intestinal inflammation and tumorigenesis. J Immunol 186(12):7187–7194

Chen LC, Wang LJ, Tsang NM, Ojcius DM, Chen CC, Ouyang CN, Hsueh C, Liang Y, Chang KP, Chen CC, Chang YS (2012) Tumour inflammasome-derived

IL-1beta recruits neutrophils and improves local recurrence-free survival in EBV-induced nasopharyngeal carcinoma. EMBO Mol Med 4(12):1276–1293

Cherfils-Vicini J, Platonova S, Gillard M, Laurans L, Validire P, Caliandro R, Magdeleinat P, Mami-Chouaib F, Dieu-Nosjean MC, Fridman WH, Damotte D, Sautes-Fridman C, Cremer I (2010) Triggering of TLR7 and TLR8 expressed by human lung cancer cells induces cell survival and chemoresistance. J Clin Invest 120(4):1285–1297

Chew V, Chen J, Lee D, Loh E, Lee J, Lim KH, Weber A, Slankamenac K, Poon RT, Yang H, Ooi LL, Toh HC, Heikenwalder M, Ng IO, Nardin A, Abastado JP (2012) Chemokine-driven lymphocyte infiltration: an early intratumoural event determining long-term survival in resectable hepatocellular carcinoma. Gut 61(3):427–438

Choubey D, Walter S, Geng Y, Xin H (2000) Cytoplasmic localization of the interferon-inducible protein that is encoded by the AIM2 (absent in melanoma) gene from the 200-gene family. FEBS Lett 474(1):38–42

Choubey D, Deka R, Ho SM (2008) Interferon-inducible IFI16 protein in human cancers and autoimmune diseases. Front Biosci 13:598–608

Chow MT, Sceneay J, Paget C, Wong CS, Duret H, Tschopp J, Moller A, Smyth MJ (2012) NLRP3 suppresses NK cell-mediated responses to carcinogen-induced tumors and metastases. Cancer Res 72(22):5721–5732

Chung HY, Cesari M, Anton S, Marzetti E, Giovannini S, Seo AY, Carter C, Yu BP, Leeuwenburgh C (2009) Molecular inflammation: underpinnings of aging and age-related diseases. Ageing Res Rev 8(1):18–30

Chung H, Watanabe T, Kudo M, Chiba T (2010) Hepatitis C virus core protein induces homotolerance and cross-tolerance to toll-like receptor ligands by activation of toll-like receptor 2. J Infect Dis 202(6):853–861

Chung H, Watanabe T, Kudo M, Chiba T (2011) Correlation between hyporesponsiveness to toll-like receptor ligands and liver dysfunction in patients with chronic hepatitis C virus infection. J Viral Hepat 18(10):e561–e567

Clark AS, West K, Streicher S, Dennis PA (2002) Constitutive and inducible Akt activity promotes resistance to chemotherapy, trastuzumab, or tamoxifen in breast cancer cells. Mol Cancer Ther 1(9):707–717

Cohen PA, Ko JS, Storkus WJ, Spencer CD, Bradley JM, Gorman JE, McCurry DB, Zorro-Manrique S, Dominguez AL, Pathangey LB, Rayman PA, Rini BI, Gendler SJ, Finke JH (2012) Myeloid-derived suppressor cells adhere to physiologic STAT3- vs STAT5-dependent hematopoietic programming, establishing diverse tumor-mediated mechanisms of immunologic escape. Immunol Invest 41(6–7):680–710

Cole JE, Navin TJ, Cross AJ, Goddard ME, Alexopoulou L, Mitra AT, Davies AH, Flavell RA, Feldmann M, Monaco C (2011) Unexpected protective role for toll-like receptor 3 in the arterial wall. Proc Natl Acad Sci U S A 108(6):2372–2377

Coley FC (1894) A pseudo-hypertrophic family. Br Med J 1(1730):399–400

Combrinck MI, Perry VH, Cunningham C (2002) Peripheral infection evokes exaggerated sickness behaviour in pre-clinical murine prion disease. Neuroscience 112(1):7–11

Corbett NP, Blimkie D, Ho KC, Cai B, Sutherland DP, Kallos A, Crabtree J, Rein-Weston A, Lavoie PM, Turvey SE, Hawkins NR, Self SG, Wilson CB, Hajjar AM, Fortuno ES III, Kollmann TR (2010) Ontogeny of toll-like receptor mediated cytokine responses of human blood mononuclear cells. PLoS One 5(11):e15041

Corsini E, Vismara L, Lucchi L, Viviani B, Govoni S, Galli CL, Marinovich M, Racchi M (2006) High interleukin-10 production is associated with low antibody response to influenza vaccination in the elderly. J Leukoc Biol 80(2):376–382

Creely SJ, McTernan PG, Kusminski CM, Fisher fM, Da Silva NF, Khanolkar M, Evans M, Harte AL, Kumar S (2007) Lipopolysaccharide activates an innate immune system response in human adipose tissue in obesity and type 2 diabetes. Am J Physiol Endocrinol Metab 292(3):E740–E747

Cribbs DH, Berchtold NC, Perreau V, Coleman PD, Rogers J, Tenner AJ, Cotman CW (2012) Extensive innate immune gene activation accompanies brain aging, increasing vulnerability to cognitive decline and neurodegeneration: a microarray study. J Neuroinflammation 9:179

Cunningham C, Wilcockson DC, Campion S, Lunnon K, Perry VH (2005) Central and systemic endotoxin challenges exacerbate the local inflammatory response and increase neuronal death during chronic neurodegeneration. J Neurosci 25(40):9275–9284

D'Souza G, Kreimer AR, Viscidi R, Pawlita M, Fakhry C, Koch WM, Westra WH, Gillison ML (2007) Case–control study of human papillomavirus and oropharyngeal cancer. N Engl J Med 356(19):1944–1956

Dang Y, Wagner WM, Gad E, Rastetter L, Berger CM, Holt GE, Disis ML (2012) Dendritic cell-activating vaccine adjuvants differ in the ability to elicit antitumor immunity due to an adjuvant-specific induction of immunosuppressive cells. Clin Cancer Res 18(11):3122–3131

Dangaj D, Abbott KL, Mookerjee A, Zhao A, Kirby PS, Sandaltzopoulos R, Powell DJ Jr, Lamaziere A, Siegel DL, Wolf C, Scholler N (2011) Mannose receptor (MR) engagement by mesothelin GPI anchor polarizes tumor-associated macrophages and is blocked by anti-MR human recombinant antibody. PLoS One 6(12):e28386

Dasari P, Zola H, Nicholson IC (2011) Expression of toll-like receptors by neonatal leukocytes. Pediatr Allergy Immunol 22(2):221–228

Dasu MR, Jialal I (2011) Free fatty acids in the presence of high glucose amplify monocyte inflammation via toll-like receptors. Am J Physiol Endocrinol Metab 300(1):E145–E154

Dasu MR, Devaraj S, Zhao L, Hwang DH, Jialal I (2008) High glucose induces toll-like receptor expression in human monocytes: mechanism of activation. Diabetes 57(11):3090–3098

Dasu MR, Devaraj S, Park S, Jialal I (2010) Increased toll-like receptor (TLR) activation and TLR ligands in recently diagnosed type 2 diabetic subjects. Diabetes Care 33(4):861–868

Dasu MR, Ramirez S, Isseroff RR (2012) Toll-like receptors and diabetes: a therapeutic perspective. Clin Sci 122(5):203–214

Davis JE, Gabler NK, Walker-Daniels J, Spurlock ME (2008) Tlr-4 deficiency selectively protects against obesity induced by diets high in saturated fat. Obesity 16(6):1248–1255

Davis JE, Braucher DR, Walker-Daniels J, Spurlock ME (2011) Absence of Tlr2 protects against high-fat diet-induced inflammation and results in greater insulin-stimulated glucose transport in cultured adipocytes. J Nutr Biochem 22(2):136–141

De Cesare M, Calcaterra C, Pratesi G, Gatti L, Zunino F, Menard S, Balsari A (2008) Eradication of ovarian tumor xenografts by locoregional administration of targeted immunotherapy. Clin Cancer Res 14(17):5512–5518

De Nardo D, Latz E (2011) NLRP3 inflammasomes link inflammation and metabolic disease. Trends Immunol 32(8):373–379

de Oliveira JG, Silva AE (2012) Polymorphisms of the TLR2 and TLR4 genes are associated with risk of gastric cancer in a Brazilian population. World J Gastroenterol 18(11):1235–1242

de Rivero Vaccari JP, Lotocki G, Alonso OF, Bramlett HM, Dietrich WD, Keane RW (2009) Therapeutic neutralization of the NLRP1 inflammasome reduces the innate immune response and improves histopathology after traumatic brain injury. J Cereb Blood Flow Metab 29(7):1251–1261

Delgado MA, Deretic V (2009) Toll-like receptors in control of immunological autophagy. Cell DeathDiffer 16(7):976–983

Della BS, Bierti L, Presicce P, Arienti R, Valenti M, Saresella M, Vergani C, Villa ML (2007) Peripheral blood dendritic cells and monocytes are differently regulated in the elderly. Clin Immunol 122(2):220–228

Deretic V (2012) Autophagy as an innate immunity paradigm: expanding the scope and repertoire of pattern recognition receptors. Curr Opin Immunol 24(1):21–31

DeYoung KL, Ray ME, Su YA, Anzick SL, Johnstone RW, Trapani JA, Meltzer PS, Trent JM (1997) Cloning a novel member of the human interferon-inducible gene family associated with control of tumorigenicity in a model of human melanoma. Oncogene 15(4):453–457

Diebold SS, Kaisho T, Hemmi H, Akira S, Sousa R (2004) Innate antiviral responses by means of TLR7-mediated recognition of single-stranded RNA. Science 303(5663):1529–1531

Diego VP, Curran JE, Charlesworth J, Peralta JM, Voruganti VS, Cole SA, Dyer TD, Johnson MP, Moses EK, Goring HH, Williams JT, Comuzzie AG, Almasy L, Blangero J, Williams-Blangero S (2012) Systems genetics of the nuclear factor-kappaB signal transduction network. I. Detection of several quantitative trait loci potentially relevant to aging. Mech Ageing Dev 133(1):11–19

Dixit VD (2012) Impact of immune-metabolic interactions on age-related thymic demise and T cell senescence. Semin Immunol 24(5):321–330

Dixit E, Kagan JC (2013) Intracellular pathogen detection by RIG-I-like receptors. Adv Immunol 117:99–125

Doan HQ, Bowen KA, Jackson LA, Evers BM (2009) Toll-like receptor 4 activation increases Akt phosphorylation in colon cancer cells. Anticancer Res 29(7):2473–2478

Dolganiuc A, Chang S, Kodys K, Mandrekar P, Bakis G, Cormier M, Szabo G (2006) Hepatitis C virus (HCV) core protein-induced, monocyte-mediated mechanisms of reduced IFN-alpha and plasmacytoid dendritic cell loss in chronic HCV infection. J Immunol 177(10):6758–6768

Dong B, Qi D, Yang L, Huang Y, Xiao X, Tai N, Wen L, Wong FS (2012) TLR4 regulates cardiac lipid accumulation and diabetic heart disease in the nonobese diabetic mouse model of type 1 diabetes. Am J Physiol Heart Circ Physiol 303(6):H732–H742

Dostert C, Ludigs K, Guarda G (2013) Innate and adaptive effects of inflammasomes on T cell responses. Curr Opin Immunol 25(3):359–365

Doyle SL, Campbell M, Ozaki E, Salomon RG, Mori A, Kenna PF, Farrar GJ, Kiang AS, Humphries MM, Lavelle EC, O'Neill LA, Hollyfield JG, Humphries P (2012) NLRP3 has a protective role in age-related macular degeneration through the induction of IL-18 by drusen components. Nat Med 18(5):791–798

Droemann D, Albrecht D, Gerdes J, Ulmer AJ, Branscheid D, Vollmer E, Dalhoff K, Zabel P, Goldmann T (2005) Human lung cancer cells express functionally active toll-like receptor 9. Respir Res 6:1

Du J, Huo J, Shi J, Yuan Z, Zhang C, Fu W, Jiang H, Yi Q, Hou J (2011) Polymorphisms of nuclear factor-kappaB family genes are associated with development of multiple myeloma and treatment outcome in patients receiving bortezomib-based regimens. Haematologica 96(5):729–737

Duan X, Ponomareva L, Veeranki S, Choubey D (2011a) IFI16 induction by glucose restriction in human fibroblasts contributes to autophagy through activation of the ATM/AMPK/p53 pathway. PLoS One 6(5):e19532

Duan X, Ponomareva L, Veeranki S, Panchanathan R, Dickerson E, Choubey D (2011b) Differential roles for the interferon-inducible IFI16 and AIM2 innate immune sensors for cytosolic DNA in cellular senescence of human fibroblasts. Mol Cancer Res 9(5):589–602

Duewell P, Kono H, Rayner KJ, Sirois CM, Vladimer G, Bauernfeind FG, Abela GS, Franchi L, Nunez G, Schnurr M, Espevik T, Lien E, Fitzgerald KA, Rock KL, Moore KJ, Wright SD, Hornung V, Latz E (2010) NLRP3 inflammasomes are required for atherogenesis and activated by cholesterol crystals. Nature 464(7293):1357–1361

Dupaul-Chicoine J, Yeretssian G, Doiron K, Bergstrom KS, McIntire CR, LeBlanc PM, Meunier C, Turbide

C, Gros P, Beauchemin N, Vallance BA, Saleh M (2010) Control of intestinal homeostasis, colitis, and colitis-associated colorectal cancer by the inflammatory caspases. Immunity 32(3):367–378

Dzopalic T, Rajkovic I, Dragicevic A, Colic M (2012) The response of human dendritic cells to co-ligation of pattern-recognition receptors. Immunol Res 52(1–2):20–33

Dzumhur A, Zibar L, Wagner J, Simundic T, Dembic Z, Barbic J (2012) Association studies of gene polymorphisms in toll-like receptors 2 and 4 in Croatian patients with acute myocardial infarction. Scand J Immunol 75(5):517–523

Edfeldt K, Bennet AM, Eriksson P, Frostegard J, Wiman B, Hamsten A, Hansson GK, de Faire U, Yan ZQ (2004) Association of hypo-responsive toll-like receptor 4 variants with risk of myocardial infarction. Eur Heart J 25(16):1447–1453

Egen JG, Kuhns MS, Allison JP (2002) CTLA-4: new insights into its biological function and use in tumor immunotherapy. Nat Immunol 3(7):611–618

Ehses JA, Meier DT, Wueest S, Rytka J, Boller S, Wielinga PY, Schraenen A, Lemaire K, Debray S, Van Lommel L, Pospisilik JA, Tschopp O, Schultze SM, Malipiero U, Esterbauer H, Ellingsgaard H, Rutti S, Schuit FC, Lutz TA, Boni-Schnetzler M, Konrad D, Donath MY (2010) Toll-like receptor 2-deficient mice are protected from insulin resistance and beta cell dysfunction induced by a high-fat diet. Diabetologia 53(8):1795–1806

Eisenbarth SC, Colegio OR, O'Connor W, Sutterwala FS, Flavell RA (2008) Crucial role for the Nalp3 inflammasome in the immunostimulatory properties of aluminium adjuvants. Nature 453(7198):1122–1126

El MR, El GM, Myer R, High KP (2009) Aging-dependent upregulation of IL-23p19 gene expression in dendritic cells is associated with differential transcription factor binding and histone modifications. Aging Cell 8(5):553–565

Elankumaran S, Chavan V, Qiao D, Shobana R, Moorkanat G, Biswas M, Samal SK (2010) Type I interferon-sensitive recombinant newcastle disease virus for oncolytic virotherapy. J Virol 84(8):3835–3844

Elinav E, Strowig T, Henao-Mejia J, Flavell RA (2011a) Regulation of the antimicrobial response by NLR proteins. Immunity 34(5):665–679

Elinav E, Strowig T, Kau AL, Henao-Mejia J, Thaiss CA, Booth CJ, Peaper DR, Bertin J, Eisenbarth SC, Gordon JI, Flavell RA (2011b) NLRP6 inflammasome regulates colonic microbial ecology and risk for colitis. Cell 145(5):745–757

Erridge C (2009) The roles of toll-like receptors in atherosclerosis. J Innate Immun 1(4):340–349

Erridge C, Samani NJ (2009) Saturated fatty acids do not directly stimulate toll-like receptor signaling. Arterioscler Thromb Vasc Biol 29(11):1944–1949

Esplin BL, Shimazu T, Welner RS, Garrett KP, Nie L, Zhang Q, Humphrey MB, Yang Q, Borghesi LA, Kincade PW (2011) Chronic exposure to a TLR ligand injures hematopoietic stem cells. J Immunol 186(9):5367–5375

Fabbri M, Paone A, Calore F, Galli R, Gaudio E, Santhanam R, Lovat F, Fadda P, Mao C, Nuovo GJ, Zanesi N, Crawford M, Ozer GH, Wernicke D, Alder H, Caligiuri MA, Nana-Sinkam P, Perrotti D, Croce CM (2012) MicroRNAs bind to toll-like receptors to induce prometastatic inflammatory response. Proc Natl Acad Sci U S A 109(31): E2110–E2116

Fabelo N, Martin V, Marin R, Santpere G, Aso E, Ferrer I, Diaz M (2012) Evidence for premature lipid raft aging in APP/PS1 double-transgenic mice, a model of familial Alzheimer disease. J Neuropathol Exp Neurol 71(10):868–881

Favre J, Musette P, Douin-Echinard V, Laude K, Henry JP, Arnal JF, Thuillez C, Richard V (2007) Toll-like receptors 2-deficient mice are protected against postischemic coronary endothelial dysfunction. Arterioscler Thromb Vasc Biol 27(5):1064–1071

Fernandes-Alnemri T, Yu JW, Datta P, Wu J, Alnemri ES (2009) AIM2 activates the inflammasome and cell death in response to cytoplasmic DNA. Nature 458(7237):509–513

Fernandez-Velasco M, Prieto P, Terron V, Benito G, Flores JM, Delgado C, Zaragoza C, Lavin B, Gomez-Parrizas M, Lopez-Collazo E, Martin-Sanz P, Bosca L (2012) NOD1 activation induces cardiac dysfunction and modulates cardiac fibrosis and cardiomyocyte apoptosis. PLoS One 7(9):e45260

Ferreira AV, Mario EG, Porto LC, Andrade SP, Botion LM (2011) High-carbohydrate diet selectively induces tumor necrosis factor-alpha production in mice liver. Inflammation 34(2):139–145

Field R, Campion S, Warren C, Murray C, Cunningham C (2010) Systemic challenge with the TLR3 agonist poly I:C induces amplified IFNalpha/beta and IL-1beta responses in the diseased brain and exacerbates chronic neurodegeneration. Brain Behav Immun 24(6):996–1007

Fischer H, Ellstrom P, Ekstrom K, Gustafsson L, Gustafsson M, Svanborg C (2007) Ceramide as a TLR4 agonist; a putative signalling intermediate between sphingolipid receptors for microbial ligands and TLR4. Cell Microbiol 9(5):1239–1251

Fortin CF, Larbi A, Lesur O, Douziech N, Fulop T Jr (2006) Impairment of SHP-1 down-regulation in the lipid rafts of human neutrophils under GM-CSF stimulation contributes to their age-related, altered functions. J Leukoc Biol 79(5):1061–1072

Fortin CF, Lesur O, Fulop T Jr (2007a) Effects of aging on triggering receptor expressed on myeloid cells (TREM)-1-induced PMN functions. FEBS Lett 581(6):1173–1178

Fortin CF, Lesur O, Fulop T Jr (2007b) Effects of TREM-1 activation in human neutrophils: activation of signaling pathways, recruitment into lipid rafts and association with TLR4. Int Immunol 19(1):41–50

Fournier P, Arnold A, Wilden H, Schirrmacher V (2012a) Newcastle disease virus induces pro-inflammatory conditions and type I interferon for counter-acting Treg activity. Int J Oncol 40(3):840–850

Fournier P, Wilden H, Schirrmacher V (2012b) Importance of retinoic acid-inducible gene I and of receptor for type I interferon for cellular resistance to infection by Newcastle disease virus. Int J Oncol 40(1):287–298

Franceschi C, Capri M, Monti D, Giunta S, Olivieri F, Sevini F, Panourgia MP, Invidia L, Celani L, Scurti M, Cevenini E, Castellani GC, Salvioli S (2007) Inflammaging and anti-inflammaging: a systemic perspective on aging and longevity emerged from studies in humans. Mech Ageing Dev 128(1):92–105

Franchini M, Monnais E, Seboek D, Radimerski T, Zini E, Kaufmann K, Lutz T, Reusch C, Ackermann M, Muller B, Linscheid P (2010) Insulin resistance and increased lipolysis in bone marrow derived adipocytes stimulated with agonists of toll-like receptors. Horm Metab Res 42(10):703–709

Frank S, Copanaki E, Burbach GJ, Muller UC, Deller T (2009) Differential regulation of toll-like receptor mRNAs in amyloid plaque-associated brain tissue of aged APP23 transgenic mice. Neurosci Lett 453(1):41–44

Frasca D, Blomberg BB (2011) Aging affects human B cell responses. J Clin Immunol 31(3):430–435

Frederich RC, Hamann A, Anderson S, Lollmann B, Lowell BB, Flier JS (1995) Leptin levels reflect body lipid content in mice: evidence for diet-induced resistance to leptin action. Nat Med 1(12):1311–1314

Frenkel D, Maron R, Burt DS, Weiner HL (2005) Nasal vaccination with a proteosome-based adjuvant and glatiramer acetate clears beta-amyloid in a mouse model of Alzheimer disease. J Clin Invest 115(9):2423–2433

Frenkel D, Puckett L, Petrovic S, Xia W, Chen G, Vega J, Dembinsky-Vaknin A, Shen J, Plante M, Burt DS, Weiner HL (2008) A nasal proteosome adjuvant activates microglia and prevents amyloid deposition. Ann Neurol 63(5):591–601

Friedman JM (2009) Obesity: causes and control of excess body fat. Nature 459(7245):340–342

Fukata M, Chen A, Vamadevan AS, Cohen J, Breglio K, Krishnareddy S, Hsu D, Xu R, Harpaz N, Dannenberg AJ, Subbaramaiah K, Cooper HS, Itzkowitz SH, Abreu MT (2007) Toll-like receptor-4 promotes the development of colitis-associated colorectal tumors. Gastroenterology 133(6):1869–1881

Fulop T, Larbi A, Douziech N, Fortin C, Guerard KP, Lesur O, Khalil A, Dupuis G (2004) Signal transduction and functional changes in neutrophils with aging. Aging Cell 3(4):217–226

Garaude J, Blander JM (2012) Attacking tumor cells with a dual ligand for innate immune receptors. Oncotarget 3(4):361–362

Garay RP, Viens P, Bauer J, Normier G, Bardou M, Jeannin JF, Chiavaroli C (2007) Cancer relapse under chemotherapy: why TLR2/4 receptor agonists can help. Eur J Pharmacol 563(1–3):1–17

Garcia-Vallejo JJ, van Kooyk Y (2009) Endogenous ligands for C-type lectin receptors: the true regulators of immune homeostasis. Immunol Rev 230(1):22–37

Garg NJ (2011) Inflammasomes in cardiovascular diseases. Am J Cardiovasc Dis 1(3):244–254

Geijtenbeek TB, Gringhuis SI (2009) Signalling through C-type lectin receptors: shaping immune responses. Nat Rev Immunol 9(7):465–479

GeurtsvanKessel CH, Lambrecht BN (2008) Division of labor between dendritic cell subsets of the lung. Mucosal Immunol 1(6):442–450

Ghiringhelli F, Apetoh L, Tesniere A, Aymeric L, Ma Y, Ortiz C, Vermaelen K, Panaretakis T, Mignot G, Ullrich E, Perfettini JL, Schlemmer F, Tasdemir E, Uhl M, Genin P, Civas A, Ryffel B, Kanellopoulos J, Tschopp J, Andre F, Lidereau R, McLaughlin NM, Haynes NM, Smyth MJ, Kroemer G, Zitvogel L (2009) Activation of the NLRP3 inflammasome in dendritic cells induces IL-1beta-dependent adaptive immunity against tumors. Nat Med 15(10): 1170–1178

Giacconi R, Caruso C, Lio D, Muti E, Cipriano C, Costarelli L, Saba V, Gasparini N, Malavolta M, Mocchegiani E (2007) CD14 C (−260)T polymorphism, atherosclerosis, elderly: role of cytokines and metallothioneins. Int J Cardiol 120(1):45–51

Gibbings DJ, Ciaudo C, Erhardt M, Voinnet O (2009) Multivesicular bodies associate with components of miRNA effector complexes and modulate miRNA activity. Nat Cell Biol 11(9):1143–1149

Glenn JV, Mahaffy H, Wu K, Smith G, Nagai R, Simpson DA, Boulton ME, Stitt AW (2009) Advanced glycation end product (AGE) accumulation on Bruch's membrane: links to age-related RPE dysfunction. Invest Ophthalmol Vis Sci 50(1):441–451

Godbout JP, Johnson RW (2004) Interleukin-6 in the aging brain. J Neuroimmunol 147(1–2):141–144

Gold MC, Donnelly E, Cook MS, Leclair CM, Lewinsohn DA (2006) Purified neonatal plasmacytoid dendritic cells overcome intrinsic maturation defect with TLR agonist stimulation. Pediatr Res 60(1):34–37

Gondois-Rey F, Dental C, Halfon P, Baumert TF, Olive D, Hirsch I (2009) Hepatitis C virus is a weak inducer of interferon alpha in plasmacytoid dendritic cells in comparison with influenza and human herpesvirus type-1. PLoS One 4(2):e4319

Gonzalez-Navajas JM, Lee J, David M, Raz E (2012) Immunomodulatory functions of type I interferons. Nat Rev Immunol 12(2):125–135

Gonzalez-Reyes S, Fernandez JM, Gonzalez LO, Aguirre A, Suarez A, Gonzalez JM, Escaff S, Vizoso FJ (2011) Study of TLR3, TLR4, and TLR9 in prostate carcinomas and their association with biochemical recurrence. Cancer Immun Immunother 60(2):217–226

Goossens GH, Blaak EE, Theunissen R, Duijvestijn AM, Clement K, Tervaert JW, Thewissen MM (2012) Expression of NLRP3 inflammasome and T cell population markers in adipose tissue are associated with insulin resistance and impaired glucose metabolism in humans. Mol Immunol 50(3):142–149

Gorden KK, Qiu XX, Binsfeld CC, Vasilakos JP, Alkan SS (2006) Cutting edge: activation of murine TLR8 by a combination of imidazoquinoline immune response modifiers and polyT oligodeoxynucleotides. J Immunol 177(10):6584–6587

Goriely S, Vincart B, Stordeur P, Vekemans J, Willems F, Goldman M, De WD (2001) Deficient IL-12(p35) gene expression by dendritic cells derived from neonatal monocytes. J Immunol 166(3):2141–2146

Gorina R, Font-Nieves M, Marquez-Kisinousky L, Santalucia T, Planas AM (2011) Astrocyte TLR4 activation induces a proinflammatory environment through the interplay between MyD88-dependent NFkappaB signaling, MAPK, and Jak1/Stat1 pathways. Glia 59(2):242–255

Goto Y, Arigami T, Kitago M, Nguyen SL, Narita N, Ferrone S, Morton DL, Irie RF, Hoon DS (2008) Activation of toll-like receptors 2, 3, and 4 on human melanoma cells induces inflammatory factors. Mol Cancer Ther 7(11):3642–3653

Gris D, Ye Z, Iocca HA, Wen H, Craven RR, Gris P, Huang M, Schneider M, Miller SD, Ting JP (2010) NLRP3 plays a critical role in the development of experimental autoimmune encephalomyelitis by mediating Th1 and Th17 responses. J Immunol 185(2):974–981

Gugliesi F, Mondini M, Ravera R, Robotti A, de Andrea M, Gribaudo G, Gariglio M, Landolfo S (2005) Up-regulation of the interferon-inducible IFI16 gene by oxidative stress triggers p53 transcriptional activity in endothelial cells. J Leukoc Biol 77(5):820–829

Guha M (2012) Anticancer TLR agonists on the ropes. Nat Rev Drug Discov 11(7):503–505

Ha T, Hu Y, Liu L, Lu C, McMullen JR, Kelley J, Kao RL, Williams DL, Gao X, Li C (2010) TLR2 ligands induce cardioprotection against ischaemia/reperfusion injury through a PI3K/Akt-dependent mechanism. Cardiovasc Res 87(4):694–703

Hageman GS, Luthert PJ, Victor Chong NH, Johnson LV, Anderson DH, Mullins RF (2001) An integrated hypothesis that considers drusen as biomarkers of immune-mediated processes at the RPE-Bruch's membrane interface in aging and age-related macular degeneration. Prog Retin Eye Res 20(6):705–732

Halle A, Hornung V, Petzold GC, Stewart CR, Monks BG, Reinheckel T, Fitzgerald KA, Latz E, Moore KJ, Golenbock DT (2008) The NALP3 inflammasome is involved in the innate immune response to amyloid-beta. Nat Immunol 9(8):857–865

Hao Y, O'Neill P, Naradikian MS, Scholz JL, Cancro MP (2011) A B-cell subset uniquely responsive to innate stimuli accumulates in aged mice. Blood 118(5):1294–1304

Hardison SE, Brown GD (2012) C-type lectin receptors orchestrate antifungal immunity. Nat Immunol 13(9):817–822

Hardy OT, Kim A, Ciccarelli C, Hayman LL, Wiecha J (2013) Increased toll-like receptor (TLR) mRNA expression in monocytes is a feature of metabolic syndrome in adolescents. Pediatric obesity 8(1):e19–e23

Harmey JH, Bucana CD, Lu W, Byrne AM, McDonnell S, Lynch C, Bouchier-Hayes D, Dong Z (2002) Lipopolysaccharide-induced metastatic growth is associated with increased angiogenesis, vascular permeability and tumor cell invasion. Int J Cancer 101(5):415–422

He W, Liu Q, Wang L, Chen W, Li N, Cao X (2007) TLR4 signaling promotes immune escape of human lung cancer cells by inducing immunosuppressive cytokines and apoptosis resistance. Mol Immunol 44(11):2850–2859

He S, Chu J, Wu LC, Mao H, Peng Y, Alvarez-Breckenridge CA, Hughes T, Wei M, Zhang J, Yuan S, Sandhu S, Vasu S, Benson DM Jr, Hofmeister CC, He X, Ghoshal K, Devine SM, Caligiuri MA, Yu J (2013) MicroRNAs activate natural killer cells through toll-like receptor signaling. Blood 121(23):4663–4671

Heneka MT, Kummer MP, Stutz A, Delekate A, Schwartz S, Vieira-Saecker A, Griep A, Axt D, Remus A, Tzeng TC, Gelpi E, Halle A, Korte M, Latz E, Golenbock DT (2013) NLRP3 is activated in Alzheimer's disease and contributes to pathology in APP/PS1 mice. Nature 493(7434):674–678

Herber DL, Mercer M, Roth LM, Symmonds K, Maloney J, Wilson N, Freeman MJ, Morgan D, Gordon MN (2007) Microglial activation is required for Abeta clearance after intracranial injection of lipopolysaccharide in APP transgenic mice. J Neuroimmune Pharmacol 2(2):222–231

Himes RW, Smith CW (2010) Tlr2 is critical for diet-induced metabolic syndrome in a murine model. FASEB J 24(3):731–739

Hinojosa E, Boyd AR, Orihuela CJ (2009) Age-associated inflammation and toll-like receptor dysfunction prime the lungs for pneumococcal pneumonia. J Infect Dis 200(4):546–554

Hoebe K, Du X, Georgel P, Janssen E, Tabeta K, Kim SO, Goode J, Lin P, Mann N, Mudd S, Crozat K, Sovath S, Han J, Beutler B (2003) Identification of Lps2 as a key transducer of MyD88-independent TIR signalling. Nature 424(6950):743–748

Hoffmann O, Braun JS, Becker D, Halle A, Freyer D, Dagand E, Lehnardt S, Weber JR (2007) TLR2 mediates neuroinflammation and neuronal damage. J Immunol 178(10):6476–6481

Holloway JW, Yang IA, Ye S (2005) Variation in the toll-like receptor 4 gene and susceptibility to myocardial infarction. Pharmacogenet Genomics 15(1):15–21

Hommelberg PP, Plat J, Langen RC, Schols AM, Mensink RP (2009) Fatty acid-induced NF-kappaB activation and insulin resistance in skeletal muscle are chain length dependent. Am J Physiol Endocrinol Metab 296(1):E114–E120

Hornung V, Ablasser A, Charrel-Dennis M, Bauernfeind F, Horvath G, Caffrey DR, Latz E, Fitzgerald KA (2009) AIM2 recognizes cytosolic dsDNA and forms a caspase-1-activating inflammasome with ASC. Nature 458(7237):514–518

Hosoi T, Yokoyama S, Matsuo S, Akira S, Ozawa K (2010) Myeloid differentiation factor 88 (MyD88)-deficiency increases risk of diabetes in mice. PLoS One 5(9)

Hotamisligil GS (2006) Inflammation and metabolic disorders. Nature 444(7121):860–867

Hsu RY, Chan CH, Spicer JD, Rousseau MC, Giannias B, Rousseau S, Ferri LE (2011) LPS-induced TLR4 signaling in human colorectal cancer cells increases beta1 integrin-mediated cell adhesion and liver metastasis. Cancer Res 71(5):1989–1998

Hu B, Elinav E, Huber S, Booth CJ, Strowig T, Jin C, Eisenbarth SC, Flavell RA (2010) Inflammation-induced tumorigenesis in the colon is regulated by caspase-1 and NLRC4. Proc Natl Acad Sci USA 107(50):21635–21640

Hu J, He Y, Yan M, Zhu C, Ye W, Zhu H, Chen W, Zhang C, Zhang Z (2013) Dose dependent activation of retinoic acid-inducible gene-I promotes both proliferation and apoptosis signals in human head and neck squamous cell carcinoma. PLoS One 8(3):e58273

Hua D, Liu MY, Cheng ZD, Qin XJ, Zhang HM, Chen Y, Qin GJ, Liang G, Li JN, Han XF, Liu DX (2009) Small interfering RNA-directed targeting of toll-like receptor 4 inhibits human prostate cancer cell invasion, survival, and tumorigenicity. Mol Immunol 46(15):2876–2884

Huang B, Zhao J, Li H, He KL, Chen Y, Chen SH, Mayer L, Unkeless JC, Xiong H (2005) Toll-like receptors on tumor cells facilitate evasion of immune surveillance. Cancer Res 65(12):5009–5014

Huang B, Zhao J, Shen S, Li H, He KL, Shen GX, Mayer L, Unkeless J, Li D, Yuan Y, Zhang GM, Xiong H, Feng ZH (2007) Listeria monocytogenes promotes tumor growth via tumor cell toll-like receptor 2 signaling. Cancer Res 67(9):4346–4352

Huang CC, Liu K, Pope RM, Du P, Lin S, Rajamannan NM, Huang QQ, Jafari N, Burke GL, Post W, Watson KE, Johnson C, Daviglus ML, Lloyd-Jones DM (2011) Activated TLR signaling in atherosclerosis among women with lower Framingham risk score: the multi-ethnic study of atherosclerosis. PLoS One 6(6):e21067

Huang CY, Chen JJ, Shen KY, Chang LS, Yeh YC, Chen IH, Chong P, Liu SJ, Leng CH (2012a) Recombinant lipidated HPV E7 induces a Th-1-biased immune response and protective immunity against cervical cancer in a mouse model. PLoS One 7(7):e40970

Huang Y, Cai B, Xu M, Qiu Z, Tao Y, Zhang Y, Wang J, Xu Y, Zhou Y, Yang J, Han X, Gao Q (2012b) Gene silencing of toll-like receptor 2 inhibits proliferation of human liver cancer cells and secretion of inflammatory cytokines. PLoS One 7(7):e38890

Huleatt JW, Nakaar V, Desai P, Huang Y, Hewitt D, Jacobs A, Tang J, McDonald W, Song L, Evans RK, Umlauf S, Tussey L, Powell TJ (2008) Potent immunogenicity and efficacy of a universal influenza vaccine candidate comprising a recombinant fusion protein linking influenza M2e to the TLR5 ligand flagellin. Vaccine 26(2):201–214

Hutton MJ, Soukhatcheva G, Johnson JD, Verchere CB (2010) Role of the TLR signaling molecule TRIF in beta-cell function and glucose homeostasis. Islets 2(2):104–111

Ilvesaro JM, Merrell MA, Swain TM, Davidson J, Zayzafoon M, Harris KW, Selander KS (2007) Toll like receptor-9 agonists stimulate prostate cancer invasion in vitro. Prostate 67(7):774–781

Ilvesaro JM, Merrell MA, Li L, Wakchoure S, Graves D, Brooks S, Rahko E, Jukkola-Vuorinen A, Vuopala KS, Harris KW, Selander KS (2008) Toll-like receptor 9 mediates CpG oligonucleotide-induced cellular invasion. Mol Cancer Res 6(10):1534–1543

Imran M, Waheed Y, Manzoor S, Bilal M, Ashraf W, Ali M, Ashraf M (2012) Interaction of Hepatitis C virus proteins with pattern recognition receptors. Virol J 9:126

in t' Veld BA, Ruitenberg A, Hofman A, Launer LJ, van Duijn CM, Stijnen T, Breteler MM, Stricker BH (2001) Nonsteroidal antiinflammatory drugs and the risk of Alzheimer's disease. N Engl J Med 345(21):1515–1521

Into T, Inomata M, Takayama E, Takigawa T (2012) Autophagy in regulation of Toll-like receptor signaling. Cell Signal 24(6):1150–1162

Ioannou S, Voulgarelis M (2010) Toll-like receptors, tissue injury, and tumourigenesis. Mediators Inflamm 2010

Iribarren P, Chen K, Hu J, Gong W, Cho EH, Lockett S, Uranchimeg B, Wang JM (2005) CpG-containing oligodeoxynucleotide promotes microglial cell uptake of amyloid beta 1–42 peptide by up-regulating the expression of the G-protein- coupled receptor mFPR2. FASEB J 19(14):2032–2034

Ishii KJ, Kawakami K, Gursel I, Conover J, Joshi BH, Klinman DM, Puri RK (2003) Antitumor therapy with bacterial DNA and toxin: complete regression of established tumor induced by liposomal CpG oligodeoxynucleotides plus interleukin-13 cytotoxin. Clin Cancer Res 9(17):6516–6522

Iwasaki A, Medzhitov R (2010) Regulation of adaptive immunity by the innate immune system. Science 327(5963):291–295

Iyer SS, Pulskens WP, Sadler JJ, Butter LM, Teske GJ, Ulland TK, Eisenbarth SC, Florquin S, Flavell RA, Leemans JC, Sutterwala FS (2009) Necrotic cells trigger a sterile inflammatory response through the Nlrp3 inflammasome. Proc Natl Acad Sci U S A 106(48):20388–20393

Janeway CA Jr (1989) Approaching the asymptote? Evolution and revolution in immunology. Cold Spring Harb Symp Quant Biol 54(Pt 1):1–13

Janeway CA Jr, Medzhitov R (2002) Innate immune recognition. Annu Rev Immunol 20:197–216

Jang HJ, Kim HS, Hwang DH, Quon MJ, Kim JA (2013) Toll-like receptor 2 mediates high-fat diet-induced impairment of vasodilator actions of insulin. Am J Physiol Endocrinol Metab 304(10):E1077–E1088

Jego G, Bataille R, Geffroy-Luseau A, Descamps G, Pellat-Deceunynck C (2006) Pathogen-associated molecular patterns are growth and survival factors for human myeloma cells through toll-like receptors. Leukemia 20(6):1130–1137

Jha S, Srivastava SY, Brickey WJ, Iocca H, Toews A, Morrison JP, Chen VS, Gris D, Matsushima GK, Ting JP (2010) The inflammasome sensor, NLRP3, regulates CNS inflammation and demyelination via caspase-1 and interleukin-18. J Neurosci 30(47):15811–15820

Jialal I, Huet BA, Kaur H, Chien A, Devaraj S (2012) Increased toll-like receptor activity in patients with metabolic syndrome. Diabetes Care 35(4):900–904

Jiang H, Van DV, Satwani P, Baxi LV, Cairo MS (2004) Differential gene expression patterns by oligonucleotide microarray of basal versus lipopolysaccharide-activated monocytes from cord blood versus adult peripheral blood. J Immunol 172(10):5870–5879

Jiang Z, Georgel P, Du X, Shamel L, Sovath S, Mudd S, Huber M, Kalis C, Keck S, Galanos C, Freudenberg M, Beutler B (2005) CD14 is required for MyD88-independent LPS signaling. Nat Immunol 6(6):565–570

Jing Y, Shaheen E, Drake RR, Chen N, Gravenstein S, Deng Y (2009) Aging is associated with a numerical and functional decline in plasmacytoid dendritic cells, whereas myeloid dendritic cells are relatively unaltered in human peripheral blood. Hum Immunol 70(10):777–784

Johansen T, Lamark T (2011) Selective autophagy mediated by autophagic adapter proteins. Autophagy 7(3):279–296

Johnson BD, Kip KE, Marroquin OC, Ridker PM, Kelsey SF, Shaw LJ, Pepine CJ, Sharaf B, Bairey Merz CN, Sopko G, Olson MB, Reis SE (2004) Serum amyloid A as a predictor of coronary artery disease and cardiovascular outcome in women: the National Heart, Lung, and Blood Institute-Sponsored Women's Ischemia Syndrome Evaluation (WISE). Circulation 109(6):726–732

Johnson KE, Chikoti L, Chandran B (2013) Herpes simplex virus 1 infection induces activation and subsequent inhibition of the IFI16 and NLRP3 inflammasomes. J Virol 87(9):5005–5018

Johnstone RW, Wei W, Greenway A, Trapani JA (2000) Functional interaction between p53 and the interferon-inducible nucleoprotein IFI 16. Oncogene 19(52):6033–6042

Jones SC, Brahmakshatriya V, Huston G, Dibble J, Swain SL (2010) TLR-activated dendritic cells enhance the response of aged naive CD4 T cells via an IL-6-dependent mechanism. J Immunol 185(11):6783–6794

Jounai N, Takeshita F, Kobiyama K, Sawano A, Miyawaki A, Xin KQ, Ishii KJ, Kawai T, Akira S, Suzuki K, Okuda K (2007) The Atg5 Atg12 conjugate associates with innate antiviral immune responses. Proc Natl Acad Sci U S A 104(35):14050–14055

Juliana C, Fernandes-Alnemri T, Kang S, Farias A, Qin F, Alnemri ES (2012) Non-transcriptional priming and deubiquitination regulate NLRP3 inflammasome activation. J Biol Chem 287(43):36617–36622

Junjie X, Songyao J, Minmin S, Yanyan S, Baiyong S, Xiaxing D, Jiabin J, Xi Z, Hao C (2012) The association between toll-like receptor 2 single-nucleotide polymorphisms and hepatocellular carcinoma susceptibility. BMC Cancer 12:57

Kadl A, Sharma PR, Chen W, Agrawal R, Meher AK, Rudraiah S, Grubbs N, Sharma R, Leitinger N (2011) Oxidized phospholipid-induced inflammation is mediated by toll-like receptor 2. Free Radic Biol Med 51(10):1903–1909

Kagan JC, Iwasaki A (2012) Phagosome as the organelle linking innate and adaptive immunity. Traffic 9999(9999)

Karin M (2006) Nuclear factor-kappaB in cancer development and progression. Nature 441(7092):431–436

Katsargyris A, Tsiodras S, Theocharis S, Giaginis K, Vasileiou I, Bakoyiannis C, Georgopoulos S, Bastounis E, Klonaris C (2011) Toll-like receptor 4 immunohistochemical expression is enhanced in macrophages of symptomatic carotid atherosclerotic plaques. Cerebrovasc Dis 31(1):29–36

Kauppinen A, Niskanen H, Suuronen T, Kinnunen K, Salminen A, Kaarniranta K (2012) Oxidative stress activates NLRP3 inflammasomes in ARPE-19 cells–implications for age-related macular degeneration (AMD). Immunol Lett 147(1–2):29–33

Kawaguchi M, Takahashi M, Hata T, Kashima Y, Usui F, Morimoto H, Izawa A, Takahashi Y, Masumoto J, Koyama J, Hongo M, Noda T, Nakayama J, Sagara J, Taniguchi S, Ikeda U (2011) Inflammasome activation of cardiac fibroblasts is essential for myocardial ischemia/reperfusion injury. Circulation 123(6):594–604

Kawai T, Akira S (2011) Toll-like receptors and their crosstalk with other innate receptors in infection and immunity. Immunity 34(5):637–650

Kawanishi N, Yano H, Yokogawa Y, Suzuki K (2010) Exercise training inhibits inflammation in adipose tissue via both suppression of macrophage infiltration and acceleration of phenotypic switching from M1 to M2 macrophages in high-fat-diet-induced obese mice. Exerc Immunol Rev 16:105–118

Kelly MG, Alvero AB, Chen R, Silasi DA, Abrahams VM, Chan S, Visintin I, Rutherford T, Mor G (2006) TLR-4 signaling promotes tumor growth and paclitaxel chemoresistance in ovarian cancer. Cancer Res 66(7):3859–3868

Kerur N, Veettil MV, Sharma-Walia N, Bottero V, Sadagopan S, Otageri P, Chandran B (2011) IFI16 acts as a nuclear pathogen sensor to induce the inflammasome in response to Kaposi Sarcoma-associated herpesvirus infection. Cell Host Microbe 9(5):363–375

Kierdorf K, Fritz G (2013) RAGE regulation and signaling in inflammation and beyond. J Leukoc Biol 94(1):55–68

Kigerl KA, Lai W, Rivest S, Hart RP, Satoskar AR, Popovich PG (2007) Toll-like receptor (TLR)-2 and TLR-4 regulate inflammation, gliosis, and myelin sparing after spinal cord injury. J Neurochem 102(1):37–50

Killeen SD, Wang JH, Andrews EJ, Redmond HP (2009) Bacterial endotoxin enhances colorectal cancer cell adhesion and invasion through TLR-4 and NF-kappaB-dependent activation of the urokinase plasminogen activator system. Br J Cancer 100(10): 1589–1602

Kim F, Pham M, Luttrell I, Bannerman DD, Tupper J, Thaler J, Hawn TR, Raines EW, Schwartz MW (2007a) Toll-like receptor-4 mediates vascular inflammation and insulin resistance in diet-induced obesity. Circ Res 100(11):1589–1596

Kim HS, Han MS, Chung KW, Kim S, Kim E, Kim MJ, Jang E, Lee HA, Youn J, Akira S, Lee MS (2007b) Toll-like receptor 2 senses beta-cell death and contributes to the initiation of autoimmune diabetes. Immunity 27(2):321–333

Kim WY, Lee JW, Choi JJ, Choi CH, Kim TJ, Kim BG, Song SY, Bae DS (2008) Increased expression of toll-like receptor 5 during progression of cervical neoplasia. Int J Gynecol Cancer 18(2):300–305

Kim S, Takahashi H, Lin WW, Descargues P, Grivennikov S, Kim Y, Luo JL, Karin M (2009a) Carcinoma-produced factors activate myeloid cells through TLR2 to stimulate metastasis. Nature 457(7225):102–106

Kim YS, Park ZY, Kim SY, Jeong E, Lee JY (2009b) Alteration of toll-like receptor 4 activation by 4-hydroxy-2-nonenal mediated by the suppression of receptor homodimerization. Chem Biol Interact 182(1):59–66

Kim KA, Gu W, Lee IA, Joh EH, Kim DH (2012) High fat diet-induced gut microbiota exacerbates inflammation and obesity in mice via the TLR4 signaling pathway. PLoS One 7(10):e47713

Kim MJ, Choi NY, Koo JE, Kim SY, Joung SM, Jeong E, Lee JY (2013) Suppression of toll-like receptor 4 activation by endogenous oxidized phosphatidylcholine, KOdiA-PC by inhibiting LPS binding to MD2. Inflamm Res 62(6):571–580

Kleinridders A, Schenten D, Konner AC, Belgardt BF, Mauer J, Okamura T, Wunderlich FT, Medzhitov R, Bruning JC (2009) MyD88 signaling in the CNS is required for development of fatty acid-induced leptin resistance and diet-induced obesity. Cell Metab 10(4):249–259

Knapp S, Matt U, Leitinger N, van der Poll T (2007) Oxidized phospholipids inhibit phagocytosis and impair outcome in gram-negative sepsis in vivo. J Immunol 178(2):993–1001

Koliaraki V, Kollias G (2011) A new role for myeloid HO-1 in the innate to adaptive crosstalk and immune homeostasis. Adv Exp Med Biol 780:101–111

Kollmann TR, Levy O, Montgomery RR, Goriely S (2012) Innate immune function by toll-like receptors: distinct responses in newborns and the elderly. Immunity 37(5):771–783

Kondo Y, Nagai K, Nakahata S, Saito Y, Ichikawa T, Suekane A, Taki T, Iwakawa R, Enari M, Taniwaki M, Yokota J, Sakoda S, Morishita K (2012) Overexpression of the DNA sensor proteins, absent in melanoma 2 and interferon-inducible 16, contributes to tumorigenesis of oral squamous cell carcinoma with p53 inactivation. Cancer Sci 103(4):782–790

Kong KF, Delroux K, Wang X, Qian F, Arjona A, Malawista SE, Fikrig E, Montgomery RR (2008) Dysregulation of TLR3 impairs the innate immune response to West Nile virus in the elderly. J Virol 82(15):7613–7623

Kong X, Thimmulappa R, Kombairaju P, Biswal S (2010) NADPH oxidase-dependent reactive oxygen species mediate amplified TLR4 signaling and sepsis-induced mortality in Nrf2-deficient mice. J Immunol 185(1):569–577

Konner AC, Bruning JC (2011) Toll-like receptors: linking inflammation to metabolism. Trends Endocrinol Metab 22(1):16–23

Kopp A, Buechler C, Neumeier M, Weigert J, Aslanidis C, Scholmerich J, Schaffler A (2009) Innate immunity and adipocyte function: ligand-specific activation of multiple toll-like receptors modulates cytokine, adipokine, and chemokine secretion in adipocytes. Obesity 17(4):648–656

Kopp A, Buechler C, Bala M, Neumeier M, Scholmerich J, Schaffler A (2010) Toll-like receptor ligands cause proinflammatory and prodiabetic activation of adipocytes via phosphorylation of extracellular signal-regulated kinase and c-Jun N-terminal kinase but not interferon regulatory factor-3. Endocrinology 151(3):1097–1108

Kotas ME, Jurczak MJ, Annicelli C, Gillum MP, Cline GW, Shulman GI, Medzhitov R (2013) Role of caspase-1 in regulation of triglyceride metabolism. Proc Natl Acad Sci U S A 110(12):4810–4815

Kovacs EJ, Palmer JL, Fortin CF, Fulop T Jr, Goldstein DR, Linton PJ (2009) Aging and innate immunity in the mouse: impact of intrinsic and extrinsic factors. Trends Immunol 30(7):319–324

Krieg AM (2008) Toll-like receptor 9 (TLR9) agonists in the treatment of cancer. Oncogene 27(2):161–167

Kundu SD, Lee C, Billips BK, Habermacher GM, Zhang Q, Liu V, Wong LY, Klumpp DJ, Thumbikat P (2008) The toll-like receptor pathway: a novel mechanism of infection-induced carcinogenesis of prostate epithelial cells. Prostate 68(2):223–229

Kunzli BM, Bernlochner MI, Rath S, Kaser S, Csizmadia E, Enjyoji K, Cowan P, d'Apice A, Dwyer K, Rosenberg R, Perren A, Friess H, Maurer CA, Robson SC (2011) Impact of CD39 and purinergic signalling on the growth and metastasis of colorectal cancer. Purinergic Signal 7(2):231–241

Kuo LH, Tsai PJ, Jiang MJ, Chuang YL, Yu L, Lai KT, Tsai YS (2011) Toll-like receptor 2 deficiency improves insulin sensitivity and hepatic insulin signalling in the mouse. Diabetologia 54(1):168–179

Kutikhin AG (2011a) Association of polymorphisms in TLR genes and in genes of the toll-like receptor signaling pathway with cancer risk. Hum Immunol 72(11):1095–1116

Kutikhin AG (2011b) Impact of toll-like receptor 4 polymorphisms on risk of cancer. Hum Immunol 72(2):193–206

Kutikhin AG, Yuzhalin AE (2012a) C-type lectin receptors and RIG-I-like receptors: new points on the oncogenomics map. Cancer Manage Res 4:39–53

Kutikhin AG, Yuzhalin AE (2012b) Inherited variation in pattern recognition receptors and cancer: dangerous liaisons? Cancer Manage Res 4:31–38

Lagos D, Vart RJ, Gratrix F, Westrop SJ, Emuss V, Wong PP, Robey R, Imami N, Bower M, Gotch F, Boshoff C (2008) Toll-like receptor 4 mediates innate immunity to Kaposi sarcoma herpesvirus. Cell Host Microbe 4(5):470–483

Lambrecht BN, Hammad H (2012) The airway epithelium in asthma. Nat Med 18(5):684–692

Lawrie CH, Gal S, Dunlop HM, Pushkaran B, Liggins AP, Pulford K, Banham AH, Pezzella F, Boultwood J, Wainscoat JS, Hatton CS, Harris AL (2008) Detection of elevated levels of tumour-associated microRNAs in serum of patients with diffuse large B-cell lymphoma. Br J Haematol 141(5):672–675

Leach DR, Krummel MF, Allison JP (1996) Enhancement of antitumor immunity by CTLA-4 blockade. Science 271(5256):1734–1736

LeBouder E, Rey-Nores JE, Raby AC, Affolter M, Vidal K, Thornton CA, Labeta MO (2006) Modulation of neonatal microbial recognition: TLR-mediated innate immune responses are specifically and differentially modulated by human milk. J Immunol 176(6):3742–3752

Lee JY, Sohn KH, Rhee SH, Hwang D (2001) Saturated fatty acids, but not unsaturated fatty acids, induce the expression of cyclooxygenase-2 mediated through toll-like receptor 4. J Biol Chem 276(20):16683–16689

Lee JW, Choi JJ, Seo ES, Kim MJ, Kim WY, Choi CH, Kim TJ, Kim BG, Song SY, Bae DS (2007) Increased toll-like receptor 9 expression in cervical neoplasia. Mol Carcinog 46(11):941–947

Lee JY, Park AK, Lee KM, Park SK, Han S, Han W, Noh DY, Yoo KY, Kim H, Chanock SJ, Rothman N, Kang D (2009) Candidate gene approach evaluates association between innate immunity genes and breast cancer risk in Korean women. Carcinogenesis 30(9):1528–1531

Lee J, Giordano S, Zhang J (2012) Autophagy, mitochondria and oxidative stress: cross-talk and redox signalling. Biochem J 441(2):523–540

Lefebvre JS, Maue AC, Eaton SM, Lanthier PA, Tighe M, Haynes L (2012) The aged microenvironment contributes to the age-related functional defects of CD4 T cells in mice. Aging Cell 11(5):732–740

Lehnardt S, Lachance C, Patrizi S, Lefebvre S, Follett PL, Jensen FE, Rosenberg PA, Volpe JJ, Vartanian T (2002) The toll-like receptor TLR4 is necessary for lipopolysaccharide-induced oligodendrocyte injury in the CNS. J Neurosci 22(7):2478–2486

Lehnardt S, Massillon L, Follett P, Jensen FE, Ratan R, Rosenberg PA, Volpe JJ, Vartanian T (2003) Activation of innate immunity in the CNS triggers neurodegeneration through a toll-like receptor 4-dependent pathway. Proc Natl Acad Sci U S A 100(14):8514–8519

Lemke G, Rothlin CV (2008) Immunobiology of the TAM receptors. Nat Rev Immunol 8(5):327–336

Letiembre M, Hao W, Liu Y, Walter S, Mihaljevic I, Rivest S, Hartmann T, Fassbender K (2007) Innate immune receptor expression in normal brain aging. Neuroscience 146(1):248–254

Letiembre M, Liu Y, Walter S, Hao W, Pfander T, Wrede A, Schulz-Schaeffer W, Fassbender K (2009) Screening of innate immune receptors in neurodegenerative diseases: a similar pattern. Neurobiol Aging 30(5):759–768

Levy O (2005) Innate immunity of the human newborn: distinct cytokine responses to LPS and other toll-like receptor agonists. J Endotoxin Res 11(2):113–116

Levy O (2007) Innate immunity of the newborn: basic mechanisms and clinical correlates. Nat Rev Immunol 7(5):379–390

Levy O, Zarember KA, Roy RM, Cywes C, Godowski PJ, Wessels MR (2004) Selective impairment of TLR-mediated innate immunity in human newborns: neonatal blood plasma reduces monocyte TNF-alpha induction by bacterial lipopeptides, lipopolysaccharide, and imiquimod, but preserves the response to R-848. J Immunol 173(7):4627–4634

Levy O, Coughlin M, Cronstein BN, Roy RM, Desai A, Wessels MR (2006) The adenosine system selectively inhibits TLR-mediated TNF-alpha production in the human newborn. J Immunol 177(3):1956–1966

Levy E, Xanthou G, Petrakou E, Zacharioudaki V, Tsatsanis C, Fotopoulos S, Xanthou M (2009) Distinct roles of TLR4 and CD14 in LPS-induced inflammatory responses of neonates. Pediatr Res 66(2):179–184

Li J, Song W, Czerwinski DK, Varghese B, Uematsu S, Akira S, Krieg AM, Levy R (2007a) Lymphoma immunotherapy with CpG oligodeoxynucleotides requires TLR9 either in the host or in the tumor itself. J Immunol 179(4):2493–2500

Li Y, Chu N, Hu A, Gran B, Rostami A, Zhang GX (2007b) Increased IL-23p19 expression in multiple sclerosis lesions and its induction in microglia. Brain 130(Pt 2):490–501

Li XD, Chiu YH, Ismail AS, Behrendt CL, Wight-Carter M, Hooper LV, Chen ZJ (2011) Mitochondrial antiviral signaling protein (MAVS) monitors commensal bacteria and induces an immune response that prevents experimental colitis. Proc Natl Acad Sci U S A 108(42):17390–17395

Li K, Li NL, Wei D, Pfeffer SR, Fan M, Pfeffer LM (2012a) Activation of chemokine and inflammatory cytokine response in hepatitis C virus-infected hepatocytes depends on toll-like receptor 3 sensing of hepatitis C virus double-stranded RNA intermediates. Hepatology 55(3):666–675

Li Q, Li X, Guo Z, Xu F, Xia J, Liu Z, Ren T (2012b) MicroRNA-574-5p was pivotal for TLR9 signaling enhanced tumor progression via down-regulating checkpoint suppressor 1 in human lung cancer. PLoS One 7(11):e48278

Liao JB (2006) Viruses and human cancer. Yale J Biol Med 79(3–4):115–122

Lifshitz V, Weiss R, Benromano T, Kfir E, Blumenfeld-Katzir T, Tempel-Brami C, Assaf Y, Xia W, Wyss-Coray T, Weiner HL, Frenkel D (2012) Immunotherapy of cerebrovascular amyloidosis in a transgenic mouse model. Neurobiol Aging 33(2):432 e431–432 e413

Lin L, Park S, Lakatta EG (2009) RAGE signaling in inflammation and arterial aging. Front Biosci 14:1403–1413

Lin H, Hua F, Hu ZW (2012) Autophagic flux, supported by toll-like receptor 2 activity, defends against the carcinogenesis of hepatocellular carcinoma. Autophagy 8(12):1859–1861

Lin H, Yan J, Wang Z, Hua F, Yu J, Sun W, Li K, Liu H, Yang H, Lv Q, Xue J, Hu ZW (2013a) Loss of immunity-supported senescence enhances suscepti-bility to hepatocellular carcinogenesis and progres-sion in toll-like receptor 2-deficient mice. Hepatology 57(1):171–182

Lin T, Walker GB, Kurji K, Fang E, Law G, Prasad SS, Kojic L, Cao S, White V, Cui JZ, Matsubara JA (2013b) Parainflammation associated with advanced glycation endproduct stimulation of RPE in vitro: implications for age-related degenerative diseases of the eye. Cytokine 62(3):369–381

Lisciandro JG, Prescott SL, Nadal-Sims MG, Devitt CJ, Pomat W, Siba PM, Tulic MC, Holt PG, Strickland D, van den Biggelaar AH (2012) Ontogeny of toll-like and NOD-like receptor-mediated innate immune responses in Papua New Guinean infants. PLoSOne 7(5):e36793

Liu HM, Gale M (2010) Hepatitis C virus evasion from RIG-I-dependent hepatic innate immunity. Gastroenterol Res Pract 2010:548390

Liu X, Xu Q, Chen W, Cao H, Zheng R, Li G (2009) Hepatitis B virus DNA-induced carcinogenesis of human normal liver cells by virtue of nonmethylated CpG DNA. Oncol Rep 21(4):941–947

Liu J, Radler D, Illi S, Klucker E, Turan E, Von Mutius ME, Kabesch M, Schaub B (2011) TLR2 polymor-phisms influence neonatal regulatory T cells depend-ing on maternal atopy. Allergy 66(8):1020–1029

Liu ML, Scalia R, Mehta JL, Williams KJ (2012) Cholesterol-induced membrane microvesicles as novel carriers of damage-associated molecular patterns: mechanisms of formation, action, and detoxification. Arterioscler Thromb Vasc Biol 32(9):2113–2121

Lokeshwar VB, Cerwinka WH, Isoyama T, Lokeshwar BL (2005) HYAL1 hyaluronidase in prostate can-cer: a tumor promoter and suppressor. Cancer Res 65(17):7782–7789

Long TM, Chakrabarti A, Ezelle HJ, Brennan-Laun SE, Raufman JP, Polyakova I, Silverman RH, Hassel BA (2013) RNase-L deficiency exacerbates experimental colitis and colitis-associated cancer. Inflamm Bowel Dis 19(6):1295–1305

Longobardo MT, Cefalu AB, Pezzino F, Noto D, Emmanuele G, Barbagallo CM, Fiore B, Monastero R, Castello A, Molini V, Notarbartolo A, Travali S, Averna MR (2003) The C(−260)>T gene polymor-phism in the promoter of the CD14 monocyte receptor gene is not associated with acute myocardial infarc-tion. Clin Exp Med 3(3):161–165

Lowe EL, Crother TR, Rabizadeh S, Hu B, Wang H, Chen S, Shimada K, Wong MH, Michelsen KS, Arditi M (2010) Toll-like receptor 2 signaling protects mice from tumor development in a mouse model of colitis-induced cancer. PLoS One 5(9):e13027

Lu H, Wagner WM, Gad E, Yang Y, Duan H, Amon LM, Van Denend N, Larson ER, Chang A, Tufvesson H, Disis ML (2010) Treatment failure of a TLR-7 agonist occurs due to self-regulation of acute inflammation and can be overcome by IL-10 blockade. J Immunol 184(9):5360–5367

Lu S, Bevier M, Huhn S, Sainz J, Lascorz J, Pardini B, Naccarati A, Vodickova L, Novotny J, Hemminki K, Vodicka P, Forsti A (2013) Genetic variants in C-type lectin genes are associated with colorectal cancer sus-ceptibility and clinical outcome. Int J Cancer. May 3 doi:10.1002/ijc.28251. [Epub ahead of print]

Luo JL, Maeda S, Hsu LC, Yagita H, Karin M (2004) Inhibition of NF-kappaB in cancer cells converts inflammation- induced tumor growth mediated by TNFalpha to TRAIL-mediated tumor regression. Cancer Cell 6(3):297–305

Lust JA, Lacy MQ, Zeldenrust SR, Dispenzieri A, Gertz MA, Witzig TE, Kumar S, Hayman SR, Russell SJ, Buadi FK, Geyer SM, Campbell ME, Kyle RA, Rajkumar SV, Greipp PR, Kline MP, Xiong Y, Moon-Tasson LL, Donovan KA (2009) Induction of a chronic disease state in patients with smoldering or indolent multiple myeloma by targeting interleukin 1{beta}-induced interleukin 6 production and the myeloma pro-liferative component. Mayo Clin Proc 84(2):114–122

Ma Y, Aymeric L, Locher C, Mattarollo SR, Delahaye NF, Pereira P, Boucontet L, Apetoh L, Ghiringhelli F, Casares N, Lasarte JJ, Matsuzaki G, Ikuta K, Ryffel B, Benlagha K, Tesniere A, Ibrahim N, Dechanet-Merville J, Chaput N, Smyth MJ, Kroemer G, Zitvogel L (2011) Contribution of IL-17-producing gamma delta T cells to the efficacy of anticancer chemother-apy. J Exp Med 208(3):491–503

Malathi K, Dong B, Gale M Jr, Silverman RH (2007) Small self-RNA generated by RNase L amplifies anti-viral innate immunity. Nature 448(7155):816–819

Manicassamy S, Pulendran B (2009) Modulation of adap-tive immunity with toll-like receptors. Semin Immunol 21(4):185–193

Marker T, Sell H, Zillessen P, Glode A, Kriebel J, Ouwens DM, Pattyn P, Ruige J, Famulla S, Roden M, Eckel J, Habich C (2012) Heat shock protein 60 as a mediator of adipose tissue inflammation and insulin resistance. Diabetes 61(3):615–625

Marshall NA, Galvin KC, Corcoran AM, Boon L, Higgs R, Mills KH (2012) Immunotherapy with PI3K inhibitor and toll-like receptor agonist induces IFN-gamma+IL-17+ polyfunctional T cells that mediate rejection of murine tumors. Cancer Res 72(3):581–591

Marta M, Andersson A, Isaksson M, Kampe O, Lobell A (2008) Unexpected regulatory roles of TLR4 and TLR9 in experimental autoimmune encephalomyeli-tis. Eur J Immunol 38(2):565–575

Martin V, Fabelo N, Santpere G, Puig B, Marin R, Ferrer I, Diaz M (2010) Lipid alterations in lipid rafts from Alzheimer's disease human brain cortex. Alzheimer's Dis 19(2):489–502

Martinez-Vicente M, Cuervo AM (2007) Autophagy and neurodegeneration: when the cleaning crew goes on strike. Lancet Neurol 6(4):352–361

Martino G, Pluchino S (2007) Neural stem cells: guard-ians of the brain. Nat Cell Biol 9(9):1031–1034

Martins I, Tesniere A, Kepp O, Michaud M, Schlemmer F, Senovilla L, Seror C, Metivier D, Perfettini JL, Zitvogel L, Kroemer G (2009) Chemotherapy induces

ATP release from tumor cells. Cell Cycle 8(22):3723–3728

Masters SL, Dunne A, Subramanian SL, Hull RL, Tannahill GM, Sharp FA, Becker C, Franchi L, Yoshihara E, Chen Z, Mullooly N, Mielke LA, Harris J, Coll RC, Mills KH, Mok KH, Newsholme P, Nunez G, Yodoi J, Kahn SE, Lavelle EC, O'Neill LA (2010) Activation of the NLRP3 inflammasome by islet amyloid polypeptide provides a mechanism for enhanced IL-1beta in type 2 diabetes. Nat Immunol 11(10):897–904

Matijevic T, Pavelic J (2011) The dual role of TLR3 in metastatic cell line. Clin Exp Metastasis 28(7):701–712

Matijevic T, Marjanovic M, Pavelic J (2009) Functionally active toll-like receptor 3 on human primary and metastatic cancer cells. Scand J Immunol 70(1):18–24

Mattson MP (2004) Pathways towards and away from Alzheimer's disease. Nature 430(7000):631–639

Maue AC, Eaton SM, Lanthier PA, Sweet KB, Blumerman SL, Haynes L (2009) Proinflammatory adjuvants enhance the cognate helper activity of aged CD4 T cells. J Immunol 182(10):6129–6135

Mawhinney LJ, de Rivero Vaccari JP, Dale GA, Keane RW, Bramlett HM (2011) Heightened inflammasome activation is linked to age-related cognitive impairment in Fischer 344 rats. BMC Neurosci 12:123

Medzhitov R (2009) Approaching the asymptote: 20 years later. Immunity 30(6):766–775

Menu P, Pellegrin M, Aubert JF, Bouzourene K, Tardivel A, Mazzolai L, Tschopp J (2011) Atherosclerosis in ApoE-deficient mice progresses independently of the NLRP3 inflammasome. Cell Death Dis 2:e137

Merrell MA, Ilvesaro JM, Lehtonen N, Sorsa T, Gehrs B, Rosenthal E, Chen D, Shackley B, Harris KW, Selander KS (2006) Toll-like receptor 9 agonists promote cellular invasion by increasing matrix metalloproteinase activity. Mol Cancer Res 4(7):437–447

Mezzaroma E, Toldo S, Farkas D, Seropian IM, Van Tassell BW, Salloum FN, Kannan HR, Menna AC, Voelkel NF, Abbate A (2011) The inflammasome promotes adverse cardiac remodeling following acute myocardial infarction in the mouse. Proc Natl Acad Sci U S A 108(49):19725–19730

Miao EA, Leaf IA, Treuting PM, Mao DP, Dors M, Sarkar A, Warren SE, Wewers MD, Aderem A (2010) Caspase-1-induced pyroptosis is an innate immune effector mechanism against intracellular bacteria. Nat Immunol 11(12):1136–1142

Michaud M, Martins I, Sukkurwala AQ, Adjemian S, Ma Y, Pellegatti P, Shen S, Kepp O, Scoazec M, Mignot G, Rello-Varona S, Tailler M, Menger L, Vacchelli E, Galluzzi L, Ghiringhelli F, di Virgilio F, Zitvogel L, Kroemer G (2011) Autophagy-dependent anticancer immune responses induced by chemotherapeutic agents in mice. Science 334(6062):1573–1577

Michelsen KS, Wong MH, Shah PK, Zhang W, Yano J, Doherty TM, Akira S, Rajavashisth TB, Arditi M (2004) Lack of toll-like receptor 4 or myeloid differentiation factor 88 reduces atherosclerosis and alters

plaque phenotype in mice deficient in apolipoprotein E. Proc Natl Acad Sci U S A 101(29):10679–10684

Miller YI, Choi SH, Wiesner P, Fang L, Harkewicz R, Hartvigsen K, Boullier A, Gonen A, Diehl CJ, Que X, Montano E, Shaw PX, Tsimikas S, Binder CJ, Witztum JL (2011) Oxidation-specific epitopes are danger-associated molecular patterns recognized by pattern recognition receptors of innate immunity. Circ Res 108(2):235–248

Miller YI, Choi SH, Wiesner P, Bae YS (2012) The SYK side of TLR4: signalling mechanisms in response to LPS and minimally oxidized LDL. Br J Pharmacol 167(5):990–999

Minoretti P, Gazzaruso C, Vito CD, Emanuele E, Bianchi M, Coen E, Reino M, Geroldi D (2006) Effect of the functional toll-like receptor 4 Asp299Gly polymorphism on susceptibility to late-onset alzheimer's disease. Neurosci Lett 391(3):147–149

Mistry AM, Swick AG, Romsos DR (1997) Leptin rapidly lowers food intake and elevates metabolic rates in lean and ob/ob mice. J Nutr 127(10):2065–2072

Mitchell PS, Parkin RK, Kroh EM, Fritz BR, Wyman SK, Pogosova-Agadjanyan EL, Peterson A, Noteboom J, O'Briant KC, Allen A, Lin DW, Urban N, Drescher CW, Knudsen BS, Stirewalt DL, Gentleman R, Vessella RL, Nelson PS, Martin DB, Tewari M (2008) Circulating microRNAs as stable blood-based markers for cancer detection. Proc Natl Acad Sci U S A 105(30):10513–10518

Moghimpour Bijani F, Vallejo JG, Rezaei N (2012) Toll-like receptor signaling pathways in cardiovascular diseases: challenges and opportunities. Int Rev Immunol 31(5):379–395

Mokdad AH, Ford ES, Bowman BA, Dietz WH, Vinicor F, Bales VS, Marks JS (2003) Prevalence of obesity, diabetes, and obesity-related health risk factors, 2001. JAMA 289(1):76–79

Mollaki V, Georgiadis T, Tassidou A, Ioannou M, Daniil Z, Koutsokera A, Papathanassiou AA, Zintzaras E, Vassilopoulos G (2009) Polymorphisms and haplotypes in TLR9 and MYD88 are associated with the development of Hodgkin's lymphoma: a candidate-gene association study. J Hum Genet 54(11):655–659

Monroy CM, Cortes AC, Lopez MS, D'Amelio AM Jr, Etzel CJ, Younes A, Strom SS, El-Zein RA (2011) Hodgkin disease risk: role of genetic polymorphisms and gene-gene interactions in inflammation pathway genes. Mol Carcinog 50(1):36–46

Morales A, Eidinger D, Bruce AW (1976) Intracavitary Bacillus Calmette-Guerin in the treatment of superficial bladder tumors. J Urol 116(2):180–183

Moumad K, Lascorz J, Bevier M, Khyatti M, Ennaji MM, Benider A, Huhn S, Lu S, Chouchane L, Corbex M, Hemminki K, Forsti A (2013) Genetic polymorphisms in host innate immune sensor genes and the risk of nasopharyngeal carcinoma in north Africa. G3 3(6):971–977

Mullins RF, Russell SR, Anderson DH, Hageman GS (2000) Drusen associated with aging and age-related macular degeneration contain proteins common to extracellular deposits associated with atherosclerosis, elastosis, amyloidosis, and dense deposit disease. FASEB J 14(7):835–846

Nakahira K, Haspel JA, Rathinam VA, Lee SJ, Dolinay T, Lam HC, Englert JA, Rabinovitch M, Cernadas M, Kim HP, Fitzgerald KA, Ryter SW, Choi AM (2011) Autophagy proteins regulate innate immune responses by inhibiting the release of mitochondrial DNA mediated by the NALP3 inflammasome. Nat Immunol 12(3):222–230

Nebel A, Flachsbart F, Schafer A, Nothnagel M, Nikolaus S, Mokhtari NE, Schreiber S (2007) Role of the toll-like receptor 4 polymorphism Asp299Gly in longevity and myocardial infarction in German men. Mech Ageing Dev 128(5–6):409–411

Netea MG, Wijmenga C, O'Neill LA (2012) Genetic variation in toll-like receptors and disease susceptibility. Nat Immunol 13(6):535–542

Ng LK, Rich AM, Hussaini HM, Thomson WM, Fisher AL, Horne LS, Seymour GJ (2011) Toll-like receptor 2 is present in the microenvironment of oral squamous cell carcinoma. Br J Cancer 104(3):460–463

Nguyen MT, Favelyukis S, Nguyen AK, Reichart D, Scott PA, Jenn A, Liu-Bryan R, Glass CK, Neels JG, Olefsky JM (2007) A subpopulation of macrophages infiltrates hypertrophic adipose tissue and is activated by free fatty acids via toll-like receptors 2 and 4 and JNK-dependent pathways. J Biol Chem 282(48):35279–35292

Nguyen M, Leuridan E, Zhang T, De WD, Willems F, Van DP, Goldman M, Goriely S (2010) Acquisition of adult-like TLR4 and TLR9 responses during the first year of life. PLoS One 5(4):e10407

Niemi K, Teirila L, Lappalainen J, Rajamaki K, Baumann MH, Oorni K, Wolff H, Kovanen PT, Matikainen S, Eklund KK (2011) Serum amyloid A activates the NLRP3 inflammasome via P2X7 receptor and a cathepsin B-sensitive pathway. J Immunol 186(11):6119–6128

Nieters A, Beckmann L, Deeg E, Becker N (2006) Gene polymorphisms in toll-like receptors, interleukin-10, and interleukin-10 receptor alpha and lymphoma risk. Genes Immun 7(8):615–624

Nijnik A, Woodbine L, Marchetti C, Dawson S, Lambe T, Liu C, Rodrigues NP, Crockford TL, Cabuy E, Vindigni A, Enver T, Bell JI, Slijepcevic P, Goodnow CC, Jeggo PA, Cornall RJ (2007) DNA repair is limiting for haematopoietic stem cells during ageing. Nature 447(7145):686–690

Nischalke HD, Coenen M, Berger C, Aldenhoff K, Muller T, Berg T, Kramer B, Korner C, Odenthal M, Schulze F, Grunhage F, Nattermann J, Sauerbruch T, Spengler U (2012) The toll-like receptor 2 (TLR2) -196 to −174 del/ins polymorphism affects viral loads and susceptibility to hepatocellular carcinoma in chronic hepatitis C. Int J Cancer 130(6):1470–1475

Nixon RA, Yang DS (2011) Autophagy failure in Alzheimer's disease–locating the primary defect. Neurobiol Dis 43(1):38–45

Nogueira-Machado JA, Volpe CM, Veloso CA, Chaves MM (2011) HMGB1, TLR and RAGE: a functional tripod that leads to diabetic inflammation. Expert Opin Ther Targets 15(8):1023–1035

Nomi N, Kodama S, Suzuki M (2010) Toll-like receptor 3 signaling induces apoptosis in human head and neck cancer via survivin associated pathway. Oncol Rep 24(1):225–231

Normand S, Delanoye-Crespin A, Bressenot A, Huot L, Grandjean T, Peyrin-Biroulet L, Lemoine Y, Hot D, Chamaillard M (2011) Nod-like receptor pyrin domain-containing protein 6 (NLRP6) controls epithelial self-renewal and colorectal carcinogenesis upon injury. Proc Natl Acad Sci U S A 108(23):9601–9606

Nyugen J, Agrawal S, Gollapudi S, Gupta S (2010) Impaired functions of peripheral blood monocyte subpopulations in aged humans. J Clin Immunol 30(6):806–813

O'Neill LA, Golenbock D, Bowie AG (2013) The history of toll-like receptors - redefining innate immunity. Nat Rev Immunol 13(6):453–460

Obici S, Zhang BB, Karkanias G, Rossetti L (2002) Hypothalamic insulin signaling is required for inhibition of glucose production. Nat Med 8(12):1376–1382

Oka T, Hikoso S, Yamaguchi O, Taneike M, Takeda T, Tamai T, Oyabu J, Murakawa T, Nakayama H, Nishida K, Akira S, Yamamoto A, Komuro I, Otsu K (2012) Mitochondrial DNA that escapes from autophagy causes inflammation and heart failure. Nature 485(7397):251–255

Okun E, Griffioen KJ, Lathia JD, Tang SC, Mattson MP, Arumugam TV (2009) Toll-like receptors in neurodegeneration. Brain Res Rev 59(2):278–292

Okun E, Griffioen K, Barak B, Roberts NJ, Castro K, Pita MA, Cheng A, Mughal MR, Wan R, Ashery U, Mattson MP (2010) Toll-like receptor 3 inhibits memory retention and constrains adult hippocampal neurogenesis. Proc Natl Acad Sci U S A 107(35):15625–15630

Okun E, Griffioen KJ, Mattson MP (2011) Toll-like receptor signaling in neural plasticity and disease. Trends Neurosci 34(5):269–281

Oliveira AG, Carvalho BM, Tobar N, Ropelle ER, Pauli JR, Bagarolli RA, Guadagnini D, Carvalheira JB, Saad MJ (2011) Physical exercise reduces circulating lipopolysaccharide and TLR4 activation and improves insulin signaling in tissues of DIO rats. Diabetes 60(3):784–796

Olivieri F, Antonicelli R, Cardelli M, Marchegiani F, Cavallone L, Mocchegiani E, Franceschi C (2006) Genetic polymorphisms of inflammatory cytokines and myocardial infarction in the elderly. Mech Ageing Dev 127(6):552–559

Palin K, Bluthe RM, McCusker RH, Levade T, Moos F, Dantzer R, Kelley KW (2009) The type 1 TNF receptor and its associated adapter protein, FAN, are required for TNFalpha-induced sickness behavior. Psychopharmacology 201(4):549–556

Palm NW, Medzhitov R (2009) Immunostimulatory activity of haptenated proteins. Proc Natl Acad Sci U S A 106(12):4782–4787

Panda A, Arjona A, Sapey E, Bai F, Fikrig E, Montgomery RR, Lord JM, Shaw AC (2009) Human innate immunosenescence: causes and consequences for immunity in old age. Trends Immunol 30(7):325–333

Panda A, Qian F, Mohanty S, Van DD, Newman FK, Zhang L, Chen S, Towle V, Belshe RB, Fikrig E, Allore HG, Montgomery RR, Shaw AC (2010) Age-associated decrease in TLR function in primary human dendritic cells predicts influenza vaccine response. J Immunol 184(5):2518–2527

Pandey S, Mittal RD, Srivastava M, Srivastava K, Singh S, Srivastava S, Mittal B (2009) Impact of toll-like receptors [TLR] 2 (−196 to −174 del) and TLR 4 (Asp299Gly, Thr399Ile) in cervical cancer susceptibility in North Indian women. Gynecol Oncol 114(3):501–505

Park JH, Yoon HE, Kim DJ, Kim SA, Ahn SG, Yoon JH (2011) Toll-like receptor 5 activation promotes migration and invasion of salivary gland adenocarcinoma. J Oral Pathol Med 40(2):187–193

Pasare C, Medzhitov R (2005) Control of B-cell responses by toll-like receptors. Nature 438(7066):364–368

Patel MR, Kratzke RA (2013) Oncolytic virus therapy for cancer: the first wave of translational clinical trials. Transl Res 161(4):355–364

Paul-Clark MJ, McMaster SK, Sorrentino R, Sriskandan S, Bailey LK, Moreno L, Ryffel B, Quesniaux VF, Mitchell JA (2009) Toll-like receptor 2 is essential for the sensing of oxidants during inflammation. Am J Respir Crit Care Med 179(4):299–306

Peng G, Guo Z, Kiniwa Y, Voo KS, Peng W, Fu T, Wang DY, Li Y, Wang HY, Wang RF (2005) Toll-like receptor 8-mediated reversal of CD4+ regulatory T cell function. Science 309(5739):1380–1384

Peters T, Weiss JM, Sindrilaru A, Wang H, Oreshkova T, Wlaschek M, Maity P, Reimann J, Scharffetter-Kochanek K (2009) Reactive oxygen intermediate-induced pathomechanisms contribute to immunosenescence, chronic inflammation and autoimmunity. Mech Ageing Dev 130(9):564–587

Pikarsky E, Ben-Neriah Y (2006) NF-kappaB inhibition: a double-edged sword in cancer? Eur J Cancer 42(6):779–784

Pikarsky E, Porat RM, Stein I, Abramovitch R, Amit S, Kasem S, Gutkovich-Pyest E, Urieli-Shoval S, Galun E, Ben-Neriah Y (2004) NF-kappaB functions as a tumour promoter in inflammation-associated cancer. Nature 431(7007):461–466

Pimentel-Nunes P, Afonso L, Lopes P, Roncon-Albuquerque R Jr, Goncalves N, Henrique R, Moreira-Dias L, Leite-Moreira AF, Dinis-Ribeiro M (2011) Increased expression of toll-like receptors (TLR) 2, 4 and 5 in gastric dysplasia. Pathology Oncol Res 17(3):677–683

Pimentel-Nunes P, Goncalves N, Boal-Carvalho I, Afonso L, Lopes P, Roncon-Albuquerque R Jr, Henrique R, Moreira-Dias L, Leite-Moreira AF, Dinis-Ribeiro M (2013) Helicobacter pylori induces increased expression of toll-like receptors and decreased Toll-interacting protein in gastric mucosa that persists throughout gastric carcinogenesis. Helicobacter 18(1):22–32

Plum L, Belgardt BF, Bruning JC (2006) Central insulin action in energy and glucose homeostasis. J Clin Invest 116(7):1761–1766

Poggi M, Bastelica D, Gual P, Iglesias MA, Gremeaux T, Knauf C, Peiretti F, Verdier M, Juhan-Vague I, Tanti JF, Burcelin R, Alessi MC (2007) C3H/HeJ mice carrying a toll-like receptor 4 mutation are protected against the development of insulin resistance in white adipose tissue in response to a high-fat diet. Diabetologia 50(6):1267–1276

Pontillo A, Catamo E, Arosio B, Mari D, Crovella S (2012) NALP1/NLRP1 genetic variants are associated with Alzheimer disease. Alzheimer Dis Assoc Disord 26(3):277–281

Prakash S, Agrawal S, Cao JN, Gupta S, Agrawal A (2012) Impaired secretion of interferons by dendritic cells from aged subjects to influenza: role of histone modifications. Age (Dordr) Sep 25. [Epub ahead of print]

Purdue MP, Lan Q, Wang SS, Kricker A, Menashe I, Zheng TZ, Hartge P, Grulich AE, Zhang Y, Morton LM, Vajdic CM, Holford TR, Severson RK, Leaderer BP, Cerhan JR, Yeager M, Cozen W, Jacobs K, Davis S, Rothman N, Chanock SJ, Chatterjee N, Armstrong BK (2009) A pooled investigation of toll-like receptor gene variants and risk of non-Hodgkin lymphoma. Carcinogenesis 30(2):275–281

Qian F, Wang X, Zhang L, Lin A, Zhao H, Fikrig E, Montgomery RR (2011) Impaired interferon signaling in dendritic cells from older donors infected in vitro with West Nile virus. J Infect Dis 203(10):1415–1424

Qian F, Wang X, Zhang L, Chen S, Piecychna M, Allore H, Bockenstedt L, Malawista S, Bucala R, Shaw AC, Fikrig E, Montgomery RR (2012) Age-associated elevation in TLR5 leads to increased inflammatory responses in the elderly. Aging Cell 11(1):104–110

Qian F, Bolen CR, Jing C, Wang X, Zheng W, Zhao H, Fikrig E, Bruce RD, Kleinstein SH, Montgomery RR (2013) Impaired toll-like receptor 3-mediated immune responses from macrophages of patients chronically infected with hepatitis C virus. Clin Vaccine Immunol 20(2):146–155

Rajamaki K, Lappalainen J, Oorni K, Valimaki E, Matikainen S, Kovanen PT, Eklund KK (2010) Cholesterol crystals activate the NLRP3 inflammasome in human macrophages: a novel link between cholesterol metabolism and inflammation. PLoS One 5(7):e11765

Rajaraman P, Brenner AV, Butler MA, Wang SS, Pfeiffer RM, Ruder AM, Linet MS, Yeager M, Wang Z, Orr N, Fine HA, Kwon D, Thomas G, Rothman N, Inskip PD, Chanock SJ (2009) Common variation in genes related to innate immunity and risk of adult glioma. Cancer Epidemiol Biomarkers Prev 18(5):1651–1658

Rajaraman P, Brenner AV, Neta G, Pfeiffer R, Wang SS, Yeager M, Thomas G, Fine HA, Linet MS, Rothman N, Chanock SJ, Inskip PD (2010) Risk of meningioma and common variation in genes related to innate immunity. Cancer Epidemiol Biomarkers Prev 19(5):1356–1361

Rakoff-Nahoum S, Medzhitov R (2007) Regulation of spontaneous intestinal tumorigenesis through the adaptor protein MyD88. Science 317(5834):124–127

Rathinam VA, Fitzgerald KA (2011) Cytosolic surveillance and antiviral immunity. Curr Opin Virol 1(6):455–462

Rathinam VA, Jiang Z, Waggoner SN, Sharma S, Cole LE, Waggoner L, Vanaja SK, Monks BG, Ganesan S, Latz E, Hornung V, Vogel SN, Szomolanyi-Tsuda E, Fitzgerald KA (2010) The AIM2 inflammasome is essential for host defense against cytosolic bacteria and DNA viruses. Nat Immunol 11(5):395–402

Ray ME, Su YA, Meltzer PS, Trent JM (1996) Isolation and characterization of genes associated with chromosome-6 mediated tumor suppression in human malignant melanoma. Oncogene 12(12):2527–2533

Raynor J, Lages CS, Shehata H, Hildeman DA, Chougnet CA (2012) Homeostasis and function of regulatory T cells in aging. Curr Opin Immunol 24(4):482–487

Reed-Geaghan EG, Savage JC, Hise AG, Landreth GE (2009) CD14 and toll-like receptors 2 and 4 are required for fibrillar A{beta}-stimulated microglial activation. J Neurosci 29(38):11982–11992

Reed-Geaghan EG, Reed QW, Cramer PE, Landreth GE (2010) Deletion of CD14 attenuates Alzheimer's disease pathology by influencing the brain's inflammatory milieu. J Neurosci 30(46):15369–15373

Ren T, Wen ZK, Liu ZM, Qian C, Liang YJ, Jin ML, Cai YY, Xu L (2008) Targeting toll-like receptor 9 with CpG oligodeoxynucleotides enhances antitumor responses of peripheral blood mononuclear cells from human lung cancer patients. Cancer Invest 26(5):448–455

Ren T, Xu L, Jiao S, Wang Y, Cai Y, Liang Y, Zhou Y, Zhou H, Wen Z (2009) TLR9 signaling promotes tumor progression of human lung cancer cell in vivo. Pathol Oncol Res 15(4):623–630

Renshaw M, Rockwell J, Engleman C, Gewirtz A, Katz J, Sambhara S (2002) Cutting edge: impaired toll-like receptor expression and function in aging. J Immunol 169(9):4697–4701

Reyna SM, Ghosh S, Tantiwong P, Meka CS, Eagan P, Jenkinson CP, Cersosimo E, Defronzo RA, Coletta DK, Sriwijitkamol A, Musi N (2008) Elevated toll-like receptor 4 expression and signaling in muscle from insulin-resistant subjects. Diabetes 57(10):2595–2602

Reynolds CM, McGillicuddy FC, Harford KA, Finucane OM, Mills KH, Roche HM (2012) Dietary saturated fatty acids prime the NLRP3 inflammasome via TLR4 in dendritic cells-implications for diet-induced insulin resistance. Mol Nutr Food Res 56(8):1212–1222

Rietschel ET, Brade H, Brade L, Brandenburg K, Schade U, Seydel U, Zahringer U, Galanos C, Luderitz O, Westphal O et al (1987) Lipid A, the endotoxic center of bacterial lipopolysaccharides: relation of chemical structure to biological activity. Prog Clin Biol Res 231:25–53

Rolls A, Shechter R, London A, Ziv Y, Ronen A, Levy R, Schwartz M (2007) Toll-like receptors modulate adult hippocampal neurogenesis. Nat Cell Biol 9(9):1081–1088

Roncon-Albuquerque R Jr, Moreira-Rodrigues M, Faria B, Ferreira AP, Cerqueira C, Lourenco AP, Pestana M, von Hafe P, Leite-Moreira AF (2008) Attenuation of the cardiovascular and metabolic complications of obesity in CD14 knockout mice. Life Sci 83(13–14):502–510

Rosenbaum JT (2012) Eyeing macular degeneration–few inflammatory remarks. N Engl J Med 367(8):768–770

Roth GA, Moser B, Roth-Walter F, Giacona MB, Harja E, Papapanou PN, Schmidt AM, Lalla E (2007) Infection with a periodontal pathogen increases mononuclear cell adhesion to human aortic endothelial cells. Atherosclerosis 190(2):271–281

Russell SJ, Peng KW, Bell JC (2012) Oncolytic virotherapy. Nat Biotechnol 30(7):658–670

Saberi M, Woods NB, de Luca C, Schenk S, Lu JC, Bandyopadhyay G, Verma IM, Olefsky JM (2009) Hematopoietic cell-specific deletion of toll-like receptor 4 ameliorates hepatic and adipose tissue insulin resistance in high-fat-fed mice. Cell Metab 10(5):419–429

Sadeghi K, Berger A, Langgartner M, Prusa AR, Hayde M, Herkner K, Pollak A, Spittler A, Forster-Waldl E (2007) Immaturity of infection control in preterm and term newborns is associated with impaired toll-like receptor signaling. J Infect Dis 195(2):296–302

Saitoh T, Fujita N, Jang MH, Uematsu S, Yang BG, Satoh T, Omori H, Noda T, Yamamoto N, Komatsu M, Tanaka K, Kawai T, Tsujimura T, Takeuchi O, Yoshimori T, Akira S (2008) Loss of the autophagy protein Atg16L1 enhances endotoxin-induced IL-1beta production. Nature 456(7219):264–268

Salagianni M, Galani IE, Lundberg AM, Davos CH, Varela A, Gavriil A, Lyytikainen LP, Lehtimaki T, Sigala F, Folkersen L, Gorgoulis V, Lenglet S, Montecucco F, Mach F, Hedin U, Hansson GK, Monaco C, Andreakos E (2012) Toll-like receptor 7 protects from atherosclerosis by constraining "inflammatory" macrophage activation. Circulation 126(8):952–962

Salaun B, Coste I, Rissoan MC, Lebecque SJ, Renno T (2006) TLR3 can directly trigger apoptosis in human cancer cells. J Immunol 176(8):4894–4901

Salminen A, Ojala J, Suuronen T, Kaarniranta K, Kauppinen A (2008) Amyloid-beta oligomers set fire to inflammasomes and induce Alzheimer's pathology. J Cell Mol Med 12(6A):2255–2262

Salminen A, Kaarniranta K, Kauppinen A (2012) Inflammaging: disturbed interplay between autophagy and inflammasomes. Aging (AlbanyNY) 4(3):166–175

Sandanger O, Ranheim T, Vinge LE, Bliksoen M, Alfsnes K, Finsen AV, Dahl CP, Askevold ET, Florholmen G, Christensen G, Fitzgerald KA, Lien E, Valen G, Espevik T, Aukrust P, Yndestad A (2013) The NLRP3 inflammasome is up-regulated in cardiac fibroblasts and mediates myocardial ischaemia-reperfusion injury. Cardiovasc Res 99(1):164–174

Sandoval D, Cota D, Seeley RJ (2008) The integrative role of CNS fuel-sensing mechanisms in energy balance and glucose regulation. Annu Rev Physiol 70:513–535

Schaefer L, Babelova A, Kiss E, Hausser HJ, Baliova M, Krzyzankova M, Marsche G, Young MF, Mihalik D, Gotte M, Malle E, Schaefer RM, Grone HJ (2005) The matrix component biglycan is proinflammatory and signals through toll-like receptors 4 and 2 in macrophages. J Clin Invest 115(8):2223–2233

Schaeffler A, Gross P, Buettner R, Bollheimer C, Buechler C, Neumeier M, Kopp A, Schoelmerich J, Falk W (2009) Fatty acid-induced induction of toll-like receptor-4/nuclear factor-kappaB pathway in adipocytes links nutritional signalling with innate immunity. Immunology 126(2):233–245

Scheibner KA, Lutz MA, Boodoo S, Fenton MJ, Powell JD, Horton MR (2006) Hyaluronan fragments act as an endogenous danger signal by engaging TLR2. J Immunol 177(2):1272–1281

Schindowski K, Frohlich L, Maurer K, Muller WE, Eckert A (2002) Age-related impairment of human T lymphocytes' activation: specific differences between CD4(+) and CD8(+) subsets. Mech Ageing Dev 123(4):375–390

Schlapbach LJ, Mattmann M, Thiel S, Boillat C, Otth M, Nelle M, Wagner B, Jensenius JC, Aebi C (2010) Differential role of the lectin pathway of complement activation in susceptibility to neonatal sepsis. Clin Infect Dis 51(2):153–162

Schneider-Ohrum K, Giles BM, Weirback HK, Williams BL, DeAlmeida DR, Ross TM (2011) Adjuvants that stimulate TLR3 or NLPR3 pathways enhance the efficiency of influenza virus-like particle vaccines in aged mice. Vaccine 29(48):9081–9092

Scholtes VP, Versteeg D, de Vries JP, Hoefer IE, Schoneveld AH, Stella PR, Doevendans PA, van Keulen KJ, de Kleijn DP, Moll FL, Pasterkamp G (2011) Toll-like receptor 2 and 4 stimulation elicits an enhanced inflammatory response in human obese patients with atherosclerosis. Clin Sci 121(5):205–214

Schon MP, Schon M (2008) TLR7 and TLR8 as targets in cancer therapy. Oncogene 27(2):190–199

Schwartz EA, Zhang WY, Karnik SK, Borwege S, Anand VR, Laine PS, Su Y, Reaven PD (2010) Nutrient modification of the innate immune response: a novel mechanism by which saturated fatty acids greatly amplify monocyte inflammation. Arterioscler Thromb Vasc Biol 30(4):802–808

Sen G, Chen Q, Snapper CM (2006) Immunization of aged mice with a pneumococcal conjugate vaccine combined with an unmethylated CpG-containing oligodeoxynucleotide restores defective immunoglobulin G antipolysaccharide responses and specific CD4+−T-cell priming to young adult levels. Infect Immun 74(4):2177–2186

Senn JJ (2006) Toll-like receptor-2 is essential for the development of palmitate-induced insulin resistance in myotubes. J Biol Chem 281(37):26865–26875

Seya T, Azuma M, Matsumoto M (2013) Targeting TLR3 with no RIG-I/MDA5 activation is effective in immunotherapy for cancer. Expert Opin Ther Targets 17(5):533–544

Sharma S, Dominguez AL, Hoelzinger DB, Lustgarten J (2008) CpG-ODN but not other TLR-ligands restore the antitumor responses in old mice: the implications for vaccinations in the aged. Cancer Immunol Immunother 57(4):549–561

Sharma MD, Hou DY, Baban B, Koni PA, He Y, Chandler PR, Blazar BR, Mellor AL, Munn DH (2010) Reprogrammed foxp3(+) regulatory T cells provide essential help to support cross-presentation and CD8(+) T cell priming in naive mice. Immunity 33(6):942–954

Shaw AC, Panda A, Joshi SR, Qian F, Allore HG, Montgomery RR (2011) Dysregulation of human toll-like receptor function in aging. Ageing Res Rev 10(3):346–353

Shi H, Kokoeva MV, Inouye K, Tzameli I, Yin H, Flier JS (2006) TLR4 links innate immunity and fatty acid-induced insulin resistance. J Clin Invest 116(11): 3015–3025

Shi CS, Shenderov K, Huang NN, Kabat J, Abu-Asab M, Fitzgerald KA, Sher A, Kehrl JH (2012) Activation of autophagy by inflammatory signals limits IL-1beta production by targeting ubiquitinated inflammasomes for destruction. Nat Immunol 13(3):255–263

Shimada K, Crother TR, Karlin J, Dagvadorj J, Chiba N, Chen S, Ramanujan VK, Wolf AJ, Vergnes L, Ojcius DM, Rentsendorj A, Vargas M, Guerrero C, Wang Y, Fitzgerald KA, Underhill DM, Town T, Arditi M (2012) Oxidized mitochondrial DNA activates the NLRP3 inflammasome during apoptosis. Immunity 36(3):401–414

Shojaei H, Oberg HH, Juricke M, Marischen L, Kunz M, Mundhenke C, Gieseler F, Kabelitz D, Wesch D (2009) Toll-like receptors 3 and 7 agonists enhance tumor cell lysis by human gammadelta T cells. Cancer Res 69(22):8710–8717

Siegemund S, Sauer K (2012) Balancing pro- and anti-inflammatory TLR4 signaling. Nat Immunol 13(11):1031–1033

Siegmund B, Lehr HA, Fantuzzi G, Dinarello CA (2001) IL-1 beta -converting enzyme (caspase-1) in intestinal inflammation. Proc Natl Acad Sci U S A 98(23): 13249–13254

Simons MP, O'Donnell MA, Griffith TS (2008) Role of neutrophils in BCG immunotherapy for bladder cancer. Urol Oncol 26(4):341–345

Skountzou I, Martin Mdel P, Wang B, Ye L, Koutsonanos D, Weldon W, Jacob J, Compans RW (2010) Salmonella flagellins are potent adjuvants for intranasally administered whole inactivated influenza vaccine. Vaccine 28(24):4103–4112

Sloane JA, Batt C, Ma Y, Harris ZM, Trapp B, Vartanian T (2010) Hyaluronan blocks oligodendrocyte progenitor maturation and remyelination through TLR2. Proc Natl Acad Sci U S A 107(25):11555–11560

Sluyter R, Dalitz JG, Wiley JS (2004a) P2X7 receptor polymorphism impairs extracellular adenosine 5'-triphosphate-induced interleukin-18 release from human monocytes. Genes Immun 5(7):588–591

Sluyter R, Shemon AN, Wiley JS (2004b) Glu496 to Ala polymorphism in the P2X7 receptor impairs ATP-induced IL-1 beta release from human monocytes. J Immunol 172(6):3399–3405

Soares JB, Pimentel-Nunes P, Afonso L, Rolanda C, Lopes P, Roncon-Albuquerque R Jr, Goncalves N, Boal-Carvalho I, Pardal F, Lopes S, Macedo G, Lara-Santos L, Henrique R, Moreira-Dias L, Goncalves R, Dinis-Ribeiro M, Leite-Moreira AF (2012) Increased hepatic expression of TLR2 and TLR4 in the hepatic inflammation-fibrosis-carcinoma sequence. Innate Immun 18(5):700–708

Solana R, Tarazona R, Gayoso I, Lesur O, Dupuis G, Fulop T (2012) Innate immunosenescence: effect of aging on cells and receptors of the innate immune system in humans. Semin Immunol 24(5):331–341

Song X, Krelin Y, Dvorkin T, Bjorkdahl O, Segal S, Dinarello CA, Voronov E, Apte RN (2005) CD11b+/Gr-1+ immature myeloid cells mediate suppression of T cells in mice bearing tumors of IL-1beta-secreting cells. J Immunol 175(12):8200–8208

Song MJ, Kim KH, Yoon JM, Kim JB (2006) Activation of toll-like receptor 4 is associated with insulin resistance in adipocytes. Biochem Biophys Res Commun 346(3):739–745

Song LL, Alimirah F, Panchanathan R, Xin H, Choubey D (2008) Expression of an IFN-inducible cellular senescence gene, IFI16, is up-regulated by p53. Mol Cancer Res 6(11):1732–1741

Song LL, Ponomareva L, Shen H, Duan X, Alimirah F, Choubey D (2010) Interferon-inducible IFI16, a negative regulator of cell growth, down-regulates expression of human telomerase reverse transcriptase (hTERT) gene. PLoS One 5(1):e8569

Song M, Jin J, Lim JE, Kou J, Pattanayak A, Rehman JA, Kim HD, Tahara K, Lalonde R, Fukuchi K (2011) TLR4 mutation reduces microglial activation, increases Abeta deposits and exacerbates cognitive deficits in a mouse model of Alzheimer's disease. J Neuroinflammation 8:92

Sotomayor EM, Borrello I, Tubb E, Allison JP, Levitsky HI (1999) In vivo blockade of CTLA-4 enhances the priming of responsive T cells but fails to prevent the induction of tumor antigen-specific tolerance. Proc Natl Acad Sci U S A 96(20):11476–11481

Spaner DE, Shi Y, White D, Shaha S, He L, Masellis A, Wong K, Gorczynski R (2010) A phase I/II trial of TLR-7 agonist immunotherapy in chronic lymphocytic leukemia. Leukemia 24(1):222–226

Spirig R, Tsui J, Shaw S (2012) The emerging role of TLR and innate immunity in cardiovascular disease. Cardiol Res Prac 2012:181394

Sridharan A, Esposo M, Kaushal K, Tay J, Osann K, Agrawal S, Gupta S, Agrawal A (2011) Age-associated impaired plasmacytoid dendritic cell functions lead to decreased CD4 and CD8 T cell immunity. Age 33(3):363–376

Srivastava K, Srivastava A, Kumar A, Mittal B (2010) Significant association between toll-like receptor gene polymorphisms and gallbladder cancer. Liver Int 30(7):1067–1072

Stagg J, Smyth MJ (2010) Extracellular adenosine triphosphate and adenosine in cancer. Oncogene 29(39):5346–5358

Stewart WF, Kawas C, Corrada M, Metter EJ (1997) Risk of Alzheimer's disease and duration of NSAID use. Neurology 48(3):626–632

Stienstra R, Joosten LA, Koenen T, van Tits B, van Diepen JA, van den Berg SA, Rensen PC, Voshol PJ, Fantuzzi G, Hijmans A, Kersten S, Muller M, van den Berg WB, van Rooijen N, Wabitsch M, Kullberg BJ, van der Meer JW, Kanneganti T, Tack CJ, Netea MG (2010) The inflammasome-mediated caspase-1 activation controls adipocyte differentiation and insulin sensitivity. Cell Metab 12(6):593–605

Stienstra R, van Diepen JA, Tack CJ, Zaki MH, van de Veerdonk FL, Perera D, Neale GA, Hooiveld GJ, Hijmans A, Vroegrijk I, van den Berg S, Romijn J, Rensen PC, Joosten LA, Netea MG, Kanneganti TD (2011) Inflammasome is a central player in the induction of obesity and insulin resistance. Proc Natl Acad Sci U S A 108(37):15324–15329

Stout-Delgado HW, Yang X, Walker WE, Tesar BM, Goldstein DR (2008) Aging impairs IFN regulatory factor 7 up-regulation in plasmacytoid dendritic cells during TLR9 activation. J Immunol 181(10):6747–6756

Stout-Delgado HW, Du W, Shirali AC, Booth CJ, Goldstein DR (2009) Aging promotes neutrophil-induced mortality by augmenting IL-17 production during viral infection. Cell Host Microbe 6(5):446–456

Stout-Delgado HW, Vaughan SE, Shirali AC, Jaramillo RJ, Harrod KS (2012) Impaired NLRP3 inflammasome function in elderly mice during influenza infection is rescued by treatment with nigericin. J Immunol 188(6):2815–2824

Sun Z, Luo Q, Ye D, Chen W, Chen F (2012) Role of toll-like receptor 4 on the immune escape of human oral squamous cell carcinoma and resistance of cisplatin-induced apoptosis. Mol Cancer 11:33

Sutton CE, Lalor SJ, Sweeney CM, Brereton CF, Lavelle EC, Mills KH (2009) Interleukin-1 and IL-23 induce innate IL-17 production from gammadelta T cells, amplifying Th17 responses and autoimmunity. Immunity 31(2):331–341

Szajnik M, Szczepanski MJ, Czystowska M, Elishaev E, Mandapathil M, Nowak-Markwitz E, Spaczynski M, Whiteside TL (2009) TLR4 signaling induced by lipopolysaccharide or paclitaxel regulates tumor survival and chemoresistance in ovarian cancer. Oncogene 28(49):4353–4363

Szczepanski M, Stelmachowska M, Stryczynski L, Golusinski W, Samara H, Mozer-Lisewska I, Zeromski J (2007) Assessment of expression of toll-like receptors 2, 3 and 4 in laryngeal carcinoma. Eur Arch Otorhinolaryngol 264(5):525–530

Szczepanski MJ, Czystowska M, Szajnik M, Harasymczuk M, Boyiadzis M, Kruk-Zagajewska A, Szyfter W,

Zeromski J, Whiteside TL (2009) Triggering of toll-like receptor 4 expressed on human head and neck squamous cell carcinoma promotes tumor development and protects the tumor from immune attack. Cancer Res 69(7):3105–3113

Tahara K, Kim HD, Jin JJ, Maxwell JA, Li L, Fukuchi K (2006) Role of toll-like receptor signalling in Abeta uptake and clearance. Brain 129(Pt 11):3006–3019

Tahara T, Arisawa T, Wang F, Shibata T, Nakamura M, Sakata M, Hirata I, Nakano H (2007) Toll-like receptor 2–196 to 174del polymorphism influences the susceptibility of Japanese people to gastric cancer. Cancer Sci 98(11):1790–1794

Tal MC, Sasai M, Lee HK, Yordy B, Shadel GS, Iwasaki A (2009) Absence of autophagy results in reactive oxygen species-dependent amplification of RLR signaling. Proc Natl Acad Sci USA 106(8):2770–2775

Tan L, Schedl P, Song HJ, Garza D, Konsolaki M (2008) The Toll–>NFkappaB signaling pathway mediates the neuropathological effects of the human Alzheimer's Abeta42 polypeptide in Drosophila. PLoS One 3(12):e3966

Tanaka S, Ide M, Shibutani T, Ohtaki H, Numazawa S, Shioda S, Yoshida T (2006) Lipopolysaccharide-induced microglial activation induces learning and memory deficits without neuronal cell death in rats. J Neurosci Res 83(4):557–566

Tanaka T, Oh-Hashi K, Shitara H, Hirata Y, Kiuchi K (2008) NF-kappaB independent signaling pathway is responsible for LPS-induced GDNF gene expression in primary rat glial cultures. Neurosci Lett 431(3):262–267

Tanaka J, Sugimoto K, Shiraki K, Tameda M, Kusagawa S, Nojiri K, Beppu T, Yoneda K, Yamamoto N, Uchida K, Kojima T, Takei Y (2010) Functional cell surface expression of toll-like receptor 9 promotes cell proliferation and survival in human hepatocellular carcinomas. Int J Oncol 37(4):805–814

Tang SC, Arumugam TV, Xu X, Cheng A, Mughal MR, Jo DG, Lathia JD, Siler DA, Chigurupati S, Ouyang X, Magnus T, Camandola S, Mattson MP (2007) Pivotal role for neuronal toll-like receptors in ischemic brain injury and functional deficits. Proc Natl Acad Sci U S A 104(34):13798–13803

Tang SC, Lathia JD, Selvaraj PK, Jo DG, Mughal MR, Cheng A, Siler DA, Markesbery WR, Arumugam TV, Mattson MP (2008) Toll-like receptor-4 mediates neuronal apoptosis induced by amyloid beta-peptide and the membrane lipid peroxidation product 4-hydroxynonenal. Exp Neurol 213(1):114–121

Tarallo V, Hirano Y, Gelfand BD, Dridi S, Kerur N, Kim Y, Cho WG, Kaneko H, Fowler BJ, Bogdanovich S, Albuquerque RJ, Hauswirth WW, Chiodo VA, Kugel JF, Goodrich JA, Ponicsan SL, Chaudhuri G, Murphy MP, Dunaief JL, Ambati BK, Ogura Y, Yoo JW, Lee DK, Provost P, Hinton DR, Nunez G, Baffi JZ, Kleinman ME, Ambati J (2012) DICER1 loss and Alu RNA induce age-related macular degeneration via the NLRP3 inflammasome and MyD88. Cell 149(4):847–859

Tauber SC, Ebert S, Weishaupt JH, Reich A, Nau R, Gerber J (2009) Stimulation of toll-like receptor 9 by chronic intraventricular unmethylated cytosine-guanine DNA infusion causes neuroinflammation and impaired spatial memory. J Neuropathol Exp Neurol 68(10):1116–1124

Tesar BM, Walker WE, Unternaehrer J, Joshi NS, Chandele A, Haynes L, Kaech S, Goldstein DR (2006) Murine [corrected] myeloid dendritic cell-dependent toll-like receptor immunity is preserved with aging. Aging Cell 5(6):473–486

Ting JP, Lovering RC, Alnemri ES, Bertin J, Boss JM, Davis BK, Flavell RA, Girardin SE, Godzik A, Harton JA, Hoffman HM, Hugot JP, Inohara N, Mackenzie A, Maltais LJ, Nunez G, Ogura Y, Otten LA, Philpott D, Reed JC, Reith W, Schreiber S, Steimle V, Ward PA (2008) The NLR gene family: a standard nomenclature. Immunity 28(3):285–287

Tomita T, Kanai T, Fujii T, Nemoto Y, Okamoto R, Tsuchiya K, Totsuka T, Sakamoto N, Akira S, Watanabe M (2008) MyD88-dependent pathway in T cells directly modulates the expansion of colitogenic CD4+ T cells in chronic colitis. J Immunol 180(8):5291–5299

Touil T, Fitzgerald D, Zhang GX, Rostami A, Gran B (2006) Cutting Edge: TLR3 stimulation suppresses experimental autoimmune encephalomyelitis by inducing endogenous IFN-beta. J Immunol 177(11):7505–7509

Tripathy D, Mohanty P, Dhindsa S, Syed T, Ghanim H, Aljada A, Dandona P (2003) Elevation of free fatty acids induces inflammation and impairs vascular reactivity in healthy subjects. Diabetes 52(12):2882–2887

Tseng WA, Thein T, Kinnunen K, Lashkari K, Gregory MS, D'Amore PA, Ksander BR (2013) NLRP3 inflammasome activation in retinal pigment epithelial cells by lysosomal destabilization: implications for age-related macular degeneration. Invest Ophthalmol Vis Sci 54(1):110–120

Tsukumo DM, Carvalho-Filho MA, Carvalheira JB, Prada PO, Hirabara SM, Schenka AA, Araujo EP, Vassallo J, Curi R, Velloso LA, Saad MJ (2007) Loss-of-function mutation in toll-like receptor 4 prevents diet-induced obesity and insulin resistance. Diabetes 56(8):1986–1998

Tu S, Bhagat G, Cui G, Takaishi S, Kurt-Jones EA, Rickman B, Betz KS, Penz-Oesterreicher M, Bjorkdahl O, Fox JG, Wang TC (2008) Overexpression of interleukin-1beta induces gastric inflammation and cancer and mobilizes myeloid-derived suppressor cells in mice. Cancer Cell 14(5):408–419

Turnbaugh PJ, Ley RE, Mahowald MA, Magrini V, Mardis ER, Gordon JI (2006) An obesity-associated gut microbiome with increased capacity for energy harvest. Nature 444(7122):1027–1031

Tzima S, Victoratos P, Kranidioti K, Alexiou M, Kollias G (2009) Myeloid heme oxygenase-1 regulates innate immunity and autoimmunity by modulating IFN-beta production. J Exp Med 206(5):1167–1179

Unterholzner L, Keating SE, Baran M, Horan KA, Jensen SB, Sharma S, Sirois CM, Jin T, Latz E, Xiao TS, Fitzgerald KA, Paludan SR, Bowie AG (2010) IFI16 is an innate immune sensor for intracellular DNA. Nat Immunol 11(11):997–1004

Upham JW, Lee PT, Holt BJ, Heaton T, Prescott SL, Sharp MJ, Sly PD, Holt PG (2002) Development of interleukin-12-producing capacity throughout childhood. Infect Immun 70(12):6583–6588

Uysal KT, Wiesbrock SM, Marino MW, Hotamisligil GS (1997) Protection from obesity-induced insulin resistance in mice lacking TNF-alpha function. Nature 389(6651):610–614

Vaknin I, Blinder L, Wang L, Gazit R, Shapira E, Genina O, Pines M, Pikarsky E, Baniyash M (2008) A common pathway mediated through toll-like receptors leads to T- and natural killer-cell immunosuppression. Blood 111(3):1437–1447

Valadi H, Ekstrom K, Bossios A, Sjostrand M, Lee JJ, Lotvall JO (2007) Exosome-mediated transfer of mRNAs and microRNAs is a novel mechanism of genetic exchange between cells. Nat Cell Biol 9(6):654–659

van Deventer HW, Burgents JE, Wu QP, Woodford RM, Brickey WJ, Allen IC, McElvania-TeKippe E, Serody JS, Ting JP (2010) The inflammasome component NLRP3 impairs antitumor vaccine by enhancing the accumulation of tumor-associated myeloid-derived suppressor cells. Cancer Res 70(24):10161–10169

van Diepen JA, Stienstra R, Vroegrijk IO, van den Berg SA, Salvatori D, Hooiveld GJ, Kersten S, Tack CJ, Netea MG, Smit JW, Joosten LA, Havekes LM, van Dijk KW, Rensen PC (2013) Caspase-1 deficiency in mice reduces intestinal triglyceride absorption and hepatic triglyceride secretion. J Lipid Res 54(2):448–456

Van DD, Shaw AC (2007) Toll-like receptors in older adults. J Am Geriatr Soc 55(9):1438–1444

Van DD, Allore HG, Mohanty S, Ginter S, Newman FK, Belshe RB, Medzhitov R, Shaw AC (2007a) Prevaccine determination of the expression of costimulatory B7 molecules in activated monocytes predicts influenza vaccine responses in young and older adults. JInfect Dis 195(11):1590–1597

Van DD, Mohanty S, Thomas V, Ginter S, Montgomery RR, Fikrig E, Allore HG, Medzhitov R, Shaw AC (2007b) Age-associated defect in human TLR-1/2 function. J Immunol 178(2):970–975

Vandanmagsar B, Youm YH, Ravussin A, Galgani JE, Stadler K, Mynatt RL, Ravussin E, Stephens JM, Dixit VD (2011) The NLRP3 inflammasome instigates obesity-induced inflammation and insulin resistance. Nat Med 17(2):179–188

Veeranki S, Duan X, Panchanathan R, Liu H, Choubey D (2011) IFI16 protein mediates the anti-inflammatory actions of the type-I interferons through suppression of activation of caspase-1 by inflammasomes. PLoS One 6(10):e27040

Vincent IE, Zannetti C, Lucifora J, Norder H, Protzer U, Hainaut P, Zoulim F, Tommasino M, Trepo C, Hasan U, Chemin I (2011) Hepatitis B virus impairs TLR9 expression and function in plasmacytoid dendritic cells. PLoS One 6(10):e26315

Vollmar P, Kullmann JS, Thilo B, Claussen MC, Rothhammer V, Jacobi H, Sellner J, Nessler S, Korn T, Hemmer B (2010) Active immunization with amyloid-beta 1–42 impairs memory performance through TLR2/4-dependent activation of the innate immune system. J Immunol 185(10):6338–6347

Voronov E, Shouval DS, Krelin Y, Cagnano E, Benharroch D, Iwakura Y, Dinarello CA, Apte RN (2003) IL-1 is required for tumor invasiveness and angiogenesis. Proc Natl Acad Sci U S A 100(5):2645–2650

Walker VP, Zhang X, Rastegar I, Liu PT, Hollis BW, Adams JS, Modlin RL (2011) Cord blood vitamin D status impacts innate immune responses. J Clin Endocrinol Metab 96(6):1835–1843

Walter S, Letiembre M, Liu Y, Heine H, Penke B, Hao W, Bode B, Manietta N, Walter J, Schulz-Schuffer W, Fassbender K (2007) Role of the toll-like receptor 4 in neuroinflammation in Alzheimer's disease. Cell Physiol Biochem 20(6):947–956

Wang JH, Manning BJ, Wu QD, Blankson S, Bouchier-Hayes D, Redmond HP (2003) Endotoxin/lipopolysaccharide activates NF-kappa B and enhances tumor cell adhesion and invasion through a beta 1 integrin-dependent mechanism. J Immunol 170(2):795–804

Wang H, Rayburn ER, Wang W, Kandimalla ER, Agrawal S, Zhang R (2006a) Chemotherapy and chemosensitization of non-small cell lung cancer with a novel immunomodulatory oligonucleotide targeting toll-like receptor 9. Mol Cancer Ther 5(6):1585–1592

Wang H, Rayburn ER, Wang W, Kandimalla ER, Agrawal S, Zhang R (2006b) Immunomodulatory oligonucleotides as novel therapy for breast cancer: pharmacokinetics, in vitro and in vivo anticancer activity, and potentiation of antibody therapy. Mol Cancer Ther 5(8):2106–2114

Wang Y, Zhang HX, Sun YP, Liu ZX, Liu XS, Wang L, Lu SY, Kong H, Liu QL, Li XH, Lu ZY, Chen SJ, Chen Z, Bao SS, Dai W, Wang ZG (2007) Rig-I–/– mice develop colitis associated with downregulation of G alpha i2. Cell Res 17(10):858–868

Wang N, Liang Y, Devaraj S, Wang J, Lemon SM, Li K (2009a) Toll-like receptor 3 mediates establishment of an antiviral state against hepatitis C virus in hepatoma cells. J Virol 83(19):9824–9834

Wang SS, Bratti MC, Rodriguez AC, Herrero R, Burk RD, Porras C, Gonzalez P, Sherman ME, Wacholder S, Lan ZE, Schiffman M, Chanock SJ, Hildesheim A (2009b) Common variants in immune and DNA repair genes and risk for human papillomavirus persistence and progression to cervical cancer. J Infect Dis 199(1):20–30

Wang SS, Purdue MP, Cerhan JR, Zheng T, Menashe I, Armstrong BK, Lan Q, Hartge P, Kricker A, Zhang Y, Morton LM, Vajdic CM, Holford TR, Severson RK, Grulich A, Leaderer BP, Davis S, Cozen W, Yeager M, Chanock SJ, Chatterjee N, Rothman N (2009c) Common gene variants in the tumor necrosis factor

(TNF) and TNF receptor superfamilies and NF-kB transcription factors and non-Hodgkin lymphoma risk. PLoS One 4(4):e5360

Wang LZ, Yu JT, Miao D, Wu ZC, Zong Y, Wen CQ, Tan L (2011) Genetic association of TLR4/11367 polymorphism with late-onset alzheimer's disease in a Han Chinese population. Brain Res 1381:202–207

Wang C, Fei G, Liu Z, Li Q, Xu Z, Ren T (2012) HMGB1 was a pivotal synergistic effecor for CpG oligonucleotide to enhance the progression of human lung cancer cells. Cancer Biol Ther 13(9):727–736

Wang Y, Li J, Wang X, Ye L, Zhou Y, Thomas RM, Ho W (2013a) Hepatitis C virus impairs TLR3 signaling and inhibits IFN-lambda 1 expression in human hepatoma cell line. Innate Immun. Mar 25. [Epub ahead of print]

Wang Z, Lin H, Hua F, Hu ZW (2013b) Repairing DNA damage by XRCC6/KU70 reverses TLR4-deficiency-worsened HCC development via restoring senescence and autophagic flux. Autophagy 9(6):925–927

Wang Z, Yan J, Lin H, Hua F, Wang X, Liu H, Lv X, Yu J, Mi S, Wang J, Hu ZW (2013c) Toll-like receptor 4 activity protects against hepatocellular tumorigenesis and progression by regulating expression of DNA repair protein Ku70 in mice. Hepatology 57(5):1869–1881

Watson MB, Costello DA, Carney DG, McQuillan K, Lynch MA (2010) SIGIRR modulates the inflammatory response in the brain. Brain Behav Immun 24(6):985–995

Weiner HL, Frenkel D (2006) Immunology and immunotherapy of Alzheimer's disease. Nat Rev Immunol 6(5):404–416

Weisberg SP, McCann D, Desai M, Rosenbaum M, Leibel RL, Ferrante AW Jr (2003) Obesity is associated with macrophage accumulation in adipose tissue. J Clin Invest 112(12):1796–1808

Weismann D, Binder CJ (2012) The innate immune response to products of phospholipid peroxidation. Biochim Biophys Acta 1818(10):2465–2475

Wen H, Gris D, Lei Y, Jha S, Zhang L, Huang MT, Brickey WJ, Ting JP (2011) Fatty acid-induced NLRP3-ASC inflammasome activation interferes with insulin signaling. Nat Immunol 12(5):408–415

Wen H, Ting JP, O'Neill LA (2012) A role for the NLRP3 inflammasome in metabolic diseases–did Warburg miss inflammation? Nat Immunol 13(4):352–357

West XZ, Malinin NL, Merkulova AA, Tischenko M, Kerr BA, Borden EC, Podrez EA, Salomon RG, Byzova TV (2010) Oxidative stress induces angiogenesis by activating TLR2 with novel endogenous ligands. Nature 467(7318):972–976

West AP, Brodsky IE, Rahner C, Woo DK, Erdjument-Bromage H, Tempst P, Walsh MC, Choi Y, Shadel GS, Ghosh S (2011) TLR signalling augments macrophage bactericidal activity through mitochondrial ROS. Nature 472(7344):476–480

Willingham SB, Ting JP (2008) NLRs and the dangers of pollution and aging. Nat Immunol 9(8):831–833

Winter RN, Kramer A, Borkowski A, Kyprianou N (2001) Loss of caspase-1 and caspase-3 protein expression in human prostate cancer. Cancer Res 61(3):1227–1232

Woerner SM, Kloor M, Schwitalle Y, Youmans H, Doeberitz M, Gebert J, Dihlmann S (2007) The putative tumor suppressor AIM2 is frequently affected by different genetic alterations in microsatellite unstable colon cancers. Genes Chromosomes Cancer 46(12):1080–1089

Wolchok JD, Hodi FS, Weber JS, Allison JP, Urba WJ, Robert C, O'Day SJ, Hoos A, Humphrey R, Berman DM, Lonberg N, Korman AJ (2013) Development of ipilimumab: a novel immunotherapeutic approach for the treatment of advanced melanoma. Ann N Y Acad Sci 1291(1):1–13

Wright SD, Ramos RA, Tobias PS, Ulevitch RJ, Mathison JC (1990) CD14, a receptor for complexes of lipopolysaccharide (LPS) and LPS binding protein. Science 249(4975):1431–1433

Xie W, Wang Y, Huang Y, Yang H, Wang J, Hu Z (2009) Toll-like receptor 2 mediates invasion via activating NF-kappaB in MDA-MB-231 breast cancer cells. Biochem Biophys Res Commun 379(4):1027–1032

Xie W, Huang Y, Xie W, Guo A, Wu W (2010) Bacteria peptidoglycan promoted breast cancer cell invasiveness and adhesiveness by targeting toll-like receptor 2 in the cancer cells. PLoS One 5(5):e10850

Xin H, Curry J, Johnstone RW, Nickoloff BJ, Choubey D (2003) Role of IFI 16, a member of the interferon-inducible p200-protein family, in prostate epithelial cellular senescence. Oncogene 22(31):4831–4840

Xin H, Pereira-Smith OM, Choubey D (2004) Role of IFI 16 in cellular senescence of human fibroblasts. Oncogene 23(37):6209–6217

Xu H, Barnes GT, Yang Q, Tan G, Yang D, Chou CJ, Sole J, Nichols A, Ross JS, Tartaglia LA, Chen H (2003) Chronic inflammation in fat plays a crucial role in the development of obesity-related insulin resistance. J Clin Invest 112(12):1821–1830

Xu Y, Zhao Y, Huang H, Chen G, Wu X, Wang Y, Chang W, Zhu Z, Feng Y, Wu D (2010) Expression and function of toll-like receptors in multiple myeloma patients: toll-like receptor ligands promote multiple myeloma cell growth and survival via activation of nuclear factor-kappaB. Br J Haematol 150(5):543–553

Xu H, Wu Q, Dang S, Jin M, Xu J, Cheng Y, Pan M, Wu Y, Zhang C, Zhang Y (2011) Alteration of CXCR7 expression mediated by TLR4 promotes tumor cell proliferation and migration in human colorectal carcinoma. PLoS One 6(12):e27399

Xu N, Yao HP, Lv GC, Chen Z (2012) Downregulation of TLR7/9 leads to deficient production of IFN-alpha from plasmacytoid dendritic cells in chronic hepatitis B. Inflamm Res 61(9):997–1004

Xu L, Wen Z, Zhou Y, Liu Z, Li Q, Fei G, Luo J, Ren T (2013) MicroRNA-7-regulated TLR9 signaling-enhanced growth and metastatic potential of human lung cancer cells by altering the phosphoinositide-3-kinase, regulatory subunit 3/Akt pathway. Mol Biol Cell 24(1):42–55

Yamada Y, Ishibashi K, Ishibashi K, Bhutto IA, Tian J, Lutty GA, Handa JT (2006) The expression of advanced glycation endproduct receptors in rpe cells associated with basal deposits in human maculas. Exp Eye Res 82(5):840–848

Yanagisawa S, Koarai A, Sugiura H, Ichikawa T, Kanda M, Tanaka R, Akamatsu K, Hirano T, Matsunaga K, Minakata Y, Ichinose M (2009) Oxidative stress augments toll-like receptor 8 mediated neutrophilic responses in healthy subjects. Respir Res 10:50

Yang H, Zhou H, Feng P, Zhou X, Wen H, Xie X, Shen H, Zhu X (2010) Reduced expression of toll-like receptor 4 inhibits human breast cancer cells proliferation and inflammatory cytokines secretion. J Exp Clin Cancer Res 29:92

Yao D, Brownlee M (2010) Hyperglycemia-induced reactive oxygen species increase expression of the receptor for advanced glycation end products (RAGE) and RAGE ligands. Diabetes 59(1):249–255

Ye SM, Johnson RW (2001) An age-related decline in interleukin-10 may contribute to the increased expression of interleukin-6 in brain of aged mice. Neuroimmunomodulation 9(4):183–192

Yerkovich ST, Wikstrom ME, Suriyaarachchi D, Prescott SL, Upham JW, Holt PG (2007) Postnatal development of monocyte cytokine responses to bacterial lipopolysaccharide. PediatrRes 62(5):547–552

Yin Y, Yan Y, Jiang X, Mai J, Chen NC, Wang H, Yang XF (2009) Inflammasomes are differentially expressed in cardiovascular and other tissues. Int J Immunopathol Pharmacol 22(2):311–322

Youm YH, Adijiang A, Vandanmagsar B, Burk D, Ravussin A, Dixit VD (2011) Elimination of the NLRP3-ASC inflammasome protects against chronic obesity-induced pancreatic damage. Endocrinology 152(11):4039–4045

Youm YH, Kanneganti TD, Vandanmagsar B, Zhu X, Ravussin A, Adijiang A, Owen JS, Thomas MJ, Francis J, Parks JS, Dixit VD (2012) The Nlrp3 inflammasome promotes age-related thymic demise and immunosenescence. Cell reports 1(1):56–68

Zaki MH, Boyd KL, Vogel P, Kastan MB, Lamkanfi M, Kanneganti TD (2010a) The NLRP3 inflammasome protects against loss of epithelial integrity and mortality during experimental colitis. Immunity 32(3): 379–391

Zaki MH, Vogel P, Body-Malapel M, Lamkanfi M, Kanneganti TD (2010b) IL-18 production downstream of the Nlrp3 inflammasome confers protection against colorectal tumor formation. J Immunol 185(8): 4912–4920

Zaki MH, Vogel P, Malireddi RK, Body-Malapel M, Anand PK, Bertin J, Green DR, Lamkanfi M, Kanneganti TD (2011) The NOD-like receptor NLRP12 attenuates colon inflammation and tumorigenesis. Cancer Cell 20(5):649–660

Zanoni I, Ostuni R, Marek LR, Barresi S, Barbalat R, Barton GM, Granucci F, Kagan JC (2011) CD14 controls the LPS-induced endocytosis of toll-like receptor 4. Cell 147(4):868–880

Zee RY, Lindpaintner K, Struk B, Hennekens CH, Ridker PM (2001) A prospective evaluation of the CD14 C(−260)T gene polymorphism and the risk of myocardial infarction. Atherosclerosis 154(3):699–702

Zee RY, Hegener HH, Gould J, Ridker PM (2005) Toll-like receptor 4 Asp299Gly gene polymorphism and risk of atherothrombosis. Stroke 36(1):154–157

Zhang Z, Schluesener HJ (2006) Mammalian toll-like receptors: from endogenous ligands to tissue regeneration. Cell Mol Life Sci 63(24):2901–2907

Zhang CF, Cao BW, Lu ZM, Xing HP, Cui JG, Ning T, Ke Y (2004) Relationship between polymorphism of IRF-3 gene codon 427 and esophageal cancer in Anyang population of China. Beijing Da Xue Xue Bao 36(4):345–347

Zhang Y, Luo F, Cai Y, Liu N, Wang L, Xu D, Chu Y (2011) TLR1/TLR2 agonist induces tumor regression by reciprocal modulation of effector and regulatory T cells. J Immunol 186(4):1963–1969

Zhang K, Zhou B, Wang Y, Rao L, Zhang L (2013) The TLR4 gene polymorphisms and susceptibility to cancer: a systematic review and meta-analysis. Eur J Cancer 49(4):946–954

Zhao P, Wang J, He L, Ma H, Zhang X, Zhu X, Dolence EK, Ren J, Li J (2009) Deficiency in TLR4 signal transduction ameliorates cardiac injury and cardiomyocyte contractile dysfunction during ischemia. J Cell Mol Med 13(8A):1513–1525

Zheng L, Kagedal K, Dehvari N, Benedikz E, Cowburn R, Marcusson J, Terman A (2009) Oxidative stress induces macroautophagy of amyloid beta-protein and ensuing apoptosis. Free Radic Biol Med 46(3):422–429

Zheng L, Terman A, Hallbeck M, Dehvari N, Cowburn RF, Benedikz E, Kagedal K, Cedazo-Minguez A, Marcusson J (2011) Macroautophagy-generated increase of lysosomal amyloid beta-protein mediates oxidant-induced apoptosis of cultured neuroblastoma cells. Autophagy 7(12):1528–1545

Zheng L, Cedazo-Minguez A, Hallbeck M, Jerhammar F, Marcusson J, Terman A (2012) Intracellular distribution of amyloid beta peptide and its relationship to the lysosomal system. Transl neurodegeneration 1(1):19

Zhou M, McFarland-Mancini MM, Funk HM, Husseinzadeh N, Mounajjed T, Drew AF (2009) Toll-like receptor expression in normal ovary and ovarian tumors. Cancer Immunol Immunother 58(9):1375–1385

Zhou R, Yazdi AS, Menu P, Tschopp J (2011) A role for mitochondria in NLRP3 inflammasome activation. Nature 469(7329):221–225

Zitvogel L, Kepp O, Kroemer G (2010) Decoding cell death signals in inflammation and immunity. Cell 140(6):798–804

Zitvogel L, Kepp O, Kroemer G (2011) Immune parameters affecting the efficacy of chemotherapeutic regimens. Nat Rev Clin Oncol 8(3):151–160

Zitvogel L, Kepp O, Galluzzi L, Kroemer G (2012) Inflammasomes in carcinogenesis and anticancer immune responses. Nat Immunol 13(4):343–351

Impact of Aging on T Cell Repertoire and Immunity

Marcia A. Blackman and David L. Woodland

9.1 Introduction

A hallmark of aging is a decline in immune function, resulting in increased susceptibility to infection and reduced vaccination efficacy. For example, elderly humans respond poorly to influenza virus infection and suffer increased morbidity and mortality. The elderly also respond poorly to vaccines, for example, for influenza virus, and fail to generate high titers of neutralizing antibodies (Vu et al. 2002) and efficient cytolytic CD8[+] T cells (McElhaney et al. 2006, 2009). In addition, previously established memory can be disrupted during aging. Many factors impact immune dysfunction, including age-associated changes in innate cells, B cells, and T cells (Miller 1996; Solana et al. 2006; Agrawal et al. 2008; Gibson et al. 2009). These include age-associated increases in numbers of T-regulatory (Treg) cells, impaired T cell function, and repertoire perturbations in both mouse and human (Nishioka et al. 2006; Lages et al. 2008; Jiang et al. 2009; Pawelec et al. 2010; Goronzy et al. 2007; Cicin-Sain et al. 2010; Ahmed et al. 2009). As it is believed that a diverse T cell repertoire to allow a broad polyclonal response to pathogens

is essential for strong cellular immunity (Yewdell and Haeryfar 2005; Messaoudi et al. 2002; Kedzierska et al. 2005), declining repertoire diversity is strongly implicated in impaired immunity associated with aging, which is the focus of this chapter.

Much of our understanding of the impact of aging on immunity has come from the experimentally amenable mouse model. Mice display key characteristics of age-associated decline in immune function that have been described in human and other models. The mouse model allows longitudinal studies and direct determination of the impact of age on the ability to respond to infection with a variety of pathogens (Murasko and Jiang 2005; Ely et al. 2007b). For example, the mouse influenza virus model is frequently used to examine the impact of aging on vaccination and immunity (Po et al. 2002; Effros and Walford 1983). The basic observation is that aged mice are more difficult to vaccinate and are more susceptible to influenza infection, often succumbing to doses that are nonlethal for young mice. Aged mice are also impaired in their ability to clear infectious virus. Although effector cells in aged mice have been shown to be highly functional on a per cell basis, they are fewer in number as a consequence of impaired T cell proliferation (Effros et al. 2003). In addition, there are profound repertoire perturbations (Yager et al. 2008; Li et al. 2002; Jiang et al. 2011; Decman et al. 2012; Valkenburg et al. 2012).

Several factors affect the diversity of the T cell repertoire in mouse and human. First, there is

M.A. Blackman, PhD (✉)
Trudeau Institute, Saranac Lake, NY 12983, USA
e-mail: mblackman@trudeauinstitute.org

D.L. Woodland, PhD
Keystone Symposia, Silverthorne, CO 80498, USA

A. Massoud, N. Rezaei (eds.), *Immunology of Aging*,
DOI 10.1007/978-3-642-39495-9_9, © Springer-Verlag Berlin Heidelberg 2014

progressive thymic involution with age, resulting in export of fewer naïve T cells. Second, with increasing antigen experience, the memory pool progressively expands, and there is a steady reversal of the naïve-memory ratio over time, with the memory pool eventually dominating the peripheral repertoire. Third, the memory compartment is further perturbed by the frequent appearance of T cell clonal expansions (TCEs) in the memory CD8[+] T cells. In humans, chronic infection with cytomegalovirus (CMV) drives the development of TCE and is strongly associated with impaired immunity. Accumulating data from studies in mouse, primate, and human support the role of repertoire perturbation in immune dysfunction associated with aging, which have directed experimental approaches to reverse immunosenescence. While it is likely that there are many contributing factors to the decline of T cell function in aging, increasing evidence suggests that a major controlling factor is the reduction in the diversity of the antigen-specific repertoire of T cells, which will be the focus of this chapter.

9.2 Influence of Age on the T Cell Repertoire

As discussed above, aging is associated with decreased T cell repertoire and it has been hypothesized that decreased repertoire diversity is associated with impaired immune function. There are constraints in both the naïve and memory T cell repertoires with age.

9.2.1 Impact of Aging on the Naïve T Cell Repertoire

In young adults, T cells in the periphery are largely naïve, with a highly diverse repertoire. The mouse is estimated to have $\sim 1\text{--}2 \times 10^8$ T cells expressing $\sim 2 \times 10^6$ different specificities, suggesting that there are ~ 50 naïve T cells of each specificity (Casrouge et al. 2000). Humans are estimated to have $\sim 3 \times 10^{11}$ T cells with $\sim 10^8$ different specificities, suggesting that the clone size for each specificity in human is $\sim 1,000$ (Arstila et al. 1999; Goronzy and Weyand 2005).

T cells mature in the thymus and seed the periphery with naïve T cells. With age, the thymus undergoes atrophy, which results in loss of thymic epithelial cells and decreased production of new, naïve T cells (Taub and Longo 2005; Heng et al. 2010). Since maintenance of the naïve pool is dependent on homeostatic proliferation in the periphery, the absence of new T cells from the thymus results in a decline in numbers and loss of diversity of naïve T cells. Importantly, the homeostatic maintenance is not random, but becomes biased toward cells capable of higher rates of homeostatic proliferation and of higher T cell receptor (TCR) avidity (Rudd et al. 2011b). With aging, the naïve T cells become more "memory-like" and the repertoire becomes more focused. In addition, the proportion of naïve-memory T cells decreases with increasing antigen experience and increasing age.

It has been shown that the number of naïve peripheral T cells declines with age. The diversity of the T cell repertoire has been measured both by genetic approaches (spectratyping, which assesses T cell receptor CDR3 length) and by directly counting antigen-specific naïve T cells. Spectratyping and sequence analysis of naïve CD8[+] T cells isolated from young and aged mice showed that aged mice had skewed spectratype profiles indicative of reduced diversity (Ahmed et al. 2009). In addition, unexpected sequence repeats in naïve T cells from aged mice suggested dysregulation in the normal homeostatic mechanisms that maintain diversity in young animals. This analysis was carried out in specific pathogen-free "naïve" mice and was not associated with the presence of clonal expansions in the CD8[+] memory pool or with chronic infection.

More recently, the decline in the size of antigen-specific naïve pools has been measured directly using the tetramer pull-down assay (Moon et al. 2007; Obar et al. 2008). In one report, the number of naïve CD8[+] T cells specific for a herpes simplex virus (HSV)-1 glycoprotein B epitope showed a decline in frequency from ~ 400 in adult, unprimed mice to ~ 125 in 22-month-old mice (Rudd et al. 2011b). Interestingly, the constriction with age was accompanied by the emergence of dominant clonotypes shared in individual aged mice, indicative of selective rather than stochastic mechanisms (Rudd et al. 2011a). In another study, the naïve repertoire was analyzed in aged and young mice, as well as herpesvirus-infected aged mice. The data showed that there was a reduction in epitope-specific naïve precursors to ovalbumin (OVA) expressed in the context of Listeria monocytogenes, determined by tetramer pull-down experiments in aged compared to young mice, which was further reduced in mice infected with murine CMV (Smithey et al. 2012). The impact of CMV infection on repertoire will be discussed in detail below.

Studies in humans have shown that the decline in diversity of the naïve T cell repertoire with age is not linear. In the case of the CD4+ T cell repertoire, it has been shown that diversity was maintained relatively stably at ~2×10^7 different T cell receptor β-chains until age 70, despite extensive loss of thymic function at that age. However, after age 70 the diversity plummeted to 2×10^5 specificities (Naylor et al. 2005). These data suggest that homeostatic proliferation, which maintains the T cell repertoire increasingly as thymic function declines, may have physiological limits, and the proliferative capacity of T cells may become greatly diminished by age 70 (Goronzy and Weyand 2005).

9.2.2 TCE Basic Parameters

One of the most profound changes in repertoire with age is the development of TCE, which are nonmalignant, monoclonal populations of CD8+ T cells, but not CD4+ T cells. These TCE were first detected in mice, using TCR Vβ antibodies (Callahan et al. 1993). The expansions varied in size and could be as great as 90 % of the population of peripheral CD8+ T cells in aged mice. TCE are found in about 60 % of mice over 2 years old (although the frequency probably varies in different animal facilities) (Clambey et al. 2007). In addition, clonal populations of CD8+ T cells in aged humans were identified in approximately one-third of individuals over 65 years of age (Posnett et al. 1994; Clambey et al. 2007). It has been hypothesized that such expansions cause perturbation of the repertoire due to "crowding out" of naïve and/or memory cells of diverse specificities and thus contributing to impaired immunity associated with aging. Data supporting this possibility are presented below.

Characteristics of TCE have been described in detail (Clambey et al. 2007, 2008). One key characteristic is that most TCE do not require antigen for their generation or maintenance. This is supported by the observations that specific pathogen-free mice develop TCE and that TCEs transferred into β$_2$ microglobulin-deficient mice maintain their proliferative function. TCE sometimes arise as a consequence of chronic stimulation in mice (Lang et al. 2008). In humans, most TCE are thought to be triggered by infection with CMV, suggesting that they are driven by chronic antigen stimulation (Khan et al. 2002; Ouyang et al. 2003). TCE can also develop from the memory pool specific for viruses that are cleared following an acute infection (Ely et al. 2007a; Kohlmeier et al. 2010; Connor et al. 2012). It is hypothesized that these acute virus-specific TCE are formed as a consequence of slight variations in the rate of homeostatic proliferation of memory cells, in agreement with previous studies assessing rates of basal proliferation of TCE compared with normal memory homeostatic proliferation (Kohlmeier et al. 2010; Connor et al. 2012; Ku et al. 2001, 1997).

Another key characteristic is that TCE are phenotypically heterogeneous and their stability varies. There is considerable variability in the phenotype of TCE perhaps reflecting heterogeneity in the types or origin of TCE. In one study, microarray analysis was used to study integrin α4-gene expression in TCE and polyclonal memory CD8+ T cells. There was variation in expression within individual TCE although levels were stable within a single TCE. Furthermore, clones with high levels of integrin α4-gene expression were found to be unstable in vivo (Clambey et al. 2008). It has also been shown in the mouse that TCE are frequently unstable, with some clones disappearing in a 2–4-month time frame and new ones developing (LeMaoult et al. 2000). In some studies, TCE have been reported that appear to be a type of central memory cell, expressing higher levels of CD122 and CD127, components of the interleukin (IL)-15R and IL-7R which regulate homeostasis (Messaoudi et al. 2006b).

Are there perturbations in the CD4$^+$ T cell repertoire? Although most of the attention has focused on CD8$^+$ TCE in CMV-infected aged individuals, high levels of CD4$^+$ CMV-specific T cells have been found in healthy seropositive individuals (Sester et al. 2002). It is unclear whether they increase with age and contribute to the immunosenescence (Pawelec et al. 2005). Infection with CMV has been shown to induce the accumulation of late-stage differentiated CD4$^+$ T cells in addition to CD8$^+$ T cells in middle-aged individuals, although in lower frequencies than CD8$^+$ T cells (Derhovanessian et al. 2011). The late-stage differentiation phenotype was CD27$^-$, CD28$^-$, and with some cells CD57$^+$, a putative senescence marker. Higher levels of anti-CMV antibody correlated exclusively with levels of late-differentiated CD4$^+$ T cells, perhaps as a consequence of the helper role CD4$^+$ T cells play in generating antibody (Derhovanessian et al. 2011). It has also been shown that accumulation of CMV-driven CD4$^+$ T cells, rather than CD8$^+$ T cells, correlated with poor humoral response to influenza vaccination (Derhovanessian et al. 2012).

There are conflicting reports of the functional capacity of TCE. Whereas in vitro studies have shown that TCE can respond in terms of cytokine secretion (Clambey et al. 2007; Ely et al. 2007a), in vivo studies of antigen-specific TCE generated from acute virus-specific memory CD8$^+$ T cells show a reduced capacity to participate in recall responses. These studies directly compared the ability of antigen-specific TCE to respond to secondary infection in an in vivo model with the ability of young, non-expanded memory cells, using a dual adoptive transfer approach in which equal numbers of antigen-specific cells were cotransferred into a young naïve recipient and then challenged with virus. The data show that the TCE generally failed to compete equally with the young memory cells, although some TCE clones had comparable responsiveness (Kohlmeier et al. 2010; Connor et al. 2012).

9.2.3 Role of Chronic Infection in the Development of TCE

How do TCE arise? Early studies in the mouse were carried out in specific pathogen-free mice and were detected using T cell receptor Vβ antibodies, so that the antigen specificity was not known (Blackman and Woodland 2011). More recent evidence shows that TCE can develop from memory cells derived from previous encounters with viruses that cause acute infections, such as influenza virus and Sendai virus (Ely et al. 2007a; Kohlmeier et al. 2010; Connor et al. 2012). However, the bulk of data in humans show that chronic infections such as CMV are important drivers of TCEs.

CMV is a β-herpesvirus that infects a majority of the world's population. The seroprevalence increases with increasing age. Following acute infection, the virus goes dormant and persists for the life of the individual. Human CMV (HCMV) responses to the initial, acute infection occupy more than 20 % of the total CD8$^+$ T cell pool (Sylwester et al. 2005). Initially there is a broad repertoire of CMV-specific cells, but with time the repertoire becomes focused on a restricted number of immunodominant epitopes (Munks et al. 2006; Day et al. 2007), and over time there is a preferential expansion of "inflationary" epitopes, and the human CD8$^+$ T cell repertoire becomes dominated by CMV-specific cells (Khan et al. 2002, 2004; Karrer et al. 2003). The clonality of the populations increases with age, perhaps a result of exhaustion and dropping out of many specificities (Hadrup et al. 2006). It is unknown whether the strong repertoire effects are due to the persistence and periodic reactivation of CMV, as reactivation events are clinically silent. With age, large oligoclonal populations of CD28$^-$CD8$^+$ T cells accumulate in the periphery, with a corresponding decrease in naïve T cells. Over time, there is a further focusing, culminating in dominance by a single specificity with a higher avidity (Schwanninger et al. 2008). It is assumed, but not proven, that other clones disappear with age, due to exhaustion or superinfection (Trautmann et al. 2005; Hansen et al. 2010). CD8$^+$CD28$^-$ T cells dominate in CMV-infected elderly individuals (Almanzar et al. 2005; Ge et al. 2002; Appay et al. 2002; Ouyang et al. 2004). CD8⁺CD28⁻ T cells are considered to be senescent T cells, with shorter telomeres, arising from chronic TCR stimulation (Effros et al. 1996; Monteiro et al. 1996). The noninflationary epitopes maintain a functional, central memory phenotype, whereas the inflationary epitopes develop an extreme effector memory phenotype. They are strong secretors of tumor necrosis factor alpha (TNF-α) and interferon gamma (IFN-γ), they maintain lytic capacity, and they are not exhausted, as has been described for LCMV (Klenerman and Dunbar 2008; Snyder et al. 2008; Waller et al. 2008). CMV not only acts through effects on T cells but also impacts proinflammatory status, as viral gene products upregulate production of IL-6, IL-1, TNF-α, IFN-γ, and a variety of chemokines (reviewed in (Varani et al. 2009)).

TCE can also arise as a consequence of chronic infection of the mouse. For example, HSV-1 was shown to elicit an acute response, which contracted but then exhibited memory inflation and an accumulation of antigen-specific cells. However, continuous treatment with an antiviral drug that prevented viral replication did not prevent the inflation, showing that continual viral replication was not required for the development of TCE (Lang et al. 2008). There is such a strong association between CMV and senescence that it has been proposed that immunosenescence is "infectious" (Pawelec et al. 2005) (reviewed in (Pawelec et al. 2009)). CMV drives the development of CD8⁺CD28⁻ dysfunctional T cells and is strongly implicated in the immune risk phenotype (Wikby et al. 2002).

9.2.4 Is CMV Unique, or Will Other Chronic Infections Induce TCE?

The strong association between CMV, TCE, and immunosenescence has raised the question as to whether there is something unique about CMV infection or whether any persistent virus can induce the same effect. Although Epstein-Barr

virus (EBV) is also a persistent herpes virus, it is not as strongly associated as CMV with accumulations of memory cells and development of TCE (Khan et al. 2004). Although the frequency of CMV-negative EBV-positive individuals is low, making an analysis of the impact of EBV in the absence of CMV is difficult, EBV memory cells have been shown to accumulate in some CMV seronegative individuals, and TCE to EBV have been demonstrated at reduced frequencies compared with CMV-specific TCE (Colonna-Romano et al. 2007; Ouyang et al. 2003; Vescovini et al. 2004). In addition, important phenotypic differences between CMV- and EBV-induced T cells have been identified. CMV drives differentiation of CD8⁺ T cells to a highly differentiated phenotype-effector memory (CCR7^{null}CD45RA^{low}) or effector (CCR7^{null}CD45RA$^+$)⁻ and to become CD28⁻, a phenotype associated with dysfunction and immunosenescence, whereas this was not the case of EBV-specific T cells (Derhovanessian et al. 2011), which maintained expression of CD28 (Pawelec et al. 2005). Although CMV and EBV elicit TCE, it appears that not all chronic viruses can do this. For example, infection with HSV, another persistent virus, does not result in clonal expansions in CMV-negative aged humans (Derhovanessian et al. 2011). In contrast, the virus does cause TCE in mice (Lang et al. 2009). One possible reason for the disparate results is that the mouse model employs systemic infection, so is different from naturally occurring infections in humans and may be more similar to CMV in terms of dissemination and latency reservoirs.

The reason that CMV apparently preferentially induces TCE is not entirely understood. One key feature of CMV is that, although infections with the three herpes viruses studied in detail (CMV, EBV, and HSV) are all persistent, the site of latency establishment differs. CMV establishes a latent infection in myeloid progenitor cells and monocytes that can serve as antigen-presenting cells and, in addition, there is a low-level chronic infection in epithelial cells of the salivary gland of the liver that may serve to continually present antigen and drive CD8⁺ T cells. In contrast, HSV resides in neurons, hidden from the immune system, reappearing only occasionally during reactivation events. Another possibility is that CMV has higher rates of reactivation, but this is difficult to assess since reactivation is asymptomatic (Derhovanessian et al. 2011). Yet another explanation may be that there is a greater degree of cross-reactivity in CMV compared to EBV-specific cells. Finally, it may be due to the nature of the primary infection, which has been understudied due to its asymptomatic nature.

9.3 Impact of Age-Associated Changes in T Cell Repertoire on Immunity

The T cell repertoire changes discussed above constitute a key contributing factor to age-associated immune dysfunction. Constriction of the naïve T cell repertoire results in impaired immunity to new infections in the elderly. In addition, perturbation over time in the memory T cell repertoire can impact protective immunity and the ability to generate recall responses to previously encountered infections.

9.3.1 Impact of Reduced Naïve Repertoire Diversity on Immunity to New Infections

As discussed, there is a reduced naïve repertoire with age. Several studies have defined an approximate 10-fold decline in precursor frequency of epitope-specific T cells in aged compared with young mice (Rudd et al. 2011b; Smithey et al. 2012). Constriction in the naïve repertoire with age is due to diminished thymic function and the generation of fewer naïve T cells, coupled with increasing antigenic experience, and/or the development of TCE resulting in a shift in the ratio of naïve to memory T cells in the periphery. Reduction in diversity of the naïve T cell repertoire profoundly impairs the ability of aged individuals to respond to new infections. This has been extensively documented in both mouse and human. In some, but not all, cases, the immune

dysfunction has been directly linked to the development of TCEs, which can dilute out the diversity of the naïve repertoire. Below we will discuss the impact of reduced naïve repertoire diversity, with or without a direct link to TCEs, on immunity to new infections.

Examination of the age-associated constriction of the naïve CD8+ T cell repertoire in the absence of large TCEs and the impact on immune function to a new virus infection was carried out in the mouse influenza virus model. Although comparable numbers of CD8+ T cells were elicited in the lung airways following primary influenza virus infection in young and aged mice, most, but not all of the aged mice showed perturbations in the repertoire of responding cells (Yager et al. 2008). There was a preferential decline in the response to the immunodominant epitope from the influenza virus nucleoprotein (NP), which varied in individual mice. In some cases there was a failure to respond to the NP epitope, with a shift to other epitopes, indicating a "hole" in the repertoire. In addition, in aged mice that retained the ability to respond to NP, the prototypical T cell receptor Vβ usage was perturbed. Development of the repertoire perturbations were accelerated in thymectomized mice, consistent with a decline in naïve T cell repertoire diversity with aging. Importantly, the decline in response to NP correlated with impaired protective immunity to challenge with heterosubtypic influenza virus that bypasses humoral immunity and is dependent on CD8+ T cell protection. In this study, efforts were made to eliminate mice that exhibited large TCE from the study.

It has also been shown that CMV-infected individuals have impaired immunity to other infections. For example, CMV infection impairs immunity to a coresident EBV infection in old age (Khan et al. 2004, 2002). Although CMV is associated with the development of TCEs, the immune dysfunction has not always been directly correlated with the presence of TCEs. Because of difficulties studying the impact of a chronic infection longitudinally in humans, many experiments have been carried out with the mouse virus, murine CMV (MCMV). The MCMV virus is well characterized and is considered an appropriate model for human CMV infection (Cicin-Sain et al. 2012). MCMV-infected mice showed inflation of CMV-specific memory cells, reduced numbers of naïve CD8+ T cells in the periphery and a perturbed repertoire assessed by T cell receptor Vβ analysis. Importantly, there was also impaired immunity to new infections with influenza virus, HSV-1, and West Nile virus in the CMV-infected, aged animals. This effect was specific for CMV, as it was not seen in aged mice chronically infected with HSV-1. Further experiments with mutant CMV viruses that lacked key immune evasion genes still caused the impairment in immune function. This impaired immunity to new infections corresponded to an observed reduction in diversity of the naïve repertoire (Smithey et al. 2012). In a related study, Mekker et al. showed that challenge infection with LCMV was more profoundly impaired in MCMV-infected mice compared with aged or thymectomized mice (Mekker et al. 2012). However, in contrast to the Smithey study mentioned above, this did not correlate with reduced numbers of naïve T cells specific for CMV (although the authors did not specifically examine the repertoire of naïve T cells), as there were similar naïve T cell numbers in MCMV-infected and noninfected mice (Mekker et al. 2012). In the Mekker study, the authors concluded that rather than reduction in the naïve repertoire, MCMV infection impairs immunity due to the increased competition between MCMV-specific memory and a "de novo" immune response in aged individuals (Mekker et al. 2012).

In other studies, the presence of TCE has been directly correlated with declining immunity to new infections. They have been shown to dilute out the repertoire diversity of naïve and other memory T cells, which results in impaired immune function. In addition, TCE may be dysfunctional and have a direct effect on immune responses. Early correlative data in humans showed that individuals with TCE have an impaired ability to respond to influenza vaccination, in terms of both humoral immunity and cellular immunity (Saurwein-Teissl et al. 2002; Trzonkowski et al. 2003; Goronzy et al. 2001; Xie and McElhaney 2007). Also, the presence of TCE predicted poor control of HIV, resulting in increased progression to AIDS (Sinicco et al. 1997).

In mice, it was directly demonstrated that TCE impair the ability to respond to a new pathogen (Messaoudi et al. 2004). Specifically, the response to HSV is known to be focused exclusively on a single epitope and dominated by T cells bearing Vβ8 or Vβ10. The study showed that a TCE in either of those two Vβ families corresponded with a poor response to HSV infection (Messaoudi et al. 2004). Development of immunity to Listeria monocytogenes in young and old mice was comparable in terms of numbers, but yet aged mice were inferior in terms of protection (Smithey et al. 2011).

Similar results have been observed in old rhesus monkeys. Old primates have been shown to develop TCEs with corresponding reductions in naïve T cells (Jankovic et al. 2003; Pitcher et al. 2002; Cicin-Sain et al. 2007). It was shown that aged monkeys with reduced proportions of naïve T cells (assessed by phenotyping) and expressing TCEs (determined by spectratyping), responded poorly to vaccination with the modified vaccinia strain Ankara (Cicin-Sain et al. 2010). Thus, the correlation between age-associated reduction in naïve repertoire diversity and poor immunity to new infections observed in mouse studies was confirmed in primate studies. These data in experimental models support the correlation between reduced repertoire diversity and impaired response to new infections and vaccination observed in elderly humans.

9.3.2 Impact of Reduced Memory Repertoire Diversity on Memory Maintenance and Recall Responses

Perturbation of the memory repertoire with age can also have profound effects on protective immunity generated to previous infections. The repertoire of memory cells is reduced during aging due to the focusing of certain clones and presumable loss of others and/or the development of TCE. In addition, memory cells may become dysfunctional over time, resulting in impaired recall function.

Previous studies in the mouse have shown that memory generated in young mice retains function, whereas memory generated in aged mice is poor, for both CD8[+] and CD4[+] T cell memory (Kapasi et al. 2002; Haynes et al. 2003). These data suggest that function depends more on the age of the naïve cell when it first encounters antigen than on the age of the memory cell when it is restimulated by antigen. This observation potentially explains one of the difficulties associated with successful vaccination of the elderly against new pathogens. Additional studies examined the functional capacity of memory cells generated in young mice with time into old age and showed that memory generated when young actually improved with age, whereas memory generated in aged mice was poorly functional. The data showed a progressive increase in the recall response to secondary pathogen challenge over time that was especially apparent in the central memory population (Roberts et al. 2005).

Recently, it has been shown that memory in aged mice was generated at a comparable magnitude to memory in young mice, although the memory in the aged mice was biased toward an effector memory/senescent phenotype, and protective immunity against viral challenge was impaired (Decman et al. 2010). The aged mice experienced morbidity and mortality after the same challenge dose from which the young mice were protected. This feature of the memory cells was "cell intrinsic," because the same defects were observed after transfer of memory cells into naïve congenic recipients and challenged. Several possible explanations for the impaired memory discussed by the authors include extended exposure to antigen during the development of memory because of delayed clearance of the initial infection, differences in the inflammatory environment during memory T cell development, and/or differences in the repertoire of T cells that develop into memory in the aged versus young mice.

Despite these data, it has been shown in both mice and humans that previously established memory can deteriorate with age, as a result of clonal expansions and reduced diversity as a consequence of "focusing" of the repertoire. In

the mouse, it has been shown that TCE can develop from the memory population. As previously discussed, in addition to TCE arising as a result of chronic infections, it has been shown that TCE can arise from memory cells established to acute (nonpersistent) viral infections (Ely et al. 2007b; Kohlmeier et al. 2010). Sendai virus- or influenza virus-infected mice developed clonal expansions in their memory pool. The cells retained function as assessed by cytokine secretion, maintained proliferative capacity, and proliferated in vitro in the absence of antigen. In addition, TCE transferred into naïve recipients were maintained for several weeks and had high rates of homeostatic proliferation. Further functional analysis, however, showed that the TCEs varied in their ability to mediate a recall response to antigen challenge, three out of the four TCE examined were functionally impaired compared with their non-expanded counterparts in responding to secondary viral challenge (Kohlmeier et al. 2010). The TCE appeared progressively with time, between 320 and 700 days postinfection. More recently it was shown using a more sensitive detection assay that the memory repertoire perturbations first started to develop within months of infection and increased over time into large TCE (Connor et al. 2012). These data suggest that the development of TCEs is a natural outcome of long-term maintenance of memory and is independent of the aging process.

Also, in the mouse LCMV model, it has been shown that the memory T cell response to LCMV is diverse and maintained for long periods of time. However, analysis over time showed that although the magnitude of the virus-specific CD8[+] T cells was maintained, the distribution of clones within the population changed dramatically. In one of two mice examined, the percentage of a single clone reached 100 %! This supports the contention that TCE can arise from memory cells (Bunztman et al. 2012), as discussed above (Ely et al. 2007a; Kohlmeier et al. 2010; Connor et al. 2012).

A similar focusing of the influenza-specific memory CD8[+] repertoire was shown in healthy elderly people (Lee et al. 2011). Using a sensitive assay to expand the population of memory

T cells, it was possible to assess responses to both dominant epitopes and subdominant influenza virus epitopes. The data showed that young individuals had a response to dominant epitopes as well as a strong response to subdominant epitopes, which was statistically significantly reduced in healthy elderly individuals, resulting in greatly diminished diversity in the influenza-specific recall response. It was speculated that perturbation of the memory repertoire in T cells specific for a virus that is not a persistent virus could be driven by multiple exposures to influenza virus.

9.4 Therapeutic Approaches

As the human population ages and anticipates an extended lifespan, there has been much emphasis on how to overcome or reverse the impact of aging on immune function. Some strategies are discussed below.

9.4.1 Vaccination Strategies

Aging is correlated with poor vaccination efficacy. Consequently, a major emphasis has been placed on developing better adjuvants or vaccine delivery systems for the elderly (Haynes and Swain 2006; Maue et al. 2009; Coler et al. 2010; Zhu et al. 2010). In addition, it has been shown that vaccination early in life when immune cells are functional and there is a highly diverse repertoire of T cells elicits strong immunity that can last into old age. Thus, early priming leads to long-term maintenance of memory T cells and preserves optimal responses in old age (Valkenburg et al. 2012). For example, in studies where mice were vaccinated at 6 weeks and then challenged at 22 months strong functional T cell responses developed that expressed the repertoire characteristic of a young mouse, whereas vaccination at 22 months had responses of the same magnitude as young mice but with reduced receptor diversity. Also, infection of aged mice with LCMV or influenza resulted in poor protective immunity, whereas if memory was established

when young, protective memory cells persisted (Kapasi et al. 2002), and memory generated in young mice against respiratory viruses actually improved with age (Roberts et al. 2005). These data have supported the idea of increased vaccinations in middle age to establish memory before immune dysfunction limits the ability to respond to new infections. However, there were concerns that there were limitations of "space" for memory T cells, and that previously established memory would be replaced with new memory cells upon new infection. These concerns were somewhat allayed by the report suggested that there is no limit to the size of the memory compartment (Vezys et al. 2008). However, it was later reported that although the memory compartment can grow in size, function can be lost (Huster et al. 2009), so limitations to memory "storage space" remain a concern.

9.4.2 Thymic Rejuvenation

The fundamental importance of the loss of new naïve T cells as a consequence of thymic involution to impaired immunity in the elderly has prompted attempts to rejuvenate the thymus. Several treatments have been tried with varying degrees of success, including modulation with sex hormones, administration of growth hormone, anti-transforming growth factor beta (TGF-β), IL-7, Flt3L, or keratinocyte growth factor (KGF) (Holland and van den Brink 2009; Lynch et al. 2009; Aspinall and Mitchell 2008; Heng et al. 2010). Recently it has been shown that IL-22 promotes thymic regeneration in mice after stress, infection, or immunodepletion (Dudakov et al. 2012). Maintenance of the naïve T cell pool in mice was shown to be almost exclusively due to thymic output, whereas homeostatic peripheral T cell proliferation was shown to play a key role in maintenance of the naïve human pool (den Braber et al. 2012), suggesting that thymectomized mice may serve as a better experimental model for humans than aged mice (Mackall and Gress 1997). The report showed that peripheral T cell division was responsible for maintaining numbers of peripheral naïve cells, even in young children with a healthy thymus. However, it was pointed that maintenance of the peripheral repertoire by homeostatic proliferation does not introduce T cells of new specificity, but merely amplifies preexisting specificities. However, with age, the loss of repertoire diversity suggests that homeostatic proliferation is unable to maintain adequate numbers of naïve T cells. Therefore, the thymus may still make an important contribution to maintaining a diverse peripheral repertoire in humans, consistent with the loss of repertoire diversity with age. It has also been shown that thymocyte development relies on a source of progenitors from the bone marrow, which also have been shown to exhibit age-related defects (Waterstrat and Van Zant 2009). New approaches, exploiting new tissue engineering and stem cell technologies and still under development in the mouse and dependent on recently-discovered thymic epithelial progenitor cells, include de novo thymus generation (Heng et al. 2010).

9.4.3 Rejuvenation of Peripheral T Cells

With increasing age, the periphery fills up with exhausted CD28− CD8+ T cells. It has been suggested that a possible approach to enhancing immune function in the elderly would be to deplete CD28− CD8+ T cells from the periphery to create space for new naïve T cells and functional memory cells. This approach has been successful with systemic lupus erythematosus (SLE) patients (Alexander et al. 2009; Brunner et al. 2010). In the mouse it has been shown that deletion of aged CD4+ T cells allowed the repopulation with cells that were functional, even in the aged host (Haynes 2005). These strategies depend on residual thymus function in the elderly.

9.4.4 Calorie Restriction

Studies in rhesus monkey studies showed that calorie restriction (CR) in CMV+ animals enhanced maintenance of naïve T cells, which were proliferatively "younger" (excision circles), had lower levels of proinflammatory cytokines IFN-γ and TNF-β, and had fewer effector memory cells (Messaoudi et al. 2006a). Although previous studies in mice and monkeys correlated CR with longer life, a recent 25-year study in rhesus monkeys fed 30 % less than control animals, failed to show a simple correlation, and instead suggested that genetics and composition of the diet predict longevity rather than simply numbers of calories (Mattison et al. 2012).

9.4.5 Targeting CMV

CMV infection strongly impacts human immunosenescence, and is a key characteristic defining the "immune risk phenotype," which describes progressive changes in the immune system associated with predicted mortality in the elderly. The immune risk phenotype includes, in addition to CMV seropositivity, an inverted CD4+/CD8+ ratio and a preponderance of CD28− CD8+ T cells (Wikby et al. 1998, 2002; Hadrup et al. 2006). Senescent CD28− CD8+ T cells are found almost exclusively in CMV seropositive individuals, and 80–90 % of the elderly population are CMV seropositive, making it difficult to separate CMV as the culprit or "an innocent bystander" (Tatum and Hill 2010). Also, elderly individuals with very high levels of CMV-specific serum immunoglobulin had the highest risk of mortality (Roberts et al. 2010). A study of individuals who attained 100 years of age showed that they did not have the hallmarks of the immune risk phenotype, in that they maintained a high CD4+ to CD8+ ratio and had low numbers of CD28− CD8+ T cells. However, most of them were positive for CMV, raising the question of what factors influence the response of individuals to CMV. Is it due to the duration of infection, the frequency of reactivation events, the genetics of the individual, or variation in the proinflammatory profile (Finch and Crimmins 2004)? It is important to note that the immune risk profile predicts mortality independently of health status (Strindhall et al. 2007).

9.4.6 Vaccination Against CMV

The strong association between CMV infection, impaired immunity, and the immune risk phenotype has raised the suggestion that approaches to prevent CMV infection or to control reactivation would improve the life expectancy of the elderly. One approach would be to develop a vaccine to prevent infection. There are two difficulties with this approach. First, it would be difficult to develop a sterilizing vaccine to prevent infection, as these viruses are masters of immune evasion. A more feasible approach would be a therapeutic vaccine that would prevent reactivation events that may be responsible for driving the development of TCEs and immunosenescence, but such a vaccine is currently not on the horizon. Second, it has been suggested that chronic herpes virus infections are beneficial (Barton et al. 2007), and it would be detrimental to vaccinate against them. Taking this possibility into account, it might be better to focus on therapeutic vaccines to be administered in healthy adults to allow the putative beneficial effects of CMV infection early in life, yet prevent the onset of dysfunction associated with CMV infection in the elderly.

9.4.7 Antiviral Therapy

It was previously shown that latent infection and viral reactivation are necessary for memory inflation (Lang et al. 2009), suggesting that antiviral therapy may be effective in controlling the development of CMV-driven immunosenescence. A recent study showed that extended antiviral therapy (for as long as 12 months) can reverse the development of CMV-associated immunosenescence in aged mice (Beswick et al. 2013). These studies supported the possibility that antiviral therapy to suppress CMV reactivation events can prevent/reverse the inflation of CMV infection. Not only was the magnitude of the CMV-specific CD8+ T cells reduced, but the remaining virus-specific T cells displayed a less-differentiated phenotype. In addition, drug-treated aged mice showed improvement in their response to influenza virus infection. It had previously been shown that transferred inflated memory cells had a short lifespan (Klenerman and Dunbar 2008) and that memory inflation was maintained by continuous stimulation of naïve T cells (Snyder et al. 2008), which probably explains the recovery. Regarding the possibility that CMV has advantages against other acute infections mentioned above (Barton et al. 2007), the authors noted both clinical and immunological differences between the drug-treated aged animals and uninfected animals. This raises the possibility that the drug treatment "may have unmasked a potential benefit of underlying MCMV infection that is otherwise lost in elderly animals due to uncontrolled memory inflation." These studies suggest that memory inflation is reversible.

9.4.8 T Cell Therapy

As it is thought that periodic viral reactivation events may be driving CMV-mediated memory inflation, a possible therapy might be adoptive T cell therapy, the transfer of CMV-specific T cell clones (Schmitt et al. 2011; Feuchtinger et al. 2010) or ex vivo-generated CMV-specific CD8+ T cells, to control reactivation events, similar to the approaches that have been successful in controlling EBV in bone marrow transplant recipients (Pawelec 2005).

Conclusion

People are living longer, and the proportion of the population considered elderly is increasing. The experimental mouse model, despite its limitations, has allowed great advances in our understanding of the impact of aging on immune function. The mouse allows longitudinal studies and in vivo functional studies not possible in human. Therapeutic strategies to prevent or reverse immune dysfunction associated with aging can be tested in the mouse model, and the fundamental principals learned then translated to primate and human studies. Although difficult, more longitudinal studies of humans are needed and CMV-negative populations need to be studied alongside the majority of the CMV-positive elderly.

References

Agrawal A, Agrawal S, Tay J et al (2008) Biology of dendritic cells in aging. J Clin Immunol 28(1):14–20

Ahmed M, Lanzer KG, Yager EJ et al (2009) Clonal expansions and loss of receptor diversity in the naive CD8+ T cell repertoire of aged mice. J Immunol 182(2):784–792

Alexander T, Thiel A, Rosen O et al (2009) Depletion of autoreactive immunologic memory followed by autologous hematopoietic stem cell transplantation in patients with refractory SLE induces long-term remission through de novo generation of a juvenile and tolerant immune system. Blood 113(1):214–223

Almanzar G, Schwaiger S, Jenewein B et al (2005) Long-term cytomegalovirus infection leads to significant changes in the composition of the CD8+ T-cell repertoire, which may be the basis for an imbalance in the cytokine production profile in elderly persons. J Virol 79(6):3675–3683

Appay V, Dunbar PR, Callan M et al (2002) Memory CD8+ T cells vary in differentiation phenotype in different persistent virus infections. Nat Med 8(4):379–385

Arstila TP, Casrouge A, Baron V et al (1999) A direct estimate of the human alphabeta T cell receptor diversity. Science 286(5441):958–961

Aspinall R, Mitchell W (2008) Reversal of age-associated thymic atrophy: treatments, delivery, and side effects. Exp Gerontol 43(7):700–705

Barton ES, White DW, Cathelyn JS et al (2007) Herpesvirus latency confers symbiotic protection from bacterial infection. Nature 447(7142):326–329

Beswick M, Pachnio A, Lauder SN et al (2013) Antiviral therapy can reverse the development of immune senescence in elderly mice with latent cytomegalovirus infection. J Virol 87(2):779–789

Blackman MA, Woodland DL (2011) The narrowing of the CD8+ T cell repertoire in old age. Curr Opin Immunol 23(4):537–542

Brunner S, Herndler-Brandstetter D, Weinberger B et al (2010) Persistent viral infections and immune aging. Ageing Res Rev 10(3):362–369

Bunztman A, Vincent BG, Krovi H et al (2012) The LCMV gp33-specific memory T cell repertoire narrows with age. Immun Ageing 9(1):17

Callahan JE, Kappler JW, Marrack P (1993) Unexpected expansions of CD8+ –bearing cells in old mice. J Immunol 151(12):6657–6669

Casrouge A, Beaudoing E, Dalle S et al (2000) Size estimate of the alpha beta TCR repertoire of naive mouse splenocytes. J Immunol 164(11):5782–5787

Cicin-Sain L, Messaoudi I, Park B et al (2007) Dramatic increase in naive T cell turnover is linked to loss of naive T cells from old primates. Proc Natl Acad Sci U S A 104(50):19960–19965

Cicin-Sain L, Smyk-Pearson S, Currier N et al (2010) Loss of naive T cells and repertoire constriction predict poor response to vaccination in old primates. J Immunol 184(12):6739–6745

Cicin-Sain L, Brien JD, Uhrlaub JL et al (2012) Cytomegalovirus infection impairs immune responses and accentuates T-cell pool changes observed in mice with aging. PLoS Pathog 8(8):e1002849

Clambey ET, Kappler JW, Marrack P (2007) CD8+ T cell clonal expansions & aging: a heterogeneous phenomenon with a common outcome. Exp Gerontol 42(5):407–411

Clambey ET, White J, Kappler JW et al (2008) Identification of two major types of age-associated CD8+ clonal expansions with highly divergent properties. Proc Natl Acad Sci U S A 105(35):12997–13002

Coler RN, Baldwin SL, Shaverdian N et al (2010) A synthetic adjuvant to enhance and expand immune responses to influenza vaccines. PLoS One 5(10):e13677

Colonna-Romano G, Akbar AN, Aquino A et al (2007) Impact of CMV and EBV seropositivity on CD8+ T lymphocytes in an old population from West-Sicily. Exp Gerontol 42(10):995–1002

Connor LM, Kohlmeier JE, Ryan L et al (2012) Early dysregulation of the memory CD8+ T cell repertoire leads to compromised immune responses to secondary viral infection in the aged. Immun Ageing 9(1):28

Day EK, Carmichael AJ, ten Berge IJ et al (2007) Rapid CD8+ T cell repertoire focusing and selection of high-affinity clones into memory following primary infection with a persistent human virus: human cytomegalovirus. J Immunol 179(5):3203–3213

Decman V, Laidlaw BJ, Dimenna LJ et al (2010) Cell-intrinsic defects in the proliferative response of antiviral memory CD8+ T cells in aged mice upon secondary infection. J Immunol 184(9):5151–5159

Decman V, Laidlaw BJ, Doering TA et al (2012) Defective CD8+ T cell responses in aged mice are due to quantitative and qualitative changes in virus-specific precursors. J Immunol 188(4):1933–1941

den Braber I, Mugwagwa T, Vrisekoop N et al (2012) Maintenance of peripheral naive T cells is sustained by thymus output in mice but not humans. Immunity 36(2):288–297

Derhovanessian E, Maier AB, Hahnel K et al (2011) Infection with cytomegalovirus but not herpes simplex virus induces the accumulation of late-differentiated CD4+ and CD8+ T-cells in humans. J Gen Virol 92(Pt 12):2746–2756

Derhovanessian E, Theeten H, Hahnel K et al (2012) Cytomegalovirus-associated accumulation of late-differentiated CD4+ T-cells correlates with poor humoral response to influenza vaccination. Vaccine 31(4):685–690

Dudakov JA, Hanash AM, Jenq RR et al (2012) Interleukin-22 drives endogenous thymic regeneration in mice. Science 336(6077):91–95

Effros RB, Walford RL (1983) Diminished T-cell response to influenza virus in aged mice. Immunology 49(2):387–392

Effros RB, Allsopp R, Chiu CP et al (1996) Shortened telomeres in the expanded CD28-CD8+ cell subset in HIV disease implicate replicative senescence in HIV pathogenesis. AIDS 10(8):F17–F22

Effros RB, Cai Z, Linton PJ (2003) CD8+ T cells and aging. Crit Rev Immunol 23(1–2):45–64

Ely KH, Ahmed M, Kohlmeier JE et al (2007a) Antigen-specific CD8+ T cell clonal expansions develop from memory T cell pools established by acute respiratory virus infections. J Immunol 179(6):3535–3542

Ely KH, Roberts AD, Kohlmeier JE et al (2007b) Aging and CD8+ T cell immunity to respiratory virus infections. Exp Gerontol 42(5):427–431

Feuchtinger T, Opherk K, Bethge WA et al (2010) Adoptive transfer of pp 65-specific T cells for the treatment of chemorefractory cytomegalovirus disease or reactivation after haploidentical and matched unrelated stem cell transplantation. Blood 116(20): 4360–4367

Finch CE, Crimmins EM (2004) Inflammatory exposure and historical changes in human life-spans. Science 305(5691):1736–1739

Ge Q, Hu H, Eisen HN et al (2002) Different contributions of thymopoiesis and homeostasis-driven proliferation to the reconstitution of naive and memory T cell compartments. Proc Natl Acad Sci U S A 99(5): 2989–2994

Gibson KL, Wu YC, Barnett Y et al (2009) B-cell diversity decreases in old age and is correlated with poor health status. Aging Cell 8(1):18–25

Goronzy JJ, Weyand CM (2005) T cell development and receptor diversity during aging. Curr Opin Immunol 17(5):468–475

Goronzy JJ, Fulbright JW, Crowson CS et al (2001) Value of immunological markers in predicting responsiveness to influenza vaccination in elderly individuals. J Virol 75(24):12182–12187

Goronzy JJ, Lee WW, Weyand CM (2007) Aging and T-cell diversity. Exp Gerontol 42(5):400–406

Hadrup SR, Strindhall J, Kollgaard T et al (2006) Longitudinal studies of clonally expanded CD8+ T cells reveal a repertoire shrinkage predicting mortality and an increased number of dysfunctional cytomegalovirus-specific T cells in the very elderly. J Immunol 176(4):2645–2653

Hansen SG, Powers CJ, Richards R et al (2010) Evasion of CD8+ T cells is critical for superinfection by cytomegalovirus. Science 328(5974):102–106

Haynes L (2005) The effect of aging on cognate function and development of immune memory. Curr Opin Immunol 17(5):476–479

Haynes L, Swain SL (2006) Why aging T cells fail: implications for vaccination. Immunity 24(6):663–666

Haynes L, Eaton SM, Burns EM et al (2003) CD4+ T cell memory derived from young naive cells functions well into old age, but memory generated from aged naive cells functions poorly. Proc Natl Acad Sci U S A 100(25):15053–15058

Heng TS, Chidgey AP, Boyd RL (2010) Getting back at nature: understanding thymic development and overcoming its atrophy. Curr Opin Pharmacol 10(4):425–433

Huster KM, Stemberger C, Gasteiger G et al (2009) Cutting edge: memory CD8+ T cell compartment grows in size with immunological experience but nevertheless can lose function. J Immunol 183(11): 6898–6902

Jankovic V, Messaoudi I, Nikolich-Zugich J (2003) Phenotypic and functional T-cell aging in rhesus macaques (Macaca mulatta): differential behavior of CD4+ and CD8+ subsets. Blood 102(9):3244–3251

Jiang J, Bennett AJ, Fisher E et al (2009) Limited expansion of virus-specific CD8+ T cells in the aged environment. Mech Ageing Dev 130(11–12):713–721

Jiang J, Fisher EM, Murasko DM (2011) CD8+ T cell responses to influenza virus infection in aged mice. Ageing Res Rev 10(4):422–427

Kapasi ZF, Murali-Krishna K, McRae ML et al (2002) Defective generation but normal maintenance of memory T cells in old mice. Eur J Immunol 32: 1567–1573

Karrer U, Sierro S, Wagner M et al (2003) Memory inflation: continuous accumulation of antiviral CD8+ T cells over time. J Immunol 170(4):2022–2029

Kedzierska K, La Gruta NL, Davenport MP et al (2005) Contribution of T cell receptor affinity to overall avidity for virus-specific CD8+ T cell responses. Proc Natl Acad Sci U S A 102(32):11432–11437

Khan N, Shariff N, Cobbold M et al (2002) Cytomegalovirus seropositivity drives the CD8+ T cell repertoire toward greater clonality in healthy elderly individuals. J Immunol 169(4):1984–1992

Khan N, Hislop A, Gudgeon N et al (2004) Herpesvirus-specific CD8+ T cell immunity in old age: cytomegalovirus impairs the response to a coresident EBV infection. J Immunol 173(12):7481–7489

Klenerman P, Dunbar PR (2008) CMV and the art of memory maintenance. Immunity 29(4):520–522

Kohlmeier JE, Connor LM, Roberts AD et al (2010) Nonmalignant clonal expansions of memory CD8+ T cells that arise with age vary in their capacity to mount recall responses to infection. J Immunol 185(6):3456–3462

Ku CC, Kotzin B, Kappler J et al (1997) CD8+ T-cell clones in old mice. Immunol Rev 160:139–144

Ku CC, Kappler J, Marrack P (2001) The growth of the very large CD8+ T cell clones in older mice is controlled by cytokines. J Immunol 166(4):2186–2193

Lages CS, Suffia I, Velilla PA et al (2008) Functional regulatory T cells accumulate in aged hosts and promote chronic infectious disease reactivation. J Immunol 181(3):1835–1848

Lang A, Brien JD, Messaoudi I et al (2008) Age-related dysregulation of CD8+ T cell memory specific for a persistent virus is independent of viral replication. J Immunol 180(7):4848–4857

Lang A, Brien JD, Nikolich-Zugich J (2009) Inflation and long-term maintenance of CD8+ T cells responding to a latent herpesvirus depend upon establishment of latency and presence of viral antigens. J Immunol 183(12):8077–8087

Lee JB, Oelke M, Ramachandra L et al (2011) Decline of influenza-specific CD8+ T cell repertoire in healthy geriatric donors. Immun Ageing 8:6

LeMaoult J, Messaoudi I, Manavalan JS et al (2000) Age-related dysregulation in CD8+ T cell homeostasis: kinetics of a diversity loss. J Immunol 165(5): 2367–2373

Li SP, Cai Z, Shi W et al (2002) Early antigen-specific response by naive CD8+ T cells is not altered with aging. J Immunol 168:6120–6127

Lynch HE, Goldberg GL, Chidgey A et al (2009) Thymic involution and immune reconstitution. Trends Immunol 30(7):366–373

Mackall CL, Gress RE (1997) Pathways of T-cell regeneration in mice and humans: implications for bone marrow transplantation and immunotherapy. Immunol Rev 157:61–72

Mattison JA, Roth GS, Beasley TM et al (2012) Impact of caloric restriction on health and survival in rhesus monkeys from the NIA study. Nature 489(7415): 318–321

Maue AC, Eaton SM, Lanthier PA et al (2009) Proinflammatory adjuvants enhance the cognate helper activity of aged CD4+ T cells. J Immunol 182(10):6129–6135

McElhaney JE, Xie D, Hager WD et al (2006) T cell responses are better correlates of vaccine protection in the elderly. J Immunol 176(10):6333–6339

McElhaney JE, Ewen C, Zhou X et al (2009) Granzyme B: correlates with protection and enhanced CTL response to influenza vaccination in older adults. Vaccine 27(18):2418–2425

Mekker A, Tchang VS, Haeberli L et al (2012) Immune senescence: relative contributions of age and cytomegalovirus infection. PLoS Pathog 8(8):e1002850

Messaoudi I, Guevara Patino JA, Dyall R et al (2002) Direct link between mhc polymorphism, T cell avidity, and diversity in immune defense. Science 298(5599): 1797–1800

Messaoudi I, Lemaoult J, Guevara-Patino JA et al (2004) Age-related CD8+ T cell clonal expansions constrict CD8+ T cell repertoire and have the potential to impair immune defense. J Exp Med 200(10):1347–1358

Messaoudi I, Warner J, Fischer M et al (2006a) Delay of T cell senescence by caloric restriction in aged long-lived nonhuman primates. Proc Natl Acad Sci U S A 103(51):19448–19453

Messaoudi I, Warner J, Nikolich-Zugich J (2006b) Age-related CD8+ T cell clonal expansions express elevated levels of CD122 and CD127 and display defects in perceiving homeostatic signals. J Immunol 177(5): 2784–2792

Miller RA (1996) The aging immune system: primer and prospectus. Science 273(5271):70–74

Monteiro J, Batliwalla F, Ostrer H et al (1996) Shortened telomeres in clonally expanded CD28-CD8+ T cells imply a replicative history that is distinct from their CD28 + CD8+ counterparts. J Immunol 156(10): 3587–3590

Moon JJ, Chu HH, Pepper M et al (2007) Naive CD4(+) T cell frequency varies for different epitopes and predicts repertoire diversity and response magnitude. Immunity 27(2):203–213

Munks MW, Gold MC, Zajac AL et al (2006) Genome-wide analysis reveals a highly diverse CD8+ T cell response to murine cytomegalovirus. J Immunol 176(6):3760–3766

Murasko DM, Jiang J (2005) Response of aged mice to primary virus infections. Immunol Rev 205:285–296

Naylor K, Li G, Vallejo AN et al (2005) The influence of age on T cell generation and TCR diversity. J Immunol 174(11):7446–7452

Nishioka T, Shimizu J, Iida R et al (2006) CD4 + CD25 + Foxp3+ T cells and CD4 + CD25-Foxp3+ T cells in aged mice. J Immunol 176(11):6586–6593

Obar JJ, Khanna KM, Lefrancois L (2008) Endogenous naive CD8+ T cell precursor frequency regulates primary and memory responses to infection. Immunity 28(6):859–869

Ouyang Q, Wagner WM, Walter S et al (2003) An age-related increase in the number of CD8+ T cells carrying receptors for an immunodominant Epstein-Barr virus (EBV) epitope is counteracted by a decreased frequency of their antigen-specific responsiveness. Mech Ageing Dev 124(4):477–485

Ouyang Q, Wagner WM, Zheng W et al (2004) Dysfunctional CMV-specific CD8(+) T cells accumulate in the elderly. Exp Gerontol 39(4):607–613

Pawelec G (2005) Immunosenescence and vaccination. Immun Ageing 2:16

Pawelec G, Akbar A, Caruso C et al (2005) Human immunosenescence: is it infectious? Immunol Rev 205: 257–268

Pawelec G, Derhovanessian E, Larbi A et al (2009) Cytomegalovirus and human immunosenescence. Rev Med Virol 19(1):47–56

Pawelec G, Larbi A, Derhovanessian E (2010) Senescence of the human immune system. J Comp Pathol 142(Suppl 1):S39–S44

Pitcher CJ, Hagen SI, Walker JM et al (2002) Development and homeostasis of T cell memory in rhesus macaque. J Immunol 168(1):29–43

Po JL, Gardner EM, Anaraki F et al (2002) Age-associated decrease in virus-specific CD8+ T lymphocytes during primary influenza infection. Mech Ageing Dev 123(8):1167–1181

Posnett DN, Sinha R, Kabak S et al (1994) Clonal populations of T cells in normal elderly humans: the T cell equivalent to "benign monoclonal gammapathy". J Exp Med 179(2):609–618

Roberts AD, Ely KH, Woodland DL (2005) Differential contributions of central and effector memory T cells to recall responses. J Exp Med 202(1):123–133

Roberts ET, Haan MN, Dowd JB et al (2010) Cytomegalovirus antibody levels, inflammation, and mortality among elderly Latinos over 9 years of follow-up. Am J Epidemiol 172(4):363–371

Rudd BD, Venturi V, Davenport MP et al (2011a) Evolution of the antigen-specific CD8+ TCR repertoire across the life span: evidence for clonal homogenization of the old TCR repertoire. J Immunol 186(4):2056–2064

Rudd BD, Venturi V, Li G et al (2011b) Nonrandom attrition of the naive CD8+ T-cell pool with aging governed by T-cell receptor:pMHC interactions. Proc Natl Acad Sci U S A 108(33):13694–13699

Saurwein-Teissl M, Lung TL, Marx F et al (2002) Lack of antibody production following immunization in old age: association with CD8(+)CD28(−) T cell clonal expansions and an imbalance in the production of Th1 and Th2 cytokines. J Immunol 168(11):5893–5899

Schmitt A, Tonn T, Busch DH et al (2011) Adoptive transfer and selective reconstitution of streptamer-selected cytomegalovirus-specific CD8+ T cells leads to virus clearance in patients after allogeneic peripheral blood stem cell transplantation. Transfusion 51(3):591–599

Schwanninger A, Weinberger B, Weiskopf D et al (2008) Age-related appearance of a CMV-specific high-avidity CD8+ T cell clonotype which does not occur in young adults. Immun Ageing 5:14

Sester M, Sester U, Gartner B et al (2002) Sustained high frequencies of specific CD4+ T cells restricted to a single persistent virus. J Virol 76(8):3748–3755

Sinicco A, Raiteri R, Sciandra M et al (1997) The influence of cytomegalovirus on the natural history of HIV infection: evidence of rapid course of HIV infection in HIV-positive patients infected with cytomegalovirus. Scand J Infect Dis 29(6):543–549

Smithey MJ, Renkema KR, Rudd BD et al (2011) Increased apoptosis, curtailed expansion and incomplete differentiation of CD8+ T cells combine to decrease clearance of L. monocytogenes in old mice. Eur J Immunol 41(5):1352–1364

Smithey MJ, Li G, Venturi V et al (2012) Lifelong persistent viral infection alters the naive T cell pool, impairing CD8+ T cell immunity in late life. J Immunol 189(11):5356–5366

Snyder CM, Cho KS, Bonnett EL et al (2008) Memory inflation during chronic viral infection is maintained by continuous production of short-lived, functional T cells. Immunity 29(4):650–659

Solana R, Pawelec G, Tarazona R (2006) Aging and innate immunity. Immunity 24(5):491–494

Strindhall J, Nilsson BO, Lofgren S et al (2007) No Immune Risk Profile among individuals who reach 100 years of age: findings from the Swedish NONA immune longitudinal study. Exp Gerontol 42(8):753–761

Sylwester AW, Mitchell BL, Edgar JB et al (2005) Broadly targeted human cytomegalovirus-specific CD4+ and CD8+ T cells dominate the memory compartments of exposed subjects. J Exp Med 202(5):673–685

Tatum A, Hill AB (2012) Chronic viral infections and immunosenescence, with a focus on CMV. Open Longevity Science 6:33–38

Taub DD, Longo DL (2005) Insights into thymic aging and regeneration. Immunol Rev 205:72–93

Trautmann L, Rimbert M, Echasserieau K et al (2005) Selection of T cell clones expressing high-affinity public TCRs within Human cytomegalovirus-specific CD8+ T cell responses. J Immunol 175(9):6123–6132

Trzonkowski P, Mysliwska J, Szmit E et al (2003) Association between cytomegalovirus infection, enhanced proinflammatory response and low level of anti-hemagglutinins during the anti-influenza vaccination–an impact of immunosenescence. Vaccine 21(25–26):3826–3836

Valkenburg SA, Venturi V, Dang TH et al (2012) Early priming minimizes the age-related immune compromise of CD8(+) T cell diversity and function. PLoS Pathog 8(2):e1002544

van den Holland AM, Brink MR (2009) Rejuvenation of the aging T cell compartment. Curr Opin Immunol 21(4):454–459

Van Waterstrat A, Zant G (2009) Effects of aging on hematopoietic stem and progenitor cells. Curr Opin Immunol 21(4):408–413

Varani S, Frascaroli G, Landini MP et al (2009) Human cytomegalovirus targets different subsets of antigen-presenting cells with pathological consequences for host immunity: implications for immunosuppression, chronic inflammation and autoimmunity. Rev Med Virol 19(3):131–145

Vescovini R, Telera A, Fagnoni FF et al (2004) Different contribution of EBV and CMV infections in very long-term carriers to age-related alterations of CD8+ T cells. Exp Gerontol 39(8):1233–1243

Vezys V, Yates A, Casey KA et al (2008) Memory CD8+ T-cell compartment grows in size with immunological experience. Nature 457(7226):196–199

Vu T, Farish S, Jenkins M et al (2002) A meta-analysis of effectiveness of influenza vaccine in persons aged 65 years and over living in the community. Vaccine 20(13–14):1831–1836

Waller EC, Day E, Sissons JG et al (2008) Dynamics of T cell memory in human cytomegalovirus infection. Med Microbiol Immunol 197(2):83–96

Wikby A, Maxson P, Olsson J et al (1998) Changes in CD8+ and CD4+ lymphocyte subsets, T cell proliferation responses and non-survival in the very old: the Swedish longitudinal OCTO-immune study. Mech Ageing Dev 102(2–3):187–198

Wikby A, Johansson B, Olsson J et al (2002) Expansions of peripheral blood CD8+ T-lymphocyte subpopulations and an association with cytomegalovirus seropositivity in the elderly: the Swedish NONA immune study. Exp Gerontol 37(2–3):445–453

Xie D, McElhaney JE (2007) Lower GrB + CD62Lhigh CD8+ TCM effector lymphocyte response to influenza virus in older adults is associated with increased CD28null CD8+ T lymphocytes. Mech Ageing Dev 128(5–6):392–400

Yager EJ, Ahmed M, Lanzer K et al (2008) Age-associated decline in T cell repertoire diversity leads to holes in the repertoire and impaired immunity to influenza virus. J Exp Med 205(3):711–723

Yewdell JW, Haeryfar SM (2005) Understanding presentation of viral antigens to CD8(+) T cells in vivo: the key to rational vaccine design. Annu Rev Immunol 23:651–682

Zhu Q, Egelston C, Gagnon S et al (2010) Using 3 TLR ligands as a combination adjuvant induces qualitative changes in T cell responses needed for antiviral protection in mice. J Clin Invest 120(2):607–616

T Cell-Mediated Immunity in the Immunosenescence Process

10

Pierre Olivier Lang

10.1 Introduction

Advances in medicine and technologies and socioeconomic development have all contributed to the well-being of mankind and an unprecedented increasing in longevity (Lang and Aspinall 2012). Consecutively, in addition to declining fertility this has also led to a continuous rise in the number and proportion of older persons worldwide (Lutz et al. 1997; Oeppen and Vaupel 2002). Presently 673 million inhabitants in the world are aged ≥60 years, among them 88 million are ≥80 years old. According to the United Nations Prospects (United Nations 2008), the expected numbers for 2050 are of 2 billion (60 and over) and 400 million (80 and over), which means a multiplication by 3 and 4.5, respectively. Today, 21 % of the European population and 17 % of the Northern American population are aged 60 and above. Those figures will increase to 35 and 27 %, respectively, by 2050. Five years from now, for the first time in the human being history, the number of people aged 65 years or older will outnumber children younger than 5 years (Shetty 2012). Moreover, one of the challenges in industrialized societies is that aging will progressively impact

on every country in the world. Indeed, whether today, 50 % of the population aged ≥80 years lives in the most developed countries (29 % of them in Europe and 13 % in Northern America); tomorrow, less-developed countries will also observe this demographic transition. By 2050, 62 % of the aged ≥60 years population will live in Asia (United Nations 2008).

Although the aging of the general population is one of humanity's greatest triumphs (Lloyd-Sherlock et al. 2012), it also confronts our societies to enormous medical challenges (Oeppen and Vaupel 2002). If aging should be considered as being a positive experience (World Health Organization 2002), lengthening lifetime is not necessarily synonymous of extending life expectancy in good health; studies demonstrated that chronic and degenerative disorders become more and more prevalent with advancing age and multimorbidity is increasing (Thorpe and Howard 2006). Thus, the optimism created by the ever-increasing life expectancy, and the expectation of many individuals that they will live longer and healthier, must be balanced by the increased number of older individuals (Lang and Aspinall 2012). Thus, one of the challenges of a "long-life society" is to ensure that the years gained with a higher life expectancy are not only healthy and disability-free years but are years offering a good quality of life. In this perspective, recent research has concentrated on identifying the factors contributing rather than hindering the healthy aging process, and among them, the age-related changes of the immune system, commonly termed immunosenescence, have

P.O. Lang, MD, MPH, PD, PhD
Nescens Centre of Preventive Medicine,
Clinique of Genolier, Genolier, Switzerland

Translational Medicine Research Group,
School of Health, Cranfield University, Cranfield, UK
e-mail: polang@nescens.com

A. Massoud, N. Rezaei (eds.), *Immunology of Aging*,
DOI 10.1007/978-3-642-39495-9_10, © Springer-Verlag Berlin Heidelberg 2014

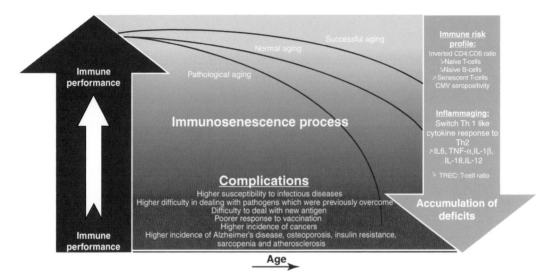

Fig. 10.1 The immunosenescence process with advancing age. This figure depicts the concept of accumulation of deficits applied to immunosenescence. Thus, an accumulation of immune deficits could be used to predict immune status of a given individual. In complex systems such as the immune system, reliability of functions being undertaken is dependent in part of the quality of the component and also on any functional overlap. Thus, reliability in the face of possible component failure can be achieved by having multiple components capable of fulfilling the same task ensuring that while some components fail the system as a whole remains functional. *CMV* cytomegalovirus, *IL* interleukin, *TNF* tumor necrosis factor, and *TREC* T cell receptor excision circles

been particularly investigated (Weiskopf et al. 2009; Ongrádi and Kövesdi 2010).

As depicted in the Fig. 10.1, immunosenescence has been implicated in the increasing state of susceptibility to pathogens previously encountered and the decline in the body's ability to mount adequate immune responses to new antigens. It also acts as a contributing factor to the increased susceptibility of older adults to develop not only infectious diseases but cancer, Alzheimer's diseases, osteoporosis, insulin resistance, diabetes, atherosclerosis and autoimmunity, and other main aged-related diseases (Lang et al. 2010c; Fulop et al. 2011; Giunta et al. 2008; Ginaldi et al. 2005). Although individuals' age seems to be a major contributor of this state of vulnerability, there is no single cause of immunosenescence, which is the consequence of a compilation of events (Govind et al. 2012; Lang et al. 2013a), including thymic involution (Aspinall et al. 2010), the continuous reshaping of the immune repertoire by persistent antigenic challenges (Virgin et al. 2009), the dysregulation

of Toll-like receptor (TLR) functions (Shaw et al. 2011), the reduced production of naïve B cells and the intrinsic defects arising in resident B cells (Frasca et al. 2011), and the impact of nutritional status and dysregulation of hormonal pathways (Lang et al. 2012a; Kelley et al. 2007). Moreover, human aging is, by itself, also inextricably linked with an ever-increasing incidence of chronic-comorbid conditions which contribute to increase the age-related chronic low-grade inflammation (i.e., inflammaging) that further impinge the immune system (Fulop et al. 2010). Effects of immunosenescence are now evident in both arms of the immune system: the innate and adaptive immune system (Lang et al. 2010b). With respect to its central role in orchestrating the immune response, this chapter will focus on the main features of T cell-mediated immunity senescence and the underlying mechanisms contributing to the age-related state of increased vulnerability. Furthermore, it will explore the means by which T cell functions could be identified and predicted by using biomarkers.

10.2   What Are the Main Features of the Senescence of T Cell Immunity?

Quantification of T cell numbers throughout the life-span shows that they are maintained in humans (Aspinall et al. 2010) even in their tenth decades at levels which are comparable to those found in younger individuals (Mitchell et al. 2010). This would imply that there is no decline in the homeostatic mechanisms which preserve the size of the peripheral T cell pool within defined boundaries. As shown in Fig. 10.1, the age-related changes in cell-mediated immunity are characterized by two major patterns: the reduction in thymic output (i.e., decrease in naïve T cells) and the increase in the number of antigen-experienced memory and in particular effector cells (i.e., increase in senescent cells) (Weiskopf et al. 2009). In addition, but not further detailed thereafter, thymic involution also leads to a decreased output of T regulatory cells (Treg) which have been reported to decline after the age of 50 and could contribute to age-related phenomena such as autoimmunity and increased inflammation as well (Tsaknaridis et al. 2003; Weiskopf et al. 2009).

10.2.1   Decreased Number of Naïve T Cells

Production and maintenance of the peripheral naïve T cell repertoire are critical to the normal function of the adaptive immune system as a whole (Ongrádi and Kövesdi 2010; Weiskopf et al. 2009). As a result of thymic involution, the output of peripheral naïve T cells is dramatically reduced with advancing age. Indeed, at birth the thymus is fully developed, its involution and the replacement of the active areas of thymopoiesis related to fat accumulation start soon after birth and continue throughout life, and it is almost complete at the age of 50 years (Aspinall et al. 2010). This leads to a reduced ability of the aged host to respond adequately to new antigens (Naylor et al. 2005), including not only pathogen but also vaccine antigens (Lang et al. 2010a). Low naïve T cell numbers have been described in

the periphery as well as lymphoid tissues (Aspinall et al. 2010). The thymic involution appears to be one of the major features of human immunosenescence (Ostan et al. 2008; Aspinall et al. 2010) because this is the single preceding event in all cases.

In the older adults, both the diversity and functional integrity of the naïve CD4$^+$ and CD8$^+$ T cells subsets are decreased, but in slightly different ways (Naylor et al. 2005; Aspinall and Andrew 2000; Weinberger et al. 2007; Effros et al. 2003; Pfister et al. 2006; Lang et al. 2013a). Although the diversity and number of naïve CD4$^+$ T cell compartment are maintained stable for a long time, a dramatic and sudden collapse of diversity occurs after the age of 70 years, considerably shrinking the repertoire. Similar changes occur, but earlier and more gradually when aged, in the naïve CD8$^+$ T cells subset (Arnold et al. 2011). In contrast with CD4$^+$, naïve CD8$^+$ T cells are more susceptible to apoptosis in aged individuals (Gupta and Gollapudi 2008). The reduced thymic output of newly generated naïve T cells seems to be compensated by different mechanisms, and among them homeostatic proliferation has been identified as playing a key role for the maintenance and restoration of the size of the naïve T cell pool (Hazenberg et al. 2003). Indeed, naive T cells are also readily detectable in elderly people (Douek et al. 1998; Chen et al. 2010), and adult thymectomy does not lead to a rapid decline in naïve T cell number. Similar data have been reported for juvenile rhesus macaques, where thymectomy did not accelerate age-related naïve T cell decline (Hazenberg et al. 2003). Thus, T cell can be produced at extra-thymic sites, such as peripheral lymph nodes and the gut.

Thymic atrophy and decreased thymopoiesis are active processes mediated by the upregulation of cytokines, i.e., interleukin (IL)-6, leukemia inhibitory factor (LIF), and oncostatin M (OSM), in aged human being and mice thymus tissue (Ongrádi and Kövesdi 2010; Sempowski et al. 2000), while IL-7 production by stromal cell is significantly decreased (Ortman et al. 2002; Andrew and Aspinall 2002). IL-7 is necessary for thymopoiesis (Surh and Sprent 2002), promoting cell survival by maintaining the antiapoptotic

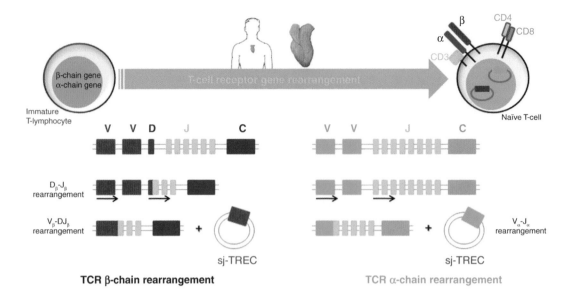

TCR β-chain rearrangement   TCR α-chain rearrangement

Fig. 10.2 Schematic representation of the somatic rearrangement process undergoing in every immature T cell TCR loci during the development from hematopoietic stem cell to mature naïve T cells. During the rearrangement process, the intervening DNA sequences, both for **α**- and **β**-chain, are deleted and circularized into episomal DNA molecules, called TCR excision circles (TRECs) (Adapted from Lang et al. (2013a))

protein B cell lymphoma 2 (Bcl-2) and inducing VDJ recombination (Fig. 10.2) (Kim et al. 1998; Jiang et al. 2005; Aspinall and Andrew 2000). The above changes result in decreased thymic output, in diminished number of circulating naïve T cells (i.e., CD45RA⁺CD28⁺ and CD45RA⁺CD28⁺CD26L) in the blood stream and lymph nodes (Aspinall et al. 2010; Ongrádi and Kövesdi 2010). Naïve T cells from aged individuals exhibit numerous functional defects which are accelerated according to the increasing homeostatic proliferation (Arnold et al. 2011). Indeed, if the naïve T cell count drops below 4 % of total T cells, homeostatic proliferation increases exponentially. This leads, for example, to accelerated telomere shortening and may lead to a memory-like phenotype (Kilpatrick et al. 2008; Cicin-Sain et al. 2007).

Restricted T cell receptor (TCR) repertoire, reduced cytokine production, and impaired expansion and differentiation into effector cells following antigen stimulation are also described (Weiskopf et al. 2009; Ferrando-Martinez et al. 2011). Thus, CD45RA⁺CD28⁺CD8⁺ in aged individuals produce larger amounts of proinflammatory cytokines such as interferon gamma (IFN-γ) and IL-2 and have a

highly restricted TCR repertoire compared to younger adults (Aspinall et al. 2010; Pfister and Savino 2008). It has been also demonstrated that the CD4⁺ subtype does not form immunologic synapses upon stimulation with peptide antigen and antigen presenting cell and this partly through age-associated defects in TCR signaling (Arnold et al. 2011). In addition, naïve T cells from aged individuals exhibit numerous functional defects in their activation, expansion, and differentiation that may also considerably affect their cognate helper function to B cells hence leading to reduced antibody-mediated immunity following antigen stimulation (Weiskopf et al. 2009; Ferrando-Martinez et al. 2011; Haynes 2005).

10.2.2 The Expansion of Dysfunctional Terminally Differentiated T Cells

Consequently to decreasing thymopoiesis, a shift in the ratio of naïve to memory T cells with an increasing number of the memory compartment in order to maintain peripheral T cell homeostasis is observed with advancing age. In contrast to naïve T cells, memory cells rely on IL-7 in concert with IL-15, cycle and self-renew in vivo three- to fourfold faster than naïve cells, and thereby are capable of vigorous proliferation (Arnold et al. 2011; Surh and Sprent 2002). Homeostatic turnover of naïve CD8$^+$ T cells that induces a memory-like phenotype further contributes in a dramatically reduced diversity of the memory T cell pool in the elderly individuals (Weinberger et al. 2007; Naylor et al. 2005).

Repeated antigenic stimulation by certain pathogens shapes the T cell pool and directly contributes to immunosenescence (Virgin et al. 2009; Ongrádi and Kövesdi 2010) by accumulating clones of certain specificities (Karrer et al. 2003; Virgin et al. 2009). Scientific evidence has indeed accumulated that persistent viral infections play a major role in driving clonal expansion, contraction, and homeostasis of the T cell compartment leading to the age-dependent accumulation of dysfunctional terminally differentiated T cells (CD8$^+$CD28$^-$) commonly named senescent cells (Brunner et al. 2011; Virgin et al. 2009). While some reports suggest that localized, niche limited, latent herpes virus including Epstein-Barr virus (EBV), varicella-zoster virus (VZV), herpes simplex viruses (HVS) 1, and HVS2 may not have any impact, persistent viral infection with HCV (Gruener et al. 2001), HIV (Pantaleo et al. 1997; Sewell et al. 2000; Shankar et al. 2000), and CMV (Pawelec et al. 2009) has been shown to cause chronic inflammation of exhausted T cells, even already early in life. Indeed, T cells are thus repeatedly stimulated by viral antigens thereby contributing to the massive accumulation of virus-specific CD4$^+$ and CD8$^+$ T cell clone. This has been observed in both mice and humans (Arnold et al. 2011). Particularly in the elderly individuals, the lifelong exposure to CMV severely impairs the T cell-mediated immune system by increasing the number of highly differentiated, exhausted CMV-specific CD4$^+$ and CD8$^+$ T cells (Pawelec et al. 2009).

One of the most robust markers in describing these exhausted T cell is the loss of the costimulatory molecule CD28 which has been furthermore reported as key predictor of immune incompetence in older individuals (Vallejo 2005;

Frasca et al. 2011). CD28 marker is expressed constitutively on >99 % of human T cells at birth. With advancing age a progressive increase in the proportion of CD28$^-$ T cells is observed and particularly within the CD8$^+$ T cell subset (Lang et al. 2010a). CD28-mediated costimulation is needed for effective primary T cell expansion and for the generation and activation of Treg cells (Hünig et al. 2010). CD28 signal transduction results in IL-2 gene transcription, expression of IL-2 receptor, and the stabilization of a variety of cytokine messenger RNAs. Consequently, memory CD8$^+$CD28$^-$ T cells generated from aged naïve T cells, compared to memory cells produced from young naïve cells, produced much less cytokine (IL-2 from T helper (Th) 1 and IL-4 and IL-5 from Th2) (Ongrádi and Kövesdi 2010). Aged CD4$^+$CD28$^-$ produced from aged naïve cells also expressed decreased CD40-ligand (CD40L or CD154) marker. The CD154 ligand has been shown to induce cytokine production and costimulate proliferation of activated T cells, and this is accompanied by production of IFN-γ, tumor necrosis factor alpha (TNF-α), and IL-2. Hence, the capacity of these cells to help in B cell proliferation and antibody production is considerably reduced contributing to the impairment of humoral response in the aged (Haynes 2005; Frasca et al. 2011).

Globally, the proliferative capacity of CD28$^-$ T cells is also limited; these cells have shortened telomeres and show increased resistance to apoptosis and restricted T cell diversity and are named senescent cells (Vallejo 2005). These cells are also able to secrete proinflammatory cytokines such as TNF-α and INF-γ through a switch from Th1- to Th2-like cytokine response that contributes to the ongoing age-related proinflammatory background observed in elderly persons (i.e., inflammaging) (Franceschi et al. 2007). Senescent cells also exert regulatory roles in vivo that further impinge the immune system capacities such as poorer immune responses to influenza vaccination (Goronzy et al. 2001; Saurwein-Teissl et al. 2002) and higher autoreactive immunologic memory (Weiskopf et al. 2009). Recently, it has been demonstrated that senescent CD8$^+$ T cells are specially enriched in niches such as the bone marrow, where they resided in a state of pre-activation and can produce cytokine upon stimulation (Herndler-Brandstetter et al. 2011). In general, the CD8+ subset is more affected by the accumulation of terminally differentiated T cell than the CD4+ compartments with advancing age (Arnold et al. 2011).

10.2.3 The Decreased Output of Regulatory T Cells

Treg, formerly known as suppressor T cells, are a special subset of T lymphocytes of which the phenotype is CD4+CD25+FOXP3+. They are generated from the thymus or from anergized peripheral CD4+ T cells under particular conditions of suboptimal antigen exposure and/or costimulation. Natural Treg cells are positively selected in the cortex through their TCR interactions with self-peptides presented by thymic stromal cells. It is likely that this high-affinity recognition results in signals rendering them anergic and able to produce antiapoptotic molecules which protect them from negative selection and results in an endogenous long-lived population of self-antigen-specific T cells in the periphery (Maggi et al. 2005).

These cells have demonstrated to mediate self-tolerance, modulate the immune response, and abrogate autoimmune disease (Korn et al. 2007).They represent the link between the two arms of the adaptive immune system by regulating the switch between Th1-like cytokine responses (IL-2, INF-γ, and TNF-α) and Th2-like cytokine responses (IL-3, IL-4, IL-5, and IL-10) that, respectively, support T and B cell-mediated immunity (CMI) (i.e., pro- and anti-inflammatory responses). Moreover, these cells seem to also play a crucial role in defense against certain pathogens including *C. albicans*, *C. neoformans*, *H. pylori*, *K. pneumoniae*, *M. tuberculosis*, and *Staphylococcus* (Peck and Mellins 2010; Lages et al. 2008). Whether Treg cell number or functions are altered with age is still controversial (Fulop et al. 2010). Some reports highlighted however that their proportion and activity were increased with advancing age, also contributing to the reduced proliferative capacity of T cells

from older adults (Tsaknaridis et al. 2003; Weiskopf et al. 2009). As this is an important issue with still rather few data available, Treg cells activity and effects on other T cell subsets activities in the elderly would be worth addressing (Fulop et al. 2010).

10.3 Progress in Understanding Underlying Mechanisms

10.3.1 Defects in Some Signaling Pathways in CD4+ T Cells

The decrease ability of aged individuals to mount adequate specific antibody response to influenza vaccination (i.e., anti-hemagglutination activity inhibition or HAI) partly results from decrease in naïve T cells (Lang et al. 2010a, b). Concomitant increase in memory/effector T cells (CD8+) (Effros 2007; Herndler-Brandstetter et al. 2011) and loss in CD28 expression (Vallejo 2005; Effros 2007), cytokine production, and T cell proliferation seem also to be affected by signal transduction defects (Sadighi Akha and Miller 2005) particularly in CD4+ (Yu et al. 2012). Recently, Yu et al. have observed that CD4+ memory cells from individuals ≥65 years displayed significant increased and sustained transcription of the dual-specific phosphatase 4 (DUSP4) that shortened expression of CD40L (Yu et al. 2012). The CD40L has been shown to induce cytokine production and costimulate proliferation of activated T cells, and this is accompanied by production of IFN-γ, TNF-α, and IL-2 (Lang et al. 2010a). The capacity of CD4+CD40L⁻ to help B cell proliferation and anti-HA production is reduced (Haynes 2005). Moreover, sustained transcription of DUSP4 also shortened inducible T cell costimulator (ICOS) and decreased production of IL-4, IL-17A, and IL-2 after in vitro activation (Yu et al. 2012). In vivo after influenza vaccination, activated CD4+ T cells from older adults had increased DUSP4 transcription, which inversely correlated with the expression of CD40L, ICOS, and IL-4 (Yu et al. 2012). These findings therefore suggest that increased DUSP4 expression in activated T cells in part accounts for defective adaptive immune responses to influenza vaccination in the elderly. Furthermore, silencing of DUPS4 expression in elderly CD4$^+$ T cells restores their ability to provide helper activity for B cell differentiation and antibody production (Yu et al. 2012).

10.3.2 The Role of the Aged Bone Marrow in Regulating Memory T Cell Functions

The homeostatic maintenance of memory T cells throughout lifetime is tightly regulated and preserves T cell repertoire diversity to combat common and emerging pathogens as well as recall response to booster vaccination (Nikolich-Zugich 2008). It is only recently that researcher has begun to understand how and where memory T cells are maintained and sheltered. In this respect, the bone marrow (BM) and its mesenchymal stromal cells (MSCs) have been paid attention (Herndler-Brandstetter et al. 2011, 2012). MSCs express proteoglycan ligands to CD44 which is present on memory T cells and mediates their local retention. They also produce IL-7 and IL-15 for the homeostatic maintenance of memory T cells (Tokoyoda et al. 2010). IL-7 has been shown to be important for the survival of memory CD4$^+$ T cells (Guimond et al. 2009; Kondrack et al. 2003), and in the BM, memory CD4$^+$ T cells with a Ly6C^{hi}CD62 ligand$^-$ phenotype are in close contact with IL-7-producing VCAM1$^+$ stromal cells (Tokoyoda et al. 2009). In contrast, memory CD8$^+$ T cell survival is mostly dependent on IL-15-mediated signaling (Zhang et al. 1998), and the BM has been shown to be a preferred site for IL-15-driven activation and proliferation of memory CD8$^+$ T cells (Becker et al. 2005). In contrast to IL-7, IL-15 is presented by IL-15Rα^+ BM cell leading to sustained IL-15-mediated signaling (Schluns et al. 2004). However, lifelong homeostatic turnover of memory T cells may lead to the accumulation of highly differentiated memory T cells in elderly persons (Weinberger et al. 2007; Nikolich-Zugich 2008). In vitro studies indicate that common γ-chain signaling in CD8$^+$CD28$^+$ T cells, in particular, mediated by IL-15, downregulates the expression of the important costimulatory molecule CD28, thereby facilitating the accumulation of CD8$^+$CD28$^-$ senescent T cells (Borthwick et al. 2000; Chiu et al. 2006). Thus, it has been proposed that memory T cell, when in contact with MSCs, is suppressed and displays reduced allogenic and mitogenic proliferation, a state of T cell anergy and reduced apoptosis as well as modulated cytokine production (Tokoyoda et al. 2010; Herndler-Brandstetter et al. 2011). Little is however known about the aged BM and its role in regulating the survival and function of memory T cells (Arnold et al. 2011).

In a recent report, Herndler-Brandstetter et al. have observed that the number of CD4$^+$ and CD8$^+$ T cells was maintained during aging into the BM (Herndler-Brandstetter et al. 2011). Similarly to what happens into the blood stream, the composition of this pool is altered with a decline of naïve and an increase in memory T cells. However, in contrast to the peripheral blood, a highly activated CD8$^+$CD28$^-$T cell population, which lacks the late differentiation marker CD57, accumulates in the BM of elderly persons. IL-6 and IL-15, which are both increased in the aged BM, efficiently induce the activation, proliferation, and differentiation of CD8$^+$ T cells in vitro, highlighting a role of these cytokines in the age-dependent accumulation of highly activated CD8$^+$CD28$^-$ T cells in the BM (Herndler-Brandstetter et al. 2012). However, these age-related changes do not impair nevertheless the maintenance of a high number of polyfunctional memory CD4$^+$ and CD8$^+$T cells. Effector CD8$^+$ T cells that reside in the BM are in a state of pre-activation and can rapidly express cytokines and CD40L upon stimulations and efficiently induce the production of high-affinity antibodies by B cells (Tokoyoda et al. 2009; Na et al. 2009). Taken together these findings demonstrate that with advancing age a highly activated CD8$^+$CD28$^-$ T cell population accumulates in the BM, which is driven by the age-related increase of IL-6 and IL-15. Terminally differentiated effector CD8$^+$ T cells may therefore represent an interesting and important line of defense to pathogens in aging and old adult population and can still fulfil important functions and compensate for the loss of regenerative capacity (Herndler-Brandstetter et al. 2012).

10.3.3 Decreasing of Memory T Cells Reactogenicity

Some interesting information about the reactogenicity of memory T cells in the aged individuals can be learnt from the experience of the herpes zoster (HZ) vaccine. Indeed, the specific VZV CMI is naturally amounted following the primary contact with the virus responsible for chickenpox. While VZV becomes permanently latent in the dorsal-root sensory nerves, the specific CMI contributes to prevent VZV reactivating and acute HZ occurrence (Lang and Michel 2011). It was, however, observed that the age-related reduction in CMI to VZV was the main cause of VZV reactivation in older individuals and in individuals who are immunocompromised as a result of diseases or its treatments (Weinberg et al. 2009; Kimberlin and Whitley 2007). CMI is, however, expected to be restored across the life-span either by subclinical VZV infections occurring periodically and a similar boost in immunocompromised hosts who experience asymptomatic VZV viremia (Lang and Michel 2011) or vaccinating individuals with the licensed HZ vaccine (Levin and Hayward 1996).

Although Oxman et al. in a large randomized controlled trial has demonstrated that the HZ vaccine markedly reduced morbidity from HZ among older adults (Oxman et al. 2005), subsequent analyses have demonstrated that the vaccine-induced boost in CMI was also a function of the age of the vaccine (Weinberg et al. 2009). Furthermore, a loss of CD4+ and CD8+ early effectors and CD4+ effector memory cells was particularly observed among poorer responders (Weinberg et al. 2012). This demonstrates that the vaccine cannot reactivate VZV CMI efficiently enough in older adults. This is moreover reinforced by the recent demonstration that risk of HZ recurrences after a first episode that was initially considered being negligible appears as frequent as rates of the first occurrence in immunocompetent individuals after the age of 50 years (Yawn et al. 2011). Thus, also the natural infection cannot properly reactivate CMI to elicit durable protection in older adult population either.

10.4 Is the Senescence of T Cell-Mediated Immunity a Quantifiable Disorder?

Predicting individual immune responsiveness using biological markers that easily distinguish between healthy and immunosenescent states is a great but desirable challenge. Since the single preceding event in all cases of immunosenescence is thymic involution (Aspinall et al. 2010), the question is: can we identify specific T cell immunity makers linked to a state of immunosenescence? The pioneering OCTO and NONA studies have resulted in the emerging concept of an Immune Risk Profile (IRP) (Strindhall et al. 2007; Wikby et al. 2005, 2008). This immune condition consists of (1) a depleted number of naïve T cells, (2) a high CD8+ and low CD4+ numbers characterized by an inverted CD4+:CD8+ ratio, (3) a poor mitogen response to concanavalin (ConA) stimulation, and (4) the expansion of dysfunctional terminally differentiated CD8+CD28- T cells (i.e., senescent cells) (Brunner et al. 2011; Pawelec et al. 2009). This IRP was identified from healthy octogenarians and nonagenarians and 2-, 4-, and 6-year mortality predicted. Hirokawa et al. have thus proposed a T cell immune score expressing the immune status as a simple score combining five T cell-related parameters (Hirokawa et al. 2009): total number of T cells, CD4+:CD8+ ratio, number of naïve T cells (CD4+CD45RA+), ratio of naïve to memory (CD4+CDRO+) T cells, and T cell proliferative index (TCPI). In patients with colorectal cancer compared to healthy age-matched controls, this T cell immune score of patients in stages I–IV was significantly decreased. Furthermore, the complex remodeling of immune system observed during aging also includes profound modifications within the cytokine network (Larbi et al. 2011). The typical feature of this phenomenon is a general increase in plasma cytokine levels and cell capability to produce proinflammatory cytokines, including a chronic, low-grade, proinflammatory condition usually termed inflammaging (Franceschi et al. 2007; Franceschi 2007; Macaulay et al. 2012). This results from a shift from a CD4+ Th cells, Th1-like cytokine response to a Th2-like response, and, furthermore, an increase in levels of proinflammatory cytokines (i.e., IL-6, TNF-α, as well as IL-1β, IL-18, and IL-12). While a wide range of factors have been claimed to contribute to this state (i.e., increased amount of adiposity, decreased production of sex steroid, and chronic health comorbid disorders) (Ostan et al. 2008; Fulop et al. 2010), this altered inflammatory response has also been attributed to the continuous exposure to CMV antigen stimulation and/or reactive oxygen species (ROS) (Pawelec et al. 2009; Larbi et al. 2011; Brunner et al. 2011). However, whether these parameters could provide a robust set of criteria for the determination of an individual's immunological status in the older old adults, further studies are still required in order to identify biomarkers that are identifiable earlier in life so that intervention strategies can be administered sooner rather than later (Govind et al. 2012).

With this aim, genomic not only may help to identify factors usable as a measure of biological aging but that may also be useful as a tool for predicting immune capabilities within the population (Ostan et al. 2008). Studies that tracked the changes in thymic output have attempted to establish the number of naïve cells and thereby provide an assessment of immune status by using an excisional by-product of TCR genes rearrangement (Govind et al. 2012; Douek et al. 1998, 2000; Mitchell et al. 2010; Hazenberg et al. 2002, 2003). These products are termed TCR-rearrangement excision circles (TRECs) (Kong et al. 1998; Livak and Schatz 1996; Takeshita et al. 1989).

10.5   Could sj-TREC Be Considered as a Biomarker of Effective Aging?

10.5.1   sj-TREC: Episomal DNA Sequences Generated During the TCR Gene Rearrangement

The ability of T lymphocytes to recognize a specific region of a particular antigen is driven by the presence of antigen receptors on the surface of each cell. The TCR is a heterodimer that consists in 95 % of T cells of an alpha (α) and beta (β)

chain, whereas in 5 % of T cells this consists of gamma and delta (γ/δ) chains. In order to create a border repertoire of TCR, an intricate process of cutting and splicing undergoes during the complex transition from hematopoietic stem cell to mature naïve T lymphocyte that leads to random joining of DNA segments from the TRC locus (Chain et al. 2005). In T cells expressing TCR-αβ, rearrangements of both TCR-α and TCR-β genes produce TRECs, as depicted in Fig. 10.2, by VJ gene recombination and by V(D)J gene recombination, respectively (Bogue and Roth 1996). Both involve a somewhat random joining of gene segments to generate the complete TCR chain, and the two rearrangement events that occur during this process are identical in 70 % of αβ T cells (Verschuren et al. 1997). The α-chain rearrangement produces a signal-joint TREC (sj-TREC) and the β-chain a coding-joint TREC (Douek et al. 1998). Thus, the TRECs generated are common to most αβ T lymphocytes and are detectable exclusively in phenotypically naïve T cells (i.e., undetectable in memory/effector T cells, B cells, and other peripheral mononuclear cells) (Aspinall and Andrew 2000; Kohler et al. 2005; Hazenberg et al. 2003). Because of the enormous diversity of TCR-α VJ and TCR-β VDJ recombination events (Siu et al. 1984; Arden et al. 1985) and thus the number of TRECs produced, no single TREC can be used as a marker to assess the overall thymic function (Douek et al. 1998; Hazenberg et al. 2003). While α- and β-TRECs possess an identical DNA sequences, respectively, and are both stable (Livak and Schatz 1996), not duplicated during subsequent mitosis (Takeshita et al. 1989), TRECs generated during α-chain rearrangement are generally preferred (Aspinall et al. 2000). Indeed they are generated after β-TRECs and are therefore less diluted out with each subsequent cellular division. Moreover, a common requirement for productive rearrangement of the TCR-α locus is the deletion of the TCR-δ locus (Fig. 10.2). Sj-TREC generated during the α-chain rearrangement can be easily quantified in clinical samples (Douek et al. 2000; Hazenberg et al. 2000, 2002, 2003; Lang et al 2011; Zubakov et al. 2010; Patel et al. 2000; Aspinall et al. 2000; Murray et al. 2003; Kohler et al. 2005).

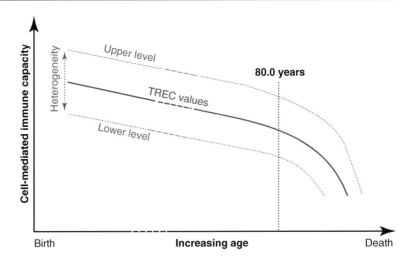

Fig. 10.3 Schematic representation of the age-related changes in TREC values across the life-span based on Zubakov et al. (2010) and Mitchell et al. (2010) study results. The red line depicts the decline in TREC value in healthy individuals, and the two dashed lines on either side the upper and lower TREC values for a given age observed within this population. Thus, the whole of the figure gives (Adapted from Lang et al. (2013a))

10.5.2 sj-TREC: A Marker of the Resting Naïve T Cell Pool

Phenotypic analyses have confirmed that the exhaustion of thymic output with advancing age was at the basis of the deficient replacing of naïve T cells lost in the periphery (i.e., by death or conversion to memory/effector cells) (Weiskopf et al. 2009; Haines et al. 2009; Ostan et al. 2008; Kohler et al. 2005). Whether this contributes to the inability of maintaining the T cell repertoire breadth in older adults, TREC values could not be immediately interpreted to reflect continuous thymic output of naïve T cells (Hazenberg et al. 2003). While, as showed in Fig. 10.3, some reports have shown age-associated decline in the sj-TREC values (Mitchell et al. 2010; Zubakov et al. 2010), Chen et al. have demonstrated that TRECs were still readily detectable in healthy nonagenarians (Chen et al. 2010). This suggests, as demonstrated by Hazenberg, that TREC T cells content should be finally more considered as a biomarker of the resting naïve T cell pools rather than a record of thymic output (Hazenberg et al. 2003). This is well illustrated by findings from studies performed in individuals suffering from different health conditions (Douek et al. 1998, 2000; Markert et al. 1999; Patel et al. 2000). Two major biological parameters that complicate the interpretation of TREC data explain this assertion: longevity of naïve T cells and TREC dilution within the two daughter cells

after each round of cell division (Hazenberg et al. 2003). Indeed, estimating that healthy adult has a steady state of 10^{11} naïve T cells and a thymic output of 10^7–10^8 naïve cells per day, it was estimated that naïve T cells have a life-span of 1,000–10,000 days (Sprent and Tough 1994). Consistently, thymectomy should not lead to rapid decline in naïve T cell numbers, and in a group of adults thymectomized three to 39 years prior to analysis, TRECs were still clearly present (Douek et al. 1998). It was thus assumed that naïve T cell division would be too low to significantly affect the TREC content (Douek et al. 1998). Whether that is true in healthy adults, it is not the case in human immunodeficiency virus (HIV)-infected individuals or in lymphopenic cancer adults (Hazenberg et al. 2000, 2002). In these two populations TREC values are significantly lower compared to healthy age-matched control, but TREC increased rapidly with highly active antiretroviral therapy (HAART) and during T cell reconstitution with stem cell transplantation, respectively, and even TREC values reached supranormal levels (Hazenberg et al. 2000, 2002). In individuals with severe combined immunodeficiency (SCID) or in congenitally athymic patients (i.e., Di George syndrome), TRECs became detectable after either haematopoietic stem cell transplantation or transplantation of cultured postnatal thymic tissue (Markert et al. 1999; Patel et al. 2000). Finally, in any case, in clinical conditions involving or influencing the

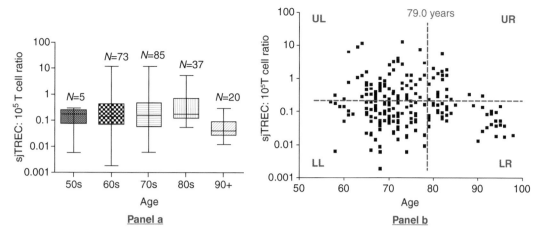

Fig. 10.4 Graphic representation of the age-related changes in TREC:10^5 T cells ratio. (**a**) (1) The slow decline in the ratio values between the sixth and nineth decades of life with a more pronounced decline seen in individuals more than 90 years of age and (2) a convergence of the sample heterogeneity observed in the TREC levels with increasing age. (**b**) An annotated diagram of the age-related changes observed in TREC measurement.

The dashed horizontal line indicates the median TREC:10^5 T cell ratios in the sample population and the dashed vertical line the average life expectancy across the study population (79.0 years). UL, LL, UR, and LR quadrants refer to different quadrants formed by the bisection of the data horizontal and vertical lines (Adapted from Lang et al (2013a))

cell-mediated immune system or with advancing age, the number of TREC and the T cell TREC content are not only determined by thymic output but also by peripheral events such as homeostatic proliferation of existing naïve T cells which replace those cells lost by death or conversion to memory/effector cells (Hazenberg et al. 2003). Thus, analyzing TREC numbers in healthy individuals, Murray et al. found a marked change in the source of naive T cells before and after 20 years of age (Murray et al. 2003). The bulk of the naive T cell pool was sustained primarily from thymic output for individuals younger than 20 years of age, whereas proliferation within the naïve phenotype was dominant for older individuals. Over 90 % of phenotypically naïve T cells in middle age were not of direct thymic origin.

10.6 Could We Identify Different Trends of Aging When Analyzing sj-TREC Values?

A possibly clearer picture the TREC decline in the oldest old was recently shown in a study analyzing blood samples from 215 healthy individuals

ranging in age from 60 to 104 years (Mitchell et al. 2010). The number of donors aged ≥70 years were 66 %, and ≥80 years were 27 %. Changes in thymic output were quantified using TREC: 10^5 T cells ratio. TREC measurements were obtained by quantitative polymerase chain reaction (QPCR), and the number of T cells was determined using fluorescence-activated cell sorter (FACS) analysis. Thus, while the absolute number of leukocytes and T lymphocytes did not change significantly across the age range studied, the authors demonstrated a slowly accelerated curvilinear decline of the TREC ratio between sixth and nineth decade of life. As shown with Fig. 10.4, the most pronounced decline was seen in those individuals more than 90 years of age. Moreover, samples from earlier decades showed a wide range of TREC values with a convergence of the sample heterogeneity observed in the TREC levels with increasing age (Fig. 10.4 – Panel a). These findings contribute to speculate for a number of interesting hypotheses presented in Fig. 10.4 –Panel b. First, are low TREC measurements reflective of an individual's immunosenescence status? If so, are the individuals in the lower left (LL) quadrant (low TREC level at younger age) at a more advanced stage of immunosenescence? The converse argument could also be inferred for individuals with the highest TREC levels (upper left (UL) quadrant). These individuals may therefore be more likely to progress to become the long-lived healthy individuals observed in the lower right (LR) quadrant. This concept lends itself to the argument that immunosenescence is not merely a measurement of chronological age but points towards immune exhaustion arising at different ages (i.e., physiological age) (Mitchell et al. 2010; Lang et al. 2010c). The downward trajectory of an individual's thymic output profile over time has been demonstrated previously by Kilpatrick et al. (Kilpatrick et al. 2008) and could be considered as part of longitudinal studies similar to the OCTA and NONA studies to investigate further the potential role of sj-TREC as predictive marker of aging (Strindhall et al. 2007; Wikby et al. 2005, 2008). Interestingly, in one study carried out in old female rhesus macaques, which were vaccinated with inactivated influenza vaccine (strain A/PR/8/34), animals with the higher HAI and best specific T cell proliferation titres against influenza antigen were among those with the highest TREC ratio levels (Aspinall et al. 2007).

Thus, whether predicting human phenotypes from genotypes is relevant both for personalized medicine and applying preventive strategies (Janssens and van Duijn 2008), additional clinical and translational studies at population, clinical, cellular, and molecular levels are still needed in order to elucidate the exact implications of the TREC values on the age-related senescence of the cell-mediated immune response (Lang et al. 2011). With these perspectives, we have recently developed and optimized a quantitative real-time polymerase chain reaction (qPCR) mono-assay measuring the TREC ratio in dried blood spot (DBS) samples (Lang et al. 2011, 2012b, 2013b). This technology (Fig. 10.5) will be applied on the DBS collected during the 2002–2011 World Health Organization's (WHO) *S*tudy on global *AG*ing and adult health (*SAGE*) project (World Health Organization 2011). The SAGE project is a longitudinal study conducted in six countries (China, Ghana, India, Mexico, Russia Federation, and South Africa) with a total sample size of nearly 50,000 respondents aged 18 years or over with an special emphasis on the population aged ≥50 years. The objective of the study is to obtain reliable, valid, and comparable health-related and well-being data over a range of key domains for younger and older adult populations in nationally representative samples. The collected data examines health, health-related outcomes and well-being, and their determinants over time. With a first whole data collection completed, a follow up will be conducted every 2 years. SAGE intends to generate large cohorts of older adult populations to be compared with cohorts of younger populations to follow up intermediate outcomes, monitoring trends, examining transitions and life events, and addressing relationships between determinants and health, well-being, and health-related outcomes (http://www.who.int/healthinfo/systems/sage/en/).

Conclusion

This chapter clearly has presented the main features of T cell-mediated immunity both related to intrinsic defects and its reduced capacity to help B cells proliferation, maturation, and specific antibody production. It has also explored some new insights in the understanding of the mechanisms underlying immunosenescence. Ongoing research in this field is very active (Govind et al. 2012), and this is not only in exploring the process itself but also more and more growing regarding how best to rejuvenate T cell-mediated immunity (Lang et al. 2013a). Nevertheless some robust markers for identifying and grading immunosenescent states and finally distinguishing between healthy and immunosenescent individuals are still and profoundly lacking. Furthermore, although age clearly imposes drastic changes in the immune physiology and contributes to render individuals more prone to develop main age-related diseases and being vulnerable facing of many pathogens, older adults also demonstrate a broad heterogeneity in their health and/or immune phenotypes (Yao et al. 2011; Mitchell et al. 2010) (Fig. 10.1). This finally poses new challenges to scientists. Research on the immunology of aging has to go beyond the simple identification of age-associated immune features.

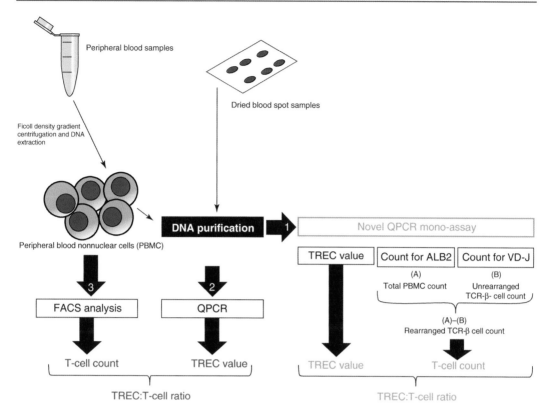

Fig. 10.5 Schematic representation of the novel QPCR mono-assay measuring the TREC:T cell ratio in blood samples including DBS samples. This QPCR mono-assay (*1*) considering DNA samples purified either from PBMCs isolated by a Ficoll-Hypaque density gradient centrifugation or from DBS samples. The prior method combined QPCR measurement for TREC measurement (*2*) and FACS analysis for the T cell count (*3*). This figure depicts how the approximation of the VD-J to T cell count is derived with the novel QPCR mono-assay (*1*). From either whole blood samples or DBS samples, the total cellular DNA is quantified by using the count for ALB2 (albumin gene) considered as a housekeeping gene (*A*). Similarly, unrearranged TCR-β count is quantified according to the VD-J level; unrearranged TCR-β cells correspond to the total germline cell number (*B*). Therefore, the unrearranged TCR-β PBMC count subtracted from the total PBMC count gives us the final rearranged TCR-β count and hence the T cell count ((A)−(B)) (Adapted from Lang et al (2011))

References

Andrew D, Aspinall R (2002) Age-associated thymic atrophy is linked to a decline in IL-7 production. Exp Gerontol 37:455–463

Arden B, Klotz JL, Siu G et al (1985) Diversity and structure of genes of the alpha family of mouse T-cell antigen receptor. Nature 316:783–787

Arnold CR, Wolf J, Brunner S et al (2011) Gain and loss of T cell subsets in old age–age-related reshaping of the T cell repertoire. J Clin Immunol 31:137–146

Aspinall R, Andrew D (2000) Thymic involution in aging. J Clin Immunol 20:250–256

Aspinall R, Pido J, Andrew D (2000) A simple method for the measurement of sjTREC levels in blood. Mech Ageing Dev 121:59–67

Aspinall R, Pido-Lopez J, Imami N et al (2007) Old rhesus macaques treated with interleukin-7 show increased TREC levels and respond well to influenza vaccination. Rejuvenation Res 10(1):5–17

Aspinall R, Pitts D, Lapenna A et al (2010) Immunity in the elderly: the role of the thymus. J Comp Pathol 142(Suppl 1):S111–S115

Becker TC, Coley SM, Wherry EJ et al (2005) Bone marrow is a preferred site for homeostatic proliferation of memory CD8 T cells. J Immunol 174:1269–1273

Bogue M, Roth DB (1996) Mechanism of V(D)J recombination. Curr Opin Immunol 8:175–180

Borthwick NJ, Lowdell M, Salmon M et al (2000) Loss of CD28 expression on CD8(+) T cells is induced by IL-2 receptor γ-chain signaling cytokines and type I IFN, and increases susceptibility to activation-induced apoptosis. Int Immunol 12:1005–1013

Brunner S, Herndler-Brandstetter D, Weinberger B et al (2011) Persistent viral infections and immune aging. Ageing Res Rev 10:362–369

Chain JL, Joachims ML, Hooker SW et al (2005) Real-time PCR method for the quantitative analysis of human T-cell receptor gamma and beta gene rearrangements. J Immunol Methods 300:12–23

Chen JC, Lim FC, Wu Q et al (2010) Maintenance of naïve CD8 T-cells in nonagerians by leptine, IGFBP3 and T3. Mech Ageing Dev 131:37–38

Chiu WK, Fann M, Weng NP (2006) Generation and growth of CD28nullCD8+ memory T cells mediated by IL-15 and its induced cytokines. J Immunol 177:7802–7810

Cicin-Sain L, Messaoudi I, Park B et al (2007) Dramatic increase in naive T cell turnover is linked to loss of naive T cells from old primates. Proc Natl Acad Sci U S A 104:19960–19965

Douek DC, McFarland RD, Keiser PH et al (1998) Changes in thymic function with age and during the treatment of HIV infection. Nature 396:690–695

Douek DC, Vescio RA, Betts MR et al (2000) Assessment of thymic output in adults after haematopoietic stem-cell transplantation and prediction of T-cell reconstruction. Lancet 355:1875–1878

Effros RB (2007) Role of T lymphocyte replicative senescence in vaccine efficacy. Vaccine 25:599–604

Effros RB, Cai Z, Linton PJ (2003) CD8 T cells and aging. Crit Rev Immunol 23:45–64

Ferrando-Martinez S, Ruiz-Mateos E, Hernandez A et al (2011) Age-related deregulation of naive T cell homeostasis in elderly humans. Age 33:197–207

Franceschi C (2007) Inflammaging as a major characteristic of old people: can it be prevented or cured? Nutr Rev 65:S173–S176

Franceschi C, Capri M, Monti D et al (2007) Inflammaging and anti-inflammaging: a systemic perspective on aging and longevity emerged from studies in humans. Mech Ageing Dev 128:92–105

Frasca D, Diaz A, Romero M et al (2011) Age effects on B cells and humoral immunity in humans. Ageing Res Rev 10:330–335

Fulop T, Larbi A, Witkowski JM et al (2010) Aging, frailty and age-related diseases. Biogerontology 11:547–563

Fulop T, Larbi A, Kotb R et al (2011) Aging, immunity, and cancer. Discov Med 11:537–550

Ginaldi L, Di Benedetto MC, De Martinis M (2005) Osteoporosis, inflammation and ageing. Immun Ageing 2:14

Giunta B, Fernandez F, Nikolic WV et al (2008) Inflammaging as a prodrome to Alzheimer's disease. J Neuroinflammation 5:51

Goronzy JJ, Fulbright JW, Crowson CS et al (2001) Value of immunological markers in predicting responsiveness to influenza vaccination in elderly individuals. J Virol 75:12182–12187

Govind S, Lapenna A, Lang PO et al (2012) Immunotherapy of immunosenescence: who, how and when? Open Longev Sci 6:56–63

Gruener NH, Lechner F, Jung MC et al (2001) Sustained dysfunction of antiviral CD8+ T lymphocytes after infection with hepatitis C virus. J Virol 75:5550–5558

Guimond M, Veenstra RG, Grindler DJ et al (2009) Interleukin 7 signaling in dendritic cells regulates the homeostatic proliferation and niche size of CD4 T cells. Nat Immunol 10:149–157

Gupta S, Gollapudi S (2008) CD95-mediated apoptosis in naïve, central and effector memory subsets of CD4+ and CD8+ T cells in aged humans. Exp Gerontol 43:266–274

Haines CJ, Giffon TD, Lu LS et al (2009) Human CD4+ T cells recent thymic emigrants are identified by protein tyrosine kinase 7 and have reduced immune function. J Exp Med 206:275–285

Haynes LES (2005) The effect of age on the cognate function of CD4+ T cells. Immunol Rev 205:220–228

Hazenberg MD, Stuart JW, Otto SA et al (2000) T-cell division in human immunodeficiency virus (HIV)-1 infection is mainly due to immune activation: a longitudinal analysis in patients before and during highly active antiretroviral therapy (HAART). Blood 95:249–255

Hazenberg MD, Otto SA, de Pauw ES et al (2002) T-cell receptor excision circle and T-cell dynamics after allogeneic stem cell transplantation are related to clinical events. Blood 99:3449–3453

Hazenberg MD, Borghans JAM, Boer RJ et al (2003) Thymic output: a bad TREC record. Nat Immunol 4:97–99

Herndler-Brandstetter D, Landgraf K, Jenewein B et al (2011) Human bone marrow hosts polyfunctional memory CD4+ and CD8+ T cells with close contact to IL-15-producing cells. J Immunol 186:6965–6971

Herndler-Brandstetter D, Landgraf K, Tzankov A et al (2012) The impact of aging on memory T cell phenotype and function in the human bone marrow. J Leukoc Biol 91:197–205

Hirokawa K, Utsuyama M, Ishikawa T et al (2009) Decline of T cell-related immune functions in cancer patients and an attempt to restore then through infusion of activated autologous T cells. Mech Ageing Dev 130:86–91

Hünig T, Lücher F, Elfein K et al (2010) CD28 and IL-4: two heavyweights controlling the balance between immunity and inflammation. Med Microbiol Immunol 199:239–246

Janssens ACJW, van Duijn CM (2008) Genome-based prediction of common diseases: advances and prospects. Hum Mol Genet 17:R166–R173

Jiang Q, Li WQ, Aiello FB et al (2005) Cell biology of IL-7, a key lymphotrophin. Cytokine Growth Factor Rev 16:513–533

Karrer U, Sierro S, Wagner M et al (2003) Memory inflation: continuous accumulation of antiviral CD8+ T cells over time. J Immunol 170:2022–2029

Kelley KW, Weigent DA, Kooijman R (2007) Protein hormones and immunity. Brain Behav Immun 21:384–392

Kilpatrick RD, Rickabaugh T, Hultin LE et al (2008) Homeostasis of the naive CD4+ T cell compartment during aging. J Immunol 180:1499–1507

Kim K, Le CK, Sayers TJ et al (1998) The trophic action of IL-7 on pro-T cells: inhibition of apoptosis of pro-T1, -T2 and -T3 cells correlates with Bcl-2 and Bax levels and is independent of Fas and p53 pathways. J Immunol 160:5735–5741

Kimberlin DW, Whitley RJ (2007) Varicella-zoster vaccine for the prevention of herpes zoster. N Eng J Med 356:1338–1343

Kohler S, Wagner U, Pierer M et al (2005) Post-thymic in vivo proliferation of naive CD4+ T cells constrains the TCR repertoire in healthy human adults. Eur J Immunol 35:1987–1994

Kondrack RM, Harbertson J, Tan JT et al (2003) Interleukin 7 regulates the survival and generation of memory CD4 cells. J Exp Med 198:1797–1806

Kong FK, Chen CL, Cooper M (1998) Thymic function can be accurately monitored by the level of recent T cell emigrants in the circulation. Immunity 8:97–104

Korn T, Oukka M, Kuchroo V et al (2007) Th17 cells: effector cells with inflammatory properties. Semin Immunol 19:362.371

Lages CS, Suffia I, Velilla PA et al (2008) Functional regulatory T cells accumulate in aged hosts and promote chronic infectious disease reactivation. J Immunol 181:1835–1848

Lang PO, Aspinall R (2012) Immunosenescence and herd immunity: with an ever increasing aging population do we need to rethink vaccine schedules? Expert Rev Vaccines 11:167–176

Lang PO, Michel JP (2011) Herpes Zoster vaccine: what are the potential benefits for the ageing and older adults? Eur Geriatr Med 2:134–139

Lang PO, Govind S, Mitchell WA et al (2010a) Influenza vaccine effectiveness in aged individuals: the role played by cell-mediated immunity. Eur Geriatr Med 1:233–238

Lang PO, Govind S, Mitchell WA et al (2010b) Vaccine effectiveness in older individuals: what has been learned from the influenza-vaccine experience. Ageing Res Rev 10:389–395

Lang PO, Mitchell WA, Lapenna A et al (2010c) Immunological pathogenesis of main age-related diseases and frailty: role of immunosenescence. Eur Geriatric Med 1:112–121

Lang PO, Mitchell WA, Govind S et al (2011) Real time-PCR assay estimating the naive T-cell pool in whole blood and dried blood spot samples: Pilot study in young adults. J Immunol Methods 369:133–140

Lang PO, Samaras D, Aspinall R et al (2012a) How important is Vitamin D in preventing infections? Osteoporos Int 24(5):1537–1553

Lang PO, Govind S, Dramé M et al (2012b) Comparison of manual and automated DNA purification for measuring TREC in dried blood spot (DBS) samples with qPCR. J Immunol Methods 384:118–127

Lang PO, Govind S, Aspinall R (2013a) Reversing T cell immunosenescence: why, who, and how. Age 35(3):609–620

Lang PO, Govind S, Dramé M et al (2013b) Measuring the TREC ratio in dried blood spot samples: intra- and inter-filter paper cards reproducibility. J Immunol Methods 389:1–8

Larbi A, Pawelec G, Wong SC et al (2011) Impact of age on T-cell signaling: a general defect or specific alteration? Ageing Res Rev 10:370–378

Levin MJ, Hayward AR (1996) The varicella vaccine. Prevention of herpes zoster. Infect Dis Clin North Am 10:657–675

Livak F, Schatz D (1996) T-cell receptor α locus V(D)J recombination by-products are abundant in thymocytes and mature T-cells. Mol Cell Biol 16:609–618

Lloyd-Sherlock P, McKee M, Ebrahim S et al (2012) Population ageing and health. Lancet 379:1295–1296

Lutz W, Sanderson W, Scherbov S (1997) Doubling of world population unlikely. Nature 387:803–805

Macaulay R, Akbar AN, Henson SM (2012) The role of the T-cell in a aged-related inflammation. Age 35(3):563–572

Maggi E, Cosmi L, Liotta F et al (2005) Thymic regulatory T cells. Autoimmun Rev 4:579–586

Markert ML, Boeck A, Hale LP et al (1999) Transplantation of thymus tissue in complete DiGeorge syndrome. N Eng J Med 341:1180–1189

Mitchell WA, Lang PO, Aspinall R (2010) Tracing thymic output in older individuals. Clin Exp Immunol 161:497–503

Murray JM, Kaufmann GR, Hodgkin PD et al (2003) Naive T cells are maintained by thymic output in early ages but by proliferation without phenotype change after age twenty. Immunol Cell Biol 81:487–495

Na IK, Letsch A, Guerreiro M et al (2009) Human bone marrow as a source to generate CMV-specific CD4+ T cells with multifunctional capacity. J Immunother 32:907–913

Naylor K, Li G, Vallejo AN et al (2005) The influence of age on T cell generation and TCR diversity. J Immunol 174:7446–7452

Nikolich-Zugich J (2008) Ageing and life-long maintenance of T-cell subsets in the face of latent persistent infections. Nat Rev Immunol 8:512–522

Oeppen J, Vaupel JW (2002) Demography. Broken limits to life expectancy. Science 296:1029–1031

Ongrádi J, Kövesdi V (2010) Factors that may impact on immunosenescence: a appraisal. Immun Ageing 7:7

Ortman CL, Dittmar KA, Witte PL et al (2002) Molecular characterization of the mouse involuted thymus: aberrations in expression of transcription regulators in thymocyte and epithelial compartments. Int Immunol 14:813–822

Ostan R, Bucci L, Capril M et al (2008) Immunosenescence and immunogenetics of human longevity. Neuroimmunomodulation 15:224–240

Oxman MN, Levin MJ, Johnson GR et al (2005) A vaccine to prevent herpes zoster and postherpetic neuralgia in older adults. N Eng J Med 352:2271–2284

Pantaleo G, Soudeyns H, Demarest JF et al (1997) Evidence for rapid disappearance of initially expanded HIV-specific CD8+ T cell clones during primary HIV infection. Proc Natl Acad Sci U S A 94:9848–9853

Patel DD, Gooding ME, Parrott RE et al (2000) Thymic function after hematopoietic stem-cell transplantation for the treatment of severe combined immunodeficiency. N Eng J Med 342:1325–1332

Pawelec G, Derhovanessian E, Larbi A et al (2009) Cytomegalovirus and human immunosenescence. Rev Med Virol 19:47–56

Peck A, Mellins ED (2010) Precarious balance: Th17 cells in host defense. Infect Immun 78:32–38

Pfister G, Savino W (2008) Can the immune system still be efficient in the elderly? An immunological and immunoendocrine therapeutic perspective. Neuro-immunomodulation 15:351–364

Pfister G, Weiskopf D, Lazuardi L et al (2006) Naive T cells in the elderly: are they still there? Ann N Y Acad Sci 1067:152–157

Sadighi Akha AA, Miller RA (2005) Signal transduction in the aging immune system. Curr Opin Immunol 17:486–491

Saurwein-Teissl M, Lung TL, Marx F et al (2002) Lack of antibody production following immunization in old age: association with CD8(+)CD28(−) T cell clonal expansions and an imbalance in the production of Th1 and Th2 cytokines. J Immunol 168:5893–5899

Schluns KS, Klonowski KD, Lefrancois L (2004) Transregulation of memory CD8 T-cell proliferation by IL-15R bone marrow-derived cells. Blood 103:988–994

Sempowski GD, Hale LP, Sundy JS et al (2000) Leukemia inhibitory factor, oncostatin M, Il-6 and stem cell factor mRNA expression in human thymus increases with age and is associated with thymic atrophy. J Immunol 164:2180–2187

Sewell AK, Price DA, Oxenius A et al (2000) Cytotoxic T lymphocyte responses to human immunodeficiency virus: control and escape. Stem Cells 18:230–244

Shankar P, Russo M, Harnisch B et al (2000) Impaired function of circulating HIV-specific CD8(+) T cells in chronic human immunodeficiency virus infection. Blood 96:3094–3101

Shaw AC, Panda A, Joshi SR et al (2011) Dysregulation of human Toll-like receptor function in aging. Ageing Res Rev 10(346–353)

Shetty P (2012) Grey matter: ageing in developing countries. Lancet 379:1285–1287

Siu G, Kronenberg M, Strauss E et al (1984) The structure, rearrangement and expression of D beta gene segments of the murine T-cell antigen receptor. Nature 311:344–350

Sprent J, Tough DF (1994) Lymphocyte life-span and memory. Science 265:1395–1400

Strindhall J, Nilsson BO, Lofgren S et al (2007) No Immune Risk Profile among individuals who reach 100 years of age: findings from the Swedish NONA immune longitudinal study. Exp Gerontol 42:753–761

Surh CD, Sprent J (2002) Regulation of naïve and memory T-cell homeostasis. Microbes Infect 4:51–56

Takeshita S, Toda M, Ymagishi H (1989) Excision products of the T cell receptor gene support a progressive rearrangement model of the α/δ locus. EMBO J 8:3261–3270

Thorpe KE, Howard DH (2006) The rise in spending among Medicare beneficiaries: the role of chronic disease prevalence and change in treatment intensity. Health Aff 25:w378–w388

Tokoyoda KZS, Hegazy AN, Albrecht I et al (2009) Professional memory CD4 T lymphocytes preferentially reside and rest in the bone marrow. Immunity 30:721–730

Tokoyoda K, Hauser AE, Nakayama T et al (2010) Organization of immunological memory by bone marrow stroma. Nat Rev Immunol 10:193–200

Tsaknaridis L, Spencer L, Culbertson N et al (2003) Functional assay for human CD4 + CD25+ Treg cells reveals an age- dependent loss of suppressive activity. J Neurosci Res 74:296–308

United Nations (UN) (2008) World population ageing: 1950–2050. http://www.un.org/esa/population/publications/worldageing19502050/

Vallejo AN (2005) CD28 extinction in human T-cells: altered functions and the program of T-cell senescence. Immunol Rev 205:158–169

Verschuren MC, Wolvers-Tettero IL, Breit TM et al (1997) Preferential rearrangements of the T cell receptor-delta-deleting elements in human T cells. J Immunol 159:4341–4349

Virgin HW, Wherry EJ, Ahmed R (2009) Redefining chronic viral infection. Cell 138:30–50

Weinberg A, Zhang JH, Oxman MN et al (2009) Varicella-zoster virus-specific immune responses to herpes zoster in elderly participants in a trial of a clinically effective zoster vaccine. J Infect Dis 200:1068–1076

Weinberg A, Huang S, Song LY et al (2012) Immune correlates of herpes zoster in HIV-infected children and youth. J Virol 86:2878–2881

Weinberger B, Lazuardi L, Weiskirchner I et al (2007) Healthy aging and latent infection with CMV lead to distinct changes in CD8 and CD4 T-cell subsets in the elderly. Hum Immunol 68:86–90

Weiskopf D, Weinberger B, Grubeck-Loebenstein B (2009) The aging of the immune system. Transpl Int 22:1041–1050

Wikby A, Ferguson F, Forsey R et al (2005) An immune risk phenotype, cognitive impairment, and survival in very late life: impact of allostatic load in Swedish octogenarian and nonagenarian humans. J Gerontol A Biol Sci Med Sci 60:556–565

Wikby A, Mansson IA, Johansson B et al (2008) The immune risk profile is associated with age and gender: findings from three Swedish population studies of individuals 20–100 years of age. Biogerontology 9:299–308

World Health Organization (WHO) (2002) Active ageing: a policy framework. http://whqlibdoc.who.int/hq/2002/who_nmh_nph_02.8.pdf

World Health Organization (WHO) (2011) Initiative of vaccine research (IVR) of the Immunization, Vaccines and Biologicals Department and the Ageing and Life Course (ALC) Department. Report on the ad-hoc Consultation on Ageing and Immunization, Geneva

Yao X, Hamilton RG, Weng NP et al (2011) Frailty is associated with impairment of vaccine-induced antibody response and increase in post-vaccination influenza infection in community-dwelling older adults. Vaccine 29:5015–5021

Yawn BP, Wollan PC, Kurland MJ et al (2011) Herpes zoster recurrences more frequent than previously reported. Mayo Clin Proc 86:88–93

Yu M, Li G, Lee WW et al (2012) Signal inhibition by the dual-specific phosphatase 4 impairs T cell-dependent B-cell responses with age. Proc Natl Acad Sci U S A 109:E879–E888

Zhang X, Sun S, Hwang I et al (1998) Potent and selective stimulation of memory-phenotype CD8 T cells in vivo by IL-15. Immunity 8:591–599

Zubakov D, Liu F, van Zelm MC et al (2010) Estimating human age from T-cell DNA rearrangements. Curr Biol 20:R970–R971

Biological and Phenotypic Alterations of T Cells in Aging

11

Ahmad Massoud and Amir Hossein Massoud

11.1 Introduction

The immune system exhibits age-related changes, collectively termed immunosenescence. The most visible of these changes is the decline in protective immunity resulting in complex immune defects and compensatory immune homeostatic mechanisms. The sum of these changes is a dysregulation of many processes that normally ensure optimal immune function. There are some evidences showing an increased susceptibility to infections in elderly individuals. Morbidity and mortality from numerous viral and bacterial diseases are increased in elderly humans and old animals.

Although it is likely that functional and structural alterations in both the entry sites and the target organs used by pathogens facilitate age-related susceptibility to some infections (e.g., impaired barrier function) (Minematsu et al. 2011), there is no doubt that the dysregulation of immunity also plays a central and critically important role in this process.

A. Massoud, PharmD, MPH, PhD (✉)
Department of Immunology, School of Medicine,
Tehran University of Medical Sciences, Tehran, Iran
e-mail: massoud.ahmad@yahoo.com

A.H. Massoud, PhD
Department of Microbiology and Immunology,
McGill University, Montreal, QC, Canada

Meakins-Christie Laboratories, McGill University,
Montreal, QC H2X-2P2, Canada

The deleterious effects of aging on the T cell compartment are well studied as they lead to increased susceptibility to infection, impaired immunosurveillance of malignant cells, leading to increased risk of cancer and autoimmunity in elders. Accordingly, responsiveness to vaccination in the elderly is also substantially diminished, and vaccine-induced protection is suboptimal (Weinberger and Grubeck-Loebenstein 2012). Aging reduces the number and T cell potential of hematopoietic precursors, and involution of the thymus renders it less capable of supporting de novo T cell development. Consequently, aging compromises the functional capacity of lymphocytes, resulting in a T cell pool with restricted receptor specificity and fewer naïve T cells (Henson and Akbar 2010). Age-related T cell compartment defects, as well as strategies to boost T cell function in aging individuals, are reviewed in this chapter.

11.2 T Cell Defects in Senescence

Aging-associated alterations in immunity occur in every component of the immune system. Alterations in T cell immunity occur with aging, affecting the function and proportions of T cell subsets, while changes in naive and memory $CD4^+$ and $CD8^+$ T cells percentages seem to be the most important alterations of T cell immunity during immunosenescence. In fact, the frequency of naive $CD4^+$ and $CD8^+$ T cells decreases with aging, whereas the frequency of memory $CD4^+$

A. Massoud, N. Rezaei (eds.), *Immunology of Aging*,
DOI 10.1007/978-3-642-39495-9_11, © Springer-Verlag Berlin Heidelberg 2014

and CD8[+] T cells increases. Also, changes in T cell proliferation, cytokine production, memory response, and cytotoxicity as well as in T regulatory (Treg) cell number and function have been reported with aging.

The age-related shortage in circulating naïve T cells is due to different changes in the immune organs. One major change during aging is a process termed "thymic involution." The thymus naturally atrophies as one of the important feature of aging. The volume of thymic tissue in a 60-year-old adult is less that 5 % that of a newborn (High et al. 2012). It seems that there is progressive decay of the thymus over the time which leads to a decrease in number and type of produced T cells. Thymic involution appears to associate with the production of sex hormones and reinforced by decreases in growth hormones (Chidgey and Boyd 2006; Goldberg et al. 2007). Importantly, this decline in new T cell production does not result in a proportional loss of naïve T cells which decline more slowly (Sempowski et al. 2002; Linton and Dorshkind 2004; Kilpatrick et al. 2008). This homeostasis is likely achieved by a set of feedback mechanisms that senses naïve CD4[+] T cell number and acts to preserve it. Hence, naïve CD4[+] T cells develop intrinsic changes by aging that includes a longer cellular lifespan.

In aged individuals, T cells shift from naïve to memory phenotypes (decreased numbers of naive T cells) (Kapasi et al. 2002; Hobbs et al. 1991). Nevertheless, numerous studies have demonstrated a deficiency in the ability of aged naïve and memory T cells to respond to antigens in respect to cell proliferation, cytokine productions, and the generation of cytotoxic CD8[+] T cells (McLeod 2000; Engwerda et al. 1996). In newborns, the ratio of naive to memory T cells is quite high; in adults the ratio is reversed because most of the naive T cells have been exposed to antigen and hence converted to memory cells. Consequently, the reserves of naive T cells become depleted, and the aged immune system cannot respond as well as a young person to new antigens.

Naïve CD4[+] cells also develop intrinsic age-associated defects. Most studies of the defects in primary naïve CD4[+] T cells have been carried out in mice. Some of the most definitive studies have used naïve CD4[+] T cells rigorously purified from T cell receptor (TCR) transgenic mice which were then studied in vitro or transferred to young hosts so that intrinsic defects in the aged naïve cells could be studied (Haynes and Swain 2006). Remarkable defects in CD4[+] T cell function are found when aged naïve CD4[+] T cells that differentiated to memory cells reencounter antigen. These memory cells generated from aged naïve CD4[+] T cells secrete a restricted pattern of cytokines and expand little after restimulation. In the mouse, in vitro studies showed that these memory cells make little interleukin (IL)-2, very low levels of T helper (Th)2 cytokines (IL-4, IL-5, and IL-13) but normal levels of interferon gamma (IFN-γ), and tumor necrosis factor alpha (TNF-α) (Haynes et al. 2003; Eaton et al. 2008).

The analysis of antigen-specific memory populations, differentiated from naïve T cells, also revealed that the helper response of memory cells generated from aged naïve cells is dramatically reduced even when the primary effector populations generated from young and aged naïve CD4[+] T cells are equivalent due to the addition of exogenous cytokines. For instance, the expansion of antigen-specific B cells, as well as the titers of immunoglobulin (Ig)G, was significantly lower when memory cells generated from aged naïve CD4[+] T cells provided help compared to memory cells generated from young naïve CD4[+] T cells (Haynes et al. 2003; Eaton et al. 2008). Interestingly, memory cells generated from young naïve CD4[+] T cells had a quite satisfactory function for at least 1 year following primary stimulation (Eaton et al. 2008), suggesting that the age of the cell at initial priming determines the quality of the resulting memory cells. This poor memory response, especially the loss of cognate helper function among CD4[+] T cells, is likely a major cause of the poor efficacy of vaccines that are given to the elderly. In human studies, following vaccination, both CD4[+] and CD8[+] memory T cells, in the elderly were less responsive than those from the young (Zhou and McElhaney 2011).

In addition, defect of T cell activation happens in the elderly at different levels. For instance, important changes occur at the cell surface of different subsets of T cells. Aged T cells do not display the CD28 antigen, a molecule critical for signal transduction and T cell activation, on the cell surface (Chou and Effros 2013). Without this protein, T cells remain quiescent and do not respond properly to foreign pathogens. Many molecules are involved in signal transduction. It seems that the presence of CD69 antigen on the cell surface is decreased during aging (Noble et al. 1999). T cells are induced to display CD69 antigen only after antigen binds to the T cell receptor. If the signal is not transmitted to the T cell, CD69 will not appear on the cell surface, and therefore less signal transduction is expected in elderly individuals.

Another defect of T cell activation among the elderly is characterized by a decrease in calcium (Lustyik and O'Leary 1989). Calcium is a vital element that is absolutely crucial for many biochemical reactions, including signal transduction. Decrease in calcium levels in T cells effectively halts signal transduction by failing to stimulate enzymes, including protein kinases, such as protein kinase C (PKC) and mitogen-activated protein kinases (MAPK), that require calcium for proper function (Douziech et al. 2002; Tamura et al. 2000).

One of the main defects of aged $CD4^+$ T cells is that they produce significantly less IL-2 upon TCR stimulation when compared to young cells. This results in the aged cells undergoing fewer rounds of cell division, exhibiting less clonal expansion and expressing a less differentiated phenotype (Haynes et al. 1999).

One cytokine that has been widely studied in aged T cells is IL-2, a cytokine produced and secreted by T cells that induces cell proliferation and supports long-term growth of T cells. As T cells age, they lose their capacity to produce and respond to IL-2. The aged $CD4^+$ effectors also have defects in cytokine production after restimulation, with a significantly reduced production of IL-2 compared with young cells (Haynes et al. 1999).

When exposed to antigen, memory T cells will rapidly divide and proliferate to make more T cell clones to fight the antigen, but only proliferate upon stimulation with IL-2. If enough IL-2 is not produced, or if the T cells cannot respond effectively to IL-2, T cell function is greatly impaired. Changes in other cytokines such as IL-4, TNF-α, and IFN-γ have also been recorded, but it is not yet known to what extent these changes influence the aging immune system (Lee et al. 2012).

Importantly, this age-related defect in the aged naïve T cells can be reversed by the addition of exogenous IL-2 (Haynes et al. 1999). This leads to proliferation of aged cells much like the young cells and subsequently exhibiting enhanced IL-2 production. In addition, aged T cells, stimulated in the presence of exogenous IL-2 also exhibit a more activated cell surface phenotype, including enhanced expression of CD25 and down regulation of CD62L when compared to aged cells stimulated without exogenous IL-2.

Aging is also reported to be associated with decline in oral and intestinal mucosal tolerance induction, which might be in part due to reduction of regulatory-type cytokines production by T cells in mucosa (Santiago et al. 2011). These results demonstrated that one functionally significant defect of aged naïve $CD4^+$ T cells was dysregulated production of cytokines in aging.

Some of the age-related defects in T cells appear to be due to genetic alterations occurring within T cells. In vitro studies of human T cells cultured for long periods have shown that the cell cycle slows and eventually stops, even when the cells are grown in the presence of IL-2; this results in defects in T cell proliferation; so T cells become too old to function properly (Effros 2003). Several problems with the genetic machinery of T cells may account for this gradual failure of the cell cycle. Following repeated stimulation with antigens, T cells eventually reach an irreversible state of cell cycle arrest; at that time, they show loss of gene expression of a key T cell-specific signaling molecule required for proliferation such as transcription factors like NFκB and the activator protein 1 (AP-1) (Ponnappan 2002; Kwon et al. 1996). Thus, it appears that aging contributes to the decline in T cell responsiveness by failing to activate the genes necessary for T cell stimulation in both human and murine systems.

Aged T cells also are more susceptible to apoptosis, partly due to the gradual loss of telomeres. Telomeres are protein-DNA complexes, which cap the ends of the chromosomes to prevent DNA degradation. Their length shortens with each cell division and correlates inversely with age (Kaszubowska 2008). It can be modified by genetic and epigenetic factors, sex hormones, reactive oxygen species (ROS), and inflammatory reactions (Kaszubowska 2008). Thus, it seems that age-related reduction in T cells lifespan is genetically programmed.

The reduced functions and lifespan of T cells in the elderly also affect B cell functions because T cells act in concert with B cells to regulate the production of antibodies. Aged helper T cells cannot interact effectively with B cells, and so in the elderly, the potential antibody repertoire is more limited than the antibody repertoire of younger people. The production of IgM, one of five classes of antibodies, is specially affected. During infection, IgM is the first class of antibodies to respond. In the elderly, the inability to defense against infections could be linked to this diminishing IgM response (Strasser et al. 1997). The rate of B cell maturation also decreases with age. Although B cells are produced in the bone marrow throughout life, the number of B cells generated declines with age (Klinman and Kline 1997). Having fewer mature B cells contributes to the observed decrease in the amount of antibody produced in response to infection.

Autoantibodies are usually hallmarks of autoimmune diseases. However, the presence of autoantibodies is often correlated with age. Although the reasons behind this phenomenon are not completely understood, autoantibody production in the elderly may be linked to the functional changes in T cells described earlier. The age-related mutations in T cell genes could lead to a group of T cells that recognize host self-antigen. Normally, such T cells would be eliminated in the thymus before they fully matured, but thymic involution allows this destructive population of T cells to persist. This theory seems to be supported by a study performed in mice demonstrating that transplantation of a fetal thymus into an aged recipient with an autoimmune disease can restore immune function and thus treat autoimmunity (Hosaka et al. 1996).

11.3 Clinical Strategies to Enhance T Cell Responses in the Elderly

The loss of T cell immunity significantly increases the risk of infections and cancer, because of a restricted capacity for immunosurveillance. Therefore, employing the strategies to enhance T cell immunity in the elderly would be beneficial to overcome these conditions.

Recent clinical studies have defined strategies that could enhance T cell immunity in aging individuals. These approaches enhance the number of T cell precursors and their functionality or promote thymopoiesis.

Thymic rejuvenation, although not yet used in clinical trials, is very promising strategy but, even if it could be achieved, probably is accompanied by significant risks. The principle would be that depletion of a substantial fraction of the peripheral naïve CD4[+] population, along with rebalancing of sex and growth hormones, can consequently facilitate the generation of newly naïve CD4[+] T cells. Aging humans have lower serum levels of growth hormones. A number of investigators have studied the possible effects of growth hormones that stimulate thymopoiesis (Chen et al. 2003, 2010; Holland and van den Brink 2009) that might enhance the generation of new naïve T cells. The Insulin Growth Factor-1 (IGF-1) receptor is expressed on thymocytes and T cells and may act directly on these cells to stimulate lymphopoiesis (Welniak et al. 2002), which could further contribute to the improved T cell reconstitution.

Contrarily sex steroids are known to negatively regulate development of immune cells and a number of studies addressed the possible effect of sex hormone ablation in boosting immune system in the elderly (Goldberg et al. 2005, 2007; Heng et al. 2010).

One of the main defects of aged T cells is that they produce significantly less IL-2 upon stimulation when compared to young cells. This results in the aged cells exhibiting less clonal expansion. Signaling induced by cytokines with common γ chain receptor (IL-2, IL-7, IL-15) supports thymocyte development and peripheral T cell survival and proliferation (von Freeden-Jeffry et al. 1997). For instance, addition of exogenous IL-2 to aged naïve T cells can reversed this defect in aged mice. Moreover, aged T cells stimulated in the presence of exogenous IL-2 also exhibit a more activated cell surface phenotype (Haynes et al. 1999). However, once these aged effectors generated in the presence of exogenous IL-2 returned to a resting state, they re-exhibited age-related defects such as reduced clonal expansion and cytokine production, indicating that the IL-2 enhancement effects were only transient (Haynes et al. 2003). Proinflammatory cytokines can also provide a third signal that enhances the costimulation of naïve CD4+ T cells (Curtsinger et al. 1999). Therefore, employing these cytokines can boost the aged CD4+ T cells responses and clonal expansion via a mechanism that involves NFκB activation (Haynes et al. 2004). Furthermore, Toll-like receptor (TLR) agonists, used as an adjuvant in vaccination, can also boost the in vivo cognate helper function of aged CD4+ T cells, leading to enhanced humoral responses (Maue et al. 2009). A recent study has shown that a TLR4 agonist adjuvant can also boost the T cell responses to influenza vaccination in older adults (Behzad et al. 2012). These findings are encouraging and have the potential to greatly improve vaccine-mediated protection against infections in the elderly.

In addition, nutrition plays a prominent role in regulation of the immune system, and reduced caloric intake is known to slow the aging process and help maintain higher numbers of naive T cells and levels of IL-2 (Alam et al. 2012). Vitamin E and zinc in particular are important nutrients for the proper functioning of the immune system (Pae et al. 2012). Long-term zinc deficiency in the elderly causes a decrease in cytokine production and impaired regulation of helper T cell activity. Vitamin E has been shown as a possible treatment for Alzheimer's disease, and it seems that vitamin E supplements may also boost the immune system (Pae et al. 2012).

Vitamin E is also an antioxidant that can protect lymphocytes, the brain, and other tissues from destructive free radicals (Alvarado et al. 2006).

Additionally there are some studies on aged mice stem cell transplantation which demonstrated improving T cell development. Hematopoietic stem cell transplantation (HSCT) can help in the reconstitution of damaged immune system in the elderly, and studies in experimental mouse models of HSCT have identified agents that are relevant for boosting T cell reconstitution not only after transplant but also potentially in aging recipients (Holland and van den Brink 2009).

References

Alam I, Larbi A, Pawelec G (2012) Nutritional status influences peripheral immune cell phenotypes in healthy men in rural Pakistan. Immun Ageing 9(1):16

Alvarado C, Alvarez P, Puerto M et al (2006) Dietary supplementation with antioxidants improves functions and decreases oxidative stress of leukocytes from prematurely aging mice. Nutrition 22(7–8):767–777

Behzad H, Huckriede AL, Haynes L et al (2012) GLA-SE, a synthetic toll-like receptor 4 agonist, enhances T-cell responses to influenza vaccine in older adults. J Infect Dis 205(3):466–473

Chen BJ, Cui X, Sempowski GD et al (2003) Growth hormone accelerates immune recovery following allogeneic T-cell-depleted bone marrow transplantation in mice. Exp Hematol 31(10):953–958

Chen BJ, Deoliveira D, Spasojevic I et al (2010) Growth hormone mitigates against lethal irradiation and enhances hematologic and immune recovery in mice and nonhuman primates. PLoS One 5(6):e11056

Chidgey AP, Boyd RL (2006) Stemming the tide of thymic aging. Nat Immunol 7(10):1013–1016

Chou JP, Effros RB (2013) T cell replicative senescence in human aging. Curr Pharm Des 19(9):1680–1698

Curtsinger JM, Schmidt CS, Mondino A et al (1999) Inflammatory cytokines provide a third signal for activation of naive CD4+ and CD8+ T cells. J Immunol 162(6):3256–3262

Douziech N, Seres I, Larbi A et al (2002) Modulation of human lymphocyte proliferative response with aging. Exp Gerontol 37(2–3):369–387

Eaton SM, Maue AC, Swain SL et al (2008) Bone marrow precursor cells from aged mice generate CD4 T cells that function well in primary and memory responses. J Immunol 181(7):4825–4831

Effros RB (2003) Genetic alterations in the ageing immune system: impact on infection and cancer. Mech Ageing Dev 124(1):71–77

Engwerda CR, Fox BS, Handwerger BS (1996) Cytokine production by T lymphocytes from young and aged mice. J Immunol 156(10):3621–3630

Goldberg GL, Sutherland JS, Hammet MV et al (2005) Sex steroid ablation enhances lymphoid recovery following autologous hematopoietic stem cell transplantation. Transplantation 80(11):1604–1613

Goldberg GL, Alpdogan O, Muriglan SJ et al (2007) Enhanced immune reconstitution by sex steroid ablation following allogeneic hemopoietic stem cell transplantation. J Immunol 178(11):7473–7484

Haynes L, Swain SL (2006) Why aging T cells fail: implications for vaccination. Immunity 24(6):663–666

Haynes L, Linton PJ, Eaton SM et al (1999) Interleukin 2, but not other common gamma chain-binding cytokines, can reverse the defect in generation of CD4 effector T cells from naive T cells of aged mice. J Exp Med 190(7):1013–1024

Haynes L, Eaton SM, Burns EM et al (2003) CD4 T cell memory derived from young naive cells functions well into old age, but memory generated from aged naive cells functions poorly. Proc Natl Acad Sci U S A 100(25):15053–15058

Haynes L, Eaton SM, Burns EM et al (2004) Inflammatory cytokines overcome age-related defects in CD4 T cell responses in vivo. J Immunol 172(9):5194–5199

Heng TS, Chidgey AP, Boyd RL (2010) Getting back at nature: understanding thymic development and overcoming its atrophy. Curr Opin Pharmacol 10(4):425–433

Henson SM, Akbar AN (2010) Memory T-cell homeostasis and senescence during aging. Adv Exp Med Biol 684:189–197

High KP, Akbar AN, Nikolich-Zugich J (2012) Translational research in immune senescence: assessing the relevance of current models. Semin Immunol 24(5):373–382

Hobbs MV, Ernst DN, Torbett BE et al (1991) Cell proliferation and cytokine production by CD4+ cells from old mice. J Cell Biochem 46(4):312–320

Holland AM, van den Brink MR (2009) Rejuvenation of the aging T cell compartment. Curr Opin Immunol 21(4):454–459

Hosaka N, Nose M, Kyogoku M et al (1996) Thymus transplantation, a critical factor for correction of autoimmune disease in aging MRL/+mice. Proc Natl Acad Sci U S A 93(16):8558–8562

Kapasi ZF, Murali-Krishna K, McRae ML et al (2002) Defective generation but normal maintenance of memory T cells in old mice. Eur J Immunol 32(6):1567–1573

Kaszubowska L (2008) Telomere shortening and ageing of the immune system. J Physiol Pharmacol 59(Suppl 9):169–186

Kilpatrick RD, Rickabaugh T, Hultin LE et al (2008) Homeostasis of the naive CD4+ T cell compartment during aging. J Immunol 180(3):1499–1507

Klinman NR, Kline GH (1997) The B-cell biology of aging. Immunol Rev 160:103–114

Kwon TK, Nagel JE, Buchholz MA et al (1996) Characterization of the murine cyclin-dependent kinase inhibitor gene p27Kip1. Gene 180(1–2):113–120

Lee N, Shin MS, Kang I (2012) T-cell biology in aging, with a focus on lung disease. J Gerontol A Biol Sci Med Sci 67(3):254–263

Linton PJ, Dorshkind K (2004) Age-related changes in lymphocyte development and function. Nat Immunol 5(2):133–139

Lustyik G, O'Leary JJ (1989) Aging and the mobilization of intracellular calcium by phytohemagglutinin in human T cells. J Gerontol 44(2):B30–B36

Maue AC, Eaton SM, Lanthier PA et al (2009) Proinflammatory adjuvants enhance the cognate helper activity of aged CD4 T cells. J Immunol 182(10):6129–6135

McLeod JD (2000) Apoptotic capability in ageing T cells. Mech Ageing Dev 121(1–3):151–159

Minematsu T, Yamamoto Y, Nagase T et al (2011) Aging enhances maceration-induced ultrastructural alteration of the epidermis and impairment of skin barrier function. J Dermatol Sci 62(3):160–168

Noble JM, Ford GA, Thomas TH (1999) Effect of aging on CD11b and CD69 surface expression by vesicular insertion in human polymorphonuclear leucocytes. Clin Sci (Lond) 97(3):323–329

Pae M, Meydani SN, Wu D (2012) The role of nutrition in enhancing immunity in aging. Ageing Dis 3(1):91–129

Ponnappan U (2002) Ubiquitin-proteasome pathway is compromised in CD45RO + and CD45RA + T lymphocyte subsets during aging. Exp Gerontol 37(2–3):359–367

Santiago AF, Alves AC, Oliveira RP et al (2011) Aging correlates with reduction in regulatory-type cytokines and T cells in the gut mucosa. Immunobiology 216(10):1085–1093

Sempowski GD, Gooding ME, Liao HX et al (2002) T cell receptor excision circle assessment of thymopoiesis in aging mice. Mol Immunol 38(11):841–848

Strasser A, Sonnek U, Niedermuller H (1997) Age-related changes in plasma IgM level after SRBC-stimulation in the rat. Arch Gerontol Geriatr 25(3):277–284

Tamura T, Kunimatsu T, Yee ST et al (2000) Molecular mechanism of the impairment in activation signal transduction in CD4(+) T cells from old mice. Int Immunol 12(8):1205–1215

von Freeden-Jeffry U, Solvason N, Howard M et al (1997) The earliest T lineage-committed cells depend on IL-7 for Bcl-2 expression and normal cell cycle progression. Immunity 7(1):147–154

Weinberger B, Grubeck-Loebenstein B (2012) Vaccines for the elderly. Clin Microbiol Infect 18(Suppl 5):100–108

Welniak LA, Sun R, Murphy WJ (2002) The role of growth hormone in T-cell development and reconstitution. J Leukoc Biol 71(3):381–387

Zhou X, McElhaney JE (2011) Age-related changes in memory and effector T cells responding to influenza A/H3N2 and pandemic A/H1N1 strains in humans. Vaccine 29(11):2169–2177

T Cells Seen from the Metabolic and Aging Perspective

12

Xavier Camous and Anis Larbi

12.1 Importance of T Cells in Immunity

The immune system is a crucial key for survival. It has evolved from a very basic mechanism in sponges, one type of cell releasing toxins and phagocyting (Hirsch 1959), to a complex meta-system in superior animals, including human, with a complex network of signalization and communication between numerous types of cells. In this present chapter, we will focus on human immunology and more particularly on adaptive immunology with T cells.

Our immune system is divided in two subsystems called innate and adaptive immunity (Dempsey et al. 2003). Innate immunity is our first line of defense against pathogens such as parasite, fungi, bacteria, or yeast. It reacts very fast but doesn't keep record of the pathogens it met and is composed of various cell types. Although there are some higher affinities for certain foreign antigens, the innate immune system as a whole is considered nonspecific. It can be sufficient by itself to eliminate threats but may require further activation by adaptive immune system.

The adaptive immunity is probably the latest evolution of the immune system (Laird et al. 2000).

It is mainly composed of highly specialized cells, the lymphocytes. Contrarily to the innate immunity, adaptive responses require a longer time to be fully efficient. This longer incubation time enable cooperation between the two types of lymphocytes, the B and the T lymphocytes that induce the humoral and the cellular responses, respectively. The B cells express the B cell receptor (BCR), CD19, and human leukocyte antigen (HLA)-DR, and their main function is the production of antibodies upon recognition of the antigen. Antibodies, or immunoglobulins, are Y-shaped proteins that bind specifically to their antigen, located on a pathogen, to neutralize it, by binding a viral protein involved in virus internalization, for example, or to make it accessible to the immune system, process called opsonization. Finally, B cells are also able to secrete various cytokines to strengthen or inhibit immune response.

The T cells are the others effectors of the adaptive immune system (Santana and Esquivel-Guadarrama 2006) and the central topic of this present chapter. These cells are produced in bone marrow from hematopoietic stem cells and then migrate to the thymus to mature and become naïve T cells ready to meet their antigen. They are segregated in two main populations, helpers and cytotoxic, who are also subdivided in various subsets that will be described deeper in the next part of this chapter. Their main role is to kill virus-infected and tumor cells recognized by their main feature, the T cell receptor (TCR). As B cells, they are able to memorize all the antigens they meet during each immune response; a few

X. Camous, PhD • A. Larbi, PhD (✉)
Singapore Immunology Network (SIgN),
Agency for Science Technology and Research,
Singapore 138648, Singapore
e-mail: anis_larbi@immunol.a-star.edu.sg

A. Massoud, N. Rezaei (eds.), *Immunology of Aging*,
DOI 10.1007/978-3-642-39495-9_12, © Springer-Verlag Berlin Heidelberg 2014

activated T (or B) cells will remain alive to mount a much more rapid response if they meet their antigen a second time, a property that is used for vaccination.

T cells have a crucial and central role in adaptive immunity as they are the main effectors of cytotoxicity (Barry and Bleackley 2002). In diseases where this response is impaired, such as acquired immunodeficiency syndrome (AIDS), reactivation of various viruses, such as herpes viruses, is often observed and clearly suggested that de novo infection or reactivation of previously encountered antigen is a daily challenge.

12.2 T Cell Homeostasis and Subsets

12.2.1 T Cell Maturation

Like every hematopoietic cell, T cells originate from pluripotent stem cells located in bone marrow (BM) called hemocytoblast or hematopoietic stem cells (HSCs) (Schwarz and Bhandoola 2006). These cells can differentiate into two different types of cell: the common myeloid progenitor (CMP) that will produce granulocytes, monocytes, and dendritic cells or a common lymphoid progenitor (CLP) that will produce B and T cells. HSCs are self-renewing as during division, at least one of the daughter cell will remain HSC, while the others will become either CLP or CMP.

Concerning the T cells lineage (Koch and Radtke 2011; Adkins et al. 1987; Bird 2009), the CLP will be influenced by several cytokines and growth factors like interleukin (IL)-2, IL-7, IL-12, stromal cell-derived factor 1 (SDF-1), FMS-like tyrosine kinase 3 ligand (FLT3-L), transforming growth factor beta (TGF-β), or tumor necrosis factor alpha (TNF-α) to differentiate into a lymphoblast then into a prolymphocyte that will leave the bone marrow to migrate into the thymus. This thymocyte will undergo lymphopoiesis in the thymic cortex. The less differentiated cell entering the thymus is called early thymocyte progenitors (ETP) and still possesses myeloid and lymphoid potential. This stage is very short as cell rapidly engages toward natural killer

(NK) or lymphocyte lineage. The second major step is the expansion and the differentiation of T cells. They undergo different steps leading them to their final differentiation. Initially, cells lack CD4 and CD8 expression; these steps are called double negative 1-2-3 (DN1-2-3) where cells start to rearrange the α and β chains of their TCR and are locked into T cell lineage. Cells that were not able to rearrange properly their TCR will be eliminated, a step called positive selection. Then, differentiation continues and cells will migrate into the thymus medulla and become CD4$^+$CD8$^+$ double positive (DP). There, they undergo the negative selection, based on elimination of cells able to recognize self-antigens, and become simple positive (SP) CD4$^+$ or CD8$^+$ depending on which major histocompatibility complex (MHC) type their TCR recognize during the selection step. If they recognize a class I MHC, they will express only CD8 and become cytotoxic T cells, and if it is a class II MHC, they will differentiate into CD4$^+$ helper T cells. Cells mature for several days in an antigen-free environment where more than 95 % of T cells will die due to thymic selection. At this point, T cells are naïve and able to recognize foreign antigens. Thymopoiesis is then a tightly regulated and resources consuming process. Cells are then released into the blood as CD3$^+$CD28$^+$CD27$^+$CD45RA$^+$CD45RO$^-$ T cells. In the circulation, the pool of naïve cells will ensure immunosurveillance for un-encountered antigens. They are retained for a significant period of time and may undergo homeostatic proliferation.

12.2.2 T Cell Activation

The population of helper T cells is heterogeneous. After meeting their antigen, CD4$^+$ cells can engage different pathways depending on the cocktail of cytokines they were stimulated with by antigen presenting cells (APC). They will differentiate into T helper 0 (Th0) cells after being activated and then secrete IL-2, IL-4, and interferon (IFN). Interleukin-2 will be responsible for the induction of their proliferation. In the context of a viral infection, Th0 cells will be driven into the Th1 profile that allow them to release IFN-γ and TGF-β that will maximize the killing ability of cytotoxic T cells and macrophages to eliminate infected cells. IFN-γ will also increase the production of IL-12 by dendritic cells and macrophages which will increase the production of IFN-γ in Th1 cells to maximize the antiviral response. If the pathogens are parasites, fungi, or bacteria, Th cells will undergo Th2 differentiation where the main molecular effectors are IL-4 and IL-6. Th2 cells are meant to support the humoral response by supporting antibody production by B cells. It is important to note that Th1 cells will secrete cytokines such as IFN-γ that inhibit Th2 differentiation and Th2 will do the same on Th1 by secreting IL-10. Thus, the type of the response is not only decided by the early events but by the cells part of the response.

More recently, two others Th differentiation profile have been discovered, the Th3 (Sakaguchi et al. 2006) and Th17 (Harrington et al. 2005) profiles. The Th3 profile is a very special type of CD4+ T cells, the T regulatory cells (Tregs). These highly immunosuppressive cells express CD4 as well as CD25 and FoxP3 and produce large amounts of IL-10 and TGF-β that inhibits both Th1 and Th2 responses. It is believed that their role is to contain the duration and intensity of the immune response to avoid internal damages. Regarding Th17 cells, their origin is still not well known. TGF-β, IL-6, IL-21, and IL-23 have been shown to be implicated into their differentiation from Th0 (Dong 2008; Manel et al. 2008). As their name suggests, Th17 cells secrete large amounts of IL-17. These cytokine is induced by IL-23 and acts as a potent mediator in delayed-type reactions by increasing chemokine production in various tissues to recruit monocytes and neutrophils to the site of inflammation, similarly to IFN-γ. Although Th17 cells may have a role in autoimmune diseases, it is believed that their main role is to disrupt the pathogen's cellular matrix.

The other family of lymphocytes, the cytotoxic T cells, expresses CD8. These are specialized in the killing of tumor and virus-infected cells. Unlike CD4+ T cells, their TCR will recognize antigens presented by a class I MHC molecule. This fact is very relevant as class I molecules are expressed on every nucleated cell, whereas class II are restricted to APC, and CD8 cells must be able to kill any cell becoming infected or malignant. Once they were activated by an APC and received correct double stimulation signal, through TCR and CD28, they will proliferate and migrate to the site of infection. Once they recognize their target using TCR, cytotoxic cells will be able to kill by releasing perforin that disintegrates the target membrane, granzyme, and granulysin that will induce apoptosis by cleaving subtracts inside the target. Once activated, CD8+ T cells also express Fas ligand at their surface. This molecule will bind to Fas on the target membrane and induce the caspase pathway leading to apoptosis.

Another way to classify T cells is not based on their functionality during the response but on their phenotype. Naïve and memory T cells comprise of several subsets. During the clonal expansion of CD4+ and CD8+ T cells following their activation, a majority will differentiate into effector cells but others, around 5 %, will become memory cells. These cells have a much longer lifespan compared to naïve T cells or other immune cells, resist to apoptosis under IL-7 stimulation (Bradley et al. 2005), and renew themselves, thanks to IL-15 (Malamut et al. 2010). They also express a range of molecules typical of activated T cells (adhesion molecules, growth factors/chemokine/cytokines receptors) and retain strong proliferation ability. As they differentiate and proliferate much faster, they accelerate greatly the response following second encounter with an antigen (called secondary immune response). They are also able to express two or three effector functions simultaneously and thus may be equivalent to two or three naïve cells. The polyfunctionality of these cells renders them essential for fighting against pathogens, controlling of persistent infections, and providing immune protection. Two distinct subsets of memory T cells have been well described (Sallusto et al. 2000): first, the central memory T cells or Tcm, found in lymph nodes which express L-selectin and chemokine receptor 7 (CCR7) and secrete IL-2, and the effector memory T cells, or Tem, that locates into peripheral tissues, more in those that were previously infected, and secrete IFN-γ and IL-4. In Tem population, a subset called Temra has been characterized (Geginat et al. 2003). These cells are the most differentiated memory cells, reexpressing CD45RA; in addition, they are very cytotoxic and also very sensitive to apoptosis. Tcm dis–play a CCR7$^+$CD45RA$^-$CD45RO$^+$ CD28^{++}CD27^{++} phenotype, while Tem display a CCR7$^-$CD45RA$^-$CD45RO$^+$CD28$^+$CD27$^+$ phenotype and Temra a CCR7$^-$CD45RA$^+$CD45RO^{low}CD 28$^{+/-}$CD27$^{+/-}$ phenotype.

12.3 Signalling Pathways That Differ in T Cell Subsets

Some of the functions and pathways described above are very specific to T cell subpopulations. The pathway conserved in all T cell subpopulations is the T cell receptor signalling. The TCR is composed, in 95 % of T cells, by one α and one β chain (or one γ and one δ chain in the other 5 %, the γ/δ T cells). These chains undergo a very specific process called the V(D)J recombination. During the maturation of T cells in the thymus, the part of the sequence coding for the area that will recognize the antigen is composed of three elements called V (for variable), D (for diverse), and J (for junction). Each step of the TCR formation is extremely monitored and any defect will lead to the apoptosis of the T cell. The TCR is anchored in the membrane but lack of truly efficient internal domain for signalling. This is the reason why it is coupled with a CD3 molecule, which is a popular maker for T cells. CD3 is a complex molecule composed of four types of chains: two ε, one δ, two ζ, and one γ. The ε, δ, and γ chains are extracellular and contain each one immunoreceptor tyrosine-based activation motif (ITAM) intracellularly, while the ζ chains possess the longest intracellular portion of the TCR/CD3 complex and contain three ITAM domains, more efficient for signalling. Following TCR ligation ITAMs are phosphorylated a kinase, Lck that induce the recruitment of ZAP-70. This molecule plays a critical role in T cell signalling as it will transmit the activation signal from TCR/CD3 to the different kinases, adaptor

molecules (e.g., LAT) that will engage either the mitogen-activated protein kinases (MAPK), c-Jun N-terminal kinase (JNK), or nuclear factor kappa-light-chain-enhancer of activated B cells (NFκB) signalling. All these events are initially tightly regulated by CD45, a phosphatize of which isoforms (CD45RA, CD45RB, and CD45RO) are also used to differentiate naïve from memory and Temra cells. Whether the expression of different isoforms directly impacts on the early events leading to T cell activation has been overlooked. The fact memory cells gain functionality with differentiation but loose proliferative capacity at the Temra stage (when CD45RA is reexpressed) suggests that the combination of signalling events (signalling cross talk) may differ with CD45 isoform expression.

TCR signalling will not lead to the same result in a Th cell compared to a Tc cell. In a Th cell, once the TCR/antigen and CD4/class II MHC molecule recognition is made, and depending on the cytokine environment, the cell will switch into Th1/2/3/17 response and secrete a wide variety of cytokines. To reach a full state of activation, all T cells need additional signals, and this is partly fulfilled by the interaction of CD28 (on T cells) and CD80 (on APC). In Th1 cells, it will leads to the secretion of antiviral molecules such as IL-12 or IL-18 that will induce and dramatically boost the IFN-γ secretion. In Th2 cells, it will induce the secretion of IL-4 which is a major mediator of humoral response. It is of note that not all T cell retain CD28 expression. The more the cell proliferates and differentiates the more CD28 expression is reduced, concomitantly to telomere length. This is true for CD4$^+$ and CD8$^+$ T cells. This suggests that other molecules may be used to keep a certain level of functionality. It is well known that differentiation of T cells also leads to loss of CD27 but is associated with expression of CD57, programmed cell death protein 1 (PD-1), killer cell lectin-like receptor subfamily G member 1 (KLRG-1), cytotoxic T lymphocyte antigen 4 (CTLA-4), and other receptors that possess immunoreceptor tyrosine-based inhibitory motifs (ITIMs) instead of ITAMs and have all been shown to have inhibitory effects on T cell proliferation. This highlights that TCR signalling may be modulated by signalling cross talk emerging from inhibitory receptors and that the steady state signalling status (phosphorylation) could be a major player determining T cell activation.

Concerning cytotoxic T cells, the TCR/CD28 activation will unlock the killing function only when the lymphocyte meets an APC, contrarily to a natural killer cell that needs no priming. The cells will then release several cytotoxic molecules using different means to kill its target. The protein, coded by the PRF1 (Fink et al. 1992), gene is located in cytotoxic cells' granules and have a structure quite similar to the C9 protein of the complement. Once secreted it will insert into the membrane and create pores that allow introduction of molecules and lysis of the cell by osmotic shock (Tschopp et al. 1986). The other mechanism used to lyse cell is the use of granzymes (Bots and Medema 2006). Granzymes are serine protein coded by several genes (GZMA/B/H/K/M), also located in granules, that will be co-secreted with perforin. They will penetrate the target and cleave their target, inducing apoptosis. It is believed that perforin creates pores to let granzymes penetrate the cells, but some researchers showed that a complex of granzyme B/perforin/granulysin can enter the targeted cell by using the mannose-6-phosphate receptor. T cells also use granulysin, a protein coded by the GNLY gene that induces apoptosis in target using mitochondrial cell death (cytochrome C and caspase pathways) (Stenger et al. 1998). Finally, the last molecule used by T cells can be assimilated with a kiss of death, the Fas/Fas ligand pathway (Andersen et al. 2006). It can induce the apoptosis of the target but also of activated T cells to prevent a too long inflammation.

12.4 T Cell Metabolism

12.4.1 General Concept in Steady State Versus During Activation

The role of T cells is to respond to a danger signal in a very specific manner and ideally in a short time with a controlled inflammatory process. To achieve this goal T cell undergoes an intense proliferation phase, the clonal expansion. This step requires an incredible amount of resources and forces T cells to alter dramatically their metabolism to fuel all the synthesis occurring during the replication process. Resting T cells, just after their release from thymus, consume low amount of nutriments to perform basic housekeeping program (Buttgereit et al. 2000). Among these nutriments, glucose is used by various metabolic processes. First, it is required for oligosaccharide synthesis for the various glycosylation reactions occurring in these cells. Then, glucose is mandatory for the lactate production during which it is broken by glycolysis and oxidized into pyruvate. Finally, after glycolysis, pyruvate is also used to fuel the Krebs cycle to produce acetyl coenzyme A (CoA) and CO_2 and the pentose phosphate pathway. To perform all of these very basal metabolic reactions, T cells must receive external survival stimuli such as cytokines or light stimulation through TCR. Without these, T cells lose their ability to import glucose and lose their homeostasis. As reported (Frauwirth and Thompson 2004), the resting T cells metabolism is limited not by nutriments but by external survival signal. It is not clear yet whether homeostatic proliferation and proliferation following activation by antigen recognition involve the same change in metabolic rate. As the signalling events are different, we can speculate that this is different.

Activated T cells have a very different metabolism (Hume et al. 1978). First, glucose uptake is dramatically increased shortly after stimulation, as well as, to a lower extent, oxygen consumption. During this metabolic event, the rate of glycolysis is much higher than oxygen consumption. This leads to an increase in lactate production and thus, energy. These processes have been named aerobic glycolysis, or Warburg effect, as oxygen supply increases, contrarily to anaerobic glycolysis occurring in muscle, where oxygen level decreases. This particular metabolism is also found in tumor cells, where it was first characterized by Otto Warburg, and may be a result of the multiple mutations leading to cancer (Warburg 1956). This is a very interesting finding because like activated lymphocytes, cancer cells must maintain an energy-demanding proliferation state, and to achieve this goal, T cells and tumor cells evolve through the same pathway. It also highlights the fact that if inhibitors of tumor cell metabolism were very efficient, they would also alter T cells.

12.4.2 The CD28/PI3K/Akt/mTOR Pathway

Glycolysis is not the only mechanism to be boosted following activation. Its alternative, the pentose phosphate pathway (PPP), that can replenish nicotinamide adenine dinucleotide phosphate-oxidase (NADPH) and pentoses cell stocks, is also increased with a peak of activity 48 h after stimulation, when protein and RNA synthesis is maximal (Sagone et al. 1974). The regulation of glucose uptake in activated T cells is very close to the one controlled by insulin. In many cell types, the binding of insulin on its receptor is followed by the activation of phosphorus triiodide (PI3)-kinase that will generate phosphatidylinositol 3,4,5-trisphosphate (PIP3). It will then recruit Akt (protein kinase B (PKB)) which will be activated by phosphoinositide-dependent kinase-1 (PDK1) leading to the expression of multiple genes involved in glucose uptake and metabolism like glucose transporter type 4 (Glut4) (Cong et al. 1997). Concerning T cells, the only change is that insulin and its receptor are substituted by TCR and CD28 (Parry et al. 1997). CD28 is an essential pathway leading to Akt phosphorylation and subsequent pathway activation. Antigen recognition as well as costimulatory signals is required to induce the metabolic switch from a "resting" to a "proliferation-fitted" metabolism. It is also interesting to know that CTLA4, a receptor that downregulates activation of immune cells, disrupts the CD28 signal on glycolysis and glucose uptake (Frauwirth et al. 2002). This clearly suggests that naïve and memory T cells, expressing different levels of CD28 and CTLA-4 may display different capacity to switch on the metabolic changes necessary for the corresponding function.

12.4.3 Lipid Metabolism in T Cells

Glucose metabolism is not the only one affected by immune activation. Lipid metabolism is crucial for T cell immunity as all the costimulatory molecules must be localized in the membrane together around the TCR to form the immune synapse and ensure a proper stimulation. To achieve this, lipid rafts organization and production is very important (Janes et al. 1999, 2000). In T cells, as in any other cells, lipid rafts are membrane microdomains that contain various specific lipids and receptors, and their composition is different from the rest of the bilayer membrane. They are composed of glycosphingolipids, such as sphingosine or sphingomyelin, and cholesterol in higher concentration than the surrounding membrane (Jin et al. 2008). This rigid structure, where certain receptors will be preferentially localized, "floats" freely into the membrane and can be recruited to the immunological synapse. Sphingolipids and cholesterol metabolisms are very complex and tightly regulated. Shortly, sphingolipids are synthesized by serine palmytolyl-transferase from serine and palmitolyl-CoA. It forms a ceramide that will be converted in sphingosine by a ceramidase or a sphingomyelin by the addition of a phosphorylcholine residue by a sphingomyelin synthase. Concerning cholesterol, the whole process contains 37 different steps. It is produced mainly in the liver but also in many others places like the intestine, adrenal glands, or reproductive organs. It begins with acetyl CoA and acetoacetyl CoA that will be reduced in 3-hydroxy-3-methylglutaryl CoA (HMG-CoA). Then, HMG-CoA reductase will transform it in mevalonate. This last step is the target of anticholesterol drugs like statins, which compete with the substrate. Then a cascade of several steps will occur to form lanosterol in the endoplasmic reticulum, and 19 other steps will convert it in cholesterol. The production of lipids is very demanding energetically.

12.4.4 Common Pathways Leading to the Nutrients/Growth Factor Hypothesis

A common pathway regulating cholesterol, glucose, and also fatty acid homeostasis is the nuclear receptors pathway, involving the liver X receptor (LXR) and peroxisome proliferator-activated receptor gamma (PPAR-γ). These transcription factors of the nuclear receptor family regulate sterol metabolism

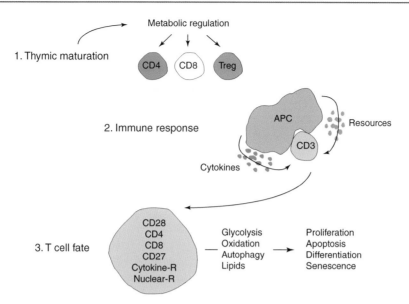

Fig. 12.1 The metabolic life of T cells. After release from the bone marrow, T cell will undergo selection/maturation in the thymus (*1*). There, a series of metabolic events will drive T cells toward the helper (CD4), cytotoxic (CD8), or Treg lineage. Once released in the circulation, T cells (CD3) display different metabolic rates due to differential metabolic pathways used (glycolysis or lipid oxidation). During the immune response APC will activate T cells by direct contact (including the CD28-B7 and CD27-CD70 axes) as well as with cytokines and provision of nutrient necessary to activate/regulate T cell metabolism (*2*). Depending on their profile (expression of coreceptors, Th/Tc lineage), T cells will utilize different metabolic pathways leading to their activation (*3*). The type, intensity, and duration of activation are dependent and regulated by these metabolic pathways and dictate the fate of T cells

during T cell activation (Pearce 2010). PPAR-γ was shown to inhibit Th17 differentiation (Klotz et al. 2009). Another study showed the regulation of the fatty acid oxidation is linked to memory in CD8⁺ T cells suggesting that availability/limitation in growth factors during the primary response may necessitate a metabolic switch (Pearce et al. 2009). Dendritic cells have a role to play in this phenomenon as amino acids and indoleamine 2,3-dioxygenase (IDO) levels are regulated by these cells in parallel to antigen presentation (Mellor and Munn 2004). The type and level of nutrient available for T cells will determine the differentiation and activation (Fig. 12.1). Studies showed that blocking the mammalian target of rapamycin (mTOR) pathway which modulates nutrient uptake and glucose metabolism is inhibiting proliferation (Delgoffe et al. 2009). Proteins are recycled in amino acids by catabolism driven by the endo- and exo-proteases and then used to fuel the Krebs cycle by amino acid catabolism or directly by tRNA to form new proteins. In activated T cells, another mechanism occurs, the macroautophagy (Hubbard et al. 2010). This mechanism is a form of

autophagy that degrades cytosolic proteins and whole organelles to furnish materials to lysosomes. It helps to maintain cellular homeostasis and ensure a sufficient energy production during the intense proliferation steps. Basically, cells would sacrifice a function to maintain others. The availability of growth factors was shown to influence autophagy (Lum et al. 2005). Basically, during resources shortage cells will eliminate unnecessary cellular component. This links extracellular nutriment-dependent metabolism, autophagy, and T cell activation (Pua et al. 2009). As a whole, the metabolic activation should been seen as the most important parameter indicating functionality of the cell rather than individuals functions.

12.4.5 Metabolism in T Cell Subsets

Because the metabolic pathways seem to be dependent on signalling pathways that are differently regulated in T cell subsets, it is very likely that during T cell differentiation steps, the cell adapts its metabolic rate (Gerriets and Rathmell 2012). While naïve and anergic cells utilize poorly glucose, the effector and autoreactive cells consume large amount of glucose for their functions.

After activation, T cells differentiate into Th1, Th2, Treg, and effector T cells and will die by apoptosis or remain as memory T cells (Fig. 12.1). Although the duration, intensity, and type of activation the cells will undergo are highly influenced by the receptors expressed by T cells, by the availability of nutrients, and by a variety of cytokines present in the milieu, the metabolic pathways involved in the numerous T cell subsets can be categorize in two. Cells needing a slow metabolism such as Tregs and memory CD8$^+$ cells will utilize lipid oxidation, while cells with higher metabolic such as memory CD4$^+$ T cells rate will utilize the glycolytic pathway. T cells that fail to upregulate glycolysis following activation may tend to differentiate into Treg based on mTOR$^{-/-}$ knockout mice which effector cells differentiation was aborted toward a Treg profile (Delgoffe et al. 2009). The difference in CD4$^+$ and CD8$^+$ memory T cell metabolism is striking and may be linked to differential coreceptor or cytokine expression. We hypothesize that the fact CD8$^+$ T cells lose CD28 expression while CD4$^+$ T cells lose CD27 expression following repeated proliferation stages may account for the metabolic difference.

12.5   Immunosenescence

Aging is a process that alters most functions, organs, and tissues of a human body. It is often considered, wrongly, as a disease because of the large number of diseases/conditions associated with aging. The human body can adapt itself to some features of aging, for example, by adjusting respiratory functions with heart capacities, but the muscle fibers and bone density loss, thymic involution, the blood vessels rigidity, the thickness of skin, and other phenomena cannot be reversed/adjusted and may contribute to morbidity and mortality. At the cellular level, there are also changes that may lead to dysfunctions. When this erosion concerns T cells, it is termed immunosenescence. The causes for immunosenescence are not yet well understood but

several theories rose and may be all partially true. The first one is the telomere shortening (Hayflick and Moorhead 1961). Telomeres are long sequences of noncoding DNA protecting genome during division. After each cycle, they are shorter until they reach a critical length where cell stop to divide and enter the senescence state. The decreased activity of telomerase is responsible for non-replacement of telomeres, and models have shown that modifying its activity can extend lifespan. Another theory claims the accumulation throughout life of mutations that modify or alter cellular functions or even induce the DNA repair system that can stop cell cycle (Edney and Gill 1968). Two other hypothesis can be reunified, the low calorie diet (caloric restriction or CR) and the free radicals theory (Schulz et al. 2007). Researcher noticed that CR could significantly extend animal models' lifespan and could also explain the prevalence of very elderly people in region of the world like Japan and Crete. The other is the free radicals theory (Harman 1981). With age, the damages induced by free radicals can lead to an arrest in cell cycle to repair damaged DNA and thus induce senescence. These two hypotheses are linked as metabolism is the main producer of free radicals and this metabolic rate is higher in people having a very rich diet. While free radicals are necessary, the excess may prove difficult to be well controlled and may lead to adverse effects.

As any other physiological process, the immune system also undergoes a so-called immunosenescence and that can be the cause of several dysfunctions with aging (Miller 1996). With aging/time, each immune cell subset undergoes changes, at the phenotypical and functional levels. The persistent stimulation of the T cells may lead to their exhaustion or their senescence. It is of note that senescent cells are considered senescent because of loss of proliferative capacities but retain the ability to produce cytokines and their cytotoxic activity. For this reasons, the senescent cells are often considered as the major source of proinflammatory cytokines associated with aging. This senescence-associated secretory phenotype is however less well understood, but future studies will be of great interest to understand to which extent senescence can go (can cells lose their polyfunctionality?) and why the secretory phenotype is initiated.

The unbalance in anti- vs. proinflammatory molecules secreted in aging will slowly provoke a loss of control on inflammation leading to inflamm-aging, which is a subclinical condition, and to proinflammatory conditions such as autoimmune diseases (e.g., rheumatoid arthritis or RA), liver/kidney/thyroid failure, and diabetes, and make the immune system less efficient against pathogens. This generalized inflammation may also be one of the causes for conditions affecting the autonomy of elderly individuals such as dementia and frailty. Frailty consists in a general and massive loss of function such as mobility, muscle strength (or sarcopenia), joint flexibility, and a fast unintentional weight loss. One component of this syndrome could be autoimmune disease, targeting, for example, muscle/bone stem cells, induced by the deregulation of the immune system. Moreover, in the bone marrow, HSCs show a decreased self-renewal ability that impair the generation of new immune cells and increase the ratio of memory cells (with higher cytotoxic/inflammatory capacities which participate to increased damages). As memory cells are in majority specific of persistent viruses like herpesviruses, it decreases the ability to respond against new pathogens or tumor cells. Other cells such as macrophage (ability to phagocyte bacteria), NK cells (impaired cytotoxicity) and B cells (reduced production and affinity of antibodies) loose functionality, suggesting that immunosenescence is not restricted to T cells. The following section will focus on the fate of T cells and how aging influences their metabolism and, thus, the immune response.

12.6 Evolution of Metabolic Pathway Linked to T Cell Functions

12.6.1 Metabol-aging: A Complex Phenomenon

During a normal healthy aging, the immune system undergo various changes that will alter its functionalities, and T cells are not an exception. As said before, HSCs number decrease in the bone marrow, leading to a diminished production of T cells precursors and thus, less naïve cells will be generated

(Chambers et al. 2007). Moreover, the thymic involution is also linked to this T cells production defect (Aspinall and Andrew 2000). After puberty, due to the lack of sex hormones, the mean weight of a human thymus is 35 g and reaches 5 g at the age of 70. As it shrinks, the educational role of the thymus can become quite impaired in advanced age, inducing troubles in T cells selection that could give rise to autoreactive/impaired lymphocytes. To date, the orphan nuclear receptor estrogen-related (ERR)-α is a promising target to modulate T cell functions as it was shown to highly influence the capacity of T cells to proliferate, induce cytokines, and differentiate (Michalek et al. 2011). Following activation, T cells upregulate ERR-α, and this impacts on the expression of genes related to glycolysis (Glut1) and metabolism in general but not linked to lipid pathways (Fig. 12.1). Even if it is not happening to T cells, the changes in dendritic cells modify the adaptive response. Early studies showed that the number of dendritic cells (DC) was decreased in tissues like corneal epithelium and skin and this suggests that the metabolic activation of T cells will be altered due to the control of nutrient availability by dendritic cells (Gilchrest et al. 1982; Thiers et al. 1984). Chakravarti et al. showed that IL-2 production was altered in elderly DC (Chakravarti and Abraham 1999), and Uyemura et al. showed that induction of Th1 cytokines was impaired, while induction of Th2 was increased, particularly IL-6 and IL-10 (Castle et al. 1997). These changes can drastically modify the immune response against a pathogen by inducing an inadequate cytokine production. This also suggests that the intrinsic metabolic regulatory role of dendritic cells may be impaired in aging. The metabolic dysregulation of T cells may readily start via APC. This highlights the complexity of studying metabolism with aging and especially in a complex system such as immunity.

12.6.2 Surface Receptors

Costimulatory molecule expression is impaired during aging especially those of CD28, the ligand for CD80 on APC. One study on centenarians showed that the decline occurs more markedly in CD8 subset and accounts largely for the decline of

T cells induction by mitogens and may be an adaptation to face the chronic stimulation and inflammation occurring in elderly (Boucher et al. 1998). Another study showed that upon activation, CD25 (IL-2Ra), CD95 (Fas), and CD28 increased, and then CD25 and CD28 start to decrease rapidly as division occurred in aged cultures on CD4 cells, whereas CD8 were already low in CD28 but constant. At the metabolic level, the loss of CD28 expression will reduce the ability to initiate the glycolytic pathway. The PI3K/Akt/mTOR activation level will be certainly different in the naïve vs. memory T cell subsets and this raises the question of the role of metabolism in the definition of senescence (Fig. 12.1). Senescent T cells are defined by loss of proliferative capacity (replicative senescence) but these cells retain a high level of functionality such as cytotoxicity and cytokine production and are more polyfunctional than naïve cells in that sense. The loss of CD28 induced by several proliferative events and associated loss of telomeres leading to arrest in proliferative capacity can also be considered as a programmed event, and it is tempting to identify this as a programmed proliferation arrest via the regulation of metabolic pathways associated with T cell activation. The importance of loss of other costimulatory molecules such as CD27 is not well understood. One study showed that late-differentiated T cells that lack CD28 but retain CD27 expression were still able to upregulate Akt^{ser473} phosphorylation (Plunkett et al. 2007). Only after the loss of CD27, the T cells were unable to upregulate CD27 and this was associated with telomerase activity shutdown. All together this suggests that although the Akt pathway has been exclusively associated with CD28, it is very likely that alternative mechanisms exist to compensate the loss of certain receptor to keep functionality. This may also be true for metabolic pathways and for other surface receptors including those inducing negative signalling such as KLRG-1, PD-1, and CD57.

12.6.3 Signalling and Membrane Components

The main T cell-specific pathway, the TCR signalization, is also impaired in the elderly. First, it has been demonstrated in mice, rats, and human that the IL-2 secretion following TCR ligation is decreased (Whisler et al. 1998). As it is a crucial cytokine for inducing and maintaining adaptive immunity, it launches the clonal proliferation step and induces the secretion of various cytokines; the immune response is impaired since its very beginning. As explained earlier, lipid metabolism is very important for TCR signalization, especially for lipid raft organization and functioning (Janes et al. 2000). During aging, the plasma membrane becomes more rigid and thus less fluid, so lipid raft cannot float freely inside (Zs-Nagy et al. 1986). This could impair the formation of TCR- and immune protein-containing lipid rafts and delay or cancel response induction (Silvius 2003). Several proteins known to be associated with lipid rafts in the TCR pathway, like linker for activation of T cells (LAT) or protein kinase C (PKC), were poorly recruited in the forming immune synapse following TCR ligation in cells from aged people (Marmor and Julius 2001). This can also impact IL-2 secretion. As cholesterol level is often increased in elderly, some studies measure the quantity of cholesterol in plasma membrane of aged people T cells. Not surprisingly, the levels were higher than in young people and this could explain the rigidity and the resulting difficulties to form a proper immune synapse (Incardona and Eaton 2000). With all these defects, the second step, the phosphorylation of ITAM and recruitment of zeta-chain-associated protein kinase 70 (ZAP-70), should also be impaired, and thus, lipid rafts could explain the decreased levels of tyrosine-phosphorylated proteins observed in elderly people (Janes et al. 1999; Fulop 1994). MAPK, a major player in TCR pathway, is also modified in aging. Its phosphorylation is one of the IL-2 production limiting steps and appears to be reduced in 50 % of elderly (Whisler et al. 1996). NFκB, another major transcription factor in immunity and also IL-2 production in T cells, is impaired during aging (Pahlavani et al. 1998). Usually, this factor is sequestrated in the cytoplasm by IkB and then released and migrate to the nucleus when it receives the adequate signals (free radicals, cytokines). It will then induce numerous genes to modulate the immune response. It is a very central and crucial transcription factor.

When IkB releases NFκB it will be phosphorylated, ubiquitinated, and then degraded in the proteasome, and so NFκB can translocate to the nucleus. But, during aging and maybe due to free radicals troubles, this degradation is impaired and thus NFκB activation decreases. The defects in TCR signalling with aging cannot be dissociated from the metabolic pathways. As described previously, cell activation will be different in the various subsets of T cells. The TCR signal transduction defects identified in elderly individuals have not been really studied in T cell subsets. It is becoming evident that dysfunctions observed in the total T cell population may actually just reflect the shift in naïve vs. memory ratio or the CD4/CD8 ratio. Because memory CD4[+] and CD8[+] T cells use different bioenergetic sources, as naïve and memory cell do, an unbalance of resource bioavailability, metabolic rate, and intrinsic (in)capacity of cells to use available resources may affect T cell ability to be activated. Whether the altered TCR signalling is a cause or a consequence of different metabolic rates is unknown. Further studies will be required to dissect these phenomena. Additionally, the use of lipid oxidation or glycolysis following activation may lead to alteration in lipid metabolism or required additional resources to concomitantly perform lipid oxidation as energetic resources and adjust lipid metabolism to cover the needs in terms of lipid production and regulation. As the majority of cholesterol resides in the membrane, it is tempting to suggest that T cell lipid raft composition and functioning (polarization) will be altered following activation due to the different metabolic pathways. We have shown that membrane rafts in CD8[+] T cells are clearly functioning differently from those of CD4[+] T cells (Larbi et al. 2006). We also have tested the possibility that changing the lipid composition in blood would directly influence T cell functions. After 2 h of intravenous infusion of a polyunsaturated fatty acids (PUFA) emulsion, T cell membrane fluidity was altered; membrane rafts were disorganized altogether leading to a reduced proliferative capacity and altered capacity for cholesterol exchange with the extracellular milieu (Larbi et al. 2005).

12.6.4 Infectious Diseases and T Cell Metabolism

One theory to explain immune defects with aging is that persistent infections are inducing exhaustion and senescence of T cells. The most studied model is cytomegalovirus (CMV). CMV is asymptomatic in healthy individuals but the virus is not cleared by the immune system and tends to reactive during physiological/metabolic weakness episodes. The persistent activation of the immune system by the virus leads to the expansion of CMV-specific T cells (CD8[+] but also CD4[+]). We have discussed above the difference in resting/activated CD4[+] and CD8[+] memory T cell metabolic pathways. Probably the most relevant study on this topic has been performed by Wherry et al. and has shown significant metabolic differences in response to latent infection. In senescent T cells, there was a significant metabolic deficiency (Wherry et al. 2007). First, several ribosome subunits were downregulated in exhausted CD8[+] T cells, while this was not the case for other memory cells compared to naïve cells. A genome-wide analysis identified several metabolic changes during CD8[+] T cell exhaustion. The genes related to metabolism identified to be different in exhausted cells are downregulated Entpd1, Car2, Gpd2, Clic4, Art3, Rrm2, Cpsf2, and Ndufa 5 or upregulated Acs2l, Impdh2, Adh5, Sdha, Atp6v0b, Adcy7, Pdha1, Mat2a, Dntt, Kctd10, Kcnn4, Hba-a1, Abce1, Acadm, Hmgcs1, Hexa, Hbb-b1, Tmc6, Prps1, and Cmah. This confirms findings from others studies suggesting that the senescence process may be programmed and driven by a metabolic adaptation. The role of persistent infections or chronic stimulation of the immune system should be seriously considered as a driving force leading to alterations of metabolic pathways in antigen-specific T cells and possibly as a bystander effect to all T cells.

12.6.5 Age-Associated Diseases Requiring Further Interest for Metabolic Changes

As showed previously, even healthy aging comes with immunological impairments. But the situation is far worse in people undergoing an "unhealthy" aging, i.e., an aging coupled with one or several age-related diseases like Alzheimer's disease (AD), RA, diabetes, or osteoporosis. Autoimmune diseases can be induced by the thymic involution. As presented before, as it shrinks, it will lower its capacity to educate naïve T cells. So, it may allow autoreactive T cells with high affinity for self to enter the blood circulation by lack of control or maybe to compensate the low number of normal naïve T cells with medium or low affinity for their foreign antigen. In RA, the disease is supposed to be induced by abnormal B-T cells interactions. Autoreactive B cells will release autoantibodies targeting joints that Fc receptor on T cells will recognize. As the HLA-DR4 allele family has been linked to RA, the TCR pathway is also involved in the pathology (Majithia and Geraci 2007). The continuous inflammation will destroy the joints capsule and cartilage leading to permanent disability. RA does trigger not only joints but also the lungs, kidney, heart, blood vessels, and skin. This disease can be one of the causes of the constant "IL-6 inflammation" observed in elder people. The metabolic pathways leading to hyperactivation can be a source for therapy. However, at first, future work is needed to identify the pathways involved and putative targets.

In osteoporosis, a condition that weakens bone structure and causes most of the hip fractures occurring in the elderly, inflammation may also play an important role as T cells are able to influence osteoclastogenesis by secreting various cytokines like IL-1, IL-6, IFN-γ, or IL-4 (Mirosavljevic et al. 2003). TNF-α production by T cell in bone marrow has also been shown to increase bone loss in "menopaused" mice (Cenci et al. 2000). Th-17 cells may have an important role also as IL-17 was demonstrated to be supporting osteoclastogenesis (Sato et al. 2006). Moreover IL-17 cells express higher levels of receptor activator of nuclear factor kappa-B ligand (RANKL) than Th1 or Th2. RANKL belongs to the TNF family and bind to osteoprotegerin, which is a decoy receptor sequestrating RANKL, to prevent generation of new osteoclasts (Sato et al. 2006). IFN-γ and IL-4 secreted by Th1 or Th2 cells are also anti-osteoclastogenesis and promote bone loss. Under normal condition, T cells can secrete osteoclastogenic cytokines such as TNF-α or RANKL; under inflammatory conditions, they can switch to an "anti-osteoclastogenic" state by secreting IL-1, IL-6, IL-17, or osteoprotegerin and even block the formation of osteoclasts by secreting IL-4, IL-10, IL-13, or IFN-γ (Wyzga et al. 2004). It is very important in elderly and frail people as the mortality rate coming from surgery can reach 10 % and, after 50, 25 % die in the year following the fracture of infections or blood clot conditions (e.g., PTE and DVT). A better understanding of the regulation of the RANK/RANKL/osteoprotegerin pathway by cytokines will certainly lead to the identification of target to modulate inflammatory-dependent bone degradation. The fact Th17 express high levels of RANK-L may indicate a metabolic regulation of this pathway.

Type 2 diabetes is a pathology occurring usually late in life, or sooner depending on your alimentation, which also has an immunological component. It affects more than 350 million people worldwide and this number will grow exponentially in the next decades. It is due to an insufficient number and renewal of β-cells in the pancreas and often coupled with insulin resistance (especially in muscles, in the liver, and in adipose tissue). Inflammation may have a role in the pathogenesis of insulin resistance component, as mice lacking JNK-1 signalling never develop it (Belgardt et al. 2010). Concerning β-cells, a study on obese mice showed that they can develop necrosis and insulin desensitization (Winer et al. 2011). Insulin results in lipolysis in adipose cells and consequently release of their content in the blood stream which may cause an inflammation mediated by B and T cells. Autoantibodies are then produced and recognized by T cells, and then the autoimmune component is set up. The inflammation occurring in adipose tissues, i.e., everywhere in an obese body, causes cells to become insulin resistant and by an unknown mechanism promote hypertension, hypertriglyceridemia, and atherosclerosis. After administration of anti-CD20 antibodies, obese mice didn't develop metabolic syndrome. It seems that it influences B cells functions and thus prevents the onset of inflammation with its consequences on metabolism. The link between obesity, diabetes, and inflammation may be metabolism and explains why it is often associated with metabolic syndrome. The functionality of B cells has not been investigated with a metabolic perspective, although they also undergo intense proliferative sequences upon activation.

Finally, another feature of aging is the increase of cholesterol levels. As explained before, this can alter dramatically the immune response by modifying the fluidness of plasma membrane and thus prevent the circulation of immune protein carrying lipid rafts. Cholesterol is transported by various molecules known as low-/high-density lipoproteins (LDL and HDL). These two molecules have an impact on immunity and inflammation, notably in atherosclerosis. HDL has been shown as anti-inflammatory (Barter et al. 2004), contrarily to LDL (Sun et al. 2009). Moreover, the adiponectin, a very important hormone in lipid metabolism, has its level correlated to body mass index (BMI) and plays a role in inflammation (Palmer et al. 2008). It is secreted only in adipose tissue and plays a role in the suppression of metabolic troubles that may result in type 2 diabetes,,obesity, or atherosclerosis. Adiponectin in combination with leptin has been shown to completely reverse insulin resistance in mice. Levels of adiponectin are reduced in diabetics compared to nondiabetics, and losing weight reduction significantly increases its circulating levels. In hepatitis C patients, obese people don't respond to therapy usually and it could be due to the decreased levels of adiponectin. A study showed that losing weight increased adiponectin that will bind to its receptor on T cells and increase hepatitis C-specific IFN-γ secretion using p38MAK. The understanding of the relationship and separated mechanisms of metabolic regulations at the organism level vs. at the T cell level will enable to identify whether specific metabolic pathways can be used for immunomodulation. This also suggests that it could be useful to lower the level of activated T cells specific for chronically infecting pathogens and thus the global inflammation in elderly people.

12.7   Animal Models: What Have We Learned from Them?

Studying such a complex process like aging requires adequate tools. That is why scientist developed several animal strains of mice that mimic human aging with its associated diseases and metabolic dysfunctions. For example, Lang et al. developed an aged mouse that is latently infected by herpes simplex virus (HSV)-1 (Lang and Nikolich-Zugich 2005). They inoculated viruses to young mice, observed a rapid increase of HSV-1 specific T cells then a decrease with around 2 % of memory T cells. Sixteen months later, they remarked an increase in HSV-1-specific central memory T cells that could be even more important than the one appearing during acute infection, and this population never contracted, even when they injected antiviral drug. Their phenotype was close to the one of spontaneously appearing T cell clones with high levels of IL-17R and IL-15R. The fact that there was no sign of acute infection showed that this accumulation was not the result of a continuous antigens presence but rather a homeostatic issue (Lang et al. 2008). Woodland et al. found that T clones, specific from Sendai virus cleared during youth, can expand during aging without any new contact with the pathogen (Ely et al. 2007). Based on these results, Lang et al. reproduced the same thing in mice with West Nile virus and found the same results (Lang et al. 2008). Taken together, these studies are very important as they suggest that all one's immune history can influence how healthy one will be later in life. Using murine CMV (MCMV), Reddehase et al. and Klenerman et al. showed that an expansion of MCMV-specific memory T cells occurring as soon as 3 months after the primo-infection produced more cells than during the first contact with the virus (Holtappels et al. 2000; Karrer et al. 2003). These animal models for infectious diseases are of great relevance to understand the impact of persistent vs. acute immune stimulation on the metabolic regulation of the immune system. It is also of interest to understand if repetitive stimulation with the same antigen leads to metabolic senescence.

Several mouse models are also used, among them, the first mammalian mutant found to have an increased average (+50 %) and maximal (+40 %) lifespan was the dwarf mouse (Bartke and Brown-Borg 2004). These mice have a recessive mutation on *Prop1* reducing production of thyrotropin, growth hormone (GH), prolactin, and gonadotropin and resulting in a pituitary hypoplasia presentation. Ames dwarf mice presenting interesting features during aging including deficiency in thyroid-stimulating hormone (TSH), insulin-like growth factor 1 (IGF-1), and GH are derived from this strain (Bartke and Brown-Borg 2004). They develop delayed aging-related renal pathology, immunosenescence, memory, learning, and locomotion problems, and also they have reduced collagen cross-link and tumor development. Snell dwarf mice also present the same phenotype, with a *Pit1* mutation resulting in a reduced GH and prolactin production (Bartke and Brown-Borg 2004). Their fibroblasts are stress resistant (ultraviolet or UV, heat, free radicals, H_2O_2, and cadmium), and senescence in their immune/joint/connective tissues is slower. Another model is the Laron mouse (Zhou et al. 1997). They are deficient in GH receptors, produce few IGF1, have low insulin and glucose levels in plasma, and present a 37 % increase in mean and a 55 % increase in maximal lifespan. Interestingly, these mice are also slightly immunodeficient. The first candidate for extending lifespan was telomerase. So mice, which carry mutations inhibiting or increasing telomerase activity, have been produced. They showed that in complex animals, the enzyme was not sufficient to really increase lifespan, but when it is absent, aging occurs in very young ages and lifespan is very short. Finally, another way to study aging in mice (or other model) is to change their nutrition intake as it has been shown that decreasing caloric intake extend lifespan by 30 % in some species (Kaeberlein et al. 2005). Other models such as the senescence-accelerated

mice (SAM) or the naked mole rats are exceptional model to study premature aging or longevity, respectively (Takeda 2009; Lewis et al. 2012). Understanding the genetic compound leading to alteration in metabolic changes at the organism level is of major interest to link genes, longevity, and metabolism.

Mice are not the only available models. Yeasts, such as *Saccharomyces cerevisiae*, are also a valuable model due to its short lifespan and the fact that it shares common genetic and cellular process with human. CR also increases its lifespan so genetic studies have been performed. They found some yeast genes that delay aging in dividing and or resting yeasts, and they were involved in oxidative stress response (Kaeberlein et al. 2007). *Caenorhabditis elegans* with its 20-day lifespan is also a very good model. Lots of studies have been performed using this model to make it live longer and even immortalized its germ line by stopping the aging process (Smelick and Ahmed 2005). Among the genetic controls studied are a series of interacting proteins that act like insulin and control reproduction and longevity. Investigators have also looked at a mechanism controlled by a group of genes called clock genes. These regulate metabolism in the roundworm and affect lifespan (Lakowski and Hekimi 1996). The roundworm genes seem to confer increased longevity by supporting resistance to external stresses, such as bacterial infections, high temperatures, radiation, and oxidative damage. Some research in roundworms has focused on the gene that regulates the activity of COQ7, a particular type of protein that plays a crucial role in electron transport within mitochondria that produce energy (Nakai et al. 2004). Investigators have discovered that mutations that diminish COQ7 lead to a modest increase in lifespan. These mutations have a bigger effect when combined with other mutations, such as those in the insulin pathway mentioned above, and influence resistance to oxidative damage. Finally, some researchers rendered the germ line of the nematode immortal by reprogramming the epigenetic memory. In *Drosophila melanogaster*, researchers showed that the Methuselah protein was able to increase flies lifespan by 30 % (Lin et al. 1998) and that silencing Sun, a factor that binds Methuselah, increased the lifespan by 50 % (Cvejic et al. 2004). Various mutations in a gene called Indy (I'm Not Dead Yet) can double lifespan without any side effect (Neretti et al. 2009). These models are useful models to identify the role of targeted pathways. However, discrepancies exist in the functionality of immune system in these models compared to humans. Thus, the data from these models should be taken with care.

Conclusions

Aging is a very complex phenomenon influence by environmental, nutritional, behavior, cognitive, genetic, immunological, and metabolic factors. For this reason it may prove difficult to find a unique solution to reverse aging or to prevent age-associated conditions. It has been shown that reversing the aging of stem cells was possible (Lapasset et al. 2011). With an adequate cocktail of gene modifications (OCT4, SOX2, KLF4, c-MYC, NANOG, and LIN28), stem cells extracted from 90-year-old people rejuvenate and lose aging characteristics. It could be a formidable breakthrough in the fight against time as it unlocks the possibility of replacing old organs by young ones. Although this seems promising and validates some theories about life extension (de Grey 2003), new organs will still have to live in an "old" environment. Also, how will the body react in presence of young organs and cells? Will it cause an imbalance between physiological processes? This is still unknown. Rather than replacing old organs, will it be more valuable to keep the environment younger? Adjusting the metabolism and inflammation is feasible and may reduce the stress cells have to cope with. At the immunological level, with the described metabolic difference between immune cells, the rejuvenation of the immune system using HSC can be envisioned, if these metabolic differences are taken into account. The regulation of T cell response during stress, acute infection, and persistent infections and in memory is highly dependent on metabolism.

References

Adkins B, Mueller C, Okada CY et al (1987) Early events in T-cell maturation. Annu Rev Immunol 5:325–365

Andersen MH, Schrama D, Thor Straten P et al (2006) Cytotoxic T cells. J Invest Dermatol 126(1):32–41

Aspinall R, Andrew D (2000) Thymic involution in aging. J Clin Immunol 20(4):250–256

Barry M, Bleackley RC (2002) Cytotoxic T lymphocytes: all roads lead to death. Nat Rev Immunol 2(6): 401–409

Barter PJ, Nicholls S, Rye KA et al (2004) Antiinflammatory properties of HDL. Circ Res 95(8): 764–772

Bartke A, Brown-Borg H (2004) Life extension in the dwarf mouse. Curr Top Dev Biol 63:189–225

Belgardt BF, Mauer J, Bruning JC (2010) Novel roles for JNK1 in metabolism. Aging (Albany NY) 2(9): 621–626

Bird L (2009) T-cell development: thymocytes run the 'gauntlet'. Nat Rev Immunol 9(1):2–2

Bots M, Medema JP (2006) Granzymes at a glance. J Cell Sci 119(Pt 24):5011–5014

Boucher N, Dufeu-Duchesne T, Vicaut E et al (1998) CD28 expression in T cell aging and human longevity. Exp Gerontol 33(3):267–282

Bradley LM, Haynes L, Swain SL (2005) IL-7: maintaining T-cell memory and achieving homeostasis. Trends Immunol 26(3):172–176

Buttgereit F, Burmester GR, Brand MD (2000) Bioenergetics of immune functions: fundamental and therapeutic aspects. Immunol Today 21(4):192–199

Castle S, Uyemura K, Wong W et al (1997) Evidence of enhanced type 2 immune response and impaired upregulation of a type 1 response in frail elderly nursing home residents. Mech Ageing Dev 94(1–3):7–16

Cenci S, Weitzmann MN, Roggia C et al (2000) Estrogen deficiency induces bone loss by enhancing T-cell production of TNF-alpha. J Clin Invest 106(10): 1229–1237

Chakravarti B, Abraham GN (1999) Aging and T-cell-mediated immunity. Mech Ageing Dev 108(3): 183–206

Chambers SM, Shaw CA, Gatza C et al (2007) Aging hematopoietic stem cells decline in function and exhibit epigenetic dysregulation. PLoS Biol 5(8):e201

Cong LN, Chen H, Li Y et al (1997) Physiological role of Akt in insulin-stimulated translocation of GLUT4 in transfected rat adipose cells. Mol Endocrinol 11(13): 1881–1890

Cvejic S, Zhu Z, Felice SJ et al (2004) The endogenous ligand Stunted of the GPCR Methuselah extends lifespan in Drosophila. Nat Cell Biol 6(6):540–546

de Grey AD (2003) The foreseeability of real anti-aging medicine: focusing the debate. Exp Gerontol 38(9): 927–934

Delgoffe GM, Kole TP, Zheng Y et al (2009) The mTOR kinase differentially regulates effector and regulatory T cell lineage commitment. Immunity 30(6):832–844

Dempsey PW, Vaidya SA, Cheng G (2003) The art of war: innate and adaptive immune responses. Cell Mol Life Sci 60(12):2604–2621

Dong C (2008) TH17 cells in development: an updated view of their molecular identity and genetic programming. Nat Rev Immunol 8(5):337–348

Edney EB, Gill RW (1968) Evolution of senescence and specific longevity. Nature 220(5164):281–282

Ely KH, Ahmed M, Kohlmeier JE et al (2007) Antigen-specific CD8+ T cell clonal expansions develop from memory T cell pools established by acute respiratory virus infections. J Immunol 179(6):3535–3542

Fink TM, Zimmer M, Weitz S et al (1992) Human perforin (PRF1) maps to 10q22, a region that is syntenic with mouse chromosome 10. Genomics 13(4): 1300–1302

Frauwirth KA, Thompson CB (2004) Regulation of T lymphocyte metabolism. J Immunol 172(8): 4661–4665

Frauwirth KA, Riley JL, Harris MH et al (2002) The CD28 signaling pathway regulates glucose metabolism. Immunity 16(6):769–777

Fulop T Jr (1994) Signal transduction changes in granulocytes and lymphocytes with ageing. Immunol Lett 40(3):259–268

Geginat J, Lanzavecchia A, Sallusto F (2003) Proliferation and differentiation potential of human CD8+ memory T-cell subsets in response to antigen or homeostatic cytokines. Blood 101(11):4260–4266

Gerriets VA, Rathmell JC (2012) Metabolic pathways in T cell fate and function. Trends Immunol 33(4): 168–173

Gilchrest BA, Murphy GF, Soter NA (1982) Effect of chronologic aging and ultraviolet irradiation on Langerhans cells in human epidermis. J Invest Dermatol 79(2):85–88

Harman D (1981) The aging process. Proc Natl Acad Sci U S A 78(11):7124–7128

Harrington LE, Hatton RD, Mangan PR et al (2005) Interleukin 17-producing CD4+ effector T cells develop via a lineage distinct from the T helper type 1 and 2 lineages. Nat Immunol 6(11):1123–1132

Hayflick L, Moorhead PS (1961) The serial cultivation of human diploid cell strains. Exp Cell Res 25:585–621

Hirsch JG (1959) Immunity to infectious diseases: review of some concepts of Metchnikoff. Bacteriol Rev 23(2): 48–60

Holtappels R, Pahl-Seibert MF, Thomas D et al (2000) Enrichment of immediate-early 1 (m123/pp 89) peptide-specific CD8 T cells in a pulmonary CD62L(lo) memory-effector cell pool during latent murine cytomegalovirus infection of the lungs. J Virol 74(24):11495–11503

Hubbard VM, Valdor R, Patel B et al (2010) Macroautophagy regulates energy metabolism during effector T cell activation. J Immunol 185(12): 7349–7357

Hume DA, Radik JL, Ferber E et al (1978) Aerobic glycolysis and lymphocyte transformation. Biochem J 174(3):703–709

Incardona JP, Eaton S (2000) Cholesterol in signal transduction. Curr Opin Cell Biol 12(2):193–203

Janes PW, Ley SC, Magee AI (1999) Aggregation of lipid rafts accompanies signaling via the T cell antigen receptor. J Cell Biol 147(2):447–461

Janes PW, Ley SC, Magee AI et al (2000) The role of lipid rafts in T cell antigen receptor (TCR) signalling. Semin Immunol 12(1):23–34

Jin ZX, Huang CR, Dong L et al (2008) Impaired TCR signaling through dysfunction of lipid rafts in sphingomyelin synthase 1 (SMS1)-knockdown T cells. Int Immunol 20(11):1427–1437

Kaeberlein M, Hu D, Kerr EO et al (2005) Increased life span due to calorie restriction in respiratory-deficient yeast. PLoS Genet 1(5):e69

Kaeberlein M, Burtner CR, Kennedy BK (2007) Recent developments in yeast aging. PLoS Genet 3(5):e84

Karrer U, Sierro S, Wagner M et al (2003) Memory inflation: continuous accumulation of antiviral CD8+ T cells over time. J Immunol 170(4):2022–2029

Klotz L, Burgdorf S, Dani I et al (2009) The nuclear receptor PPAR gamma selectively inhibits Th17 differentiation in a T cell-intrinsic fashion and suppresses CNS autoimmunity. J Exp Med 206(10):2079–2089

Koch U, Radtke F (2011) Mechanisms of T cell development and transformation. Annu Rev Cell Dev Biol 27:539–562

Laird DJ, De Tomaso AW, Cooper MD et al (2000) 50 million years of chordate evolution: seeking the origins of adaptive immunity. Proc Natl Acad Sci U S A 97(13):6924–6926

Lakowski B, Hekimi S (1996) Determination of life-span in Caenorhabditis elegans by four clock genes. Science 272(5264):1010–1013

Lang A, Nikolich-Zugich J (2005) Development and migration of protective CD8+ T cells into the nervous system following ocular herpes simplex virus-1 infection. J Immunol 174(5):2919–2925

Lang A, Brien JD, Messaoudi I et al (2008) Age-related dysregulation of CD8+ T cell memory specific for a persistent virus is independent of viral replication. J Immunol 180(7):4848–4857

Lapasset L, Milhavet O, Prieur A et al (2011) Rejuvenating senescent and centenarian human cells by reprogramming through the pluripotent state. Genes Dev 25(21):2248–2253

Larbi A, Grenier A, Frisch F et al (2005) Acute in vivo elevation of intravascular triacylglycerol lipolysis impairs peripheral T cell activation in humans. Am J Clin Nutr 82(5):949–956

Larbi A, Dupuis G, Khalil A et al (2006) Differential role of lipid rafts in the functions of CD4+ and CD8+ human T lymphocytes with aging. Cell Signal 18(7):1017–1030

Lewis KN, Mele J, Hornsby PJ et al (2012) Stress resistance in the naked mole-rat: the bare essentials - a mini-review. Gerontology 58(5):453–462

Lin YJ, Seroude L, Benzer S (1998) Extended life-span and stress resistance in the Drosophila mutant Methuselah. Science 282(5390):943–946

Lum JJ, Bauer DE, Kong M et al (2005) Growth factor regulation of autophagy and cell survival in the absence of apoptosis. Cell 120(2):237–248

Majithia V, Geraci SA (2007) Rheumatoid arthritis: diagnosis and management. Am J Med 120(11): 936–939

Malamut G, El Machhour R, Montcuquet N et al (2010) IL-15 triggers an antiapoptotic pathway in human intraepithelial lymphocytes that is a potential new target in celiac disease-associated inflammation and lymphomagenesis. J Clin Invest 120(6):2131–2143

Manel N, Unutmaz D, Littman DR (2008) The differentiation of human T(H)-17 cells requires transforming growth factor-beta and induction of the nuclear receptor RORgammat. Nat Immunol 9(6):641–649

Marmor MD, Julius M (2001) Role for lipid rafts in regulating interleukin-2 receptor signaling. Blood 98(5): 1489–1497

Mellor AL, Munn DH (2004) IDO expression by dendritic cells: tolerance and tryptophan catabolism. Nat Rev Immunol 4(10):762–774

Michalek RD, Gerriets VA, Nichols AG et al (2011) Estrogen-related receptor-alpha is a metabolic regulator of effector T-cell activation and differentiation. Proc Natl Acad Sci U S A 108(45):18348–18353

Miller RA (1996) The aging immune system: primer and prospectus. Science 273(5271):70–74

Mirosavljevic D, Quinn JM, Elliott J et al (2003) T-cells mediate an inhibitory effect of interleukin-4 on osteoclastogenesis. J Bone Miner Res 18(6):984–993

Nakai D, Shimizu T, Nojiri H et al (2004) coq7/clk-1 regulates mitochondrial respiration and the generation of reactive oxygen species via coenzyme Q. Aging Cell 3(5):273–281

Neretti N, Wang PY, Brodsky AS et al (2009) Long-lived Indy induces reduced mitochondrial reactive oxygen species production and oxidative damage. Proc Natl Acad Sci U S A 106(7):2277–2282

Pahlavani MA, Harris MD, Richardson A (1998) Activation of p21ras/MAPK signal transduction molecules decreases with age in mitogen-stimulated T cells from rats. Cell Immunol 185(1):39–48

Palmer C, Hampartzoumian T, Lloyd A et al (2008) A novel role for adiponectin in regulating the immune responses in chronic hepatitis C virus infection. Hepatology 48(2):374–384

Parry RV, Reif K, Smith G et al (1997) Ligation of the T cell co-stimulatory receptor CD28 activates the serine-threonine protein kinase protein kinase B. Eur J Immunol 27(10):2495–2501

Pearce EL (2010) Metabolism in T cell activation and differentiation. Curr Opin Immunol 22(3):314–320

Pearce EL, Walsh MC, Cejas PJ et al (2009) Enhancing CD8 T-cell memory by modulating fatty acid metabolism. Nature 460(7251):103–107

Plunkett FJ, Franzese O, Finney HM et al (2007) The loss of telomerase activity in highly differentiated CD8+CD28-CD27- T cells is associated with decreased Akt (Ser473) phosphorylation. J Immunol 178(12):7710–7719

Pua HH, Guo J, Komatsu M et al (2009) Autophagy is essential for mitochondrial clearance in mature T lymphocytes. J Immunol 182(7):4046–4055

Sagone AL Jr, LoBuglio AF, Balcerzak SP (1974) Alterations in hexose monophosphate shunt during lymphoblastic transformation. Cell Immunol 14(3): 443–452

Sakaguchi S, Ono M, Setoguchi R et al (2006) Foxp3+ CD25+ CD4+ natural regulatory T cells in dominant self-tolerance and autoimmune disease. Immunol Rev 212:8–27

Sallusto F, Langenkamp A, Geginat J et al (2000) Functional subsets of memory T cells identified by CCR7 expression. Curr Top Microbiol Immunol 251: 167–171

Santana MA, Esquivel-Guadarrama F (2006) Cell biology of T cell activation and differentiation. Int Rev Cytol 250:217–274

Sato K, Suematsu A, Okamoto K et al (2006) Th17 functions as an osteoclastogenic helper T cell subset that links T cell activation and bone destruction. J Exp Med 203(12):2673–2682

Schulz TJ, Zarse K, Voigt A et al (2007) Glucose restriction extends Caenorhabditis elegans life span by inducing mitochondrial respiration and increasing oxidative stress. Cell Metab 6(4):280–293

Schwarz BA, Bhandoola A (2006) Trafficking from the bone marrow to the thymus: a prerequisite for thymopoiesis. Immunol Rev 209:47–57

Silvius JR (2003) Role of cholesterol in lipid raft formation: lessons from lipid model systems. Biochim Biophys Acta 1610(2):174–183

Smelick C, Ahmed S (2005) Achieving immortality in the C. elegans germline. Ageing Res Rev 4(1):67–82

Stenger S, Hanson DA, Teitelbaum R et al (1998) An antimicrobial activity of cytolytic T cells mediated by granulysin. Science 282(5386):121–125

Sun L, Ishida T, Yasuda T et al (2009) RAGE mediates oxidized LDL-induced pro-inflammatory effects and atherosclerosis in non-diabetic LDL receptor-deficient mice. Cardiovasc Res 82(2):371–381

Takeda T (2009) Senescence-accelerated mouse (SAM) with special references to neurodegeneration models, SAMP8 and SAMP10 mice. Neurochem Res 34(4): 639–659

Thiers BH, Maize JC, Spicer SS et al (1984) The effect of aging and chronic sun exposure on human Langerhans cell populations. J Invest Dermatol 82(3): 223–226

Tschopp J, Masson D, Stanley KK (1986) Structural/functional similarity between proteins involved in complement- and cytotoxic T-lymphocyte-mediated cytolysis. Nature 322(6082):831–834

Warburg O (1956) On respiratory impairment in cancer cells. Science 124(3215):269–270

Wherry EJ, Ha SJ, Kaech SM et al (2007) Molecular signature of CD8+ T cell exhaustion during chronic viral infection. Immunity 27(4):670–684

Whisler RL, Newhouse YG, Bagenstose SE (1996) Age-related reductions in the activation of mitogen-activated protein kinases p44mapk/ERK1 and p42mapk/ERK2 in human T cells stimulated via ligation of the T cell receptor complex. Cell Immunol 168(2):201–210

Whisler RL, Karanfilov CI, Newhouse YG et al (1998) Phosphorylation and coupling of zeta-chains to activated T-cell receptor (TCR)/CD3 complexes from peripheral blood T-cells of elderly humans. Mech Ageing Dev 105(1–2):115–135

Winer DA, Winer S, Shen L et al (2011) B cells promote insulin resistance through modulation of T cells and production of pathogenic IgG antibodies. Nat Med 17(5):610–617

Wyzga N, Varghese S, Wikel S et al (2004) Effects of activated T cells on osteoclastogenesis depend on how they are activated. Bone 35(3):614–620

Zhou Y, Xu BC, Maheshwari HG et al (1997) A mammalian model for Laron syndrome produced by targeted disruption of the mouse growth hormone receptor/binding protein gene (the Laron mouse). Proc Natl Acad Sci U S A 94(24):13215–13220

Zs-Nagy I, Kitani K, Ohta M et al (1986) Age-dependent decrease of the lateral diffusion constant of proteins in the plasma membrane of hepatocytes as revealed by fluorescence recovery after photobleaching in tissue smears. Arch Gerontol Geriatr 5(2):131–146

Age-Related Alterations in Regulatory T Cells

13

Amir Hossein Massoud

13.1 Introduction

With recent advances in medical technology and better nutrition, the elderly population is increasing at an exceptional rate, especially in developed countries. Aging is associated with impairments in a variety of biological functions. Gradual deterioration of the immune system by aging, collectively termed immunosenescence, is considered a major contributory factor to the increased morbidity and mortality among the elderly. In humans, as well as many other species, it has been recognized that the immune system declines with age, which leads to higher incidence of infections, neoplasia, and autoimmune diseases (Pawelec 1999; Pawelec et al. 2006; Hakim et al. 2004). These dysfunctions arise from alterations in almost every component of the immune system. Aging affects different immune cell types, including hematopoietic stem cells (HSCs), lymphoid progenitors in the bone marrow and thymus, thymic stromal cells, mature lymphocytes in secondary lymphoid organs, and also elements of the innate immune system (Plackett et al. 2004; Ginaldi et al. 2004). Importantly, significant alterations are seen in the T lymphocyte compartment. CD4$^+$ T cells are key elements of the adaptive immune response. Age-related alterations are evident in all stages of T cell development, making them a significant element in immunosenescence (Linton et al. 2005).

After birth, the functional and numerical decline of different subpopulation of T cell begins with the progressive involution of the thymus, the organ responsible for T cell differentiation and development. This age-associated decrease of thymic size results in a reduction/exhaustion on the number of thymocytes (i.e., premature T cells), thus reducing output of peripheral T cells. Once matured and begun to circulate throughout the peripheral system, T cells still undergo deleterious age-related changes.

Recent work has found that T regulatory cells (Tregs), a subset of CD4$^+$ T cells with immunoregulatory activities, are also affected by aging (Chougnet et al. 2011; Chiu et al. 2007; Sharma et al. 2006). Discovered in 1990s (Sakaguchi et al. 1995), Tregs are a specialized subpopulation of T cells responsible for suppressing activation of undesirable immune responses and, thereby, maintaining immune system homeostasis and peripheral tolerance to self- and non-self-antigens (Tang and Bluestone 2008). Tregs exert their modulatory effects by suppressing the activation and function of both innate and adaptive immune cells, and therefore, the deficiency of Tregs is associated with a large spectrum of autoimmune and inflammatory conditions (Sakaguchi et al. 2010). Although the classification of Treg cells into separated lineages remains controversial, based on their developmental and functional

A.H. Massoud, PhD
Department of Microbiology and Immunology,
McGill University, Montreal, QC, Canada

Meakins-Christie Laboratories,
McGill University, Montreal, QC H2X-2P2, Canada
e-mail: massoudah_2002@yahoo.com

A. Massoud, N. Rezaei (eds.), *Immunology of Aging*,
DOI 10.1007/978-3-642-39495-9_13, © Springer-Verlag Berlin Heidelberg 2014

differences, Tregs can be categorized into two main subpopulations of naturally occurring (nTreg) and peripherally induced (iTreg) Tregs, generated in the thymus and peripheral lymphoid tissues, respectively. Both subpopulations express CD4, CD25, and the forkhead box protein 3 (FoxP3) (a transcription factor that acts as a master regulator of Tregs). The fundamental property defining Tregs is their ability to transfer immune unresponsiveness in vivo from one animal to another syngeneic one or in vitro from one culture to another (Vigouroux et al. 2004).

The age-related alterations of Treg cells were described controversially, and whether such changes explain immune dysfunction in the elderly is still unclear. Recently, it has become clear that the number of Tregs significantly increases in aged mice and humans. As Treg controls the intensity of T cell responses, their increase probably contributes to age-related immune dysfunction. In addition to their role in peripheral tolerance, Tregs play critical roles in regulating excessive immune response to acute and persistent infections (viral, bacterial, parasitic, and fungal) (Vigouroux et al. 2004). Thus, increased number of Treg may contribute substantially to inefficient T cell responses in aging. This chapter focuses on mechanisms underlying Treg homeostasis and function in aging.

13.2 Evidence of Increased Frequency of Regulatory T Cells in Aged Hosts

It has become clear that the number of Tregs significantly increases by aging (Rosenkranz et al. 2007; Lages et al. 2008; Chiu et al. 2007). The age-related increase in the number of these cells might increase susceptibility to various infectious diseases and cancers in elderly, since Tregs control the intensity of immune responses (Provinciali and Smorlesi 2005; Plackett et al. 2004). Owing to limited access to human tissues, there is not enough data showing Treg numbers in various peripheral organs in elderly, though some reports supported the age-associated accumulation of Tregs in the skin (Agius et al. 2009).

Recent studies performed in different strains of mice showed a spontaneous and age-related increase in Treg cells in peripheral blood as well as lymphoid organs, but not in the thymus and other tissues (Zhao et al. 2007; Lages et al. 2008; Sharma et al. 2006). These data emphasize that Treg frequency in the blood does not accurately represent their accumulation in the tissues. The age-related alteration of different subsets of T cells, as well as alteration of other cellular and molecular factors that impact T cell development, might together contribute to the alteration of Treg cells.

13.2.1 The Nature of Regulatory T Cells in Aging

Given the significant decrease in thymic output of T cells in aging, it remains unclear whether the increased Tregs in the elderly is due to the expansion of nTregs or because of peripheral induction of iTregs or a combination of both. Persistence of iTregs in the blood correlated with long-term protection from autoimmune destruction, as iTregs mainly suppress immune responses in an antigen-specific manner, whereas expansion of nTregs might be associated to the suppression of immune responses in an antigen-independent manner.

Recently, it has been demonstrated that the majority of Tregs in aged mice express high levels of the transcription factor Helios (a specific marker of thymic-derived nTreg cells) (Thornton et al. 2010). Moreover, increased Tregs may be the result of nonspecific clonal expansion of nTreg populations due to chronic infection and exposure to superantigens that are more prevalent in the elderly due to dysfunction of the immune system. NTregs are less flexible than iTreg, ex vivo, and do not tend to lose the expression of Foxp3 (Hoffmann et al. 2009). Aged Tregs were shown that are less prone to convert to other subsets of T cells upon culturing ex vivo (Chougnet et al. 2011). Thus, considering these data, it is suggestive that aged Treg may be derived from nTreg, although further work is required to rule out a contribution of increased peripheral Treg conversion in aging.

It is postulated that the Treg cells in aging are mainly included within the group of traditionally regarded effector-memory T cells. Treg cells with memory phenotype disproportionately increased in peripheral lymphoid tissues in elderly (Chiu et al. 2007). In aged mice also the increased Tregs have been shown to highly express CD44 (a marker of effector-memory T cells) (Han et al. 2009). Thus, the ultimately differentiated population of Treg might have a superior functionality comparing to the young counterparts. Majority of studies on Tregs functional capabilities during aging support the notion that Treg cells functions remain intact or even associated with intensified suppressive capacity during aging (Simone et al. 2008; Provinciali and Smorlesi 2005). The age-associated enhancement of Tregs functions will be discussed in a later section.

13.2.2 Mechanism Behind Increasing of Treg Cells During Aging

A series of studies assessed the contributory mechanisms to the increased number of Tregs during aging. The main mechanism is attributed to the increased resistance of these cells to apoptosis. Tregs from aged mice exhibit increased expression of B-cell lymphoma 2 (Bcl-2) and myeloid leukemia cell differentiation protein-1 (Mcl-1), the two proteins associated with decreased cell apoptosis and may play a role in the development of cancer (Wojciechowski et al. 2007). Therefore, Tregs in aged mice show better survival comparing to those from young mice, while the in vivo proliferation rate of Tregs of aged and young mice is the same (Wojciechowski et al. 2007). Treg derived from aged mice also expresses decreased level of Bim (an apoptotic activator protein) which is likely counter-regulated by Bcl-2 (Kurtulus et al. 2011). Taken together, the regulation of pro- and anti-apoptotic molecules within aged Tregs enhances their survival rate and promotes their accumulation in various organs.

In addition, cytokines or cytokine receptors that are involved in the intra and extra-thymic Treg development and homeostasis, including interleukin (IL)-2 IL-7 IL-15 and their cognate receptors, have been reportedly shown to be altered in aging, in favor to a better Treg survival (Cheng et al. 2012; Burchill et al. 2007; Bayer et al. 2008). Aged Treg cells express increased levels of IL-7 receptor alpha (IL-7Rα) and IL-2Rβ and, therefore, are giving a better proliferative response in the presence of their cognate cytokines. Moreover, all of these cytokines trigger a signaling cascade through a common γ chain receptor, and aged Tregs exhibit higher expression of this receptor comparing to the young counterparts. This can lead to the conclusion that the age-related changes in cytokine and cytokine receptor profile might act as a contributing factor for a better Treg maintenance or proliferation in the elderly.

It appears that the mechanisms implicated in cell survival are independent among different subsets of T cells, e.g., Tregs and T cells during aging. Recent reports showed that despite the age-related increase in CD95 expression (Fas receptor, a death receptor on the surface of cells involved in apoptosis) on effector T cells, Tregs show a downregulation of this receptor (Todo-Bom et al. 2012), thus remaining unsusceptible to the cell death induced by Fas-Fas ligand (FasL) pathway. The upregulation of CD95 in effector T cells also has shown to implicate in T cell senescence and tumor progress in the elderly as well (Wang et al. 2010).

13.2.3 Suppressive Capacity of Tregs During Aging

So far, few studies have investigated the functionality of Tregs in aging. In vitro studies on the capacity of human Tregs purified from blood have reported increased or similar suppressive capacity of Tregs from aged subjects versus young subjects. CD4+ effector T cell function (IL-2 or interferon gamma (IFN-γ) production) was more suppressed by Tregs from elderly than young ones, although both of them suppress the proliferation of CD4+ T cells at the same degree (Vukmanovic-Stejic et al. 2006; Hwang et al. 2009; Trzonkowski et al. 2006). The analysis of Treg cells from elderly with Alzheimer and Parkinson disease also revealed that, in addition to the increased number of Tregs, their suppressive activity was also intensified (Rosenkranz et al. 2007).

Accordingly, purified Tregs from lymph nodes of aged mice, but not from blood, suppress the proliferation response of stimulated CD4⁺ effector T cells roughly three-fold better than Tregs from their young counterparts (Hoffmann et al. 2009). This suggests that aged Tregs, accumulated in peripheral organs, might behave differently than the ones in blood circulation.

The homing property of Tregs is another factor determining the capacity of Treg to be retained within sites of inflammation, and this factor correlates to their efficiency in the suppression of inflammations. The integrin CD103 may facilitate Treg homing to nonlymphoid tissues. Interestingly, the percentage of splenic CD103⁺ Tregs increases with age in mice (Lages et al. 2008). Consistently, CD103 expression on human Tregs increases by aging and disrupts effector T cell-mediated protection (Agius et al. 2009; Macdonald et al. 2011).

13.3 Age-Related Susceptibility to Inflammatory and Neoplastic Diseases in Correlation with Treg Elevation

Emerging evidence suggests that there is a relationship between aging, inflammation, and chronic diseases (Ahmad et al. 2009). The incidence of cancers seems to be increased with age. However, it is not clear whether aging leads to the induction of inflammatory processes thereby resulting in the development and maintenance of chronic diseases or whether inflammation is the causative factor for induction of both aging and chronic diseases such as cancer. Indeed development of cancer could also lead to the induction of inflammatory processes and may cause aging.

The protective or inflammatory roles of Tregs in cancer are paradoxical and are the subject of controversy. Treg cells seem to have some functions in reducing risk of inflammation-associated cancer. However, Tregs also function to suppress protective anticancer immune responses; therefore,

the accumulation of Tregs in the elderly might play an important role in tumor immune evasion by suppressing the immune system and enhancing tumor survival (Anisimov 2009; Franceschi and La Vecchia 2001).

In numerous murine tumor models, increased frequencies of CD4⁺CD25ʰⁱᵍʰ Treg cells seem to be a hallmark of tumor progression and metastasis (Tan et al. 2011; Kortylewski et al. 2009), and moreover, it has been shown that depletion of Treg cells restores antitumor T cell cytotoxic activity in aged animals and results in the generation of a protective memory response against tumors, thus decreases the subsequent inflammation (Sharma et al. 2006). In line with that, the aged mice were capable to reject tumor when treated with anti-OX40 monoclonal antibodies (a T cell costimulatory molecule, critically involved in the survival and proliferation of activated T cells and has been identified as a key negative regulator of Foxp3⁺Tregs) (Lustgarten et al. 2004; Hamilton 1991).

In addition, increased number and activity of Tregs in aged mice has been demonstrated to reduce dendritic cell (DCs) capability to prime effector T cells via downregulation of expression of costimulatory molecules on DCs (Williams-Bey et al. 2011; Zhao et al. 2007; Nishioka et al. 2006). Depletion of Tregs in aged mice can restore the capability of DCs to the level of young mice, thus conferring long-lasting immunity against tumors as well as neurodegeneration and infections (Chiu et al. 2007).

Much of what is now known about Tregs has been learned from CD4⁺Foxp3⁺ Tregs, but it is likely that the regulatory pathways are mediated by different lineages of Treg cells that might have unique mechanisms in regulating certain T cell-driven autoimmunity. Despite the widely accepted concept of increased frequency of CD4⁺CD25⁺Foxp3⁺ Treg cells in the elderly, age-related deficiencies in specific subpopulations of Tregs that are responsible to restrain certain subsets of auto-reactive T cells during chronic inflammation have been observed. For instance although human Tregs are as competent as their young counterparts in regulating T helper (Th)-1-mediated autoimmunity, they are defective to restrain Th-17 activation; thus, the elderly might be more susceptible to develop

Th-17-mediated chronic inflammation (Sun et al. 2012). Th-17 cells are mediators of certain autoimmune diseases and promote pathologic inflammation in a number of inflammatory conditions. In line with this, recently, an unconventional subset of CD8$^+$CD45RA$^+$CCR7$^+$Foxp3$^+$Treg cells has been identified that are defective in elderly with chronic inflammatory conditions (Suzuki et al. 2012). Hence, characterizing different population of Treg cells is essential to enhance our knowledge in understanding the alteration of regulating pathways throughout different stages of life (Kapp 2008).

In accordance with this, age-related reduction of other mediators involved in the peripheral tolerance might explain certain immune dysregulation. A reduction of inhibitory cytokines by aging has been reported which might increase the susceptibility to certain inflammatory disorders in the elderly. Production of transforming growth factor beta (TGF-β) and IL-10, two inhibitory cytokines implicated in regulatory pathways in small intestine, reduces by aging although the source of these cytokines remained to be determined (Santiago et al. 2011).

13.4 Concluding Remarks

Aging affects many components of the immune system. In particular alteration in regulatory pathways in the elderly is becoming a challenge in clinical settings. Therefore, further in-depth research is critical for designing effective health care for the elderly.

Increased immune-mediated chronic diseases and the associated inflammation during aging, appear, at least in part, owing to the alterations in immunoregulatory pathways. Increased Treg proportion by aging, as the main component of the peripheral tolerance, probably contributes to age-related immunosuppression, explaining age-associated higher risk to diseases such as cancers, infections, and other chronic inflammatory disorders. In this regard, some questions remained unanswered: what maintains elevated numbers of Treg in aged hosts? Can partial Treg depletion be employed in order to enhance vaccine or antitumoral responses and/or elimination of chronic infections?

Moreover our current knowledge in treating the immune-mediated diseases of young hosts cannot be readily generalized to the elderly, due to differences between elders and young immune systems. Therefore, improving our understanding of the aged immune system is crucial for developing effective prevention and treatment programs which will facilitate healthy aging and improve the quality of life of the elderly population.

References

Agius E, Lacy KE, Vukmanovic-Stejic M et al (2009) Decreased TNF-alpha synthesis by macrophages restricts cutaneous immunosurveillance by memory CD4+ T cells during aging. J Exp Med 206(9):1929–1940

Ahmad A, Banerjee S, Wang Z et al (2009) Aging and inflammation: etiological culprits of cancer. Curr Aging Sci 2(3):174–186

Anisimov VN (2009) Carcinogenesis and aging 20 years after: escaping horizon. Mech Ageing Dev 130(1–2):105–121

Bayer AL, Lee JY, de la Barrera A et al (2008) A function for IL-7R for CD4+CD25+Foxp3+ T regulatory cells. J Immunol 181(1):225–234

Burchill MA, Yang J, Vogtenhuber C et al (2007) IL-2 receptor beta-dependent STAT5 activation is required for the development of Foxp3+ regulatory T cells. J Immunol 178(1):280–290

Cheng G, Yuan X, Tsai MS et al (2012) IL-2 receptor signaling is essential for the development of Klrg1+ terminally differentiated T regulatory cells. J Immunol 189(4):1780–1791

Chiu BC, Stolberg VR, Zhang H et al (2007) Increased Foxp3(+) Treg cell activity reduces dendritic cell co-stimulatory molecule expression in aged mice. Mech Ageing Dev 128(11–12):618–627

Chougnet CA, Tripathi P, Lages CS et al (2011) A major role for Bim in regulatory T cell homeostasis. J Immunol 186(1):156–163

Ginaldi L, De Martinis M, Monti D et al (2004) The immune system in the elderly: activation-induced and damage-induced apoptosis. Immunol Res 30(1):81–94

Hakim FT, Flomerfelt FA, Boyiadzis M et al (2004) Aging, immunity and cancer. Curr Opin Immunol 16(2):151–156

Hamilton A (1991) Trauma training. Nurs Times 87(2):42–44

Han GM, Zhao B, Jeyaseelan S et al (2009) Age-associated parallel increase of Foxp3(+)CD4(+) regulatory and CD44(+)CD4(+) memory T cells in SJL/J mice. Cell Immunol 258(2):188–196

Hoffmann P, Boeld TJ, Eder R et al (2009) Loss of FOXP3 expression in natural human CD4+CD25+ regulatory T cells upon repetitive in vitro stimulation. Eur J Immunol 39(4):1088–1097

Hwang KA, Kim HR, Kang I (2009) Aging and human CD4(+) regulatory T cells. Mech Ageing Dev 130(8): 509–517

Kapp JA (2008) Special regulatory T-cell review: suppressors regulated but unsuppressed. Immunology 123(1): 28–32

Kortylewski M, Xin H, Kujawski M et al (2009) Regulation of the IL-23 and IL-12 balance by Stat3 signaling in the tumor microenvironment. Cancer Cell 15(2):114–123

Kurtulus S, Tripathi P, Moreno-Fernandez ME et al (2011) Bcl-2 allows effector and memory CD8+ T cells to tolerate higher expression of Bim. J Immunol 186(10):5729–5737

La Franceschi S, Vecchia C (2001) Cancer epidemiology in the elderly. Crit Rev Oncol Hematol 39(3):219–226

Lages CS, Suffia I, Velilla PA et al (2008) Functional regulatory T cells accumulate in aged hosts and promote chronic infectious disease reactivation. J Immunol 181(3): 1835–1848

Linton PJ, Li SP, Zhang Y et al (2005) Intrinsic versus environmental influences on T-cell responses in aging. Immunol Rev 205:207–219

Lustgarten J, Dominguez AL, Thoman M (2004) Aged mice develop protective antitumor immune responses with appropriate costimulation. J Immunol 173(7):4510–4515

Macdonald JB, Dueck AC, Gray RJ et al (2011) Malignant melanoma in the elderly: different regional disease and poorer prognosis. J Cancer 2:538–543

Nishioka T, Shimizu J, Iida R et al (2006) CD4+CD25+Foxp3+ T cells and CD4+CD25-Foxp3+ T cells in aged mice. J Immunol 176(11):6586–6593

Pawelec G (1999) Immunosenescence: impact in the young as well as the old? Mech Ageing Dev 108(1):1–7

Pawelec G, Koch S, Franceschi C et al (2006) Human immunosenescence: does it have an infectious component? Ann N Y Acad Sci 1067:56–65

Plackett TP, Boehmer ED, Faunce DE et al (2004) Aging and innate immune cells. J Leukoc Biol 76(2):291–299

Provinciali M, Smorlesi A (2005) Immunoprevention and immunotherapy of cancer in ageing. Cancer Immunol Immunother 54(2):93–106

Rosenkranz D, Weyer S, Tolosa E et al (2007) Higher frequency of regulatory T cells in the elderly and increased suppressive activity in neurodegeneration. J Neuroimmunol 188(1–2):117–127

Sakaguchi S, Sakaguchi N, Asano M et al (1995) Immunologic self-tolerance maintained by activated T cells expressing IL-2 receptor alpha-chains (CD25). Breakdown of a single mechanism of self-tolerance causes various autoimmune diseases. J Immunol 155(3):1151–1164

Sakaguchi S, Miyara M, Costantino CM et al (2010) FOXP3+ regulatory T cells in the human immune system. Nat Rev Immunol 10(7):490–500

Santiago AF, Alves AC, Oliveira RP et al (2011) Aging correlates with reduction in regulatory-type cytokines and T cells in the gut mucosa. Immunobiology 216(10):1085–1093

Sharma S, Dominguez AL, Lustgarten J (2006) High accumulation of T regulatory cells prevents the activation of immune responses in aged animals. J Immunol 177(12):8348–8355

Simone R, Zicca A, Saverino D (2008) The frequency of regulatory CD3+CD8+CD28–CD25+ T lymphocytes in human peripheral blood increases with age. J Leukoc Biol 84(6):1454–1461

Sun L, Hurez VJ, Thibodeaux SR et al (2012) Aged regulatory T cells protect from autoimmune inflammation despite reduced STAT3 activation and decreased constraint of IL-17 producing T cells. Aging Cell 11(3): 509–519

Suzuki M, Jagger AL, Konya C et al (2012) CD8+CD45RA+CCR7+FOXP3+ T cells with immunosuppressive properties: a novel subset of inducible human regulatory T cells. J Immunol 189(5):2118–2130

Tan W, Zhang W, Strasner A et al (2011) Tumour-infiltrating regulatory T cells stimulate mammary cancer metastasis through RANKL-RANK signalling. Nature 470(7335):548–553

Tang Q, Bluestone JA (2008) The Foxp3+ regulatory T cell: a jack of all trades, master of regulation. Nat Immunol 9(3):239–244

Thornton AM, Korty PE, Tran DQ et al (2010) Expression of Helios, an Ikaros transcription factor family member, differentiates thymic-derived from peripherally induced Foxp3+ T regulatory cells. J Immunol 184(7):3433–3441

Todo-Bom A, Mota-Pinto A, Alves V et al (2012) Aging and asthma – changes in CD45RA, CD29 and CD95 T cells subsets. Allergol Immunopathol (Madr) 40(1):14–19

Trzonkowski P, Szmit E, Mysliwska J et al (2006) CD4 + CD25+ T regulatory cells inhibit cytotoxic activity of CTL and NK cells in humans-impact of immunosenescence. Clin Immunol 119(3):307–316

Vigouroux S, Yvon E, Biagi E et al (2004) Antigen-induced regulatory T cells. Blood 104(1):26–33

Vukmanovic-Stejic M, Zhang Y, Cook JE et al (2006) Human CD4+ CD25hi Foxp3+ regulatory T cells are derived by rapid turnover of memory populations in vivo. J Clin Invest 116(9):2423–2433

Wang L, Pan XD, Xie Y et al (2010) Altered CD28 and CD95 mRNA expression in peripheral blood mononuclear cells from elderly patients with primary non-small cell lung cancer. Chin Med J (Engl) 123(1):51–56

Williams-Bey Y, Jiang J, Murasko DM (2011) Expansion of regulatory T cells in aged mice following influenza infection. Mech Ageing Dev 132(4):163–170

Wojciechowski S, Tripathi P, Bourdeau T et al (2007) Bim/Bcl-2 balance is critical for maintaining naive and memory T cell homeostasis. J Exp Med 204(7): 1665–1675

Zhao L, Sun L, Wang H et al (2007) Changes of CD4+CD25+Foxp3+ regulatory T cells in aged Balb/c mice. J Leukoc Biol 81(6):1386–1394

Effects of Aging on B Cells

14

Mohammad Hossein Nicknam
and Alireza Rezaiemanesh

14.1 Introduction

A major age-related health problem is the increasing frequency and severity of infectious diseases. Aging influences the immune system, and as a result, elderly individuals are more susceptible to infections, which are the fourth most common cause of death in the elderly. In addition, immune response to vaccines and infectious agents declines with age. Global understanding is still incomplete but is thought that with aging thymus gland shrinks, and this is one of the major factors resulting in the impaired immune function (Heron and Smith 2007; Weinberger et al. 2008).

14.2 Aging and B Cell Development and Differentiation

Now, it is well established that B lymphopoiesis and consequently humoral immune response decline in elderly individuals. Age-related changes in B cell commitment and development include a decline in the frequency of precursors.

M.H. Nicknam, MD, PhD (✉)
Department of Immunology,
Molecular Immunology Research Center,
Tehran University of Medical Sciences, Tehran, Iran
e-mail: nicknam_m@yahoo.com

A. Rezaiemanesh, MSc
Department of Immunology,
Tehran University of Medical Sciences, Tehran, Iran

Recent studies showed a remarkable decline in pre-B cell numbers in aged mice without decrease in the number of mature B cells (Linton and Dorshkind 2004; Johnson et al. 2002; Miller and Cancro 2007).

Identification of factors responsible for suboptimal humoral immune response is a rapidly evolving field of research. Because by recognizing these factors as biological markers, the capability of humoral immune response can be assessed not only in elderly but also in immunocompromised individuals.

It is known that the capability of hematopoietic stem cells' (HSCs) replication decreases with increasing age (Geiger and Van 2002). Production of blood cells is a result of the balance between self-renewal HSCs and production of daughter cells. Several studies have shown the proliferation in lymphoid progeny is impaired in aged mice comparing to young mice (Sudo et al. 2000). Therefore, there is a decrease in the number of common lymphoid progenitors (CLPs) which in turn influence T and B cell immune responses (Linton and Dorshkind 2004).

Miller and Allman study on aged C57BL/6 mice showed that reduction of B lymphopoiesis in these mice is due to a loss of B-lineage precursor pools. Also, their studies revealed that the response of all B cell lineage progenitors become suboptimal by aging (Miller and Allman 2003).

A growing body of literature has provided evidence that the number or proliferation of pre-B cells in bone marrow decreases with aging. However, the number of pro-B cells in old mice is

A. Massoud, N. Rezaei (eds.), *Immunology of Aging*,
DOI 10.1007/978-3-642-39495-9_14, © Springer-Verlag Berlin Heidelberg 2014

similar to young ones suggesting that probably the transition of pro-B cell to pre-B cells in old mice bone marrow is impaired (Szabo et al. 2003).

Based on Szabo et al. studies, it can be proposed that age-associated perturbations exist in recombination of V to DJ gene segment in transition stage of pro-B cell to pre-B cells (Szabo et al. 2003). These perturbations occur as a result of alteration in transcription factors such as E47, E2A-encoded E12 (Frasca et al. 2003). These transcription factors bind to the enhancer region in immunoglobulin (Ig) heavy chain gene. It has been shown that E2A family members have an effect on expression of surrogate light chain. Age-associated changes in these factors reduce surface expression of V-pre-B and $\lambda 5$ in old mice (Sherwood et al. 2000).

Despite the reduction in pre-B cell compartment, the number of B cells in bone marrow is more than expected which can be justified by considering increased life span of immature B cell and reduced B cell entrance to circulation from bone marrow (Johnson et al. 2002).

Also, different studies have shown that the response of pro-B cell to interleukin (IL)-7, as a pre-B cell stimulator in the microenvironment of bone marrow, is impaired. It was shown that the level of IL-7 receptor α and common γ chains on the surface of pro-B cell in old mice is normal compared to young mice. Therefore, this impairment in responding to IL-7 is related to IL-7 signaling pathway (Linton and Dorshkind 2004). Also Tsuboi et al. study revealed that IL-7 mRNA expression level decreases with aging (Tsuboi et al. 2004).

Krishnamurthy et al. introduced InK4A/Arf expression as a marker of aging. InK4A/Arf locus encodes P16 [INK4a] and Arf as tumor suppressor molecules. Also, they showed that the expression of cell cycle inhibitors in all stages of B cells particularly in pro-B cells and pre-B cells increases with aging (Krishnamurthy et al. 2004).

Shahaf et al. concluded three important phenomena regarding B cell development in old mice by mathematical modeling: a decrease in the maximum number of cells in pre-B cell compartment, an increase in the rate of transition from cycling pre-B cells to resting pre-B cells, and an increase

in the fractions of static cells included in the immature B cell subset (Shahaf et al. 2006).

Linton and Dorshkind showed that aging has an effect on impairment of peripheral B cells. For instance, the duration of humoral response in old individuals is shorter than young individuals, and the affinity and titer of produced antibodies is less leading to the poor ability to mount protective humoral response (Linton and Dorshkind 2004).

There is no change in the total number of B cells in old mice. However, the number of naïve B cells decreases, and on the other hand, the population of antigen-experienced cells increases. These changes occur due to increased B cell longevity and reduction in production of B cells in bone marrow.

Mehr et al. study, with a focus on modifying factors of affinity maturation in aging, showed that selection of Ig genes is variable depending on the tissue (Mehr and Melamed 2011). Most of the B cells in these individuals produce more IgM despite isotype switching. It is understood that in recombination process, B cells in old individuals have a different V region genes from young individuals. Perhaps, these impairments in B cell functions are related to reduction in expression of costimulatory molecules such as CD86, impairment in B cell signaling, age-related changes in CD4[+] T cells, or aged microenvironment (Linton and Dorshkind 2004).

With aging, the quality and quantity of humoral immune response along with somatic hypermutation (SHM) and class switch recombination (CSR) decrease. It has been understood that the number and the size of germinal center (GC) in old mice decrease comparing to young mice. In fact, these defects in GC are because of deficiency in T cells and follicular dendritic cells (FDCs) and also self-deficiency in B cells. On the other hand, by producing the long-lived plasma cells in bone marrow, as a result of defects in GC structures, the number of these cells decreases in the bone marrow (Frasca and Blomberg 2009; Linton and Dorshkind 2004).

Considering this fact that GC is a central place for SHM and CSR process, these defects in GCs lead to impairment in antibody affinity maturation and decrease in number of plasma cells in the bone marrow. Also it is known that transcription factor E47 is important for transcriptional regulation AICDA (gene encoding for activation-induced cytidine deaminase or AID). AID has a vital role in SHM and CSR required for production of Igs from different isotypes. Different studies have been shown that CSR is impaired in follicular naïve splenic B cells. It can be explained by a decrease in E47 and consequently AID with aging.

The rate of stability of E47 mRNA has an inverse relationship with the level of phosphorylated tristetraprolin (TTP) which is the product of P38 mitogen-activated protein kinase (MAPK) signaling pathway. In fact, TTP binding to E47 mRNA 3′-untranslated region (3′-UTR) leads to a decrease in its stability and in the quantity of AID. It has been understood that TTP level in old mice is higher than young mice (Frasca and Blomberg 2009).

Telomere length also plays an important role in B cell senescence. It has been revealed that the length of telomere in lymphocytes diminishes with aging. The rate of telomere shortening for B cells is 15–19 bp/year, but this range is higher in some B cell subtypes such as naïve B cells (29 bp/year) and memory B cells (40 bp/year) (Weng 2008).

References

Frasca D, Blomberg BB (2009) Effects of aging on B cell function. Curr Opin Immunol 21(4):425–430

Frasca D, Nguyen D, Riley RL et al (2003) Decreased E12 and/or E47 transcription factor activity in the bone marrow as well as in the spleen of aged mice. J Immunol 170(2):719–726

Geiger H, Van Zant G (2002) The aging of lympho-hematopoietic stem cells. Nat Immunol 3(4):329–333

Heron MP, Smith BL (2007) Deaths: leading causes for 2003. Natl Vital Stat Rep 55(10):1–92

Johnson KM, Owen K, Witte PL (2002) Aging and developmental transitions in the B cell lineage. Int Immunol 14(11):1313–1323

Krishnamurthy J, Torrice C, Ramsey MR et al (2004) Ink4a/Arf expression is a biomarker of aging. J Clin Invest 114(9):1299–1307

Linton PJ, Dorshkind K (2004) Age-related changes in lymphocyte development and function. Nat Immunol 5(2):133–139

Mehr R, Melamed D (2011) Reversing B cell aging. Aging (Albany NY) 3(4):438–443

Miller JP, Allman D (2003) The decline in B lymphopoiesis in aged mice reflects loss of very early B-lineage precursors. J Immunol 171(5):2326–2330

Miller JP, Cancro MP (2007) B cells and aging: balancing the homeostatic equation. Exp Gerontol 42(5):396–399

Shahaf G, Johnson K, Mehr R (2006) B cell development in aging mice: lessons from mathematical modeling. Int Immunol 18(1):31–39

Sherwood EM, Xu W, King AM et al (2000) The reduced expression of surrogate light chains in B cell precursors from senescent BALB/c mice is associated with decreased E2A proteins. Mech Ageing Dev 118(1–2):45–59

Sudo K, Ema H, Morita Y et al (2000) Age-associated characteristics of murine hematopoietic stem cells. J Exp Med 192(9):1273–1280

Szabo P, Shen S, Telford W et al (2003) Impaired rearrangement of IgH V to DJ segments in bone marrow Pro-B cells from old mice. Cell Immunol 222(1):78–87

Tsuboi I, Morimoto K, Hirabayashi Y et al (2004) Senescent B lymphopoiesis is balanced in suppressive homeostasis: decrease in interleukin-7 and transforming growth factor-beta levels in stromal cells of senescence-accelerated mice. Exp Biol Med (Maywood) 229(6):494–502

Weinberger B, Herndler-Brandstetter D, Schwanninger A et al (2008) Biology of immune responses to vaccines in elderly persons. Clin Infect Dis 46(7):1078–1084

Weng NP (2008) Telomere and adaptive immunity. Mech Ageing Dev 129(1–2):60–66

The Role of MicroRNAs in Immunosenescence Process

15

Seyed Hossein Aalaei-andabili, Alireza Zare-Bidoki, and Nima Rezaei

15.1 Introduction

Human aging is a very complex process with profound changes in gene expression and bimolecular pathway actions (Spazzafumo et al. 2011; Cevenini et al. 2010). Aging is recognized to be affected via many environmental factors. Genetic factors play important roles in aging process. It is found that genetic pathways which determine lifespan act in a fashion conserved across species from yeast to humans (Friedman and Johnson 1988). In cell stage, aging affects the organism totally. The aged cells accumulate in senescing tissues and organs and lead to age-associated disorders (Baker et al. 2011). One of the most important senescent-induced abnormalities is immune system function dysregulation which names immunosenescence (Jiang et al. 2012; Frasca et al. 2008). Immunosenescence is characterized by degradation of immune system maturation, function, and responsiveness (Jiang et al. 2012; Van Duin et al. 2007).

Recently, it has been recognized that proteins and genes involved in aging process are precisely regulated by various MicroRNAs (MiRs) (Bhaumik et al. 2009). MiRs have been understood as pathway regulator in biological processes such as immune system component development and activation (O'Neill et al. 2011). MiRs are small, noncoding RNAs, 19–24 nucleotides in length, which are known as post transcriptional regulator of gene expression, targeting the 3′ untranslated region (3′ UTR) of target mRNAs to prevent protein production by translation inhibition or inducing degradation of mRNA via RNases (Liu 2008). MiRs have vital regulatory roles in development of hematopoietic lineage, maturation and differentiation of B and T lymphocytes (Rodriguez et al. 2007), proliferation of neutrophils and monocytes (Johnnidis et al. 2008), secretion of type 1 interferon (IFN) and proinflammatory cytokines/chemokine (Tili et al. 2007), and effectiveness of immune system response (Bartel 2004). These emerging evidences indicate to MiRs importance in immune system function controlling and immunosenescence regulation.

S.H. Aalaei-andabili, MD
Research Center for Immunodeficiencies,
Children's Medical Center, Tehran University of
Medical Sciences, Tehran, Iran

A. Zare-Bidoki, MSc
Department of Immunology, School of Medicine,
Tehran University of Medical Sciences,
Tehran, Iran

N. Rezaei, MD, MSc, PhD (✉)
Molecular Immunology Research Center,
Tehran University of Medical Sciences,
Tehran 14194, Iran

Department of Immunology, School of Medicine,
Tehran University of Medical Sciences,
Tehran, Iran

Research Center for Immunodeficiencies,
Children's Medical Center,
Tehran, Iran
e-mail: rezaei_nima@tums.ac.ir

A. Massoud, N. Rezaei (eds.), *Immunology of Aging*,
DOI 10.1007/978-3-642-39495-9_15, © Springer-Verlag Berlin Heidelberg 2014

15.2 MiR-146a Response to Lipopolysaccharide Stimulation Is Restricted in Macrophages of Aged Mice

Aging leads to inflammatory environment via persistent upregulation of nuclear factor kappa-light-chain-enhancer of activated B cells (NFκB) that promoted cytokines such as interleukin (IL)-6, IL-1β, and tumor necrosis factor alpha (TNF-α). This situation occurs in response to internal environment of aged bodies, without presence of any disease, and is known as "inflammaging" (Franceschi et al. 2000). It is found that MiR-146a level is highly (sixfold) upregulated in macrophages of aged mice comparing to young mice in the absence of stimulation. In contrast, MiR-146a expression increases significantly to more than 12-fold in macrophages of young mice secondary to lipopolysaccharide (LPS) stimulation, whereas the level of MiR-146a remains unchanged in macrophages of old mice. The same difference in mature MiR-146a expression between young and aged subjects was also seen in premature MiR-146a expression, indicating that aberrant expression of the MiR comes from its impaired regulation in transcriptional level (Jiang et al. 2012). At least two binding sites of NFκB (sites I and II) have been found to be necessary for induction of MiR-146a by LPS stimulation (Taganov et al. 2006). Reason of lower response of macrophages to LPS stimulation in aged subjects was found in lower ability of NFκB binding to MiR-146a promoter sites, whereas NFκB binding to both binding sites of MiR-146a promoter in young mouse significantly increases in response to LPS. Although MiR-146a expression changes not significantly in response to LSP in macrophages of aged subjects (Jiang et al. 2012), MiR-146a of macrophages of aged mice negatively regulates proinflammatory cytokine (including IL-6 and IL-1β) secretion by targeting the interleukin-1 receptor-associated kinase 1 (IRAK1) level (Ceppi et al. 2009), in non-stimulated conditions in the same manner of macrophages of young mice (Jiang et al. 2012). IRAK1 and TNF receptor-associated factor 6 (TRAF-6) are important downstream components of Toll-like receptors (TLRs) and IL-1 signaling pathways.

The presence of IRAK1 and TRAF6 activity is required for proinflammatory marker production (Akira and Takeda 2004). However, in contrast to MiR-146a function in macrophages of young subjects, MiR-146a is less responsive to proinflammatory cytokines in aged macrophages and cannot extent its negative controlling roles in response to high level of inflammatory cytokines or LPS stimulation (Jiang et al. 2012).

15.3 DNA Methylation and Histone Acetylation Alter NFκB Binding Activity and, Consequently, MiR-146a Expression

Recently, it has been discovered that administration of DNA methyltransferase (DNMT) inhibitor 5-aza-2-deoxycytidine (5-Aza-CdR) and histone deacetylase (HDAC) inhibitor trichostatin A (TSA) might be effective strategies to manipulate expression of MiR-146a in macrophages of aged mice. It is suggested that hypermethylation of some genes in NFκB signaling in macrophages of aged subject is responsible for the reduction of NFκB activity and, consequently, decreased level of MiR-146a expression. 5-Aza-CdR is found to increase MiR-146a expression by unmethylation of the mentioned genes. Also, histone deacetylation is another way to inhibit NFκB subunits translocation to the MiR-146a promoter sites in macrophages of both young and aged mice; however, this effect is stronger among aged mice versus young. Thus, TSA can increase MiR-146a expression via augmentation of NFκB binding ability to the MiR-146a promoter sites in unstimulated macrophages (Jiang et al. 2012).

Almost all 11 members of HDAC have higher level of expression in macrophages of aged mouse comparing young mice. The reduction of these members in aged subjects occurs rapidly, but at the lowest point, levels of 4 members of HDAC component are still higher than their level at the same time in young mice. These facts show why reversal effect of TSA on MiR-146a expression in macrophages of aged subjects is stronger than that in young mice after LPS stimulation (Jiang et al. 2012). It seems that lower level of histone acetylation at the promoter site leads to drastic suppression of MiR-146a transcription, and consequently, impairment of MiR-146a upregulation and negative controlling of the LPS induced inflammation (Saccani et al. 2002).

15.4 MiR-146a Expression Varies Significantly Between Human Umbilical Vein Endothelial Cells of Aged and Young Individuals

MiR-146a is upregulated during the first 3 weeks of life in neonatal. MiR-146a is significantly more expressed in stimulated monocytes from cord blood comparing those isolated from adults (Chassin et al. 2010). MiR-146a is known as marker of senescence-associated proinflammatory condition in cells participated in vascular remodeling. Cytokine and oxidative stress marker release is significantly higher in aged individuals comparing younger human umbilical vein endothelial cells (HUVECs). MiR-146a is the most upregulated MiR in senescent HUVECs. Inversely, IRAK-1 is drastically inhibited in senescent versus young HUVECs; whereas, TRAF6 level, IL-6 release, and senescence-associated β-galactosidase (SA-β-gal) are not affected through MiR-146a modulation in HUVECs (Olivieri et al. 2012a).

15.5 IL-6 Is Stronger Promoter of MiR-146a/b Expression in Aged Fibroblasts

MiR-146a/b expression increases in response to aging in fibroblasts. It is reported that senescence can occur mainly by DNA damage (Bhaumik et al. 2009). Senescence-associated secretory phenotype (SASP) is known as senescent cell reaction to DNA damage through production of cytokines such as IL-6 and IL-8 which induce microenvironmental changes in aged cells (Rodier et al. 2009). MiR-146a/b level remains almost undetectable during the interval of DNA damage and SASP (Bhaumik et al. 2009), indicating that proinflammatory cytokines are stimulators of MiR-146a/b upregulation. IL-1 receptor signaling pathway has been considered as essential promoter of IL-6, IL-8, and MiR-146a/b. IL-1 contains two ligands

including IL-1α and IL-1β (Coppe et al. 2008). High level of membrane-bound IL-1α has been detected in aged cells. Proinflammatory cytokine secretion is suppressed upon administration of neutralizing antibodies against IL-1α, but not IL-1β. Thus, IL-1α level in senescent cells is a determinant factor in production of drastic levels of IL-1R signaling system. It seems that IL-6 is more important than IL-8 for MiR-146a/b promotion because MiR-146a/b level is undetectable in cells with slight increase in IL-6 level but high expression of IL-8. Initially, it was thought that MiR-146a/b downregulates IL-6 and IL-8 secretion by targeting the IRAK1 and TRAF6 which are important members of IL-1 and TLRs signaling pathways; however, it is recognized that expression of MiR-146a/b in senescent fibroblasts leads to targeting of IRAK1, whereas TRAF6 level remains unchanged (Bhaumik et al. 2009).

15.6 MiRs Regulate Neutrophil Senesce by Targeting Genes Involved in Neutrophil Apoptosis

Neutrophils are one of the polymorphonuclear (PMN) cells that contains majority of white blood cells. The cells are crucial member of human defense against bacterial and fungal infections. Neutrophils rush to the injured tissues and try to destroy the invasion by phagocytosis (Haslett 1999), secretion of proinflammatory cytokines such as IL-8, interferon gamma-induced protein 10 (IP-10) (Scapini et al. 2000), and leukotriene B4 (Lysgaard et al. 2012). Also, neutrophils attract other inflammation-associated cells to increase inflammatory response (Ford-Hutchinson et al. 1980). On the other hand, neutrophils cannot always act in this manner because their functions are limited by senescence process (Ward et al. 2011). Senescence occurs concomitantly with upregulation of chemokine (C-X-C motif) receptor 4 (CXCR4) in neutrophil surface (Martin et al. 2003), promoting neutrophil apoptosis in bone marrow. Also, neutrophils undergo apoptosis spontaneously (Lum et al. 2005). In addition, macrophages and other phagocytic cells remove senescent neutrophils to avoid undesirable inflammation and tissue or organ hurt (Kennedy and DeLeo 2009).

TNF-α and granulocyte-macrophage colony-stim-ulating factor (GM-CSF) are two inflammatory cytokines which increase neutrophils half-life, pre-venting their senescence by delaying in apoptosis process (Colotta et al. 1992). Apoptosis has been considered as a main marker of neutrophil senes-cence (Ward et al. 2011). It is found that translation of new proteins is necessary for neutrophil func-tion and viability. Blocking in each step of protein production may contribute in neutrophil apoptosis. Protein expressions in cells are precisely regulated by various types of MiRs (Whyte et al. 1997).

Most of the neutrophils express 146 MiRs out of the 851, and MiR-223 is the most abundant one. Also, it is known that neutrophils express 44 % (11/25) MiRs clusters in human. The presented clusters regulate neutrophil function and apoptosis. Six MiRs (including MiR-491-3p, MiR-34b, MiR-595, MiR-328, MiR-1281, and MiR-483-3p) sig-nificantly but slowly upregulate in response to GM-CSF treatment. It is suggestive that MiRs upregulation secondary to GM-CSF stimulation may promote neutrophil apoptosis and prevent other inflammatory cell reaction. These MiRs are located in regions with specific sensitivity to regu-lation via DNA methylation. From 602 downregu-lated genes, 176 genes had predicted binding site for at least one of the 6 MiRs above, and 83 genes had 2 binding sites for them. Thus, neutrophil MiRs target genes involved in proinflammatory functions such as inflammation mediated by che-mokine and cytokine signaling pathways, Ras pro-tein, and actin cytoskeleton. Further, upregulated MiRs may target pathways involving in neutrophil apoptosis. BCL2L11 (BIM), BCLAF, and PAK2 are known as genes which regulate neutrophil lifes-pan and contain binding sites for MiRs (Ward et al. 2011). Some clusters/MiRs (such as MiR-27a, let-7) have antiapoptotic roles by suppression of caspase-3 function (Tsang and Kwok 2008). On the other hand, MiR-29 family members target Mcl-1 (Mott et al. 2007). However, most of the MiRs expressing in neutrophils have regulatory effects on cell cycle (Ward et al. 2011). Collectively, balance among expressing MiRs seems to be determinant factor in neutrophil function and senescence.

Although MiRs effects on neutrophil functions and senescence are stated, more investigations are required to find exact targets of MiRs, to find ways for manipulation of neutrophils MiRs, hoping to open new avenue in treatment of inflammatory diseases.

15.7 Downregulated Level of MiR-92a Leads to Reduction of CD8+ T Lymphocytes in Aged Subjects

The MiR-17-92 family is known as regulator of immune system (Xiao et al. 2008), especially development of lymphoid cells by inhibition of BIM function (Ventura et al. 2008). Suppression of MiR-92a expression leads to impairment of naïve T cells, consequently to immunological changes. It is reported that MiR-92a expression significantly decreases in CD8+ T and non-significantly in CD4+ cells by aging. Also, older subjects have significantly lower levels of CD8+ family members comparing young people (Ohyashiki et al. 2011). It is found that most of the MiR-92a in CD8+ is originated from cytotoxic T cells (Salaun et al. 2011). Downregulation of MiR-17-92 expression and reduction of naïve cytotoxic T cells fraction are the reasons for suppressed level of MiR-92a derived from naïve cytotoxic T cells. Thus, this reduction in MiRs expression is associ-ated with decreased number of naïve CD8+ T lym-phocytes among healthy subjects. In addition, it is speculated that degradation of MiR-92a level pro-motes naïve T cells apoptosis and, then, attrite naïve CD8+ T cells. It is also hypothesized that downregulated level of MiR-92a leads to severe reduction of naïve T cells receptor (TCR) expres-sion and, consequently, lack of naïve CD8+ cell function (Ohyashiki et al. 2011). However, these results indicate the importance of MiRs effects on T cell function and senescence.

15.8 MiRs Expression by Aging Inhibits Triple Negative 1 Cell Transition to More Differentiated T Cells

Entering the T cell progenitors from the bone marrow to thymus occurs when none of mature T cell markers such as CD3, CD4, and CD8 exist. On the other word, the cells are triple negative

(TN). The TN cells should pass from TN1 (CD44+CD25−), TN2 (CD44+CD25+), TN3 (CD44−CD25+), and TN4 (CD44−CD25−) steps to produce one of CD4 or CD8 single positive cells (Godfrey and Zlotnik 1993). Thymus structure and function change with age and age-associated check points suppress thymopoiesis, leading to significant reduction in thymus-dependent T cells lymphopoiesis (Li et al. 2003). A number of TN1 cells increase drastically in aged thymus, showing inhibitory effects of age-associated check points (Virts and Thoman 2010). It is clearly understood that MiRs expression influences aging process by regulating various mRNAs translation or stability (Bartel 2009). MiRs expression varies in different steps of T cell development in TN subsets. Expression level of majority of the MiRs increases in TN1 cells by aging. In contrast, only 0.8 % of MiRs downregulate in aged cells of this group. This significant upregulation of most of the MiRs in aged TN1 cells leads to striking changes in gene expression and protein production. The changes in MiRs and protein expression in aged TN1 cells result to age-associated block of thymopoiesis. Further, very fewer changes in MiRs expression have been detected among TN2-TN4 cells in aged individuals. Moreover, MiRs profile in final stage of T cell development (TN4) in aged population is a little different with young individuals' profile. According to the results above, it can be suggested that age-related upregulation of MiRs occurs in less differentiated cells to the mature T cells, leading to blockage of TN1 cell transit to the TN2/TN3 population (Virts and Thoman 2010).

15.9 MiRs Regulatory Pathway Prevents Premature Involution of Thymic

MiRs are involved in thymus involution. The absence of MiRs controlling signaling pathway or MiR-29a cluster in thymic epithelial cells (TECs) leads to upregulation of IFN-α receptor (INFAR) and, then, higher level of INF-α production. These changes increase TECs sensitivity to stimulations and also premature and chronic involution of thymus (Olivieri et al. 2012b).

15.10 B-Lymphocyte Maturation Is Influenced by Age-Induced MiRs Expression

Another feature of immunosenescence is impairment of lymphopoiesis and maturation of B lymphocytes. It has been found that MiR-181 promotes lymphopoiesis, whereas high levels of MiR-34a expression inhibit this process. Aging leads to augmentation of MiR-34a and, inversely, downregulation of MiR-181 expression level, suppressing lymphopoiesis and B-lymphocytes maturation. These changes dysregulate immune system function, promoting immunosenescence (Seeger et al. 2013).

MiRs effects on age-associated failure of immune system are emerging. Although it is accepted that MiRs have crucial roles in regulation of immunosenescence, exploring involved MiRs characteristics in detail, effects of each MiRs, and their precise targets in immunosenescence process is not clearly stated. Also, most of the reported studies concluded from animal or laboratory works indicate the necessity of more investigations in human. Further researches on approaches to control MiRs expression during immunosenescence might bring new era in prevention and treatment of age-related immunological diseases.

References

Akira S, Takeda K (2004) Toll-like receptor signalling. Nat Rev Immunol 4(7):499–511

Baker DJ, Wijshake T, Tchkonia T et al (2011) Clearance of p16Ink4a-positive senescent cells delays ageing-associated disorders. Nature 479(7372):232–236

Bartel DP (2004) MicroRNAs: genomics, biogenesis, mechanism, and function. Cell 116(2):281–297

Bartel DP (2009) MicroRNAs: target recognition and regulatory functions. Cell 136(2):215–233

Bhaumik D, Scott GK, Schokrpur S et al (2009) MicroRNAs MiR-146a/b negatively modulate the senescence-associated inflammatory mediators IL-6 and IL-8. Aging 1(4):402–411

Ceppi M, Pereira PM, Dunand-Sauthier I et al (2009) MicroRNA-155 modulates the interleukin-1 signaling pathway in activated human monocyte-derived dendritic cells. Proc Natl Acad Sci U S A 106(8):2735–2740

Cevenini E, Bellavista E, Tieri P et al (2010) Systems biology and longevity: an emerging approach to identify innovative anti-aging targets and strategies. Curr Pharm Des 16(7):802–813

Chassin C, Kocur M, Pott J et al (2010) MiR-146a mediates protective innate immune tolerance in the neonate intestine. Cell Host Microbe 8(4):358–368

Colotta F, Re F, Polentarutti N et al (1992) Modulation of granulocyte survival and programmed cell death by cytokines and bacterial products. Blood 80(8):2012–2020

Coppe JP, Patil CK, Rodier F et al (2008) Senescence-associated secretory phenotypes reveal cell-nonautonomous functions of oncogenic RAS and the p53 tumor suppressor. PLoS Biol 6(12):2853–2868

Ford-Hutchinson AW, Bray MA, Doig MV et al (1980) Leukotriene B, a potent chemokinetic and aggregating substance released from polymorphonuclear leukocytes. Nature 286(5770):264–265

Franceschi C, Bonafe M, Valensin S et al (2000) Inflammaging. An evolutionary perspective on immunosenescence. Ann N Y Acad Sci 908:244–254

Frasca D, Landin AM, Riley RL et al (2008) Mechanisms for decreased function of B cells in aged mice and humans. J Immunol 180(5):2741–2746

Friedman DB, Johnson TE (1988) A mutation in the age-1 gene in Caenorhabditis elegans lengthens life and reduces hermaphrodite fertility. Genetics 118(1):75–86

Godfrey DI, Zlotnik A (1993) Control points in early T-cell development. Immunol Today 14(11):547–553

Haslett C (1999) Granulocyte apoptosis and its role in the resolution and control of lung inflammation. Am J Respir Crit Care Med 160(5 Pt 2):S5–S11

Jiang M, Xiang Y, Wang D et al (2012) Dysregulated expression of MiR-146a contributes to age-related dysfunction of macrophages. Aging Cell 11(1):29–40

Johnnidis JB, Harris MH, Wheeler RT et al (2008) Regulation of progenitor cell proliferation and granulocyte function by microRNA-223. Nature 451(7182):1125–1129

Kennedy AD, DeLeo FR (2009) Neutrophil apoptosis and the resolution of infection. Immunol Res 43(1–3):25–61

Li L, Hsu HC, Grizzle WE et al (2003) Cellular mechanism of thymic involution. Scand J Immunol 57(5):410–422

Liu J (2008) Control of protein synthesis and mRNA degradation by microRNAs. Curr Opin Cell Biol 20(2):214–221

Lum JJ, Bren G, McClure R et al (2005) Elimination of senescent neutrophils by TNF-related apoptosis-inducing ligand. J Immunol 175(2):1232–1238

Lysgaard C, Nielsen MS, Christensen JH et al (2012) No effect of high-dose atorvastatin on leukotriene B(4) formation from neutrophils in patients treated with coronary bypass surgery: a randomized placebo-controlled double-blinded trial with a crossover design. Prostaglandins Leukot Essent Fatty Acids 87(6): 185–188

Martin C, Burdon PC, Bridger G et al (2003) Chemokines acting via CXCR2 and CXCR4 control the release of neutrophils from the bone marrow and their return following senescence. Immunity 19(4):583–593

Mott JL, Kobayashi S, Bronk SF et al (2007) MiR-29 regulates Mcl-1 protein expression and apoptosis. Oncogene 26(42):6133–6140

O'Neill LA, Sheedy FJ, McCoy CE (2011) MicroRNAs: the fine-tuners of Toll-like receptor signalling. Nat Rev Immunol 11(3):163–175

Ohyashiki M, Ohyashiki JH, Hirota A et al (2011) Age-related decrease of MiRNA-92a levels in human CD8+ T-cells correlates with a reduction of naive T lymphocytes. Immun Ageing 8(1):11

Olivieri F, Lazzarini R, Recchioni R et al (2012a) MiR-146a as marker of senescence-associated pro-inflammatory status in cells involved in vascular remodelling. Age (Dordr). doi:10.1007/s11357-012-9440-8

Olivieri F, Spazzafumo L, Santini G et al (2012b) Age-related differences in the expression of circulating microRNAs: MiR-21 as a new circulating marker of inflammaging. Mech Ageing Dev 133(11–12): 675–685

Rodier F, Coppe JP, Patil CK et al (2009) Persistent DNA damage signalling triggers senescence-associated inflammatory cytokine secretion. Nat Cell Biol 11(8): 973–979

Rodriguez A, Vigorito E, Clare S et al (2007) Requirement of bic/microRNA-155 for normal immune function. Science 316(5824):608–611

Saccani S, Pantano S, Natoli G (2002) p38-Dependent marking of inflammatory genes for increased NF-kappa B recruitment. Nat Immunol 3(1):69–75

Salaun B, Yamamoto T, Badran B et al (2011) Differentiation associated regulation of microRNA expression in vivo in human CD8+ T cell subsets. J Transl Med 9:44

Scapini P, Lapinet-Vera JA, Gasperini S et al (2000) The neutrophil as a cellular source of chemokines. Immunol Rev 177:195–203

Seeger T, Haffez F, Fischer A et al (2013) Immuno-senescence-associated microRNAs in age and heart failure. Eur J Heart Fail 15(4):385–393

Spazzafumo L, Olivieri F, Abbatecola AM et al (2011) Remodelling of biological parameters during human ageing: evidence for complex regulation in longevity and in type 2 diabetes. Age (Dordr) 35(2):419–429

Taganov KD, Boldin MP, Chang KJ et al (2006) NF-kappa B-dependent induction of microRNA MiR-146, an inhibitor targeted to signaling proteins of innate immune responses. Proc Natl Acad Sci U S A 103(33): 12481–12486

Tili E, Michaille JJ, Cimino A et al (2007) Modulation of MiR-155 and MiR-125b levels following lipopolysaccharide/TNF-alpha stimulation and their possible roles in regulating the response to endotoxin shock. J Immunol 179(8):5082–5089

Tsang WP, Kwok TT (2008) Let-7a microRNA suppresses therapeutics-induced cancer cell death by targeting caspase-3. Apoptosis 13(10):1215–1222

Van Duin D, Mohanty S, Thomas V et al (2007) Age-associated defect in human TLR-1/2 function. J Immunol 178(2):970–975

Ventura A, Young AG, Winslow MM et al (2008) Targeted deletion reveals essential and overlapping functions of the MiR-17 through 92 family of MiRNA clusters. Cell 132(5):875–886

Virts EL, Thoman ML (2010) Age-associated changes in MiRNA expression profiles in thymopoiesis. Mech Ageing Dev 131(11–12):743–748

Ward JR, Heath PR, Catto JW et al (2011) Regulation of neutrophil senescence by microRNAs. PLoS One 6(1):e15810

Whyte MK, Savill J, Meagher LC et al (1997) Coupling of neutrophil apoptosis to recognition by macrophages: coordinated acceleration by protein synthesis inhibitors. J Leukoc Biol 62(2):195–202

Xiao C, Srinivasan L, Calado DP et al (2008) Lymphoproliferative disease and autoimmunity in mice with increased MiR-17-92 expression in lymphocytes. Nat Immunol 9(4):405–414

Immunogenetics of Aging

16

Ali Akbar Amirzargar

16.1 Introduction

Old age survival has been improved substantially since 1950 in developing countries. As a result, the number of octogenarians has increased to 4-fold, the number of nonagenarians to 8-fold, and the number of centenarians has increased to 20-fold (Vaupel et al. 1998). Therefore, the study on human aging and longevity has become a very popular topic in the last decades because of the change in demography, which led to the remarkable increase in the number of people over the age of 80 years living in countries such as China, India, and Western countries (Franceschi et al. 2008).

16.2 Genetics and Longevity

The literature on gene and longevity during the last 20 years arisen from different experimental animal and human populations suggests that the pictures of the aging phenotype are controversial which could be due to several reasons: (1) few studies evaluate many parameters at the same time in the same individual, and (2)

another factor contributing to the complexity of the problem is human aging and longevity which are complex and multifactorial events that result from a combination of environmental, genetic, epigenetic, and stochastic factors, which all are important in aging and longevity (Salvioli et al. 2006; De Benedictis and Franceschi 2006; Fraga et al. 2005; Capri et al. 2006).

It is hypothesized that the importance of each component of the environment, genetics (and epigenetics), and stochasticity changes with the passing of time. According to this hypothesis, genetics is less important in the early adult phase of life and becomes more important in old age. Moreover, these different components interact with each other, specially genetics and environment (Cevenini et al. 2010).

Studies comparing life expectancy in twins and other family members have found that up to 25 % of the variation in human lifespan is heritable; the remaining 75 % is due to environmental exposures, accidents and injuries, and chance. Very long life, to beyond ages 90 or 100 years, appears to have an even stronger genetic basis. Conversely, several clinical syndromes of "accelerated aging" and death at an early age (the progeroid syndromes) have a known genetic basis. Elderly children of centenarians have much less diabetes and ischemic heart disease, and better self-rated health, than do age-matched controls. This suggests that they have inherited a longevity gene (or more likely a set of gene) from their long-lived parent that protects against these infirmities. Previous studies have reported

A.A. Amirzargar, PhD
Molecular Immunology Research Center
and Departement of Immunology,
Tehran University of Medical Sciences, Tehran, Iran
e-mail: amirzara@tums.ac.ir

A. Massoud, N. Rezaei (eds.), *Immunology of Aging*,
DOI 10.1007/978-3-642-39495-9_16, © Springer-Verlag Berlin Heidelberg 2014

that centenarian offspring (CO), like their centenarian parents, has genetic and immune system advantages, which reflect a minor risk to develop major age-related diseases, such as cardiovascular diseases, hypertension, or diabetes mellitus as well as cancer. The lower cardiovascular disease risk in CO suggests the probability that CO has some protective factors against atherosclerosis, such as a good lipid profile. Male COs have higher plasma high-density lipoprotein (HDL)-C levels and lower plasma low-density lipoprotein (LDL)-C levels. Since lipid profile is directly correlated to atherosclerotic cardiovascular diseases, this metabolic feature could preserve CO both to develop these diseases and, as consequence, to reach a healthy aging and longer survival (Terry et al. 2004).

16.3 Immunogenetics and Aging

It is well documented that the quality and the size of the humoral immune response decline with age. This change is characterized by lower antibody responses and decreased production of high-affinity antibodies. Although, a decreased B cell count was observed in CO and their age-matched controls, it has been demonstrated that naïve B cells (IgD$^+$CD27$^-$) were more abundant and (DN) B cells (IgD$^-$CD27$^-$) were significantly decreased, as looked similarly in young people. The evaluation of immunoglobulin (Ig) M secreted in CO serum shows that the values are within the range of the levels observed in young subjects (Bulati et al. 2011).

Therefore, individuals genetically enriched for longevity possess immune different signatures respect to those of the general population. In this regard, naïve T cells (CD3$^+$CD8$^+$CD45RA$^+$CCR7$^+$CD27$^+$CD28$^+$) and naïve B cells (IgD$^+$CD27$^-$) increase, while late-differentiated effector memory T cells (CD3$^+$CD8$^+$CD45RA$^-$CCR7$^-$CD27$^-$CD28$^-$) TEMRA (CD3$^+$CD8$^+$CD45RA$^+$CCR7$^-$CD27$^-$CD28$^-$) decrease in longevity. This suggests the idea of the "familiar youth" of the immune system (Colonna-Romano et al. 2010; Derhovanessian et al. 2010).

16.4 Gender and Longevity

In the more developed regions, the life expectancy at birth in 2000–2005 was 71.9 years for men and 79.3 years for women. The highest values are in Japan, which were 79.3 and 86.3 years for men and women, respectively. Females also live longer than males in many other species; for instance, in the laboratory, female Wistar rats live on average 14 % longer than males.

In fact, the difference in mortality between men and women is not only a question of biologic sex, but it is also a question of "socially constructed sex," a question of gender. Behavioral and environmental factors clearly play a role in determining excess male mortality. Beyond a slight biologic advantage for females, excess male mortality results from the emergency of typically male "man-made diseases." Work-related risks in industrial activity, alcoholism, smoking, and car accidents are the main factors contributing to excess male mortality. An aspect to be highlighted is that the attitude women generally have concerning their body, their health, and their lifestyle is very different from that of men (Abbott 2004; Franceschi et al. 2000).

The fact that this phenomenon also occurs in animals other than humans indicates that it cannot be only attributed to sociological factors but might reflect specific biological characteristics of both genders. A role for the sex hormones, testosterone in males and estrogen in females, in the gender differences in lifespan seen in mammals is widely claimed (Vina et al. 2005). The role of testosterone in decreasing males' lifespan has also been attributed to the link between this hormone and the male characteristics of aggression and competitiveness, as well as libido. Estrogens, on the other hand, have beneficial effects on the cardiovascular system, because they reduce LDL cholesterol and increase concentrations of HDL cholesterol, whereas testosterone also increases blood concentrations of LDL and decreases concentrations of HDL cholesterol, so that men are more prone than women to cardiovascular diseases and stroke (Mendelsohn and Karas 1999; Weidemann and Hanke 2002).

Estrogens also exhibit antioxidant properties in vivo by upregulating the expression of the genes encoding antioxidant enzymes. In experimental animals, estrogens are responsible for the lower mitochondrial free-radical production observed in females as compared with males. Estrogens should elicit this effect by upregulating expression of the genes encoding mitochondrial antioxidant enzymes. Besides, there is known sexual dimorphism in the immune response. There are some evidences showing that sex-associated hormones can modulate immune responses and therefore influence the outcome of infection, which consequently affect survival and longevity (Klein 2000; Roberts et al. 2001).

From a genetic prospective, human leukocyte antigen (HLA)-F has been studied in Sicilian population and supports a female-specific gene-longevity association. HFE gene, the most telomeric HLA class Ib gene, coding class I α chain, the human hemochromatosis (HFE) protein, which seemingly no longer participates in immunity. It has lost its ability to bind peptides due to a definitive closure of the antigen-binding cleft that prevents peptide binding and presentation. The HFE protein, expressed on crypt enterocytes of the duodenum, regulates the iron uptake by intestinal cells. It has the ability to form complex with the receptor for iron-binding transferrin. Mutations in HFE gene are associated with hereditary hemochromatosis, a disorder caused by excessive iron uptake. Three common mutations, C282Y, H63D, and S65C, have been identified in HFE gene. In particular, the C282Y mutation (a cysteine-to-tyrosine mutation at amino acid 282) destroys its ability to make up a heterodimer with β2-microglobulin. The defective HFE protein fails to associate to the transferring receptor, and the complex cannot be transported to the surface of the duodenal crypt cells. As a consequence, in homozygous people, two to three times the normal amount of iron is absorbed from food by the intestine, resulting in end-organ damage and reducing lifespan. Two other mutations, H63D (a histidine to aspartate at amino acid 63) and S65C (a serine to cysteine at amino acid 65), are associated with milder forms of this disease (Beutler 2007; Pietrangelo 2010).

An association between C282Y mutation and longevity in the Sicilian population has been studied. In particular, women carriers of C282Y mutation had a higher frequency among the oldest elderly compared to control women. Thus, the C282Y mutation may confer a selective advantage in terms of longevity in Sicilian women (Lio et al. 2002a).

Balistreri et al. showed the relevance of C282Y for women's survival to late age, adding another piece of evidence to the complex puzzle of genetic and environmental factors involved in control of lifespan in humans. The interaction between environmental and genetic factors differently characterizes different populations worldwide, which plays an important role in determining the gender-specific probability of attaining longevity.

Studies on cytokine gene single-nucleotide polymorphisms (SNPs) showed that a positive significant association between −1082 IL-10 polymorphism and longevity was observed in centenarian men but not in women; in accordance with previous observations on polymorphisms in tyrosine hydroxylase gene and mtDNA haplogroups (De Benedictis et al. 1999), interferon gamma (IFN-γ) gene polymorphisms have been shown to be associated with longevity in women, but not in men (Lio et al. 2002c).

Altogether, these findings point out that gender is a major variable in the genetics of longevity and suggest that men and women follow different strategies to reach longevity.

16.5   Role of HLA in Longevity

The HLA are membrane-bound glycoproteins express on the surface of nearly all nucleated cells and occupy 4 Mb of DNA on the chromosome band 6p21.3 and are extensively polymorphic with more than 7,000 alleles.

The MHC is divided into the class I, class II, and class III regions. Most HLA genes involved in the immune response fall into classes I and II, which encode highly polymorphic heterodimeric glycoproteins involved in antigen presentation to T cells. However, many genes of the class

III region are also involved in the immune and inflammatory responses. Genetic association of HLA-class I and II with immunodeficiency (Amanzadeh et al. 2012; Movahedi et al. 2008; Mohammadi et al. 2008), autoimmune (Mortazavi et al. 2013; Rabbani et al. 2012; Shams et al. 2009; Amirzargar et al. 2005a, b, 1998), infectious diseases (Amirzargar et al. 2004, 2008; Nicknam et al. 2008), and cancers (Mahmoodi et al. 2012; Hojjat-Farsangi et al. 2008; Amirzargar et al. 2007; Khosravi et al. 2007; Sarafnejad et al. 2006; Dehaghani et al. 2002; Ghaderi et al. 2001; Moazzeni et al. 1999) has been studied by several groups. Classes I and II molecules take up antigenic peptides intracellularly and express on the cell surface, where they present processed antigenic peptide to the T-lymphocyte receptor and induce T cell responses against specific antigen. These are the bases for the antigen-specific control of the immune response. The diversity of the immune response depends on the ability of HLA molecules to bind some peptides and presenting to T cells and induces and immune response, while some peptides cannot bind and elicit an immune response.

Thus, survival and longevity might be associated with a positive or negative selection of alleles that respectively confers resistance or susceptibility to infectious disease, autoimmunity, and cancer. An intriguing feature of the major histocompatibility complex (MHC) is the occurrence of particular combinations of alleles, more frequently than would be expected based on the frequencies of individual alleles. This nonrandom association of alleles gives rise to highly conserved haplotypes that appear to be derived from a common remote ancestor, so-called ancestral haplotypes (AHs). This term underlines the fact that conserved, population-specific haplotypes are continuous sequences derived with little change from an ancestor of all those now carrying all or part of the haplotype.

Studying the association between longevity and HLA is generally difficult to interpret partly due to the major methodological problems and the homogeneity of the population in terms of geographical origin. However, as reported by Caruso et al., some of these kinds of studies, well

designed and performed, suggest an HLA effect on longevity (Caruso et al. 2000, 2001).

In studies performed in Caucasians, an increase in HLA-DRB1:11 in Dutch women over 85 years were observed. The same laboratory performed a further study, and by using a "birthplace-restricted comparison," in which the origin of all the subjects was ascertained, the authors were able to confirm that aging in women was positively associated with HLA-DRB1: 11 (Lagaay et al. 1991; Izaks et al. 2000).

In two French studies, the relevance of HLA-DRB1:11 to longevity in aged populations were also confirmed. This increase in allele frequency in aging is consistent with the protective effects of this allele in viral diseases. HLA-DRB1:11 frequencies have been shown to be decreased in some viral diseases (Ivanova et al. 1998; Henon et al. 1999).

HLA-DRB1 frequencies in Sardinian (an ancient genetic isolate) centenarians and controls have been evaluated and showed that HLA-DRB1*15 was increased in centenarians, although no more significant after Bonferroni's correction and the HLA-DQA1*01, -DQB1*05 and HLA-DQA1*01, -DQB1*06 haplotypes were also increased in Sardinian centenarians, although it was not statistically significant (Lio et al. 2003a, b; Letizia et al. 2008).

Finally, an association between longevity and the AH 8.1 (or part of this haplotype, i.e., HLA-B8, -DR3) has been shown. The 8.1 AH is a common Caucasoid haplotype, unique in its association with a wide range of immunopathological diseases and in healthy subjects with a large array of immune dysfunctions (Candore et al. 2002, 2003). An increased frequency of AH in oldest-old men has been reported in French and in Northern Irish populations. This association appears to be gender-specific as this haplotype is more frequent in male old age. In a Greek study it has been shown that there was a significant decrease of 8.1 AH in aged women (Proust et al. 1982; Papasteriades et al. 1997).

So, the immune changes typical of the AH 8.1 should contribute to early morbidity and mortality in elderly women, who are more susceptible to autoimmune diseases than men, and to longevity in elderly men. Thus, these studies seem to suggest that HLA-DR11 in women and HLA-B8, -DR3 in men may be considered markers of successful aging (Rea et al. et al. 1994; Candore et al. 2003). However, in a longitudinal community-based study, in which a total of 919 subjects from the Netherlands, aged 85 years and older, were HLA-typed and followed up for at least 5 years, age- and sex-adjusted mortality rate ratios (MRR) were estimated for 79 antigens by the subject-years method. No HLA-association with mortality was found (Izaks et al. 1997).

HLA-DR typing in 120 centenarians (79 women and 41 men) and 86 controls (53 women and 33 men) from Sardinia (very homogeneous population) was performed to evaluate the associations between HLA alleles or haplotypes and longevity which were previously observed in other Caucasoid populations. No significant differences was obtained by analyzing the differences between Centenarians and controls except for HLA-DRB1*15 that was increased in centenarians. However, the significance was not maintained by multiplying p values for the number of alleles under study. Thus, in Sardinian centenarians, findings observed in the well-planned and well-designed studies performed in other Caucasoid populations were not confirmed (Lio et al. 2003a; Scola et al. 2008).

Moreover, a study set out to specifically confirm the previously reported increase in the frequency of the 8.1 AH in aged men of the Northern Irish population did not reveal any statistically significant haplotype frequency differences between the aged cohorts of individuals in comparison to the younger controls. However, a striking decrease was observed when the aged women (13.1 %) were compared to the control women (17.8 %) (Ross et al. 2003).

The Okinawan Japanese, a well-known population for their longevity, study showed that Okinawan centenarians HLADRB1*1401, HLA-DQB1*0503, HLADQA1*0101,*0104, and HLA-DQA1*05 haplotypes were significantly increased and placed them at lower risk for inflammatory and autoimmune diseases. It actually does not mean that Okinawan longevity is all genetic, but a result of complex interaction between genetic, lifestyle, and environmental factors. The Okinawans have both genetic and non-genetic longevity advantages, the best combination. Okinawan traditional way of life, the dietary habits, the physical activity, the psychological and social aspects, all play an important role in Okinawan longevity (Takata et al. 1987).

However, also taking into account well-planned and well-designed studies, discordant results have been obtained. The discordant results obtained in MHC/aging association studies might be due to distinct linkage in different cohorts or to other interacting genetic or environmental factors or to the heterogeneity of aging population and methodological aspects. Nevertheless, bearing all the reported studies in mind, there is no convincing evidence of a strong, direct association between longevity and any MHC alleles.

16.6 Cytokine Genes and Longevity

Cytokines are generally small molecules secreted by one cell to alter the behavior of itself or another cell, generally within the hematopoietic system. Production of numerous cytokines by the cells of the immune system, in response to both antigen-specific and nonspecific stimuli, plays a critical role in the generation of both pro- and anti-inflammatory immune responses.

However, cytokine functions are not limited to induce response after an immune insult; they can modulate the nature of response (cytotoxic, humoral, cell mediated, inflammatory, or allergic) or, in contrast, they may cause non-responsiveness and suppress immune response.

Cytokine genes and their polymorphisms located within promoter regions, mostly SNP, or microsatellites, have been described to affect gene transcription, causing interindividual variations in cytokine production. These polymorphisms might confer flexibility in the immune response by allowing differential production of cytokines. Cytokine gene polymorphisms have been shown to be involved in the susceptibility, severity, and clinical outcome of several diseases, including cancer (Amirzargar et al. 2005a), autoimmunity (Behniafard et al. 2012; Mahmoudi et al. 2011; Shahram et al. 2011; Khalilzadeh et al. 2010; Anvari et al. 2010; Barkhordari et al. 2010; Amirzargar et al. 2009; Shokrgozar et al. 2009; Rezaei et al. 2009; Mirahmadian et al. 2008); (Amirzargar et al. 2005b) and infections (Davoudi et al. 2006; Amirzargar et al. 2006).

A highly regulated immune function characterizing the successful aging has been found in centenarians. Different data suggest that centenarians seem to have gene polymorphisms to overcome the major age-related diseases. Polymorphisms in immune system genes have been found to be associated with longevity. Particularly, associations between both increased anti-inflammatory cytokine genotypes and longevity, differential gender longevity in males and females, and reciprocally age-related diseases have been demonstrated in different studies (Ostan et al. 2008; Sanjabi et al. 2009; Iannitti and Palmieri 2011; Ferrucci et al. 1999).

Genetic regulation of inflammatory processes might explain the reason why some people are more susceptible to age-related diseases and why some develop a greater inflammatory response than others.

Strong inflammatory response may benefit the young but may become detrimental at an older age, and longevity in individuals who achieve advanced age might be associated with anti-inflammatory cytokine gene profiles.

Chronic "proinflammatory" state promotes or exacerbates age-related pathological conditions, such as cardiovascular diseases, atherosclerosis, Alzheimer's disease, osteoarthritis, arthritis, sarcopenia, and type 2 diabetes.

Large studies have demonstrated that high plasma levels of interleukin (IL)-6 are correlated with greater disability, morbidity, and mortality in the elderly (Cesari et al. 2004). Moreover, high levels of IL-6, IL-1β, and C-reactive protein (CRP) are significantly associated with poor physical performance and muscle strength in older persons (Bruunsgaard et al. 2003a). Serum levels of tumor necrosis factor alpha (TNF-α) are considered a strong predictor of mortality in both 80-year-old people and

centenarians (Bruunsgaard et al. 2003b). Thus, if a strong inflammatory response means higher risk of life-threatening diseases, longevity should be correlated with the capability to maintain an inflammatory response of low intensity. This has been partially confirmed by findings in centenarians, who are considered the best example of longevity. Study on the polymorphism for a C to G transition at nucleotide −174 of the IL-6 gene promoter (−174 C/G locus) showed that IL-6 production was increased in G homozygotes (GG genotype), but not in C$^+$ (CC and CG genotypes) old subjects, and this phenomenon was significantly present only in males (Olivieri et al. 2002; Vasto 2006).

IL-10 is produced by macrophages, T and B cells, and is one of the major immunoregulatory cytokines, usually considered to mediate potent downregulation of inflammatory responses. Multiple SNPs have been identified in human IL-10, 5′ flanking region and some of these (i.e., −592, −819, −1082) combine with microsatellite alleles to form haplotype associated with differential IL-10 production. These three SNPs in the IL-10 proximal gene region (considered potential targets for transcription regulating factors) might be involved in genetic control of IL-10 production. In particular, the homozygous −1082 GG genotype seems to be associated with higher IL-10 production in respect to G/A heterozygous and AA homozygous genotypes. It has been demonstrated that −1082A carriers (low producers) seem likely develop a major number of chronic inflammatory diseases (Lio et al. 2004).

Data on Italian elderly population demonstrated an increase of subjects carrying the −1082G IL-10 allele in centenarian men. This allele is significantly associated with increased IL-10 production. Conversely, the frequency of −1082A allele, associated to low IL-10 production, was significantly higher in patients with myocardial infarction (MI), it is suggested that high IL-10 production seems to be protective against MI and a possible biomarker for longevity. In older ages, increased IL-10 levels might better control inflammatory responses induced by chronic vessel damage and reduce the risk for atherogenetic complications (Lio et al. 2003b).

IL-10 polymorphisms, related to high production of the cytokine, also appear to be involved in longevity in long-living subjects from Japan (Okayama et al. 2005).

The IL-10 haplotype (−1082G, −819C, and −592C) associated with high-level cytokine gene expression was significantly more prevalent among both the Bulgarian and the Turkish populations healthy elderly to young controls. Additionally, in Bulgarians the IL-10 haplotype (−1082A, −819T, and −592A), possibly related to a lower level of gene expression, was found with slightly lower frequency in the elderly. In the Turkish population, a decreased frequency of another low-level IL-10 haplotype (−1082A, −819C, and −592C) was observed in the elderly (Naumova et al. 2011).

These findings allow hypothesizing that different alleles at different cytokine gene coding for pro- (IL-6) or anti-inflammatory (IL-10) cytokines may affect the individual lifespan expectancy by influencing the type and intensity of the immune-inflammatory responses against environmental stressors.

Analysis of genotypes of anti-inflammatory transforming growth factor (TGF)-β1 also showed possible association with aging. The genotype TGF-β1 (codon 10) T/T; (codon 25) G/G, related to high levels of gene expression, was increased in elderly compared to young controls ($p < 0.05$). In contrast, there was a trend to a lower frequency of the genotype TGF-β1 (codon 10) C/C; (codon 25) G/G, associated with low protein level in elderly. Analysis of extended TGF-β1 genotypes in Bulgarians showed that genotype TGF-β1 (codon 10) C/C; (codon 25) G/G; (−988) C/C; (−800) G/G was decreased, while the genotype TGF- β1 (codon 10) T/C; (codon 25) G/G; (−988) C/C; (−800) G/A was increased in elderly compared with the controls. Based on codon 10 and 25, these genotypes are associated with low- and high-level gene expression, respectively. As the positions −988 and −800 are located in the promoter region of the gene, they could also modulate the expression of TGF- β1 (Naumova et al. 2011).

Active TGF-β1 plasma levels were significantly higher in elderly subjects when compared with younger controls. Although no relationship with TGF-β1 levels was observed, the C allele and GC genotype at the TGF-1 +915 polymorphism were significantly less common in Italian centenarians than in younger controls, suggesting that variability in the TGF-β1 gene also influences longevity (Carrieri et al. 2004).

Female Sicilian centenarians are characterized by an overexpression of +874 INF-γ allele. The INF-γ production is also influenced by hormonal control fundamentally mediated by 17β estradiol. Hormonal regulation of this cytokine has been suggested to modulate, in part, the ability of estrogens to potentiate many types of immune responses and to influence the disproportionate susceptibility of women for immune-inflammatory diseases. Thus, gene variants representing genetic advantage for one gender might not be reciprocally relevant for the other gender in terms of successful or unsuccessful aging (Lio et al. 2002b).

The TNF gene cluster located in the HLA region on chromosome 6, SNP at the −308G/A in TNF-α gene affect cytokine production, being A+ carriers high producers.

Analysis of the extended TNF-α genotypes showed significant differences between 60 elderly individuals and 100 young controls. GG genotype, possibly related to low-level expression, was more frequent among healthy elderly Bulgarians compared with young controls (Naumova et al. 2011).

Inconclusive results have been obtained on the role of this SNP in age-related diseases and longevity in Sicilian populations (Candore et al. 2006). However, by the innovative approach to study potential susceptibility genes for cardiovascular diseases, to use of centenarians as healthy controls, it has been demonstrated that A+ genotype is significantly overrepresented in cardiovascular disease patients and underrepresented in centenarians. So, these results suggest a negative effect of the A+ carrier status in longevity.

In any case, genetic variation in the −308 SNP seems to affect the clinical outcome of some infectious and autoimmune diseases (Mahmoudi et al. 2011; Barkhordari et al. 2010; Davoudi et al. 2006; Amirzargar et al. 2006).

Therefore, the −308A polymorphism at the locus of TNF-α may be one of the susceptibility factors for infectious and autoimmune diseases in old persons, particularly considering its association with the increased release of proinflammatory cytokines (Sonya et al. 2006).

Data presented by Franceschi et al. suggest the network between proinflammatory cytokines and oxidative stress, such as the superoxide dismutase (SOD1 and SOD2) and paraxonase (PON1), is responsible for "directive" interconnections inside the immune system and is important "candidate" genes for longevity and aging "remodeling." It has been observed that a typical feature of the aging process is a general increase in plasma levels of proinflammatory cytokines. This can lead to a chronic "proinflammatory" state, which promotes or exacerbates age-related pathological conditions (cardiovascular diseases, atherosclerosis, Alzheimer's disease, arthrosis and arthritis, sarcopenia, and type 2 diabetes, among others) (Miriam et al. 2006).

These results, which should be extended and replicated in different populations and cohorts, all support the concept that aging is associated with adaptation and remodeling of the immune system, but successful aging and longevity require a balance between pro- and anti-inflammatory activity.

The studies on human aging and longevity are further complicated by the fact that human populations are heterogeneous from the point of view of genetic pool, lifestyle, cultural habits, education, economic status, and social network. All these components are different from population to population, and each population is characterized by a unique combination of them. This fact renders the studies difficult to compare and the results very often discordant. Finally, all these considerations also apply to gender difference, since gender appears to be a crucial player in the cross-talk between genes, environment, and health.

References

Abbott A (2004) Ageing: growing old gracefully. Nature 428(6979):116–118

Amanzadeh A, Amirzargar AA, Mohseni N et al (2012) Association of HLA-DRB1, DQA1 and DQB1 alleles and haplotypes with common variable immunodeficiency in Iranian patients. Avicenna J Med Biotechnol 4(2):103–112

Amirzargar A, Mytilineos J, Yousefipour A et al (1998) HLA class II (DRB1, DQA1 and DQB1) associated genetic susceptibility in Iranian multiple sclerosis (MS) patients. Eur J Immunogenet 25(4):297–301

Amirzargar AA, Yalda A, Hajabolbaghi M et al (2004) The association of HLA-DRB, DQA1, DQB1 alleles and haplotype frequency in Iranian patients with pulmonary tuberculosis. Int J Tuberc Lung Dis 8(8): 1017–1021

Amirzargar AA, Bagheri M, Ghavamzadeh A et al (2005a) Cytokine gene polymorphism in Iranian patients with chronic myelogenous leukaemia. Int J Immunogenet 32(3):167–171

Amirzargar AA, Tabasi A, Khosravi F et al (2005b) Optic neuritis, multiple sclerosis and human leukocyte antigen: results of a 4-year follow-up study. Eur J Neurol 12(1):25–30

Amirzargar AA, Rezaei N, Jabbari H et al (2006) Cytokine single nucleotide polymorphisms in Iranian patients with pulmonary tuberculosis. Eur Cytokine Netw 17(2):84–89

Amirzargar AA, Khosravi F, Dianat SS et al (2007) Association of HLA class II allele and haplotype frequencies with chronic myelogenous leukemia and age-at-onset of the disease. Pathol Oncol Res 13(1): 47–51

Amirzargar AA, Mohseni N, Shokrgozar MA et al (2008) HLA-DRB1, DQA1 and DQB1 alleles and haplotypes frequencies in Iranian healthy adult responders and non-responders to recombinant hepatitis B vaccine. Iran J Immunol 5(2):92–99

Amirzargar AA, Movahedi M, Rezaei N et al (2009) Polymorphisms in IL4 and iLARA confer susceptibility to asthma. J Investig Allergol Clin Immunol 19(6): 433–438

Anvari M, Khalilzadeh O, Esteghamati A et al (2010) Graves' disease and gene polymorphism of TNF-alpha, IL-2, IL-6, IL-12, and IFN-gamma. Endocrine 37(2):344–348

Barkhordari E, Rezaei N, Mahmoudi M et al (2010) T-helper 1, T-helper 2, and T-regulatory cytokines gene polymorphisms in irritable bowel syndrome. Inflammation 33(5):281–286

Behniafard N, Gharagozlou M, Farhadi E et al (2012) TNF-alpha single nucleotide polymorphisms in atopic dermatitis. Eur Cytokine Netw 23(4):163–165

Beutler E (2007) Iron storage disease: facts, fiction and progress. Blood Cells Mol Dis 39(2):140–147

Bruunsgaard H, Andersen-Ranberg K, Hjelmborg J et al (2003a) Elevated levels of tumor necrosis factor alpha and mortality in centenarians. Am J Med 115(4): 278–283

Bruunsgaard H, Ladelund S, Pedersen AN et al (2003b) Predicting death from tumour necrosis factor-alpha and interleukin-6 in 80-year-old people. Clin Exp Immunol 132(1):24–31

Bulati M, Buffa S, Candore G et al (2011) B cells and immunosenescence: a focus on IgG+IgD-CD27- (DN)

B cells in aged humans. Ageing Res Rev 10(2):274–284

Candore G, Lio D, Colonna RG et al (2002) Pathogenesis of autoimmune diseases associated with 8.1 ancestral haplotype: effect of multiple gene interactions. Autoimmun Rev 1(1–2):29–35

Candore G, Modica MA, Lio D et al (2003) Pathogenesis of autoimmune diseases associated with 8.1 ancestral haplotype: a genetically determined defect of C4 influences immunological parameters of healthy carriers of the haplotype. Biomed Pharmacother 57(7):274–277

Candore G, Balistreri CR, Grimaldi MP et al (2006) Opposite role of pro-inflammatory alleles in acute myocardial infarction and longevity: results of studies performed in a Sicilian population. Ann N Y Acad Sci 1067:270–275

Capri M, Salvioli S, Sevini F et al (2006) The genetics of human longevity. Ann N Y Acad Sci 1067:252–263

Carrieri G, Marzi E, Olivieri F et al (2004) The G/C915 polymorphism of transforming growth factor beta1 is associated with human longevity: a study in Italian centenarians. Aging Cell 3(6):443–448

Caruso C, Candore G, Colonna Romano G et al (2000) HLA, aging, and longevity: a critical reappraisal. Hum Immunol 61(9):942–949

Caruso C, Candore G, Romano GC et al (2001) Immunogenetics of longevity. Is major histocompatibility complex polymorphism relevant to the control of human longevity? A review of literature data. Mech Ageing Dev 122(5):445–462

Cesari M, Penninx BW, Pahor M et al (2004) Inflammatory markers and physical performance in older persons: the InCHIANTI study. J Gerontol A Biol Sci Med Sci 59(3):242–248

Cevenini E, Bellavista E, Tieri P et al (2010) Systems biology and longevity: an emerging approach to identify innovative anti-aging targets and strategies. Curr Pharm Des 16(7):802–813

Colonna-Romano G, Buffa S, Bulati M et al (2010) B cells compartment in centenarian offspring and old people. Curr Pharm Des 16(6):604–608

Davoudi S, Amirzargar AA, Hajiabdolbaghi M et al (2006) Th-1 cytokines gene polymorphism in human brucellosis. Int J Immunogenet 33(5):355–359

De Benedictis G, Franceschi C (2006) The unusual genetics of human longevity. Sci Aging Knowledge Environ 2006(10):pe20

De Benedictis G, Rose G, Carrieri G et al (1999) Mitochondrial DNA inherited variants are associated with successful aging and longevity in humans. FASEB J 13(12):1532–1536

Dehaghani AS, Amirzargar A, Farjadian S et al (2002) HLA-DQB1 alleles and susceptibility to cervical squamous cell carcinoma in Southern Iranian patients. Pathol Oncol Res 8(1):58–61

Derhovanessian E, Maier AB, Beck R et al (2010) Hallmark features of immunosenescence are absent in familial longevity. J Immunol 185(8):4618–4624

Ferrucci L, Harris TB, Guralnik JM et al (1999) Serum IL-6 level and the development of disability in older persons. J Am Geriatr Soc 47(6):639–646

Fraga MF, Ballestar E, Paz MF et al (2005) Epigenetic differences arise during the lifetime of monozygotic twins. Proc Natl Acad Sci U S A 102(30): 10604–10609

Franceschi C, Motta L, Valensin S et al (2000) Do men and women follow different trajectories to reach extreme longevity? Italian Multicenter Study on Centenarians (IMUSCE). Aging (Milano) 12(2): 77–84

Franceschi C, Motta L, Motta M et al (2008) The extreme longevity: the state of the art in Italy. Exp Gerontol 43(2):45–52

Ghaderi A, Talei A, Gharesi-Fard B et al (2001) HLA-DBR 1 alleles and the susceptibility of Iranian patients with breast cancer. Pathol Oncol Res 7(1):39–41

Henon N, Busson M, Dehay-Martuchou C et al (1999) Familial versus sporadic longevity and MHC markers. J Biol Regul Homeost Agents 13(1):27–31

Hojjat-Farsangi M, Jeddi-Tehrani M, Amirzargar AA et al (2008) Human leukocyte antigen class II allele association to disease progression in Iranian patients with chronic lymphocytic leukemia. Hum Immunol 69(10):666–674

Iannitti T, Palmieri B (2011) Inflammation and genetics: an insight in the centenarian model. Hum Biol 83(4):531–559

Ivanova R, Henon N, Lepage V et al (1998) HLA-DR alleles display sex-dependent effects on survival and discriminate between individual and familial longevity. Hum Mol Genet 7(2):187–194

Izaks GJ, van Houwelingen HC, Schreuder GM et al (1997) The association between human leucocyte antigens (HLA) and mortality in community residents aged 85 and older. J Am Geriatr Soc 45(1):56–60

Izaks GJ, Remarque EJ, Schreuder GM et al (2000) The effect of geographic origin on the frequency of HLA antigens and their association with ageing. Eur J Immunogenet 27(2):87–92

Khalilzadeh O, Anvari M, Esteghamati A et al (2010) Genetic susceptibility to Graves' ophthalmopathy: the role of polymorphisms in anti-inflammatory cytokine genes. Ophthalmic Genet 31(4):215–220

Khosravi F, Amirzargar A, Sarafnejad A et al (2007) HLA class II allele and haplotype frequencies in Iranian patients with leukemia. Iran J Allergy Asthma Immunol 6(3):137–142

Klein SL (2000) The effects of hormones on sex differences in infection: from genes to behavior. Neurosci Biobehav Rev 24(6):627–638

Lagaay AM, D'Amaro J, Ligthart GJ et al (1991) Longevity and heredity in humans. Association with the human leucocyte antigen phenotype. Ann N Y Acad Sci 621:78–89

Letizia Scola, Domenico Lio a, Giuseppina Candore (2008) Analysis of HLA-DRB1, DQA1, DQB1 haplotypes in Sardinian centenarians. Experimental Gerontology 43 114–118.

Lio D, Balistreri CR, Colonna-Romano G et al (2002a) Association between the MHC class I gene HFE polymorphisms and longevity: a study in Sicilian population. Genes Immun 3(1):20–24

Lio D, Scola L, Crivello A et al (2002b) Allele frequencies of +874T–>A single nucleotide polymorphism at the first intron of interferon-gamma gene in a group of Italian centenarians. Exp Gerontol 37(2–3):315–319

Lio D, Scola L, Crivello A et al (2002c) Gender-specific association between −1082 IL-10 promoter polymorphism and longevity. Genes Immun 3(1):30–33

Lio D, Pes GM, Carru C et al (2003a) Association between the HLA-DR alleles and longevity: a study in Sardinian population. Exp Gerontol 38(3):313–317

Lio D, Scola L, Crivello A et al (2003b) Inflammation, genetics, and longevity: further studies on the protective effects in men of IL-10 −1082 promoter SNP and its interaction with TNF-alpha −308 promoter SNP. J Med Genet 40(4):296–299

Lio D, Candore G, Crivello A et al (2004) Opposite effects of interleukin 10 common gene polymorphisms in cardiovascular diseases and in successful ageing: genetic background of male centenarians is protective against coronary heart disease. J Med Genet 41(10):790–794

Mahmoodi M, Nahvi H, Mahmoudi M et al (2012) HLA-DRB1,-DQA1 and -DQB1 allele and haplotype frequencies in female patients with early onset breast cancer. Pathol Oncol Res 18(1):49–55

Mahmoudi M, Amirzargar AA, Jamshidi AR et al (2011) Association of IL1R polymorphism with HLA-B27 positive in Iranian patients with ankylosing spondylitis. Eur Cytokine Netw 22(4):175–180

Mendelsohn ME, Karas RH (1999) The protective effects of estrogen on the cardiovascular system. N Engl J Med 340(23):1801–1811

Miriam Capri, Stefano Salvioli, Federica Sevini, Silvana Valensin, Laura Celani, Daniela Monti, Graham Pawelec, Giovanna De Benedictis, E Efstathios S. Gonos, and Claudio Francesch (2006) The Genetics of Human Longevity. Ann. N.Y. Acad. Sci, 1067: 252–263

Mirahmadian M, Kalantar F, Heidari G et al (2008) Association of tumor necrosis factor-alpha and interleukin-10 gene polymorphisms in Iranian patients with pre-eclampsia. Am J Reprod Immunol 60(2): 179–185

Moazzeni SM, Amirzargar AA, Shokri F (1999) HLA antigens in Iranian patients with B-cell chronic lymphocytic leukemia. Pathol Oncol Res 5(2):142–145

Mohammadi J, Pourpak Z, Jarefors S et al (2008) Human leukocyte antigens (HLA) associated with selective IgA deficiency in Iran and Sweden. Iran J Allergy Asthma Immunol 7(4):209–214

Mortazavi H, Amirzargar AA, Esmaili N et al (2013) Association of human leukocyte antigen class I antigens in Iranian patients with pemphigus vulgaris. J Dermatol 40(4):244–248

Movahedi M, Moin M, Gharagozlou M et al (2008) Association of HLA class II alleles with childhood asthma and Total IgE levels. Iran J Allergy Asthma Immunol 7(4):215–220

Naumova E, Ivanova M, Pawelec G et al (2011) 'Immunogenetics of Aging': report on the activities of the 15th International HLA and Immunogenetics Working Group and 15th International HLA and Immunogenetics Workshop. Tissue Antigens 77(3): 187–192

Nicknam MH, Mahmoudi M, Amirzargar AA et al (2008) Determination of HLA-B27 subtypes in Iranian patients with ankylosing spondylitis. Iran J Allergy Asthma Immunol 7(1):19–24

Okayama N, Hamanaka Y, Suehiro Y et al (2005) Association of interleukin-10 promoter single nucleotide polymorphisms −819 T/C and −592 A/C with aging. J Gerontol A Biol Sci Med Sci 60(12):1525–1529

Olivieri F, Bonafe M, Cavallone L et al (2002) The −174 C/G locus affects in vitro/in vivo IL-6 production during aging. Exp Gerontol 37(2–3):309–314

Ostan R, Bucci L, Capri M et al (2008) Immunosenescence and immunogenetics of human longevity. Neuroimmunomodulation 15(4–6):224–240

Papasteriades C, Boki K, Pappa H et al (1997) HLA phenotypes in healthy aged subjects. Gerontology 43(3): 176–181

Pietrangelo A (2010) Hereditary hemochromatosis: pathogenesis, diagnosis, and treatment. Gastroenterology 139(2):393–408

Proust J, Moulias R, Fumeron F et al (1982) HLA and longevity. Tissue Antigens 19(3):168–173

Rabbani A, Abbasi F, Taghvaei M et al (2012) HLA-DRB, -DQA, and DQB alleles and haplotypes in Iranian patients with diabetes mellitus type I. Pediatr Diabetes. doi:10.1111/j.1399-5448.2012.00869.x

Rea IM, Middleton D (1994) Is the phenotypic combination A1B8Cw7DR3 a marker for male longevity? J Am Geriatr Soc 42(9):978–983

Rezaei N, Aghamohammadi A, Shakiba Y et al (2009) Cytokine gene polymorphisms in common variable immunodeficiency. Int Arch Allergy Immunol 150(1):1–7

Roberts CW, Walker W, Alexander J (2001) Sex-associated hormones and immunity to protozoan parasites. Clin Microbiol Rev 14(3):476–488

Ross OA, Curran MD, Rea IM et al (2003) HLA haplotypes and TNF polymorphism do not associate with longevity in the Irish. Mech Ageing Dev 124(4):563–567

Salvioli S, Olivieri F, Marchegiani F et al (2006) Genes, ageing and longevity in humans: problems, advantages and perspectives. Free Radic Res 40(12):1303–1323

Sanjabi S, Zenewicz LA, Kamanaka M et al (2009) Anti-inflammatory and pro-inflammatory roles of TGF-beta, IL-10, and IL-22 in immunity and autoimmunity. Curr Opin Pharmacol 9(4):447–453

Sarafnejad A, Khosravi F, Alimoghadam K et al (2006) HLA class II allele and haplotype frequencies in Iranian patients with acute myelogenous leukemia and control group. Iran J Allergy Asthma Immunol 5(3):115–119

Scola L, Lio D, Candore G et al (2008) Analysis of HLA-DRB1, DQA1, DQB1 haplotypes in Sardinian centenarians. Exp Gerontol 43(2):114–118

Shahram F, Nikoopour E, Rezaei N et al (2011) Association of interleukin-2, interleukin-4 and transforming growth factor-beta gene polymorphisms with Behcet's disease. Clin Exp Rheumatol 29(4 Suppl 67):S28–S31

Shams S, Amirzargar AA, Yousefi M et al (2009) HLA class II (DRB, DQA1 and DQB1) allele and haplotype frequencies in the patients with pemphigus vulgaris. J Clin Immunol 29(2):175–179

Shokrgozar MA, Sarial S, Amirzargar A et al (2009) IL-2, IFN-gamma, and IL-12 gene polymorphisms and susceptibility to multiple sclerosis. J Clin Immunol 29(6):747–751

Sonya Vasto, Eugenio Mocchegiani, Giuseppina Candore (2006) Florinda Listi etal Inflammation, genes and zinc in ageing and age-related diseases Biogerontology 7:315–327.

Takata H, Suzuki M, Ishii T et al (1987) Influence of major histocompatibility complex region genes on human longevity among Okinawan-Japanese centenarians and nonagenarians. Lancet 2(8563):824–826

Terry DF, McCormick M, Andersen S, Pennington J, Schoenhofen E, Palaima E, Bausero M, Ogawa K, Perls TT (2004) Asea A: Cardiovascular disease delay in centenarian offspring: role of heat shock proteins. Ann N Y Acad Sci, 1019:502–505.

Vasto S, Mocchegiani E, Candore G et al (2006) Inflammation, genes and zinc in ageing and age-related diseases. Biogerontology 7(5–6):315–327

Vaupel JW, Carey JR, Christensen K et al (1998) Biodemographic trajectories of longevity. Science 280(5365):855–860

Vina J, Borras C, Gambini J et al (2005) Why females live longer than males: control of longevity by sex hormones. Sci Aging Knowledge Environ 2005(23):pe17

Weidemann W, Hanke H (2002) Cardiovascular effects of androgens. Cardiovasc Drug Rev 20(3):175–198

Aging Immunity and Infection

17

Mehdi Shekarabi and Fatemeh Asgari

17.1 Immunosenescence and Susceptibility to Infections

Immunosenescence is defined as an age-related malfunction of the immune system usually accompanied by the increase of susceptibility to many bacterial, viral, and parasitic infections; it is evident that administration of many vaccines such as influenza virus vaccine (IFV) in elderly is not so efficient as in the young individuals. Aged individuals traveling to tropical countries are quite prone to be infected by opportunistic and endemic viral/bacterial agents. Failure of T cell responses during aging may also lead to reactivation of tuberculosis (TB).

Although many hypotheses proposed for the increased susceptibility to infections, it is almost acceptable that there is no defect in the immune cell number, and there are little data to indicate that aging is associated with increased susceptibility to all infections, and it is controversial that whether aging alone or aging-related diseases are responsible for vulnerability to infections, and to elucidate the cause and effect relationship between aging and infections depends on individual cases and is varied in different infections.

17.2 Aging Infections: Epidemiologic Perspective

Generally many infections occur more commonly in older individuals and infections with higher morbidity and mortality may appear during old ages. Bacterial pneumonia and other lower respiratory tract infections (LRTI), urethrocystitis, skin infections, sepsis with complicated unknown origin, infectious endocarditic, cholecystitis, and other intra-abdominal infection are among the most prevalent infections. Tuberculosis, varicella zoster infection, and skin and soft tissue infection with special etiologic agents are considered prevalent in elderly depending on specific epidemiologic condition. Majority of these infections affected old people with higher clinical complication and higher death rate compared with younger adults; for example, urinary tract infections (UTI) are 20-fold more prevalent in aged individuals; in addition, the elderly are mostly encountered with pyrogenic bacteria opposite young individuals who are encountered with low-virulence agents such as enteric bacteria.

The frequency of infections is high in hospitalized elderly and also elderly institutionalized in nursing houses, which is due to higher use of urethral catheters and other prosthetic devices in geriatrics. One of the most life-threatening

M. Shekarabi, PhD (✉) • F. Asgari, MSc
Department of Immunology, School of Medicine,
Iran University of Medical Sciences, Tehran, Iran
e-mail: m_shekarabi@yahoo.com

A. Massoud, N. Rezaei (eds.), *Immunology of Aging*,
DOI 10.1007/978-3-642-39495-9_17, © Springer-Verlag Berlin Heidelberg 2014

infections is pneumococcal pneumonia or meningitis, *Escherichia coli* and *Pseudomonas aeruginosa* are the most common isolated in old patients after catheterization, and staphylococcal species especially *Staphylococcus aureus* were the most common isolate associated with intravenous catheters in postsurgical wound infection.

Although viral infection is not so common, influenza and reactivated varicella zoster virus (VZV) frequently occurred; therefore, vaccination for influenza is highly recommended in elderly especially in those individuals who suffer from a chronic disease such as diabetes or cancer.

17.3 Clinical Consequences of Infection in Elderly

During senescence, changes in physiological condition result in a change in causative agents, and comorbidies of infection are more common than those occurred in younger adults.

Infections in younger adults present with several symptoms but in the elderly the same infections tend to have fewer symptoms. Atypical signs and symptoms contribute to the higher morbidity and mortality, though late diagnosis and poor response to antimicrobial therapy might also contribute.

17.4 Immune System and Aging

Increased risks of infections with severe clinical outcome occurred partly due to impairment of immune defenses that might be aggravated by chronic infections, malnutrition, and prolonged medication received during aging.

Immune decrement might involve all the functional categories of immune system including both innate and adaptive immunity.

17.4.1 Innate Immune Defect

There is no significant quantitative change in the component of innate immunity such as neutrophils, macrophage, natural killer (NK) cells, and

complement activity, but it seems that response to cytokine and their signals and cytokine production may be altered. Under normal conditions, many proinflammatory cytokines such as interleukin (IL)-10, tumor necrosis factor alpha (TNF-α), IL-1, and their receptors function as a body regulatory mediator, and imbalance and overproduction of cytokines can cause tissue destruction, microvascular damage, and impaired tissue oxygenation leading to organ dysfunction. The minor defect of phagocyte in sepsis detected by using sophisticated technique seems to have no significant impact on age-related severity of disease. It is experimentally proved that in vitro activation of leukocytes by lipopolysaccharide (LPS) in elderly causes the release of higher amount of IL-1, IL-6, IL-8, and TNF-α, but severity of disease is not proportionally related to cytokine concentration.

A prospective study of the effect of age on the circulating adhesion molecules in critically ill patients showed higher level of these molecules in the elderly but there was no clear explanation for these findings. However, it could be concluded that higher frequency of sepsis during aging might be mostly attributed to the age-related anatomic and physiological changes in the neurologic, cardiovascular, pulmonary, and renal system. The change in the cellular components of innate immunity is summarized in Table 17.1.

Although during aging, number and phagocytic capacity of neutrophils are preserved, other functional capabilities might be altered. Generally, toll-like receptor (TLR) ligation enhances phagocytosis, chemotaxis, and recruitment of other immune cells in the site of infection. During aging, receptor-related functions, leukocyte activation, and superoxide production are impaired. It has been showed that alteration in the neutrophil membrane lipid rafts is involved in aging, and this might be related to the TLR and granulocyte/macrophage colony-stimulating factor (GM-CSF) receptor signaling. Although their expression might not change in young individuals, LPS stimulation induces TLR4 reorientation in the immunological synapse. In contrast, in the elderly LPS stimulation induces changes in the TLR4 reorientation. In young people, binding of GM-CSF to its receptor induces displacement of

Table 17.1 Innate immunity and changing with age

Components of innate immunity	Changes during aging
PMN cells	Decreased chemotaxis (impaired tissue penetration), ROS production, signal transduction, TLR4 recruitment to lipid raft, action polymerization, phagocytosis function
	Impaired cAMP pathway
	Defective bactericidal function
	Delay in apoptosis during inflammation
Macrophage	Decreased chemotaxis, Apoptosis, superoxide production, phagocytosis, killing (impaired tumor lysis related to impaired response to IFN-γ or LPS), signal transduction, wound healing, MHC class II expression, surface expression of CD14, TLR pathway components, STAT-1, NF-κB
	Defective bactericidal function
	Increased production of inflammatory cytokine
NK cells	Decreased response to stimulatory cytokines (IL-2, IL-12, IFN-α, IFN-β, and IFN-γ), cytokine production, cytolytic potential, signal transduction
Dendritic cell	Decreased number of Langerhans cells, antigen uptake
	Impaired homing to secondary lymph node

Src family tyrosine phosphatase-1 (SHP-1) from lipid raft, while there is no delayed regulation of phosphatases in the elderly. SHP-1 functions as dephosphorylating protein involved in activation pathway; therefore, their presence in the lipid raft would block cell activation.

Phagocyte dysfunctions were studied in several experimental studies during aging (Gomez et al. 2008). Defects in cell surface expression of molecules such as major histocompatibility complex (MHC) II, CD4, and TLRs, which are downregulated, show defect in cell signaling pathways. Ca-dependent cellular signal transduction and actin polymerization are defected in chemokine-stimulated neutrophils and intracellular signal transducers, and activators of transcription 1 (STAT-1), phospholipase C (PLC)

phosphorylation, and nuclear factor kappa-light-chain-enhancer of activated B cell (NFκB) production are also reduced in phagocytes.

Aging is generally accompanied by chronic diseases such as cardiovascular disease, osteoporosis, arthritis, type 2 diabetes (T2DM), Alzheimer's disease, and neurodegenerative diseases, and in these conditions, the onset and outcome of disease are influenced by the level of proinflammatory cytokines. Diseases such as arthritis, periodontal diseases, and chronic obstructive pulmonary disease (COPD) are associated with abnormal exaggerated inflammatory responses that affect multiple organ system. However, many chronic inflammatory diseases in the elderly such as T2DM and atherosclerosis occurred without a specific organ involvement and not clearly caused by infectious agents, while sustained inflammation and prolonged macrophage activation is a major pathogenic event. Recruited macrophages are the major source of proinflammatory cytokines which are implicated in various disease conditions during aging.

One of the ways of improving the immune potency in aged individual is innate immune potentiation as an alternative strategy to defend against infections provided that excessive inflammatory condition is avoided.

17.4.2 Defects of Adaptive Immunity

Marked changes observed with aging in both cellular and humoral components of immunity are summarized in Table 17.2. Most T cells both in peripheral blood and secondary lymphoid organ present with a memory phenotype and their proliferation and IL-2 production are reduced. T cells in the elderly show low proliferation index to mitogen and specific antigens not explained by IL-2 production alone. Although these are individual variation due to differences in state of health and nutritional condition and probable accompanied chronic diseases. Among T cell subsets, CD4$^+$ naïve T cells are less influenced by aging than CD8$^+$ T cells. Functional impairment of CD4$^+$ T cells is demonstrated both in animal model and human. An age-related increase in

Table 17.2 Summary of aging changes in acquired immunity

Components of adaptive immunity	Changes during aging
T cells	Decrease in thymocytes, reduced number of naïve CD4+ T cells (number of effector and memory CD4+ T cells, PGE2 and IL-10)
	Decreased IL-2 and IL-2R, costimulatory molecule expression (CD28), CD8+ T cell expansion and proliferation
B cells	Increased plasma cells in marrow, memory B cell, autoantibodies, low-affinity antibodies
	Decreased naïve B cell, response to IL-7 stimulation, repertoire diversity, costimulatory molecules including MHC II, CD40, booster effect, efficacy of antibody in preventing infection

memory T cells is confirmed in several European populations (Choi 2001).

Many investigators show that aging process is associated with impairment of effector response to newly acquired antigen by both T cell and B cells possibly reflecting the phenomenon that naïve CD4+ T cells shifted to a memory phenotype (CD44^{high} CD45^{RO}) and reduction of CD44^{low} CD45^{RA} and showing depletion of naïve CD4+ T cells, and it is generally proposed that response to newly acquired antigen in aged individuals is mediated mostly by cross-reactive memory T cells.

The effects of aging on MHCII and MHCII processing pathway are not clearly defined, though diminished cytokine production may result in diminished antigen processing and presentation.

Finally B cell production of specific high-affinity antibody by cells reduced with age. This is proved by both in vitro and in vivo since relatively healthy elderly people do not respond to T-dependent antigens such as influenza virus envelope protein (Table 17.2).

17.4.3 Mucosal Immunity

Mucosal epithelial cells are more than a mechanical barrier and they function as a major source of antibacterial agents. The skin is shown to be a tight mechanical barrier as well as to have antibacterial properties due to low PH and glandular secretion by sebaceous glands. Aged skin significantly changes in both dermal thickness and subcutaneous glandular secretions; therefore, dry thin skin is very prone to break and cannot withstand shearing forces. During aging, the skin becomes avascular and susceptible to break, making it more prone to injury. Vascular disease and other coexisting illnesses may cause worse prognosis and facilitate bacterial colonization and tissue microbial invasion. There is also loss of Langerhans cells and lower cytokine production both of which affect antigen-processing pathway and decreasing specific immune response.

Mucus secretion and ciliary motion of the mucosal epithelial cells can remove the invading bacteria and prevent their invasion into deeper tissues. During aging, both secretion and ciliary action are reduced; however, it is not clear whether or not aging reduces the ability of mucosa to perform a host defense. Nevertheless, certain gastrointestinal diseases such as diverticulitis and ischemic bowel disease are more commonly observed in geriatric patients. Although mucosal immunoglobulin (Ig) A does not appear to be reduced with age, aged subjects are generally more susceptible to infections of the external mucosal surface. Few studies demonstrated elevated polyclonal serum IgA but the same increase was not reported in the intestine (Ogra 2010).

Animal studies suggested no impairment of mucosal immune functions although the number of Peyer's patch regress with age. In spite of change of T and B cells in the lymphoid organs, intestinal T and B cells seem to retain normal function and phenotypes. In an experimental study, infusion of cholera toxin develops impaired specific B cell response at mucosal surfaces (Ogra 2010). This might be due to reduction of homing cells from inductive sites to effector sites by antigen-specific B cells. Other animal studies showed qualitative and quantitative change in gut-associated lymphoid tissue (GALT)-associated T and B cells and their subpopulations. Other investigators suggest probable defect in direct cell-to-cell interaction and changes in pattern of cytokine production which may cause cellular and antibody immune abnormalities in GALT. On subcellular lines, aged T and B cells exhibit impaired transmembranous signal transduction.

Currently, information regarding innate mucosal mechanism is limited but decrease in lysozyme raised the possibility of decline of innate immunity in conjunctiva and upper airways.

The most dramatic change in the intestinal microbiota occurred in the compositions of the flora. During adulthood, under a normal food intake, usually intestinal microbial species and their quantity are almost stable unless in the use of antibiotics. During aging, this stability impairs and it is reported that bifidobacteria declined, while Lactobacilli, coliforms, and enterococci increased (Tiihonen et al. 2010). It is generally concluded that since immune function impairs in aging, it is expected that immune tolerance toward intestinal flora is disrupted leading to change in the composition of individual flora.

In spite of the many evidences reported above, mucosal immune function maintained relatively normal in aging subjects.

17.5 Common Infections During Elderly

17.5.1 Bacterial Meningitis

Atypical bacterial meningitis presents in older individuals with higher morbidity and mortality; therefore, its early diagnosis is more difficult. The most prevalent etiologic agents are *Streptococcus pneumoniae, Listeria monocytogenes, Streptococcus agalactiae, Escherichia coli, Klebsiella pneumoniae, Proteus sp, Enterobacter sp,* and *Pseudomonas aeruginosa.* Viral meningitis is not prevalent during aging. Concomitant treatment with corticosteroid and chemotherapeutic agents for chronic disease in aging such as T2DM, asthma, osteoporosis, or cancer may alter the clinical picture of meningitis, for example, fever and stiffness are not observed clinically. The underlying cause of bacterial meningitis during aging is often related to both cellular and humeral immunity.

17.5.2 Respiratory Infections

Chronic obstructive pulmonary disease (COPD), lung neoplasms, and pneumonia are relatively common in aged individuals, among them particularly pneumonia present with high mortality. Age-associated conditions that affect lung function, including defect in airway ciliary motion and airway hyper reactivity, may diminish pulmonary respiratory capacity and increase the impact of respiratory pathogens. Malnutrition, chronic cardiovascular disease, prolonged immunosuppressive therapy, and hospitalization or institutionalism enhance the clinical severity. Viral infections may also have important role for predisposing secondary bacterial infections as observed for influenza A and B and respiratory syncytial virus infections. In addition to viral infections, tuberculosis especially infection with mycobacterium avium-intracellulare seems to be increasingly prevalent which will be described later (Meyer 2001).

17.5.3 Tuberculosis

Chronic tuberculosis is especially of clinical significance in elderly. In developing countries and in endemic areas, most aged individuals are the largest reservoir for *Mycobacterium tuberculosis* (MTB). As previously described the principal route of infection of MTB is upper and lower airways, and primary infection occurred in lower middle lobes of the lungs. Alveolar macrophages as the main antigen-presenting cells (APCs) take up the inhaled pathogen and migrate to regional lymphatic organ specifically mediastinal lymph nodes. Infected macrophages are activated and process and present mycobacterial antigen to naïve CD4[+] T cells and produce chemokines that result in the recruitment of additional mononuclear cells which in turn produce significant proteolytic enzymes generating an exudative lesion finally converting to granuloma. The whole process occurs approximately after 3–4 weeks which are associated with positive skin reactivity to tuberculin skin test (TST) by standard PPD injection.

The characteristic tubercle granuloma ultimately produced and surrounded by organized epithelioid cells, CD4$^+$ T cells and $\gamma\delta$ T cells restraining the tubercle bacilli. Reactivation occurred due to uncontrolled activation of cytolytic T cells. NK cells and activated macrophages exposing to huge amount of cytokine especially interferon gamma (IFN-γ).

Besides the other underlying causes, aging is also a major predisposing factor for secondary TB infections. The increased susceptibility for TB infection in elderly might be due to impairment of cell-mediated immunity. Approximately 90 % of TB infection in the elderly are due to reactivation of primary infection while without underlying causes may occur in 30–40 % of individuals (Yoshikawa and Norman 2009). It is very rare that infected elderly individuals eventually clear the infection and convert to a skin seronegative patient; thus, it is partly concluded that aged individuals with TB are not considered as newly infected patients, and in these cases, latent and subclinical primary infections are reactivated.

17.5.4 Fungal Infections

Taking medications and comorbidities with autoimmune diseases, asthma, and cancers in old patients make them susceptible for opportunistic fungal infections with poorer outcome than those infections in young adults. The actual prevalence of mycosis in old ages depends on the geographical areas, outdoor activities, and life habits. Renal failure, use of parenteral infusion, and long-term antibiotic therapy contribute to higher risk of infection with Candida species. Cryptococcosis is a common secondary infection in acquired immunodeficiency syndrome (AIDS) patients; it is reported that 25 % of AIDS patients with cryptococcal meningitis are older than 60 years, which present with poorer prognosis and higher mortality. Although less common than Candidiasis, aspergillus infection is life-threatening in old hospitalized patients. Chronic necrotizing pulmonary infection and sinusoidal infection are the most common aspergillus infection in elderly (Table 17.3).

Table 17.3 Risk factor of systemic opportunistic fungal infections in older adults

Fungal infections	Risk factors
Candidiasis	Neutropenia, hematologic malignancy, corticosteroids, transplant, ICU, antibiotics, IV catheters, GI surgical procedure
Cryptococcosis	Lymphoma, transplant, cirrhosis, corticosteroids
Aspergillosis	Neutropenia, hematologic malignancy, transplant, corticosteroids
Mucormycosis	Hematologic malignancy, diabetes mellitus, neutropenia

17.5.5 Viral Infections

Aging impairs adaptive T cell response to influenza, Epstein–Barr virus (EBV), cytomegalovirus (CMV), and VZV infections. Many researches show that CD8$^+$ T cell specific response, IFN-γ release, and cytolytic activity decrease with aging leading to impaired CD8$^+$ T cell proliferation clonal expansion. This is partly related to lower efficiency of influenza vaccination in aging.

EBV infections are not very common, but in those cases that occurred in elderly individuals by the absence of EBV antibodies and present not prominent signs such as classical mononucleosis that are observed during adolescence.

Apart from other persistent herpesvirus infections such as EBV, herpes simplex virus (HSV), and VZV, CMV infections are unique since it is proposed that early infection with CMV is advantageous probably because of enhanced proinflammatory status in infected individuals which might have a protective effect on other pathogens. This would be yet another example of antagonistic pleiotropy which seems to be a contribution to immunosenescence (Caruso et al. 2009).

A longitudinal study performed in Swedish population and later confirmed in Finnish people established alteration in the elderly immune system described as immune risk phenotypes (IRP) as predication of decrease in 2-year survival rates (Buchholz et al. 2011). In those studies CMV seropositivity is highlighted and the phenomenon that CMV infection leads to increased rate of mortality is excluded. However, it is speculated that CD8$^+$ T cell population against CMV and expansion of CMV-specific clones have adverse effect on maintenance of T cell repertoire and make an immunocompromised condition in elderly.

VZV infection is a common illness during elderly and reactivation of dormant viruses and involvement of skin peripheral nerves are markedly seen with old ages. There does not seem to be any decline in specific antibody but VZV-specific cell-mediated immunity (CMI) is critical to prevent the viral reactivation and spread of the viruses residing in the nerve ganglia.

17.6 Autoimmunity

There are evidences in mice that the percentage of autoimmune CD8$^+$ T cell increased with reduced apoptosis; therefore, it is concluded that aging is associated with immune dysregulation which can lead in increased production of self-reactivating autoantibodies predisposing the people to develop autoimmune diseases. Most autoantibodies produced with aging are organ nonspecific including autoantibodies against DNA and membrane phospholipids such as antiphospholipid antibodies, antinuclear antibody, and rheumatoid factor. The increase in autoantibody production is not directly related to T cell proliferation since in vitro T cell proliferation to mitogens impaired in aging. The production of autoantibodies and polyclonal B cell activation might be caused by many latent infections which are common in aged individuals.

17.7 Vaccinations

During aging vaccine efficacy is reduced tremendously and most viral and bacterial vaccines administered in individuals greater than 65 years of age show diminished response and produced low protective antibodies. Old recipients of influenza, hepatitis B virus (HBV), and pneumococci vaccines develop less than half protective antibodies. Besides that the produced antibodies are of less functional activities, for example, lower capability to act as opsonins or lower ability to fix complement. For these reasons it is recommended that people older than 65 years should be vaccinated every year for pneumococci (Avelino-Silva et al. 2011).

Except for vaccines that have to be administered in special situations such as in those where old individuals are traveling to highly endemic areas or are exposed to fungal bacterial agents outdoors during vacation, routinely aged people are vaccinated against tetanus-diphtheria toxoids, influenza, and pneumococci. Recommended immunizing schedule for old ages is shown in Table 17.4 (Yoshikawa and Norman 2009).

The laboratory evaluation of vaccine efficacy is mandatory since in general in old age the response is more variable than responses by younger and in those individuals with clinical evidences of low response suggest approaches for enhancing vaccination strategies.

Of the recommended vaccines, many older people show antibody level blow the optimum against tetanus-diphtheria-acellular pertussis (Tdap) recommended to administer every 10 years although the risk for pertussis

Table 17.4 Recommended immunizing agents for persons aged ≥65 years

Vaccine type	Usual schedule	Indications
Tetanus-diphtheria, pertussis (TD/Tdap)	One dose if contact with <12-month-old child booster every 10 years	All elderly persons; tetanus prophylaxis in wound management
Influenza vaccine	One dose annually Administered IM optimal time during autumn, winter	Persons at high-risk influenza, immunosuppressed persons; all healthy elderly persons
Pneumococcal polysaccharide vaccine	One dose	Persons at high-risk pneumococcal disease, immunosuppressed persons; all healthy elderly persons
Zoster	One dose	Person who lacks documentation of vaccination or has no evidence of previous infection

during old age is not defined but it is recommended to administer Tdap every decade.

Although influenza and pneumococcal vaccine are administered routinely in old ages, it does not seem to prevent infection in general population but may attenuate the course of diseases preventing prolonged hospitalization and presenting the spread of infection among institutionalized elderly people. Besides the scheduled vaccine program given, recently these are great concern on other pathogens which are of major risk in aging, for example, varicella zoster vaccine (VZV) which reactivates as painful skin lesions in old age when the cell-mediated immune function is impaired. It has been shown that vaccination with live attenuated form of VZV elicits prominent IFN-γ release and had protectivity in post-herpetic neuralgia. Together with influenza, respiratory syncytial virus (RSV) accounts for a substantial majority of pediatric and young adult respiratory infection. In aging people, the T cell response and in vitro IFN-γ production are reduced; on the other hand, stable attenuation of RSV has been difficult to achieve and vaccine safety concern result is their cautious in advancement of clinical evaluation. However, the immune correlates of protection against RSV are not clearly defined.

CMV is also becoming increasingly important as a vaccine in elderly. Many studies have identified latent CMV infection as a major contributing factor for the previously described phenomenon so-called immune risk phenotype for early mortality and immunologically marked as high $CD8^+$ T cells, many of them are specific for CMV. Therefore, maintenance of latency and prevention of fatal reactivation over time require active immunization. For this reason, it is proposed that childhood vaccination against CMV might be practically effective for preventing senescent CMV-specific $CD8^+$ cells in old age (Effros 2007).

References

Avelino-Silva VI, Ho YL, Avelino-Silva TJ et al (2011) Aging and HIV infection. Ageing Res Rev 10(1): 163–172

Buchholz VR, Neuenhahn M, Busch DH (2011) $CD8^+$ T cell differentiation in the aging immune system: until the last clone standing. Curr Opin Immunol 23(4):549–554

Caruso C, Buffa S, Candore G et al (2009) Mechanisms of immunosenescence. Immun Ageing 6(10)

Choi C (2001) Bacterial meningitis in aging adults. Clin infect dis 33(8):1380–1385

Effros RB (2007) Role of T lymphocyte replicative senescence in vaccine efficacy. Vaccine 25(4):599–604

Gomez CR, Nomellini V, Faunce DE et al (2008) Innate immunity and aging. Exp Gerontol 43(8):718–728

Meyer KC (2001) The role of immunity in susceptibility to respiratory infection in the aging lung. Respir Physiol 128(1):23

Ogra PL (2010) Ageing and its possible impact on mucosal immune responses. Ageing Res Rev 9(2):101–106

Tiihonen K, Ouwehand AC, Rautonen N (2010) Human intestinal microbiota and healthy ageing. Ageing Res Rev 9(2):107

Yoshikawa T, Norman D (2009) Infectious disease in the aging: a clinical handbook. Humana Press, New York

Influenza Infection in the Elderly

18

Kasra Moazzami, Janet E. McElhaney, and Nima Rezaei

18.1 Introduction

Influenza, a febrile respiratory illness, causes more than 200,000 hospitalizations and 36,000 deaths in the United States (US) every year and is the seventh leading cause of death in the country (Thompson et al. 2003, 2004). Most influenza infections are associated with a mild acute self-limited illness. However, certain risk factors are associated with severity of the disease and the occurrence of influenza-related complications. Age is considered among the most important factors associated with the severity of disease. While patients at the extremes of age (less than 6 months or more than 65 years) are at the highest risk for developing complications, up to 90 % of influenza-related deaths occur in persons aged 65 years or older (Thompson et al. 2003). Therefore, understanding the significance of influenza infection in this population group as well as designing strategies to decrease the morbidity and mortality of elderly patients affected by influenza is of utmost importance.

18.2 Impact of Influenza in Older Adults

Aging is associated with a general increase in the susceptibility to infectious diseases. However, influenza infection has shown to be foremost among all infectious diseases in its association with an age-related increase in the incidence of serious complications.

18.2.1 Clinical Presentations

In comparison to the younger population (children and young adults), the clinical course of influenza infection shows dramatic differences among the elderly. Fever, which is considered to be among the most classical presentations in young adults, is less commonly seen in the elderly (Drinka et al. 2003; Loeb 2003). In more than 80 % of cases, cough is the most common presenting feature in the older population. Also, other lower respiratory tract symptoms including wheeze and chest pain are more often observed in these patients. The incidence of secondary bacterial pneumonia is also higher in this age group.

K. Moazzami, MD, MPH
Cardiovascular Research Center,
Massachusetts General Hospital,
Harvard Medical School, Charlestown, MA, USA

J.E. McElhaney, MD, FRCPC, FACP
Vancouver Coastal Health Research Institute,
University of British Columbia,
Vancouver, BC, Canada

N. Rezaei, MD, MSc, PhD (✉)
Research Center for Immunodeficiencies,
Children's Medical Center,
Tehran University of Medical Sciences, Tehran, Iran

Department of Immunology, School of Medicine,
Tehran University of Medical Sciences, Tehran, Iran

Molecular Immunology Research Center,
Tehran University of Medical Sciences, Tehran, Iran
e-mail: rezaei_nima@tums.ac.ir

A. Massoud, N. Rezaei (eds.), *Immunology of Aging*,
DOI 10.1007/978-3-642-39495-9_18, © Springer-Verlag Berlin Heidelberg 2014

Finally, gastrointestinal symptoms are more frequently seen in the elderly than in younger adults (McElhaney 2005).

18.2.2 Morbidity and Mortality

In the older population, influenza has been associated with a substantial increase in the rate of hospitalization, contributing to approximately 180,000 hospitalizations each year in the US (Thompson et al. 2003, 2004). In a study done in the United Kingdom (UK), the combined average hospital stay for influenza and pneumonia was 11.5 days in which 71 % of patients were in the age group of more than 60 years. Also, around 5 % of these patients remained in the hospital for as long as 28 days (Turner et al. 2006). Moreover, for patients between 65 and 74 years of age with a preexisting medical condition, the risk increases sharply (around seven times), in comparison to those who do not have a medical condition (Whitley and Monto 2006).

Disability, defined as a loss of three or more basic activities of daily living in older adults, has been recognized as a major complication of influenza and influenza-related hospitalizations (Barker et al. 1998; Falsey et al. 2005). An acute influenza infection could be a trigger for catastrophic disability. Nearly one-third of older adults in the US, who have been hospitalized, are discharged with a higher level of disability compared to before they became ill, and one-half of these individuals never recover to their previous baseline (Covinsky et al. 2003). Older patients may lose up to 5 % of muscle power (Aspinall et al. 2004) and 1 % of aerobic capacity per day of bed rest (Lalvani et al. 1997). Therefore, patients hospitalized with influenza illness may lose up to 50 % of lower limb muscle strength; their reduced functional capacity may result in a significant and permanent disability following an acute influenza illness.

Exacerbations of underlying medical conditions are also an important cause of morbidity and mortality in influenza-affected patients (Blasco et al. 1995). Influenza is often considered the underlying cause of acute coronary syndromes, strokes, and exacerbations of congestive heart failure in the older population.

Regarding mortality, influenza is associated with nearly 90 % of the 31,000–51,000 excess deaths from all causes in older adults (Thompson et al. 2003). Patients with underlying chronic disease are further susceptible to higher death rates. Influenza has been specifically associated with increased mortality from ischemic heart disease, cerebrovascular disease, and diabetes (Reichert et al. 2004). Influenza has been identified as the probable cause of most of the excess deaths due to these complications in the population age 70 years and older during the winter months (Reichert et al. 2004; Govaert et al. 1994). Finally, mortality rates due to influenza have raised and almost doubled in the period 1990–1999, compared to the period 1976–1990 (Thompson et al. 2004).

In addition to the significant medical burden of disease, influenza poses a considerable economic burden, mainly due to high hospitalization rates as well as lost lives. Older adults have been responsible for over 60 % of the total economic burden of influenza, which averages $10.4 billion per year in direct medical costs in the US (Molinari et al. 2007). However, it should be noted that the estimated burden of disease has not considered the financial burden of disability associated with influenza infection in this population, which further increases the societal cost of influenza.

18.3 The Aging Respiratory and the Immune Systems

18.3.1 Respiratory System

Aging results in a progressive decline in lung performance (Janssens and Krause 2004). First of all, functional residual capacity of the lungs is increased as a result of a decrease in the elastic recoil of the lung and also a decrease in the compliance of the chest wall. Therefore, in order to maintain adequate respiratory volumes, older adults have to breathe at higher lung volumes which increases the workload imposed on respiratory muscles (Janssens and Krause 2004). However, aging also negatively affects the respiratory muscle performance. Stiffening of the chest wall as a result of rib cage calcification, flattening of the diaphragm as a consequence of dorsal kyphosis, and increased anteroposterior diameter of the thorax all result in the diminished force-generating capabilities of the respiratory muscles. Moreover, underlying medical conditions, such as chronic heart failure and cerebral vascular disease (which are frequently observed in the older population), further decrease the respiratory muscle strength (Evans et al. 1995; Brown 1994). Finally, nutritional deficiencies which are common in the older population directly decrease the muscle strength (Tolep and Kelsen 1993). Therefore, in the setting of clinical conditions such as influenza and associated pneumonias, the additional load placed on the respiratory muscles may compromise lung function and lead to hypoventilation and the development of respiratory failure.

The intrinsic respiratory defense mechanisms also show decreased responsiveness to foreign agents such as infections with advanced age. The forced expiratory volumes and peak expiratory flow are significantly reduced in the elderly due to structural changes and chronic low-grade inflammation in peripheral airways (Meyer et al. 1996). The decreased expiratory force therefore diminishes the capability of pulmonary system to clear airway secretions by coughing. Therefore, the increased incidence of coughing in the elderly following influenza infection may be due to less effective clearance mechanisms of the lung parenchyma which necessitates more frequent coughing reflexes in order to clear the secretions.

Finally, in older patients, the respiratory centers are less sensitive to hypoxia. This age-related dysfunction leads to delays in important clinical symptoms and signs such as dyspnea and tachypnea, which are among the most important diagnostic clues to influenza-related infections and appreciation of the severity of the associated respiratory impairment (Kronenberg and Drage 1973).

18.3.2 The Immune System

A decrease in immune function is a hallmark of aging that imposes negative effects in its ability to resist influenza virus infection and its response to vaccination. It has been recognized that the aging process affects both branches of the immune system, namely, the innate and adaptive immune systems. While most detrimental age-dependent changes have been attributed to observed defects in the adaptive immune system (Franceschi et al. 2000), defects in various components of the innate immune system further compromise defense mechanisms that are important for suppression of viral replication, thus increasing the susceptibility to severe influenza disease in older people.

18.3.2.1 Innate Immune System

The innate immune responses constitute the first line of host defense to pathogens, are less specific, and lack immunologic memory. The immune response is activated within a few hours of infection and lasts for 1–2 days before the transition to the adaptive immune response. The immunity provided by this system is mediated by a variety of cells including neutrophils, monocytes/macrophages, dendritic cells, natural killer (NK) cells, eosinophils, and basophils and by the secretion of various cytokines and interferons (IFNs) which provide the basis for an adequate response to pathogens. With the progressive age-related decline in lung function, pathogens more easily invade mucosal tissues challenging the aged innate immune system to eradicate pathogens from the body (Gomez et al. 2005; Nomellini et al. 2008).

Neutrophils

Neutrophils are short-lived cells that play an important role in host defense during acute inflammation. Studies have not shown any significant changes in the number of neutrophils in the blood and their precursors in the bone marrow in elderly patients (Chatta et al. 1993). Moreover, neutrophil's ability to be recruited from the periphery along a gradient of chemotactic factors produced at the site of infection through processes of adhesion to vascular endothelial cells and migration into the affected tissue has been shown not to be altered with advanced age (Butcher et al. 2000).

The most important decline in neutrophil function in aged individuals has been attributed to its decreased ability to phagocytize opsonized bacteria, including *Escherichia coli* and *Staphylococcus aureus* (Wenisch et al. 2000). In addition, Fc receptor-mediated superoxide production is significantly reduced in elderly persons (Fulop et al. 1985). This reduced response of neutrophils could be particularly important in the increased propensity of older patients to acquire secondary bacterial pneumonia following an influenza infection and their reduced ability to eradicate the pathogens.

Macrophages

Macrophages have important roles in numerous mechanisms of innate immunity as well as their regulatory effects on the adaptive immune response. They can act directly to destroy invading pathogens or indirectly by initiating inflammatory responses and releasing mediators such as interleukin (IL)-1 and tumor necrosis factor alpha (TNFα) which can activate other inflammatory cells. Additionally, macrophages have an important role in processing antigens and presenting them to T cells.

A number of macrophage functions have been shown to be affected during the aging process. The levels of major histocompatibility complex (MHC) class II molecules in human and rodent macrophages appear to be reduced with aging (Plowden et al. 2004). This, in turn, may contribute to poor CD4$^+$ T cell responses. Also, the respiratory burst induced by IFN-γ has shown to be decreased from aged animals (Plackett et al. 2004). Therefore, impaired respiratory burst in elderly results in diminished intercellular killing ability of bacteria which may elongate the duration of infection (Plackett et al. 2004). Finally, the phagocytic ability of macrophages to ingest bacteria declines with age. These age-related changes in the function of macrophages may thus have an impact on innate as well as adaptive immunity.

Dendritic Cells

Dendritic cells are the most potent of antigen-presenting cells and play an important role in bridging innate immunity with the adaptive immunity (Banchereau and Steinman 1998). These cells have intricate innate properties that account for their roles in the immune system.

First of all, they possess special mechanisms for antigen capture and processing. Also, their unique capacity to migrate to T cell areas and their rapid differentiation or maturation in response to a variety of stimuli render dendritic cells crucial in the defense against pathogens. Finally, they are capable of secreting a variety of cytokines which dictates the nature of T helper responses (Granucci et al. 2003). For instance, while secretion of IL-12 from dendritic cells induces T cells to secrete IFN-γ, the production of IL-10 by dendritic cells induces either a T helper 2 (Th2) or a T regulatory type of response (Dumont et al. 1998).

Advancing age has been associated with a reduced capacity of dendritic cells to take up, process, and present antigens to generate effective T cell responses. Also, dendritic cells isolated from older adults show decreased phagocytic capacity of apoptotic cells compared to that of younger adults (Agrawal et al. 2007). Since phagocytosis of apoptotic cells is considered an important mechanism to prevent inflammation, the decreased phagocytic ability of these cells may be responsible for the observed pro-inflammatory background observed in older individuals (Fadok et al. 1998). Finally, aging is associated with a diminished trafficking capability of dendritic cells to draining lymph nodes, as a result of impaired expression of the lymph node homing markers (Grolleau-Julius et al. 2008). Thus, the age-related impairments in antigen presentation, phagocytosis, and migration of dendritic cells contribute to impairments in immunity in old age.

Natural Killer Cells

NK cells are large granular lymphocytes that play a major role in the MHC unrestricted recognition of virally infected cells. Following influenza infection of the epithelial cells in the lower respiratory system, viral peptides become presented on MHCI. NK cells are then able to detect these cells and become activated through binding to the MHC I-viral peptide complex. This leads to the activation of NK cells, which are then able to directly kill infected cells by releasing perforin and granzymes. These enzymes activate caspases and induce apoptosis of the target cell. A direct association has been recognized between low NK cytotoxicity and increased morbidity and mortality as a result of influenza infection, as well as poor response to influenza vaccination (Solana and Mariani 2000; Molling et al. 2005).

The number and functional capacities of NK cells change through aging. Unlike other lymphocytes, the absolute number of NK cells is increased in aged individuals (Miyaji et al. 2000; Borrego et al. 1999). Regarding functional parameters, cytotoxicity and production of IFN-γ are decreased in old age (Borrego et al. 1999). Also the proliferation rate, levels of CD69 (a stimulatory receptor on NK cell surface), and cytotoxic properties of NK cells in response to IL-2 are also decreased in aging (Solana et al. 1999). However, it should be noted that none of these age-related functional changes have been associated with the impact of influenza, and, for the most part, functional capacity of NK cells appears to be maintained in older adults (McElhaney 2005). This could be attributed in part to the compensatory increase in the number of NK cells in older adults, which could compensate for the diminished activity on a "per cell" basis.

18.3.2.2 The Adaptive Immune System
Humoral Immunity

Influenza infection occurs when there is inadequate antibody to neutralize the virus and prevent entry into the host cells. Following an influenza infection, an antibody response in B cells results in humoral immunity. Aging has been shown to influence the humoral immune response both quantitatively and qualitatively which in turn contributes to the decreased antibody production as well as reduced duration of protective immunity following immunization (Steger et al. 1996). These changes significantly contribute to the increased susceptibility of the elderly to influenza infection and reduce the protective effects of vaccination (McElhaney and Effros 2009).

Regarding quantitative changes in different compartments of the humoral immune system, there are conflicting reports regarding the absolute numbers of human B cell precursors in the bone marrow (McKenna et al. 2001) or not. However, the numbers of mature human B cells

significantly decrease with age (Frasca et al. 2008). Moreover, the total numbers of immunoglobulin M (IgM)-producing memory B cells are reduced in the elderly population which account for the reduction in specific antibody titers in those vaccinated against pneumococcal polysaccharides or exposed to Streptococcus pneumonia infection (Shi et al. 2005). Finally, total switched memory B cells decrease in both percentage and number with age.

The age-related decline in the functional capabilities of B cells is considered more significant than the quantitative abnormalities related to humoral immunity. Following influenza infection, stimulated B cells are induced to differentiate and produce antibodies that are specific for the infecting virus or vaccine strains (Virelizier et al. 1974). These specific antibodies bind to the surface glycoproteins, hemagglutinin (HA), and neuraminidase (NA) to neutralize the viral particle. While serum immunoglobulin levels are shown to be stable during aging, the antibodies generated in old age are of lower affinity. Moreover, the specificity and class of antibody produced are changed; both extrinsic and intrinsic defects account for the diminished humoral response in the elderly.

Interactions with other immune cells are essential for B cell activation and antibody production (extrinsic pathways). Aging has been associated with dysregulated interactions with other cell types of the immune system. First of all, follicular dendritic cells isolated from older individuals have reduced ability to stimulate B cells due to decreased expression of co-stimulatory molecules on dendritic cells (Aydar et al. 2002; Colonna-Romano et al. 2003). Also the production of IL-2 and expression of CD40L by CD4+ T cells decline with aging. This dysregulated interaction between B and T cells leads to a reduced B cell expansion and differentiation in response to antigens as well as to decreased antibody production and germinal center formation (Lazuardi et al. 2005; Miller and Kelsoe 1995).

Intrinsic changes in B cells also occur in aging and have a significant impact on antibody production. During an immune response, B cells switch the expression of surface immunoglobulins from IgM to IgG, IgE, or IgA. This class switch recombination (CSR) is crucial for an effective humoral immune response because it generates antibodies of the same specificity but with different effector functions. One of the recognized defects in B cells from older individuals is their impaired ability to produce secondary isotypes through CSR. This defect accounts for the decreased IgG response to influenza vaccination in adults over age 65 years old. Other intrinsic defects associated with aging include decreases in the E2A-encoded transcription factor E47 and activation-induced cytidine deaminase (AID) (Frasca et al. 2011). Recently, AID has been proposed as an effective tool to assess B cell function and influenza vaccine responses. Measuring AID in stimulated B cells has been shown to predict the ability to generate an optimal influenza vaccine response (Frasca et al. 2011).

The hemagglutination inhibition assay has been considered as the gold standard for determining the protective efficacy of influenza vaccination among the normal population. However, studies of the vaccinated older population have revealed the inaccuracy of this assay in distinguishing between those who subsequently develop influenza illness from those who do not (McElhaney et al. 2006). As a consequence of impaired B cell functions, adequate antibody titers may not be sufficient indicators of sterilizing immunity in this population (McElhaney et al. 2006). Moreover, increased antibody titers in response to influenza vaccination, which correlates with protection in younger adults, may not translate to clinically important improvements in outcomes in older adults (Gorse et al. 2004). Therefore, antibody titers should not be considered as a sole measure of influenza vaccine efficacy in this population (Rock and Shen 2005; Demotz et al. 1990; Shahid et al. 2010).

Cell-Mediated Immunity

Influenza virus stimulates an antiviral response to T cells resulting in cell-mediated immunity. T cells are activated after the antigen-presenting cells (APC) take up and process the virus and present the resulting peptides on MHC. The resulting immune response then plays a key role in both humoral and cytotoxic T lymphocyte (CTL)

responses to influenza infection (McElhaney and Dutz 2008). Studies have shown that this branch of the immune system is mostly affected by age and plays the most important role in the increased susceptibility of older patients to influenza and its complications.

One of the most striking changes following aging is the involution of the thymus, where the maturation of T cells takes place. With aging, a decline in thymic output and a reduction in the naïve T cell pool (McElhaney and Effros 2009) occur. The remaining naïve T cells exhibit numerous functional defects, such as shorter telomeres, a restricted T cell receptor repertoire, reduced IL-2 production, and impaired expansion and differentiation into effector cells (Kohler et al. 2005). These changes reduce the ability to respond to new infections and create memory T cells to combat subsequent infections. Since the size of the T cell pool is preserved with aging, the constituent cells proliferate to maintain the T cell pool and result in a relative increase in the proportion of memory T cells. However, aging is also accompanied with a delayed and diminished response of memory T cells to influenza infection, which in turn increases the risk for complicated influenza illness (Wagar et al. 2011; Zhou and McElhaney 2011).

T Helper Cells

Th cell compartment maintains its diversity for decades in spite of thymic involution; however, in individuals older than 70 years, a dramatic decline of diversity occurs, leading to a severely contracted repertoire (Goronzy and Weyand 2005). A balance between Th type 1 (Th1) and type 2 (Th2) cytokines appears to be important for viral clearance and recovery from influenza illness (van der Sluijs et al. 2004; Doherty et al. 1997). Th1 cells are mostly involved in stimulating antibody responses, IFN-γ production, and CTL memory, whereas Th2 cells stimulate antibody responses. IL-10 is produced by T cells including regulatory T cells (Treg) and suppresses the Th1 response. Aging results in a reduced ratio of IFN-γ:IL-10 due to a decline in IFN-γ relative to IL-10 production in response to influenza challenge (Skowronski 2011). This transition from Th1 to Th2 cytokines has been correlated with an increased risk for influenza illness (McElhaney et al. 2006), a decline in CTL activity and an increased risk of pneumococcal pneumonia (van der Sluijs et al. 2004) in older adults. Other functional impairments associated with aging in Th cells are reduced production of IL-2, poor proliferative and differentiation capacity following antigen stimulation, reduced CD40 ligand expression, shortened telomeres, and increased resistance to programmed cell death (Vallejo 2005; Spaulding et al. 1999).

Cytotoxic T Lymphocytes

The CTL response to influenza infection is crucial for its recovery even in the absence of adequate antibody response to the infecting virus strain (McMichael et al. 1983). Production of IFN-γ through a Th1 response recruits CTLs to influenza-infected lungs. CTLs recognize the MHC I-viral peptide complex expressed on the surface of infected cells and destroy the host cells that have become the factories for viral replication. Aging results in diminished CTL responses to influenza challenge, delays in peak CTL activity, and a loss of cross-reactive responses that delay recovery from illness (Bender and Small 1993). Also, the expression of CD28, a co-stimulatory molecule on CTLs, is permanently suppressed with aging which correlates with poor antibody responses to influenza vaccination (Goronzy et al. 2001; Saurwein-Teissl et al. 2002).

Virus-infected cells are killed by CTLs largely through perforin-/granule-mediated killing (Pasternack and Eisen 1985; Bleackley et al. 1988; Jenne and Tschopp 1988); although fas-mediated killing may be an alternate mechanism (Ito et al. 1991; Rouvier et al. 1993), the granule-mediated mechanism seems to be more crucial for the control of respiratory viral infections. Following binding of CTL to the viral peptide-MHC I complex, granules containing granzymes and perforin migrate to the "immune synapse" between the activated CTL and the virus-infected target cell and are released into the cytoplasm of the target cell. The cytolytic mediator, granzyme B (GrzB), initiates an enzymatic cascade, which eventually leads to the induction of apoptosis of the virus-infected cell. A progressive decline in the levels of GrzB is seen from younger to older adults. Moreover, low levels of GrzB are associated with increased risk of influenza illness (McElhaney 2005). This has led to the introduction of the GrzB assay as a laboratory method for challenging human peripheral blood mononuclear cells with live virus, a "test tube" method for determining a critical component of antiviral immunity (McElhaney et al. 2001, 2009; Ewen et al. 2003).

In addition to diminished cytotoxic activity, CTLs of older individuals produce high levels of certain pro-inflammatory cytokines, such as TNFα and IL-6 (Effros et al. 2005), which directly causes dysregulation of the cell-mediated immune response (Vescovini et al. 2007). Paradoxically, adjuvants, when combined with influenza vaccine to stimulate dendritic cells to produce high levels of these inflammatory cytokines, have been shown to improve the CTL response to influenza virus challenge (McElhaney 2011).

18.4   Vaccination

Vaccination against influenza virus remains the most effective method of preventing influenza infection (Fiore et al. 2009). Current vaccination programs have been able to prevent influenza complications such as pneumonia, heart attacks, strokes, and exacerbations of congestive heart failure in this population. Current influenza vaccination programs have shown a 30–40 % reduction in influenza-related hospitalization rates and have been demonstrated to be cost-effective due to a reduction in medical care costs of managing influenza and pneumonia (Mullooly et al. 1994; Nichol et al. 1994). Also, when considering the reduction in hospitalizations with exacerbations of other chronic cardiac and pulmonary conditions, influenza vaccination is associated with significant cost savings in the older population (Mullooly et al. 1994; Deans et al. 2010). Despite the importance of vaccination in the elderly population, the effectiveness of current influenza vaccines is only 30–40 % in preventing laboratory-confirmed influenza illness among healthy adults aged 60 years or older (McElhaney and Dutz 2008). Thus, there is a considerable margin for improvement in this high-risk population (McElhaney 2008; Sambhara and McElhaney 2009). The reduced vaccine response has been attributed mostly to the waning immune system with aging as well antigenic mismatch between the vaccine strains and the circulating strains in this population.

18.5 Role of Immunosenescence

The well-known defects in both branches of the immune system, namely, innate and adaptive immune systems, as discussed previously are major contributors to the poor vaccine efficacy in the older population. The challenge to increase vaccine efficiency and develop new strategies for older adults is to stimulate the senescent immune response (Monto et al. 2009; McElhaney 2009).

Measuring antibody titers against influenza has been the mainstay of predicting influenza vaccine efficacy. In the only published randomized, placebo-controlled trial of influenza vaccine in older adults, antibody responses to influenza vaccine failed to correlate with protection against laboratory-confirmed influenza illness (Govaert et al. 1994). Other observational studies have shown similar antibody titers following vaccination in younger and older adults, suggesting comparable antibody-mediated protection. However, these results are in sharp contrast to the observed clinical outcomes in older adults emphasizing the importance of T cell immunity in influenza and highlighting the importance of including cellular immune measures in studying the impact of immune senescence on vaccine responsiveness (Effros 2007; McElhaney et al. 2006). This may be due to the different roles of protective humoral and cell-mediated immune responses to influenza infections. While antibody responses are mostly important in preventing infection and providing sterilizing immunity, T cell-mediated responses are responsible for clearance of the virus once infection occurs and providing clinical protection against disease.

Following influenza vaccine administration, the inflammatory response to the vaccine recruits APCs to the site of inflammation. The viral peptides are then presented on MHC I and II of APCs, which stimulate Th cells and CTLs in order to produce antibody and CTL responses, respectively. Current influenza vaccines contain split virus particles, which mostly stimulate Th cells but only weakly influence CTLs. The net effect is the production of vaccine strain-specific antibodies. Therefore, while antibodies are considered an important defense mechanism against influenza, the current influenza vaccines are inadequate in enhancing the CTL activity against influenza infection (Rimmelzwaan and McElhaney 2008).

18.6 Role of Antigenic Mismatch

Antigenic mismatch between the vaccine virus strains and the circulating virus strains is another contributing factor that can negatively impact vaccine effectiveness (Carrat and Flahault 2007). Antigenic mismatch is caused by antigenic drift between the composition of the administered vaccine and subsequent exposure to the circulating strain. Following B cell stimulation, the specific antibodies produced against the vaccine strain bind to the surface glycoproteins HA and NA to neutralize the viral particle. Antigenic drift occurs as a result of selective pressure by the immune system against the native virus, which constantly changes the peptide sequences at the antibody-binding site on the outer surfaces of HA and NA. In the older population, antigenic mismatch has been associated with a 30 % reduction in vaccine effectiveness during seasons when a drifted influenza strain circulates (Nordin et al. 2001).

While the antibody responses of B cells to influenza vaccines are strain specific, the antigenic determinants of Th cells and CTLs are more conserved across different strains of influenza, and their immunologic response does not degrade with antigenic drift (Effros et al. 1977; Marcelin et al. 2012). This effect is due to conserved internal peptide sequences of HA and NA within subtypes of influenza, which stimulate Th cells, and the internal proteins including matrix and nucleoproteins, which stimulate a cross-reactive CTL responses across all influenza A strains. Thus, increasing CTL responses could potentially overcome the issue with antigenic mismatch and provide protective responses in the elderly population.

18.7 Future Prospective

Vaccination provides the most effective means of protection against influenza and its various complications although there is clearly a margin for improvement. New vaccine formulations are required to stimulate the senescent immune response of the older person and to reverse age-related changes at multiple levels of the cellular immune response that are critical to protect against influenza (McElhaney et al. 2012). New influenza vaccines are currently in various stages of development in order to address the unmet need of improved vaccines in older adults (Behzad et al. 2012).

References

Agrawal A, Agrawal S, Gupta S (2007) Dendritic cells in human aging. Exp Gerontol 42(5):421–426

Aspinall R, Henson S, Pido-Lopez J et al (2004) Interleukin-7: an interleukin for rejuvenating the immune system. Ann N Y Acad Sci 1019:116–122

Aydar Y, Balogh P, Tew JG et al (2002) Age-related depression of FDC accessory functions and CD21 ligand-mediated repair of co-stimulation. Eur J Immunol 32(10):2817–2826

Banchereau J, Steinman RM (1998) Dendritic cells and the control of immunity. Nature 392(6673):245–252

Barker WH, Borisute H, Cox C (1998) A study of the impact of influenza on the functional status of frail older people. Arch Intern Med 158(6):645–650

Behzad H, Huckriede AL, Haynes L et al (2012) GLA-SE, a synthetic toll-like receptor 4 agonist, enhances T-cell responses to influenza vaccine in older adults. J Infect Dis 205(3):466–473

Bender BS, Small PA Jr (1993) Heterotypic immune mice lose protection against influenza virus infection with senescence. J Infect Dis 168(4):873–880

Blasco MA, Funk W, Villeponteau B et al (1995) Functional characterization and developmental regulation of mouse telomerase RNA. Science 269(5228):1267–1270

Bleackley RC, Lobe CG, Duggan B et al (1988) The isolation and characterization of a family of serine protease genes expressed in activated cytotoxic T lymphocytes. Immunol Rev 103:5–19

Borrego F, Alonso MC, Galiani MD et al (1999) NK phenotypic markers and IL2 response in NK cells from elderly people. Exp Gerontol 34(2):253–265

Brown LK (1994) Respiratory dysfunction in Parkinson's disease. Clin Chest Med 15(4):715–727

Butcher S, Chahel H, Lord JM (2000) Review article: ageing and the neutrophil: no appetite for killing? Immunology 100(4):411–416

Carrat F, Flahault A (2007) Influenza vaccine: the challenge of antigenic drift. Vaccine 25(39–40):6852–6862

Chatta GS, Andrews RG, Rodger E et al (1993) Hematopoietic progenitors and aging: alterations in granulocytic precursors and responsiveness to recombinant human G-CSF, GM-CSF, and IL-3. J Gerontol 48(5):M207–M212

Colonna-Romano G, Bulati M, Aquino A et al (2003) B cells in the aged: CD27, CD5, and CD40 expression. Mech Ageing Dev 124(4):389–393

Covinsky KE, Palmer RM, Fortinsky RH et al (2003) Loss of independence in activities of daily living in older adults hospitalized with medical illnesses: increased vulnerability with age. J Am Geriatr Soc 51(4):451–458

Deans GD, Stiver HG, McElhaney JE (2010) Influenza vaccines provide diminished protection but are cost-saving in older adults. J Intern Med 267(2):220–227

Demotz S, Grey HM, Sette A (1990) The minimal number of class II MHC-antigen complexes needed for T cell activation. Science 249(4972):1028–1030

Doherty PC, Topham DJ, Tripp RA et al (1997) Effector CD4+ and CD8+ T-cell mechanisms in the control of respiratory virus infections. Immunol Rev 159:105–117

Drinka PJ, Krause P, Nest L (2003) Clinical features of influenza a virus infection in older hospitalized persons. J Am Geriatr Soc 51(8):1184

Dumont FJ, Staruch MJ, Fischer P et al (1998) Inhibition of T cell activation by pharmacologic disruption of the MEK1/ERK MAP kinase or calcineurin signaling pathways results in differential modulation of cytokine production. J Immunol 160(6):2579–2589

Effros RB (2007) Role of T lymphocyte replicative senescence in vaccine efficacy. Vaccine 25(4):599–604

Effros RB, Doherty PC, Gerhard W et al (1977) Generation of both cross-reactive and virus-specific T-cell populations after immunization with serologically distinct influenza A viruses. J Exp Med 145(3):557–568

Effros RB, Dagarag M, Spaulding C et al (2005) The role of CD8+ T-cell replicative senescence in human aging. Immunol Rev 205:147–157

Evans SA, Watson L, Hawkins M et al (1995) Respiratory muscle strength in chronic heart failure. Thorax 50(6): 625–628

Ewen C, Kane KP, Shostak I et al (2003) A novel cytotoxicity assay to evaluate antigen-specific CTL responses using a colorimetric substrate for Granzyme B. J Immunol Methods 276(1–2):89–101

Fadok VA, Bratton DL, Konowal A et al (1998) Macrophages that have ingested apoptotic cells in vitro inhibit proinflammatory cytokine production through autocrine/paracrine mechanisms involving TGF-beta, PGE2, and PAF. J Clin Invest 101(4):890–898

Falsey AR, Hennessey PA, Formica MA et al (2005) Respiratory syncytial virus infection in elderly and high-risk adults. N Engl J Med 352(17):1749–1759

Fiore AE, Shay DK, Broder K et al (2009) Prevention and control of seasonal influenza with vaccines: recommendations of the Advisory Committee on Immunization Practices (ACIP), 2009. MMWR Recomm Rep 58(RR-8):1–52

Franceschi C, Bonafe M, Valensin S (2000) Human immunosenescence: the prevailing of innate immunity, the failing of clonotypic immunity, and the filling of immunological space. Vaccine 18(16):1717–1720

Frasca D, Landin AM, Lechner SC et al (2008) Aging down-regulates the transcription factor E2A, activation-induced cytidine deaminase, and Ig class switch in human B cells. J Immunol 180(8):5283–5290

Frasca D, Diaz A, Romero M et al (2011) Age effects on B cells and humoral immunity in humans. Ageing Res Rev 10(3):330–335

Fulop T Jr, Foris G, Worum I et al (1985) Age-dependent alterations of Fc gamma receptor-mediated effector functions of human polymorphonuclear leucocytes. Clin Exp Immunol 61(2):425–432

Gomez CR, Boehmer ED, Kovacs EJ (2005) The aging innate immune system. Curr Opin Immunol 17(5):457–462

Goronzy JJ, Weyand CM (2005) T cell development and receptor diversity during aging. Curr Opin Immunol 17(5):468–475

Goronzy JJ, Fulbright JW, Crowson CS et al (2001) Value of immunological markers in predicting responsiveness to influenza vaccination in elderly individuals. J Virol 75(24):12182–12187

Gorse GJ, O'Connor TZ, Newman FK et al (2004) Immunity to influenza in older adults with chronic obstructive pulmonary disease. J Infect Dis 190(1):11–19

Govaert TM, Thijs CT, Masurel N et al (1994) The efficacy of influenza vaccination in elderly individuals. A randomized double-blind placebo-controlled trial. JAMA 272(21):1661–1665

Granucci F, Zanoni I, Feau S et al (2003) Dendritic cell regulation of immune responses: a new role for interleukin 2 at the intersection of innate and adaptive immunity. EMBO J 22(11):2546–2551

Grolleau-Julius A, Harning EK, Abernathy LM et al (2008) Impaired dendritic cell function in aging leads to defective antitumor immunity. Cancer Res 68(15):6341–6349

Ito T, Gorman OT, Kawaoka Y et al (1991) Evolutionary analysis of the influenza A virus M gene with comparison of the M1 and M2 proteins. J Virol 65(10):5491–5498

Janssens JP, Krause KH (2004) Pneumonia in the very old. Lancet Infect Dis 4(2):112–124

Jenne DE, Tschopp J (1988) Granzymes, a family of serine proteases released from granules of cytolytic T lymphocytes upon T cell receptor stimulation. Immunol Rev 103:53–71

Kohler S, Wagner U, Pierer M et al (2005) Post-thymic in vivo proliferation of naive CD4+ T cells constrains the TCR repertoire in healthy human adults. Eur J Immunol 35(6):1987–1994

Kronenberg RS, Drage CW (1973) Attenuation of the ventilatory and heart rate responses to hypoxia and hypercapnia with aging in normal men. J Clin Invest 52(8):1812–1819

Lalvani A, Dong T, Ogg G et al (1997) Optimization of a peptide-based protocol employing IL-7 for in vitro restimulation of human cytotoxic T lymphocyte precursors. J Immunol Methods 210(1):65–77

Lazuardi L, Jenewein B, Wolf AM et al (2005) Age-related loss of naive T cells and dysregulation of T-cell/B-cell interactions in human lymph nodes. Immunology 114(1):37–43

Loeb M (2003) Pneumonia in older persons. Clin Infect Dis 37(10):1335–1339

Marcelin G, DuBois R, Rubrum A et al (2012) A contributing role for anti-neuraminidase antibodies on immunity to pandemic H1N1 2009 influenza A virus. PLoS One 6(10):26335

McElhaney JE (2005) The unmet need in the elderly: designing new influenza vaccines for older adults. Vaccine 23(Suppl 1):S10–S25

McElhaney JE (2008) Influenza vaccination in the elderly: seeking new correlates of protection and improved vaccines. Aging health 4(6):603–613

McElhaney JE (2009) Prevention of infectious diseases in older adults through immunization: the challenge of the senescent immune response. Expert Rev Vaccines 8(5):593–606

McElhaney JE (2011) Influenza vaccine responses in older adults. Ageing Res Rev 10(3):379–388

McElhaney JE, Dutz JP (2008) Better influenza vaccines for older people: what will it take? J Infect Dis 198(5):632–634

McElhaney JE, Effros RB (2009) Immunosenescence: what does it mean to health outcomes in older adults? Curr Opin Immunol 21(4):418–424

McElhaney JE, Gravenstein S, Upshaw CM et al (2001) Granzyme B: a marker of risk for influenza in institutionalized older adults. Vaccine 19(27):3744–3751

McElhaney JE, Xie D, Hager WD et al (2006) T cell responses are better correlates of vaccine protection in the elderly. J Immunol 176(10):6333–6339

McElhaney JE, Ewen C, Zhou X et al (2009) Granzyme B: correlates with protection and enhanced CTL response to influenza vaccination in older adults. Vaccine 27(18):2418–2425

McElhaney JE, Zhou X, Talbot HK et al (2012) The unmet need in the elderly: how immunosenescence, CMV infection, co-morbidities and frailty are a challenge for the development of more effective influenza vaccines. Vaccine 30(12):2060–2067

McKenna RW, Washington LT, Aquino DB et al (2001) Immunophenotypic analysis of hematogones (B-lymphocyte precursors) in 662 consecutive bone marrow specimens by 4-color flow cytometry. Blood 98(8):2498–2507

McMichael AJ, Gotch FM, Noble GR et al (1983) Cytotoxic T-cell immunity to influenza. N Engl J Med 309(1):13–17

Meyer KC, Ershler W, Rosenthal NS et al (1996) Immune dysregulation in the aging human lung. Am J Respir Crit Care Med 153(3):1072–1079

Miller C, Kelsoe G (1995) Ig VH hypermutation is absent in the germinal centers of aged mice. J Immunol 155(7):3377–3384

Miyaji C, Watanabe H, Toma H et al (2000) Functional alteration of granulocytes, NK cells, and natural killer T cells in centenarians. Hum Immunol 61(9):908–916

Molinari NA, Ortega-Sanchez IR, Messonnier ML et al (2007) The annual impact of seasonal influenza in the US: measuring disease burden and costs. Vaccine 25(27):5086–5096

Molling JW, Kolgen W, van der Vliet HJ et al (2005) Peripheral blood IFN-gamma-secreting Valpha24 + Vbeta11+ NKT cell numbers are decreased in cancer patients independent of tumor type or tumor load. Int J Cancer 116(1):87–93

Monto AS, Ansaldi F, Aspinall R et al (2009) Influenza control in the 21st century: optimizing protection of older adults. Vaccine 27(37):5043–5053

Mullooly JP, Bennett MD, Hornbrook MC et al (1994) Influenza vaccination programs for elderly persons: cost-effectiveness in a health maintenance organization. Ann Intern Med 121(12):947–952

Nichol KL, Margolis KL, Wuorenma J et al (1994) The efficacy and cost effectiveness of vaccination against influenza among elderly persons living in the community. N Engl J Med 331(12):778–784

Nomellini V, Gomez CR, Kovacs EJ (2008) Aging and impairment of innate immunity. Contrib Microbiol 15:188–205

Nordin J, Mullooly J, Poblete S et al (2001) Influenza vaccine effectiveness in preventing hospitalizations and deaths in persons 65 years or older in Minnesota, New York, and Oregon: data from 3 health plans. J Infect Dis 184(6):665–670

Pasternack MS, Eisen HN (1985) A novel serine esterase expressed by cytotoxic T lymphocytes. Nature 314(6013):743–745

Plackett TP, Boehmer ED, Faunce DE et al (2004) Aging and innate immune cells. J Leukoc Biol 76(2):291–299

Plowden J, Renshaw-Hoelscher M, Engleman C et al (2004) Innate immunity in aging: impact on macrophage function. Aging Cell 3(4):161–167

Reichert TA, Simonsen L, Sharma A et al (2004) Influenza and the winter increase in mortality in the United States, 1959–1999. Am J Epidemiol 160(5):492–502

Rimmelzwaan GF, McElhaney JE (2008) Correlates of protection: novel generations of influenza vaccines. Vaccine 26(Suppl 4):D41–D44

Rock KL, Shen L (2005) Cross-presentation: underlying mechanisms and role in immune surveillance. Immunol Rev 207:166–183

Rouvier E, Luciani MF, Golstein P (1993) Fas involvement in Ca(2+)-independent T cell-mediated cytotoxicity. J Exp Med 177(1):195–200

Sambhara S, McElhaney JE (2009) Immunosenescence and influenza vaccine efficacy. Curr Top Microbiol Immunol 333:413–429

Saurwein-Teissl M, Lung TL, Marx F et al (2002) Lack of antibody production following immunization in old age: association with CD8(+)CD28(−) T cell clonal expansions and an imbalance in the production of Th1 and Th2 cytokines. J Immunol 168(11):5893–5899

Shahid Z, Kleppinger A, Gentleman B et al (2010) Clinical and immunologic predictors of influenza illness among vaccinated older adults. Vaccine 28(38):6145–6151

Shi Y, Yamazaki T, Okubo Y et al (2005) Regulation of aged humoral immune defense against pneumococcal bacteria by IgM memory B cell. J Immunol 175(5):3262–3267

Skowronski DM, Hottes TS, McElhaney JE et al (2011) Immuno-epidemiologic correlates of pandemic H1N1 surveillance observations: higher antibody and lower cell-mediated immune responses with advanced age. J Infect Dis 203(2):158–167

Solana R, Mariani E (2000) NK and NK/T cells in human senescence. Vaccine 18(16):1613–1620

Solana R, Alonso MC, Pena J (1999) Natural killer cells in healthy aging. Exp Gerontol 34(3):435–443

Spaulding C, Guo W, Effros RB (1999) Resistance to apoptosis in human CD8+ T cells that reach replicative senescence after multiple rounds of antigen-specific proliferation. Exp Gerontol 34(5):633–644

Steger MM, Maczek C, Berger P et al (1996) Vaccination against tetanus in the elderly: do recommended vaccination strategies give sufficient protection. Lancet 348(9029):762

Thompson WW, Shay DK, Weintraub E et al (2003) Mortality associated with influenza and respiratory syncytial virus in the United States. JAMA 289(2):179–186

Thompson WW, Shay DK, Weintraub E et al (2004) Influenza-associated hospitalizations in the United States. JAMA 292(11):1333–1340

Tolep K, Kelsen SG (1993) Effect of aging on respiratory skeletal muscles. Clin Chest Med 14(3):363–378

Turner DA, Wailoo AJ, Cooper NJ et al (2006) The cost-effectiveness of influenza vaccination of healthy adults 50–64 years of age. Vaccine 24(7):1035–1043

Vallejo AN (2005) CD28 extinction in human T cells: altered functions and the program of T-cell senescence. Immunol Rev 205:158–169

Van der Sluijs KF, van Elden LJ, Nijhuis M et al (2004) IL-10 is an important mediator of the enhanced susceptibility to pneumococcal pneumonia after influenza infection. J Immunol 172(12):7603–7609

Vescovini R, Biasini C, Fagnoni FF et al (2007) Massive load of functional effector CD4+ and CD8+ T cells against cytomegalovirus in very old subjects. J Immunol 179(6):4283–4291

Virelizier JL, Allison AC, Schild GC (1974) Antibody responses to antigenic determinants of influenza virus hemagglutinin. II. Original antigenic sin: a bone marrow-derived lymphocyte memory phenomenon modulated by thymus-derived lymphocytes. J Exp Med 140(6):1571–1578

Wagar LE, Gentleman B, Pircher H et al (2011) Influenza-specific T cells from older people are enriched in the late effector subset and their presence inversely correlates with vaccine response. PLoS One 6(8):e23698

Wenisch C, Patruta S, Daxbock F et al (2000) Effect of age on human neutrophil function. J Leukoc Biol 67(1):40–45

Whitley RJ, Monto AS (2006) Prevention and treatment of influenza in high-risk groups: children, pregnant women, immunocompromised hosts, and nursing home residents. J Infect Dis 194(Suppl 2):S133–S138

Zhou X, McElhaney JE (2011) Age-related changes in memory and effector T cells responding to influenza A/H3N2 and pandemic A/H1N1 strains in humans. Vaccine 29(11):2169–2177

Optimizing Response to Vaccination in the Elderly

19

Diana Boraschi, Rino Rappuoli,
and Giuseppe Del Giudice

19.1 The Aging of the Human Population

Life expectancy has impressively increased during the last century worldwide. This increase is linear (except for drops due to the World Wars and to the Spanish flu pandemics in 1918–1919) and is evident in all countries in the world, including developing countries where the rate of increase is slower, possibly due to the effects of acquired immunodeficiency syndrome (AIDS) (The World Bank 2004). The United Nations expects that about 25 % of the world population will be >65 years of age (a goal already reached in Europe and Japan) by 2050 and that 75 % of this elderly population will be living in developing countries (United Nations 2002).

Better nutrition, health care, and preventive measures have contributed to reducing mortality at birth and early childhood and to prolonging life expectancy. A very interesting hypothesis is that life expectancy is affected by the significant decrease in infectious disease burden at young age resulting in reduced inflammation, increased body growth, and eventually longer life span (Crimmins and Finch 2006). The introduction of

D. Boraschi, PhD (✉)
Lab Innate Immunity and Cytokines,
National Research Council,
Via G. Moruzzi, 156124 Pisa, Italy
e-mail: diana.boraschi@itb.cnr.it

R. Rappuoli, PhD • G. Del Giudice, MD, PhD
Research Center, Novartis Vaccines and Diagnostics,
53100 Siena, Italy

mass vaccination has undoubtedly contributed to the decrease of the infectious disease burden in children and even to eradicate the disease, as in the case of smallpox (eradicated), poliomyelitis, and measles (expected in the near future).

19.2 The Aging of the Immune Responsiveness

The elderly population is more susceptible to infectious diseases, with a slower and less efficient recovery (Gavazzi and Krause 2002), and to chronic diseases as compared to young and adults (Wagner and Groves 2002). This is mostly due to a decline in immunological functions known as immunosenescence, responsible not only of hampered response to infectious and pathological challenges but also of the inadequate protective response upon vaccination.

Innate and inflammatory responses are anomalous in the elderly in large part due to the changing microenvironment and only in part to intrinsic senescence of response (Shaw et al. 2010). The changes occurring in the aging body (increased cellular death, increased oxidative events, etc.), often in parallel with concurring infections or diseases, contribute to creating a constitutively inflamed microenvironment (inflammaging) that maintains the basal innate/inflammatory response of immune cells, in particular monocytes and macrophages, to a level of permanent activation (Franceschi 2007). This situation may cause excessive inflammation and tissue damage upon infectious challenges.

A. Massoud, N. Rezaei (eds.), *Immunology of Aging*,
DOI 10.1007/978-3-642-39495-9_19, © Springer-Verlag Berlin Heidelberg 2014

The functions of dendritic cells (the cells that present antigen thereby bridging innate and adaptive immunity) also appear to be constitutively activated in people >65 years of age but, at variance with young cells, are less reactive to Toll-like receptor (TLR) stimuli (Panda et al. 2010).

The function of T cells is also impaired in elderly people, with an overall inability of renewal of the naïve T cell compartment. In fact, the ability of naïve T cells to respond to stimuli and the overall balance of the different T cell subsets appears altered (Nikolich-Zugich and Rudd 2010), with a preponderance of memory T cells as opposed to naïve T cells. Regarding CD4$^+$ T cells, T cell receptor (TCR) signalling (but not TCR expression) is reduced in old cells, in part as consequence of the higher activity of the inhibitory phosphatases dual specificity phosphatase 4 (DUSP4) and DUSP6, which impair T helper (Th) polarization (Li et al. 2012; Yu et al. 2012). The CD8$^+$ T cell compartment in the elderly is strongly unbalanced towards effector memory cells as opposed to naïve cells. This may be due both to age-long stimulation with viruses and also as a compensatory mechanism to balance the decreased proliferative capacity of naïve cells (Herndler-Brandstetter et al. 2012). The direct consequence of all these alterations is a reduced ability of old T cells to mount primary responses to newly introduced antigens, such as novel vaccines. Memory and effector T cells in aged individuals do not express the co-stimulatory molecules CD28 (Goronzy et al 2012) and CD40 ligand (CD40L)/CD154 (Yu et al. 2012), resulting in a reduced capacity to provide help for B cell proliferation and differentiation for antibody production.

Similar anomalies have been observed for B lymphocytes, with a significant reduction of naïve B cells and a parallel increase of memory B cells (Johnson and Cambier 2004), which however show a limited repertoire diversity (Gibson et al. 2009). In this context, the antibody response in elderly individuals to new antigens is quantitatively reduced, short-lived, and with poor isotype switching, resulting in antibodies with lower avidity and efficacy (Weinberger et al. 2008).

19.3 Increased Susceptibility to Infections in the Elderly

The increased susceptibility of the elderly to viral and bacterial infections is due to a concurrence of conditions that include, besides intrinsic immunosenescence, the anatomical modifications in organs (e.g., genitourinary and gastrointestinal tract, lung), chronic diseases (e.g., diabetes, cardiovascular diseases), and malnutrition (Flicker et al. 2010).

In the United States (US), over 86 % of the 15,573 deaths associated to seasonal influenza occurred in people of ≥65 years of age in the influenza season 2006–2007 (Centers for Disease Control 2010). Elderly individuals living in communities, in particular those with chronic diseases, are prone to pneumonia caused by respiratory syncytial virus (RSV) with excessive mortality as compared to adults (Falsey 2007). Herpes zoster is also a major problem in the elderly, who are particularly susceptible to reactivation of latent infection with varicella zoster virus (VSV). Reactivation is due to the age-related waning of cell-mediated immunity to the virus, both in CD4$^+$ and CD8$^+$ effector and memory cells, and can result in severe and disabilitating neuralgia. The estimate is that around 50 % of herpes zoster cases occur in people aged >85 years (Schmader 2001). The elderly population is also significantly more susceptible to many bacterial infections, such as those by *Streptococcus pneumonia* (causing pneumonia, bacteremia, and meningitis) and by invasive group B *streptococci* (GBS), primarily affecting the aged population (40 %) with a death rate of >50 % (Edwards and Baker 2005).

19.4 Reduced Response to Influenza Vaccination in the Elderly: How to Improve It?

To ensure healthy aging, a global strategy is required to prevent or delay immune senescence, including physical and mental exercise, adequate and balanced nutrition, and living in a healthy environment. As this is unfeasible in many circumstances, health protection in the elderly relies mostly on vaccination against the most frequent infections. Several vaccines are available that are recommended for the elderly, to counteract their increased susceptibility to infections and ensure a healthier aging. However, the current vaccines have been developed for preventing infections mainly in childhood and in immunologically mature individuals, and therefore, they may not be optimally effective in the elderly who are immunologically inadequate. Therefore, the need for specifically designed vaccines is becoming urgent for facing the unprecedented health protection challenges posed by our fast-aging society (Rappuoli et al. 2011). To understand the features of vaccine efficacy in the elderly as opposed to healthy adults, the huge amount of information accumulated with the vaccine against influenza offers an excellent paradigm.

Influenza is still a major cause of hospitalization and mortality in the elderly also in developed countries, despite vaccination is strongly recommended and largely implemented. This can be attributed both to a suboptimal coverage (Blank et al. 2008) and to a reduced efficacy of the existing vaccines in the elderly population, despite the generally recognized decrease of morbidity and mortality following vaccination. During the influenza season 1991–1992, a randomized placebo-controlled efficacy study was carried out in an aged cohort and resulted in 50 % efficacy, with better protection evident in people that had been already vaccinated in the past (Govaert et al. 1994). Later studies have shown a significant vaccine-dependent reduction of hospitalization (48 %) and death (27 %) in community-dwelling aged people (Nichol et al. 2007).

However, the observed benefits are limited, and the current influenza vaccines do not confer full protection to the aging population. In a longitudinal study, it has been shown that the efficacy of influenza vaccination against three different flu viruses (H1N1, H3N2, and B) goes down from 55, 58, and 41 % (for the three viruses) in subjects aged 65–74 years to 32, 46, and 29 % in individuals above 75 years of age, with over 30 % of older subjects not reaching the protective antibody titer (Goodwin et al. 2006).

Therefore, it is obvious that new vaccines are needed, specifically designed for conferring optimal protective immunity in the elderly. This is important for some vaccines that should be administered yearly, such as the seasonal influenza vaccine, for restimulation of memory to increase their efficacy (generated by both previous vaccination and previous natural exposure). However, it is even more important for vaccines given for the first time for infections to which the subject has never been previously exposed (as often is the case for yellow fever, tick-borne encephalitis, pandemic flu, etc.), because the decreased number of naïve T and B cells and their limited repertoire imply the inability of mounting an effective protective response, unless the vaccine is specifically designed for overcoming the immunological inadequacy of the host.

The strategies for designing vaccines for the elderly is reviewed below, again by taking seasonal influenza as an example, given the wealth of data available. In addition, the threat posed by the influenza pandemics has boosted research in the field, and many lessons were learnt in those occasions that are being applied to improving seasonal influenza vaccines.

Since the understanding of the mechanistic basis of immune senescence is still partial, no current vaccination strategy is based on such knowledge and the approaches have been exclusively empirical. Those that have better developed include the use of higher and repeated doses of influenza antigens, the choice of different administration routes, and the use of adjuvants.

19.4.1 Increasing the Vaccine Antigen Dosages

The most reliable and widely accepted correlate of protection in influenza vaccination is the titer of anti-hemagglutinin antibodies, which is measured with a classical assay of inhibition of hemagglutination (HI) (Potter and Oxford 1979). The threshold for protection has been set at a titer of 1:40 (if serum diluted 1:40 or more, still inhibits hemagglutination and there is protection; however, if at the same titer, inhibition is lost, there is no protection), because higher HI titers correlate with increased protection. It has been long known that by increasing the dose of antigen in the vaccine inoculums, the HI titer increases. In an old study, a split monovalent H1N1 vaccine was administered at increasing dosages to healthy adults and yielded a dose-dependent increase in the HI titer both in subjects with low pre-vaccination titers (16–35×) and in those with high pre-vaccination titers (3–7×) (Keitel et al. 1994). The same monovalent H1N1 split vaccine was later administered to healthy subjects aged ≥65 years. Also in this case, higher dosages could induce a significant increase in the HI titers (2–3× HI increase by increasing the antigen dose up to 9×) (Keitel et al. 1996). However, if this increase is of clinical significance is doubtful. The recent experience obtained with the pandemic H5N1 vaccine (avian flu) has shown that two inocula of antigen (amounting to a 6× increase vs. normal vaccine dosage) yielded neutralizing and protective HI antibody titers in 53–57 % of the vaccines, which were healthy adults (Treanor et al. 2006), thus implying an even less satisfactory protection in immunologically frail elderly, in particular when considering that they are most probably never been exposed previously to the avian flu virus. Therefore, it is concluded that increasing the antigen dosage is not the optimal strategy for improving vaccine efficacy in the elderly (without considering the increased costs).

19.4.2 Alternative Routes of Administration

The possibility that vaccine administration by routes other than the classical intramuscular route could improve immunogenicity and protection has been empirically investigated, focussing in particular on the intradermal route.

The intradermal delivery of antigens should favor the local uptake by Langerhans cells (LC) and dendritic cells (DC), which then migrate to the tissue-draining lymph nodes where they mature and present the antigen to T cells thereby initiating the adaptive immune response. The highly efficient immunization pathway that can be obtained by intradermal antigen delivery should also, in theory, allow for a reduction of the antigen dose required to obtain optimal protective response. By delivering the antigen at an anatomical site, rich in professional antigen-presenting cells, the intradermal vaccination has also the theoretical potential of allowing to reducing the amount of vaccine antigen to achieve protection. However, the efficacy of intradermal vaccination in the elderly may be influenced by the age-related changes in skin integrity and physiology, including the decreased number of LC and DC (Panda et al. 2009).

Intradermal vaccination has been routinely used for several vaccines, including those for smallpox and rabies. In the case of rabies, the intradermal antigen dose yielding protection is fivefold lower than by intramuscular administration, so the World Health Organization (WHO) has approved this dosage/route approach with the current cell culture-based rabies vaccines (World Health Organization 2005).

The intradermal route has been considered for the influenza vaccination since the 1940s (Halperin et al. 1979), but it has received particular attention during the 1976 pandemics of swine influenza virus A/New Jersey/76 H1N1. The use of a 5× lower dose intradermally (compared to intramuscularly) would allow a substantial dose sparing that is of key importance in the case of pandemics, where global vaccine shortage may become an issue of public health protection. Several studies showed that intradermal vaccination with lower doses of influenza vaccines induced antibody titers comparable to those induced by the full-dose intramuscular vaccine (Brown et al. 1977; Herbert et al. 1979). The effect however was not as evident in aged people >50 years, suggesting that senescence of skin immunity may hamper intradermal vaccine efficacy (Belshe et al. 2004). Thus, more recent studies have compared the response to intradermal influenza vaccines throughout all ages. The results showed that a decrease of 2.5-fold in antigen dose (as compared to the full-dose vaccines) is possible in the elderly to achieve good response by the intradermal route, while in adults the dose could be further decreased to one fifth of the full dose (Belshe et al. 2004; Kenney et al. 2004). The intramuscular route of administration appeared to achieve better results in aged people >60 years, further underlining the issue of senescence of skin immunity (Belshe et al. 2004). However, in these studies, direct comparison of the same vaccine dosages by the two delivery routes was missing, which made interpretation of the results doubtful. Indeed, a subsequent study with the direct comparison of different vaccine doses by the two delivery routes showed that all doses (from the full 15 mg dose down to the 3 mg dose) could induce optimal response by both routes in healthy adults (Belshe et al. 2007b). Another study has reevaluated the efficacy of intradermal influenza vaccination in 1,107 elderly subjects (>60 years) of age (Holland et al. 2008). Antigen dose was either full (15 mg) or higher (21 mg). The response to intradermal vaccination (at both dosages) was found to be superior to that of old subjects vaccinated by the intramuscular route without adjuvant. In the case of seasonal flu vaccine, there are claims that the intradermal route could achieve better response as compared to the adjuvanted intramuscular vaccine, although results are inconsistent (Van Damme et al. 2010). However, vaccine reactogenicity is consistently higher by the intradermal route.

The conclusion from years of intradermal vaccination is that the intradermal route is a good one, but it is not superior to the intramuscular vaccination in adults. Also for the elderly, there is no evidence that the intradermal route may offer advantages in terms of dose sparing or overcoming immune senescence as opposed to the intramuscular delivery. It is evident that a deeper knowledge of the mechanisms of immunity and immune senescence in the skin is required, with particular attention to the function of professional antigen-presenting cells like DC, in order to design effective intradermal vaccines for the elderly.

19.4.3 Amplification of the Immune Response: Adjuvants and Immunostimulation Strategies

The principle of adjuvanticity implies the amplification of the specific, antigen-induced immune response by different immunostimulation strategies. Among the most efficient approaches for enhancing immunity, we will consider the use of cytokines, the use of live microorganisms, and the use of agents able to trigger innate immunity.

19.4.3.1 Cytokines

Cytokines can be used to enhance immune responses at different levels, and their use in vaccination for the elderly may improve their hampered immune responses. Cytokines like interleukin (IL)-7 are involved in survival of T cells and may be useful in maintaining a pool of naïve T cells in the elderly, thereby allowing a more efficient response to new vaccines. Experiments in old macaques have yielded promising results, with 50 % of animals showing an increased thymic output and a restored response to influenza vaccination (Aspinall et al. 2007). However, no attempt has been done in humans to use IL-7 to amplify the response to vaccines.

IL-2 can induce an increase of peripheral T cells and their responsiveness to antigen. In healthy young adults, administration of liposome-formulated influenza vaccine and IL-2 induced higher HI antibody titers against the vaccine antigens and higher seroconversion rates as compared to unadjuvanted vaccine (Ben-Yehuda et al. 2003b). The same vaccine was administered to elderly people in nursing homes and it could induce higher seroconversion and seroprotection rates against the virus antigens significantly as compared to aged subjects receiving the non-adjuvanted vaccine (Ben-Yehuda et al. 2003a). Whether the good results observed were due to the presence of IL-2 or to the liposome formulation of the vaccine (known to have an adjuvant effect because of their particulate nature), it is not known and would require a thorough investigation.

In another study, the antiviral and immuno-modulatory cytokine interferon alpha (IFN-α) has been used as adjuvant (by sublingual administration) immediately before intramuscular influenza vaccination in institutionalized old subjects. The treatment resulted to be actually detrimental, with a significant decrease in the HI antibody response to the vaccine antigen and overall of the circulating and salivary antibody levels (Launay et al. 2008).

These results should recommend extreme caution in the use of cytokines, which are immune-signalling proteins with huge specific activity, as if they were drugs. The delicate balance of the cytokine networks needs first to be known in detail before attempting to exploit these molecules for restoring/rebalancing the altered immune reactivity of aged people.

19.4.3.2 Live Attenuated Influenza Vaccines

The use of live attenuated influenza vaccines (LAIV) instead of inactivated or subunit vaccines is an interesting approach to improving vaccine immunogenicity in the elderly. No data are available in this age group, and in fact LAIV are not currently licensed in the US for older people. In young children, an immunologically immature population, it appears that LAIV are more efficacious than inactivated vaccines (Belshe et al. 2007a), but this is not the case in immunologically competent adults (Ohmit et al. 2006). An improved response could be obtained, both in adults and in the elderly, by combining intranasal LAIV administration with intramuscular inactivated vaccination (Betts and Treanor 2000; Treanor et al. 1992). However, in an efficacy trial carried out in South Africa in more than 3,200 elderly subjects (>60 years), the efficacy of the vaccine against matched viruses strains was only 42.3 % (De Villiers et al. 2009).

The poor outcome of LAIV in the elderly may be linked to the intranasal route of administration, since the homeostasis and immunological function of the mucosal surfaces in the elderly are impaired (Fujihashi and Kiyono 2009). Again, only the deeper basic knowledge of the age-related functional changes would allow the rational design and implementation of effective vaccination strategies of this age group.

19.4.3.3 Adjuvants to Enhance Immunogenicity and Efficacy of Vaccines in the Elderly

The use of adjuvants is by far the best known way to enhance the immune response to vaccines. Adjuvants are molecules that stimulate the innate immune response, which is the required starting point for obtaining an adequate specific immune response to the vaccine antigens. The majority of vaccines currently on the market contain adjuvants. The most used adjuvant, and the only one licensed for human use for many years, is based on aluminum salts (aluminum hydroxide or aluminum phosphate). Vaccine antigens are adsorbed on the aluminum particles, and their immunogenicity is increased both by the slower release/higher persistence of the antigens and by the innate immunity enhancement provoked by the particulate matter.

The influenza vaccine is an exception, as the presence of aluminum salt adjuvants does not improve the response to the vaccine. The reason probably lies in the fact that most individuals already have memory cells for the influenza virus (due to previous vaccinations and to previous exposure), so the vaccine is sufficient for the efficient expansion of the memory cell pool without the need of adjuvants. However, the use of non-metabolizable mineral oil adjuvants appeared to have an enhancing effect, by allowing significant dose sparing and persistent antibody response and, despite immediate reactogenicity, no long-term pathological sequel (Beebe et al. 1972).

The high frequency of local side effects prevented for many years the development of oil emulsion-based adjuvants, until the development of the first oil-in-water adjuvant, MF59. The new oil-in-water adjuvant included a lower amount of oil (4–5 % *vs.* the 50 % of the old mineral oil emulsions) and replaced the mineral oil with the fully metabolizable and physiological squalene (a precursor of cholesterol, steroid hormones, and vitamin D) (Podda et al. 2005).

After very encouraging data in small and large animals with a series of different vaccines and an extensive clinical development phase (including >20,000 elderly subjects), MF59 was licensed in Italy in 1997, and later in more than 20 countries worldwide, in association with the seasonal inactivated subunit influenza virus vaccine for individuals >65 years of age. The use of MF59 yielded a very good safety profile (Pellegrini et al. 2009) and a significant enhancement of vaccine immunogenicity in terms of extension and persistence of the specific antibody response, with the MF59-adjuvanted vaccine resulting effective also in the subpopulation with chronic diseases and significantly reducing hospitalization for influenza, pneumonia, and cardiovascular and cerebrovascular emergency events in the elderly (Puig-Barberà et al. 2007).

The protective efficacy of influenza vaccines is strongly affected by the rate of antigenic mismatch between the vaccine strain (as recommended by WHO) and the circulating viruses to which people get exposed. Indeed, a study over the period 1995–2005 showed that the vaccine effectiveness in elderly people (>65 years) can drop from >80 % against the original virus strain to values <30 % against the antigenically drifted circulating strains (Legrand et al. 2006). In this context, a particularly important observation is that immunization with MF59-adjuvanted flu vaccine can induce a powerful antibody response not only against the immunizing virus but also to variant strains, which implies the capacity to overcome the problem of decreased protection against antigenically drifted virus in the elderly (Del Giudice et al. 2006; Ansaldi et al. 2008, 2010; Camilloni et al. 2009). More recently, MF59-adjuvanted vaccines have been also used for the H5N1 avian influenza virus and for the H1N1 pandemic flu virus in all age groups, including people >65 years. Again, the key finding is that the adjuvant could induce cross-reactivity to other antigenically drifted influenza viruses. Also, boosting with H5N1 clade 1 virus 6–8 years after priming with MF59-adjuvanted H5N3 (a very different virus) could rapidly induce high neutralizing antibody titers against all drifted clade 1 variants and all

clade 2 subclades, besides the boosting strain (Stephenson et al. 2008; Galli et al. 2009). Based on the success of MF59, other oil-in-water adjuvants based on squalene have been developed more recently (Vogel et al. 2009).

The mechanism at the basis of the adjuvant activity of MF59 is only partially understood. Studies in mice and in vitro with human cells have shown that MF59 induces monocyte recruitment and macrophage trafficking, promotes monocyte differentiation to DC, and enhances antigen uptake by macrophages and DC (Dupuis et al. 1998, 2001; Seubert et al. 2008; Mosca et al. 2008). Notably, in a genome-wide microarray analysis in the mouse, MF59 was shown to upregulate a wide variety of genes involved in the initiation of the innate/inflammatory reaction, as compared to GpG or aluminum salts (Mosca et al. 2008). Among the genes that are upregulated by MF59 but also by the other adjuvants, there is *Il1b*, the gene coding for the inflammatory cytokine IL-1β that is a key player in the induction of the innate immune amplification necessary for adjuvanticity. It is noteworthy that, at variance with the other adjuvants, MF59 can also induce in parallel the expression of genes encoding a series of other IL-1-related regulators of inflammation, such as the pro-inflammatory IL-1 receptor type I (IL1R1), IL-18Rβ, and IL-36γ and the anti-inflammatory IL-1 receptor antagonist (IL-1Ra), IL-1RII, interleukin-18-binding protein (IL18BP), and ST2 (Mosca et al. 2008). This enhancement of innate/inflammatory activities together with the concomitant expression of regulatory factors leads to the hypothesis that MF59, better than other adjuvants, can induce a potent innate/inflammatory reaction (which is fundamental for the adjuvant effect) but that it can efficiently control its development and termination, thereby avoiding immunosuppressive persistence of inflammation and achieving optimal efficacy. MF59 does not activate the Nlrp3 inflammasome, nor does it bind/activate TLR receptors, and its activity is independent of the IL-1β-maturing enzyme caspase-1, but its activity depends on ASC (a component of the inflammasome) and MyD88 (a signalling intermediate of TLR), suggesting the use of novel pathways of innate enhancement (Seubert et al. 2011; Ellebedy et al. 2011).

The general approach to adjuvanticity is that of increasing immune stimulation by using particulate antigens, which achieve optimal stimulation of innate immunity. This is true for aluminum salts and for the oil-in-water emulsions. In this kind of approach, we can include the use of live attenuated viruses (LAIV, see above) and the use of virosomes, viral envelope particles that maintain the morphology and entry mechanism of the entire virus (Huckriede et al. 2005). Virosome-based influenza vaccines have shown a better performance in the elderly as compared to the non-adjuvanted vaccine (de Bruijn et al. 2005), while its outcome in comparison to MF59-adjuvanted vaccination is unclear (de Bruijn et al. 2006; Baldo et al. 2010).

Conclusions

The impressive success of vaccination in preventing the spread of many infectious diseases has contributed to the global improvement of the health conditions of the human population and, consequently, to its fast-increasing life expectancy. The world population is rapidly aging, thereby posing a totally different future scenario in public health. Preventive strategies will need to target not only newborn children and adults but most significantly the elderly population, intrinsically more susceptible to infections due to their immunological senescence. Delaying or slowing down immune senescence is one of the strategies to be adopted and includes a series of nonmedical actions (physical exercise, balanced nutrition, intellectual challenges) that not always are feasible. In many territories where infrastructures, living conditions, and lifestyle are not optimal (both in developing and in developed world), vaccination offers an affordable alternative.

However, developing vaccines that are effective and can protect the elderly is a totally new challenge for vaccinologists. Immune senescence is a complex scenario, which remains largely unknown to immunologists because of the wealth of variables affecting immune responses in aged people, starting from their individual past history of exposure and immunity. In general, aged people are more susceptible to common infectious diseases (*e.g.,* lung infections), due to both inadequate immune reactivity and acquired immunosuppression (other diseases, malnutrition). Likewise, their response to vaccination is suboptimal, thereby annihilating large part of the current preventive vaccination strategies. The best way of designing new vaccines specifically tailored for the aged population is gaining basic knowledge on the mechanisms of protective immunity against the different pathogens and, particularly, identifying the features of the age-related anomalies in mounting protective immune responses both in healthy and in diseased conditions in the elderly. However, currently, our knowledge gaps are very wide, and the current approaches are still very empirical. As summarized above, the most promising approaches imply "forcing" the immune response by the use of immunostimulants (adjuvants), which trigger the innate/inflammatory mechanism of immune amplification. These triggering agents should be particularly potent, to overcome the higher activation threshold generally present in older people, due to adaptation to their increasingly inflamed body's "normal" microenvironment (inflammaging). The possible drawback of potent adjuvant strategies may be increased reactogenicity, but inducing inflammation is key to the efficacy of adjuvants and to the overall vaccine efficacy and therefore cannot, should not, be avoided. However, the line discriminating between a transient inflammatory event (as it should take place locally at the vaccine inoculation site) and a more widespread and more persistent inflammatory reaction is becoming increasingly clear to immunologists, who can now provide us with "maps" of normal *vs.* pathological inflammation, which will help vaccinologists in selecting the most effective and safer adjuvant strategy for vaccinating the elderly.

Using alternative administration routes for delivering antigens and adjuvants is an interesting approach, as currently known the regulation of local tissue immunity follows rules that are very different from those of systemic immunity. Again, however, the basic knowledge is largely missing and therefore the possibility of exploiting the peculiarities of local immunity for increasing vaccine efficacy in the elderly is far from being at hand. An additional drawback is that until few years ago most of the studies on the regulation of immune responses were performed in animal models, mostly in mice, and it is now clear that in too many cases, the results obtained cannot be generalized to the human population.

Most of our experience in strategies for vaccination in the elderly originates from the work carried out in the field of influenza. It is of utmost importance that the progress made with the influenza vaccines be applied to other vaccines. New vaccines against infectious diseases are being designed to target the elderly population (*e.g.*, to TBE, HBV, RSV, pneumococci). However, other noninfectious chronic and degenerative diseases, such as Alzheimer's disease, diabetes, and rheumatoid arthritis, should likewise be targeted by preventive strategies preferably directed to the molecules causing the disease (when known) (Wisniewski and Konietzko 2008) or to associated risk factors (smoke, high blood pressure, alcohol abuse, etc.) (Bachmann and Jennings 2011). The first studies in this direction suggest that this can become a reality.

References

Ansaldi F, Bacilieri S, Durando P et al (2008) Cross-protection by MF59-adjuvanted influenza vaccine: neutralizing and hemagglutination-inhibiting antibody activity against A(H3N2) drifted influenza viruses. Vaccine 26:1525–1529

Ansaldi F, Zancolli F, Durando P et al (2010) Antibody response against heterogeneous circulating influenza virus strains elicited by MF59- and non-adjuvanted vaccines during seasons with good or partial matching between vaccine strain and clinical isolates. Vaccine 28:4123–4129

Aspinall R, Pido-Lopez J, Imami N et al (2007) Old rhesus macaques treated with interleukin-7 show increased TREC levels and respond well to influenza vaccination. Rejuvenation Res 10:5–17

Bachmann MF, Jennings GT (2011) Therapeutic vaccines for chronic diseases: successes and technical challenges. Philos Trans R Soc Lond B Biol Sci 366:2815–2822

Baldo V, Baldovin T, Pellegrini M et al (2010) Immunogenicity of three different influenza vaccines against homologous and heterologous strains in nursing home elderly residents. Clin Dev Immunol. doi:10.1155/2010/517198

Beebe GW, Simon AH, Vivona S (1972) Long-term mortality follow-up of Army recruits who received adjuvant influenza virus vaccine in 1951–1953. Am J Epidemiol 95:337–346

Belshe RB, Newman FK, Cannon J et al (2004) Serum antibody responses after intradermal vaccination against influenza. N Engl J Med 351:2286–2294

Belshe RB, Edwards KM, Vesikari T et al (2007a) Live attenuated versus inactivated influenza vaccine in infants and young children. N Engl J Med 356:685–696

Belshe RB, Newman FK, Wilkins K et al (2007b) Comparative immunogenicity of trivalent influenza vaccine administered by intradermal or intramuscular route in healthy adults. Vaccine 25:6755–6763

Ben-Yehuda A, Joseph A, Barenholz Y et al (2003a) Immunogenicity and safety of a novel IL-2-supplemented liposomal influenza vaccine (INFLUSOME-VAC) in nursing-home residents. Vaccine 21:3169–3178

Ben-Yehuda A, Joseph A, Zeira E et al (2003b) Immunogenicity and safety of a novel liposomal influenza subunit vaccine (INFLUSOME-VAC) in young adults. J Med Virol 69:560–567

Betts RF, Treanor JJ (2000) Approaches to improved influenza vaccination. Vaccine 18:1690–1695

Blank PR, Schwenkglenks M, Szucs TD (2008) Influenza vaccination coverage rates in five European countries during season 2006/07 and trends over six consecutive seasons. BMC Public Health 8:272

Brown H, Kasel JA, Freeman DM et al (1977) The immunizing effect of influenza A/New Jersey/76 (Hsw1N1) virus vaccine administered intradermally and intramuscularly to adults. J Infect Dis 136:S466–S471

Camilloni B, Neri M, Lepri E et al (2009) Cross-reactive antibodies in middle-aged and elderly volunteers after MF59-adjuvanted subunit trivalent influenza vaccine against B viruses of the B/Victoria or B/Yamagata lineages. Vaccine 27:4099–4103

Centers for Disease Control and Prevention (2010) Estimates of deaths associated with seasonal influenza Unites States, 1976–2007. MMWR 59:1057–1062

Crimmins EM, Finch CE (2006) Infection, inflammation, height, and longevity. Proc Natl Acad Sci U S A 103:498–503

de Bruijn IA, Nauta J, Cramer WC et al (2005) Clinical experience with inactivated, virosomal influenza vaccine. Vaccine 23(Suppl 1):S39–S49

de Bruijn IA, Nauta J, Gerez L et al (2006) The virosomal influenza vaccine Invivac: immunogenicity and tolerability compared to an adjuvanted influenza vaccine (Fluad®) in elderly subjects. Vaccine 24:6629–6631

De Villiers PJT, Steele AD, Hiemstra LA et al (2009) Efficacy and safety of a live attenuated influenza vaccine in adults 60 years of age and older. Vaccine 28:228–234

Del Giudice G, Hilbert AK, Bugarini R et al (2006) An MF59-adjuvanted inactivated influenza vaccine containing A/Panama/1999 (H3N2) induced broader serological protection against heterovariant influenza virus strain A/Fujian/2002 than a subunit and a split influenza vaccine. Vaccine 24:3063–3065

Dupuis M, Murphy TJ, Higgins D et al (1998) Dendritic cells internalize vaccine adjuvant after intramuscular injection. Cell Immunol 186:18–27

Dupuis M, Denis-Mize K, LaBarbara A et al (2001) Immunization with the adjuvant MF59 induces macrophage trafficking and apoptosis. Eur J Immunol 31:2910–2918

Edwards MS, Baker CJ (2005) Group B streptococcal infections in elderly adults. Clin Infect Dis 41:839–847

Ellebedy AH, Lupfer C, Ghoneim HE et al (2011) Inflammasome-independent role of the apoptosis-associated speck-like protein containing CARD (ASC)in the adjuvant effect of MF59. Proc Natl Acad Sci U S A 108:2927–2932

Falsey AR (2007) Respiratory syncytial virus in adults. Semin Respir Crit Care Med 28:171–181

Flicker L, McCaul KA, Hankey GJ et al (2010) Body mass index and survival in men and women aged 70 to 75. J Am Geriatr Soc 58:234–241

Franceschi C (2007) Inflammaging as a major characteristic of old people: can it be prevented or cured? Nutr Rev 65:S173–S176

Fujihashi K, Kiyono H (2009) Mucosal immunosenescence: new developments and vaccines to control infectious diseases. Trends Immunol 30:334–343

Galli G, Medini D, Borgogni E et al (2009) Adjuvanted H5N1 vaccine induces early CD4+ T cell response that predicts long-term persistence of protective antibody levels. Proc Natl Acad Sci U S A 106:3877–3882

Gavazzi G, Krause KH (2002) Ageing and infection. Lancet Infect Dis 2:659–666

Gibson KL, Wu YC, Barnett Y et al (2009) B-cell diversity decreases in old age and is correlated with poor health status. Aging Cell 8:18–25

Goodwin K, Viboud C, Simonsen L (2006) Antibody response to influenza vaccination in the elderly: a quantitative review. Vaccine 24:1159–1169

Goronzy J, Li G, Yu M et al (2012) Signaling pathways in aged T cells – A reflection of T cell differentiation, cell senescence and host environment. Semin Immunol 24(5):365–372

Govaert TM, Thijs CT, Masurel N et al (1994) The efficacy of influenza vaccination in elderly individuals. A randomized double-blind placebo-controlled trial. JAMA 272:1662–1665

Halperin W, Weiss WI, Altman R et al (1979) A comparison of the intradermal and subcutaneous routes of influenza vaccination with A/New Jersey/76 (Swine flu) and A/Victoria/75: report of a study and review of the literature. Am J Public Health 69:1247–1250

Herbert FA, Larke RP, Markstad EL (1979) Comparison of responses to influenza A/New Jersey/76-A/Victoria/75 virus vaccine administered intradermally or subcutaneously to adults with chronic respiratory disease. J Infect Dis 140:234–238

Herndler-Brandstetter D, Landgraf K, Tzankov A et al (2012) The impact of aging on memory T cell phenotype and function in the human bone marrow. J Leukoc Biol 91:197–205

Holland D, Booy R, De Looze F et al (2008) Intradermal influenza vaccine administered using a new microinjection system produces superior immunogenicity in elderly adults: a randomized controlled trial. J Infect Dis 198:650–658

Huckriede A, Bungener L, Stegmann T et al (2005) The virosome concept for influenza vaccines. Vaccine 23(Suppl 1):S26–S38

Johnson SA, Cambier JC (2004) Ageing, autoimmunity and arthritis: senescence of the B cell compartment. Implications for humoral immunity. Arthritis Res Ther 6:131–139

Keitel WA, Couch RB, Cate TR et al (1994) High doses of purified influenza A virus hemagglutinin significantly augment serum and nasal secretion antibody responses in healthy young adults. J Clin Microbiol 32:2468–2473

Keitel WA, Cate TR, Atmar RL et al (1996) Increasing doses of purified influenza virus hemagglutinin and subvirion vaccines enhance antibody responses in the elderly. Clin Diagn Lab Immunol 3:507–510

Kenney RT, Frech SA, Muenz LR et al (2004) Dose sparing with intradermal injection of influenza vaccine. N Engl J Med 351:2295–2301

Launay O, Grabar S, Bloch F et al (2008) Effect of sublingual administration of IFN-α on the immune response to influenza vaccination in institutionalized elderly individuals. Vaccine 26:4073–4079

Legrand J, Vergu E, Flahault A (2006) Real-time monitoring of the influenza vaccine field effectiveness. Vaccine 24:6605–6611

Li G, Yu M, Lee W-W et al (2012) Decline in miR-181a expression with age impairs T cell receptor sensitivity by increasing DUSP6 activity. Nat Med 18:1518–1524

Mosca F, Tritto E, Muzzi A et al (2008) Molecular and cellular signatures of human vaccine adjuvants. Proc Natl Acad Sci USA 105:10501–10506

Nichol KL, Nordin JD, Nelson DB et al (2007) Effectiveness of influenza vaccine in the community-dwelling elderly. N Engl J Med 357:1373–1381

Nikolich-Zugich J, Rudd BD (2010) Immune memory and aging: an infinite or finite resource? Curr Opin Immunol 22:535–540

Ohmit SE, Victor JC, Rotthoff JR et al (2006) Prevention of antigenically drifted influenza by inactivated and live attenuated vaccines. N Engl J Med 355:2513–2522

Panda A, Arjona A, Sapey E et al (2009) Human innate immunosenescence: causes and consequences for immunity in old age. Trends Immunol 30:325–333

Panda A, Qian F, Mohanty S et al (2010) Age-associated decrease in TLR function in primary human dendritic cells predicts influenza vaccine response. J Immunol 184:2518–2527

Pellegrini M, Nicolay U, Lindert K et al (2009) MF59-adjuvanted versus non-adjuvanted influenza vaccines: integrated analysis from a large safety database. Vaccine 27:6959–6965

Podda A, Del Giudice G, O'Hagan DT (2005) Chapter 9. MF59: a safe and potent adjuvant for human use. In: Schijns V, O'Hagan DT (eds) Immunopotentiators in modern medicines. Elsevier Press, Amsterdam

Potter CW, Oxford JS (1979) Determinants of immunity to influenza in man. Br Med Bull 35:69–75

Puig-Barberà J, Díez-Domingo J, Varea AB et al (2007) Effectiveness of the MF59™-adjuvanted subunit influenza vaccine in preventing hospitalizations for cardiovascular disease, cerebrovascular disease and pneumonia in the elderly. Vaccine 25:7313–7321

Rappuoli R, Mandl CW, Black S et al (2011) Vaccines for the twenty-first century society. Nat Rev Immunol 11:865–872

Schmader K (2001) Herpes zoster in older adults. Clin Infect Dis 32:1481–1486

Seubert A, Monaci E, Pizza M et al (2008) The adjuvants aluminum hydroxide and MF59 induce monocyte and granulocyte chemoattractants and enhance monocyte differentiation toward dendritic cells. J Immunol 180:5402–5412

Seubert A, Calabro S, Santini L et al (2011) Adjuvanticity of the oil-in-water emulsion MF59 is independent of Nlrp3 inflammasome but requires the adaptor protein MyD88. Proc Natl Acad Sci U S A 108:11169–11174

Shaw AC, Joshi S, Greenwood H et al (2010) Aging of the innate immune system. Curr Opin Immunol 22:507–513

Stephenson I, Nicholson KG, Hoschler K et al (2008) Antigenically distinct MF59-adjuvanted vaccine to boost immunity to H5N1. N Engl J Med 359:1631–1633

Treanor JJ, Mattison HR, Dumyati G et al (1992) Protective efficacy of combined live intranasal and inactivated influenza A virus vaccines in the elderly. Ann Intern Med 117:625–633

Treanor JJ, Campbell JD, Zangwill KM et al (2006) Safety and immunogenicity of an inactivated subvirion influenza A (H5N1) vaccine. N Engl J Med 354:1343–1351

United Nations, Department of Economic and Social Affairs, Population Division (2002) World population ageing 1950–2050. United Nations Publishing. http://www.un.org/esa/population/publications/worldageing19502050/. Accessed 19 May 2009

Van Damme P, Arnou R, Kafeja F et al (2010) Evaluation of non-inferiority of intradermal versus adjuvanted seasonal influenza vaccine using two serological techniques: a randomized comparative study. BMC Infect Dis 10:134

Vogel FR, Caillet C, Kusters IC et al (2009) Emulsion-based adjuvants for influenza vaccines. Expert Rev Vaccines 8:483–492

Wagner EH, Groves T (2002) Care for chronic diseases. Br Med J 325:913–914

Weinberger B, Herndler-Brandstetter D, Schwanninger A et al (2008) Biology of the immune response to vaccines in elderly persons. Clin Infect Dis 46:1078–1084

Wisniewski T, Konietzko U (2008) Amyloid-beta immunisation for Alzheimer's disease. Lancet Neurol 7:805–811

World Bank (2004) World development indicators 2004. World Bank, Washington DC

World Health Organization (2005) Expert consultation on rabies. World Health Organ Tech Rep Ser 931:1–88

Yu M, Li G, Lee W-W et al (2012) Signal inhibition by the Dual-Specific Phosphatase 4 impairs T cell-dependent B cell responses with age. Proc Natl Acad Sci U S A 109:E879–E888

Nutrition, Immunity, and Aging

20

Armin Hirbod-Mobarakeh, Maryam Mahmoudi, and Nima Rezaei

20.1 Nutrition and Immunosenescence

Immunosenescence or age-related changes of the immune system are a complex process leading to dysregulation in the function of the immune system (Weksler 1995). This dysregulation is responsible for poor responses to immunization, increased rates of infections, prolonged recovery from infections, autoimmunity, and cancer in the elderly (Castle 2000; Lesourd 2006; Pae et al. 2012; Roberts-Thomson et al. 1974). The extent of immunosenescence varies among individuals

A. Hirbod-Mobarakeh, MPH
Molecular Immunology Research Center,
Tehran University of Medical Sciences,
Tehran, Iran

M. Mahmoudi, MD, PhD (✉)
School of Nutrition and Dietetics,
Tehran University of Medical Sciences,
Tehran, Iran
e-mail: mahmoodi_maryam@yahoo.com

N. Rezaei, MD, MSc, PhD
Research Center for Immunodeficiencies,
Children's Medical Center,
Tehran, Iran

Department of Immunology, School of Medicine,
Tehran University of Medical Sciences,
Tehran, Iran

Molecular Immunology Research Center,
Tehran University of Medical Sciences,
Tehran, Iran

depending on several factors including genetics, environment, lifestyle, and nutrition (BM 2001; Chandra 2002; Pae et al. 2012).

Throughout the history, food resources have always been a determining factor for victory in wars. Similarly, body reserves and nutritional intake have a central role in host defense in the battlefield against infectious agents and malignant cells (Field et al. 2002). The immune system is a large organ consisting of millions of cells with high cellular turnover. So, appropriate nutrition by providing adequate energy and nutrition for this high rate of cell renewal has a central role in improving efficiency of the immune system (Marcos et al. 2003; Lesourd 2004; Pae et al. 2012).

In the last four decades, the concept of nutrition as a modifiable factor with widespread influence on the immune system established the foundation of the immunonutrition (Rymkiewicz et al. 2012; Pae et al. 2012; Grimm and Calder 2002). Nutritional deficiencies particularly micronutrient deficits are prevalent among the elderly not only in developing world but also in developed countries (Grimm and Calder 2002; Lesourd 2006). In England, 16 % of the elderly over 65 years old had nutrition deficiency (Ahmed and Haboubi 2010; Office of National Statistics 2011). The presence of undernutrition in the elderly staying in hospitals or nursing homes reaches to 30–65 % (Volkert 2002). Undernutrition results in impaired immune system and impaired host resistance to infectious agents. Infections lead to further consumption

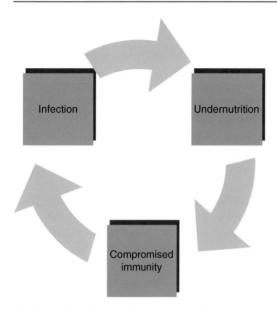

Fig. 20.1 The vicious cycle of undernutrition, immunodeficiency, and infectious diseases

of body reserve which in turn results in further compromised immune function thus setting up a vicious cycle (Fig. 20.1) (Grimm and Calder 2002; Marcos et al. 2003). The immune system in the elderly is more sensitive to nutrition deficits (Meydani 2001).

Today, there is no debate on the vital role of nutritional status on the phenomena of immunosenescence. Indeed, several previously described characteristics of immunosenescence like impairment of cellular arm of the immune system, diminished delayed hypersensitivity, impaired neutrophil function, and decreased interleukin-2 production are similar to the changes occurring during PEM and may be related to secondary immunodeficiency due to undiagnosed nutritional deficiencies (Lesourd and Mazari 1999; Bogden and Louria 1999). Having this concept in mind, immunosenescence can be classified into 3 categories in regard to nutritional status (Lesourd and Mazari 1999; Bogden and Louria 1999; Lesourd 2006):

1. Primary immunosenescence or successful immunosenescence which can be observed in very healthy elderly with no nutritional deficit.
2. Secondary immunosenescence occurring in apparently healthy elderly with subopti-

mal nutritional statue, i.e., deficiencies in one or more micronutrient or subclinical macronutrient deficiency. This type of immunosenescence is termed as common immunosenescence, since this nutritional statue is very common among the elderly.
3. Tertiary immunosenescence or pathological immunosenescence can be seen in diseased elderly individuals suffering from major undernutrition such as protein–energy malnutrition (PEM).

20.1.1 Primary Immunosenescence

Primary immunosenescence or successful immunosenescence was defined as age-related natural changes in the immune system observed in individuals with no macronutrient or micronutrient deficiencies and optimal reserves of nutrients in the body (Lesourd and Mazari 1999; Bogden and Louria 1999; Lesourd 2006). During the last decades, several strict inclusion criteria have been developed for studies on the phenomena of primary immunosenescence. The aim of these criteria was exclusion of any subclinical ongoing disease or nutritional deficiency which can lead to deviation of the natural process of immunosenescence. The first criteria were proposed by European Community's Concerted Action Program on Aging (EURAGE) in 1984 which named SENIEUR protocol (Ligthart et al. 1984). Three factors of living conditions, laboratory values, and drug intake were considered in this protocol. In 1988, inclusion criterion of serum albumin value of more than 35 g/l was added to SENIEUR criteria in order to exclude presence of PEM (Reibnegger et al. 1988). Finally, in 1999, Lesourd and Mazari added several inclusion conditions to the previous criteria which significantly decreased the presence of confounding biases in studies on primary immunosenescence (Lesourd et al. 1998). The new criteria were as follows (Lesourd 2006):

1. Good health with no ongoing, developing, or degenerative diseases
2. Normal adult values for laboratory variables
3. No drugs acting on the immune system

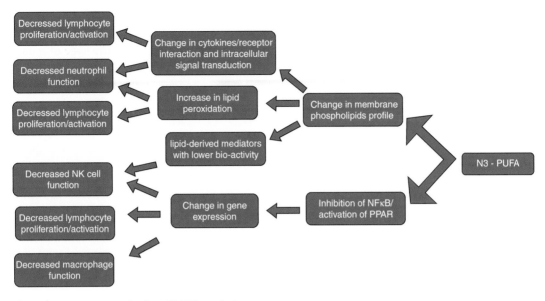

Fig. 20.2 Mechanisms of action of PUFA on the immune system

4. No disease in the past 5 years
5. No motor skill difficulties
6. Normal physical activity (defined as more than 4 km walk per day)
7. No drug treatment for cardiac, neurological, or psychotropical diseases (including depression)
8. Normal mental status (defined as minimental status of Folstein of 28/30)
9. Serum albumin level of more than 39 g/l
10. Normal values for trace elements or vitamins
11. No major acute-phase response (defined as serum C-reactive protein level of less than 30 mg/l)

Studies on the elderly, who fulfilled these inclusion criteria, provided a large body of information on the natural changes occurring in the immune system by aging. These changes will be discussed in other chapters of this book. These studies also suggest that primary immunosenescence can be modified by addition of dietary lipids such as n-3 polyunsaturated fatty acids (PUFA), micronutrients such as vitamin E above the recommended dietary intake, and probiotics. In addition, total calorie control or caloric restriction (CR) has been shown to have beneficiary effect on primary immunosenescence (Meydani

2001; Pae et al. 2012). Probably, in the future, the inclusion criteria for studies on primary immunosenescence will be stricter so that effects of these dietary modifications are excluded from primary immune aging.

20.1.1.1 Polyunsaturated Fatty Acids

N-3 PUFA found mainly in marine fish oils has been long known for its anti-inflammatory role in the immune system (Wahrburg 2004). Several mechanisms are responsible for anti-inflammatory effect of n-3 PUFA (Galli and Calder 2009) (Fig. 20.2). Increased intake of n-3 PUFA results in change in composition of membrane phospholipids fatty acid which in turn can interfere with binding of cytokines to their receptor. Different membrane phospholipid profiles lead to change in intracellular signal transduction due to the different second messengers, and signaling molecules resulted from the change in acylation patterns and fatty acyl chains (Sijben and Calder 2007). A high n-3 PUFA in membranes results in production of lipid-derived mediators like prostaglandins (PG) and leukotrienes (LT) with lower bioactivity. They can also directly change the expression of inflammatory genes through activating peroxisomal proliferator-activated receptors (PPAR) pathway and inhibiting nuclear factor kappa-light-chain-enhancer of activated B cells (NFκB) pathway (Grimble 2005). Last but not least, n-3 PUFA are more sensitive to peroxidation resulting in more production of toxic lipid peroxides which are toxic for the immune cells (Field et al. 2002). Studies have shown that n-3 PUFA can decrease production of PGE2, proinflammatory cytokines, chemokines, and adhesion molecules and inhibit T-cell proliferation and neutrophil respiratory burst (Kim et al. 2010; Shaikh and Edidin 2006). These effects are larger in the elderly comparing to young adults (Pae et al. 2012).

Overall, these mechanisms lead to decreased systemic inflammatory response and suppression of both innate and adaptive immunity especially T-cell-mediated immunity. These effects make n-3 PUFA a good candidate for alleviation of inflammatory and autoimmune diseases such as rheumatoid arthritis, asthma, inflammatory bowel disease, cardiovascular disease, and degenerative neurological diseases. But these effects also make n-3 PUFA like a double-edged sword as it impairs host's resistance to a number of pathogens (Pae et al. 2012). However, some studies showed moderate amounts of n-3 PUFA can enhance immune functions and even increase protection against infection (Pae et al. 2012; Field et al. 2002).

20.1.1.2 Probiotics

Probiotics are beneficial microorganisms from genera of *Lactobacillus* (*L.*), *Bifidobacterium* (*B.*), and *Streptococcus* (*S.*) which settle in the gastrointestinal (GI) tract and modulate both the GI immune system, as the largest immune organ, and systemic immune system (Guarner and Schaafsma 1998). Several changes like decrease in beneficial microbes and secretory immunoglobulin (Ig) A and reduction of gut-associated lymphoreticular tissues (GALT) occurring naturally by aging in the GI immune system can be improved by probiotics consumption (de Moreno de LeBlanc et al. 2008; Pae et al. 2012; Delcenserie et al. 2008). Animal studies have shown increased production of interleukin (IL)-2 and interferon gamma (IFN-γ), tumor necrosis factors alpha (TNF-α), and IL-6 and increased number of T lymphocytes specially CD4+ cells and antibody-secreting cells

as a result of probiotics consumption (Baba et al. 2009; Calder and Kew 2002; Pae et al. 2012). Human studies have shown enhanced phagocytosis and cytotoxicity in monocytes, NK cells, and neutrophils with certain strains of probiotics (Calder and Kew 2002; Bengmark 2006). The improved humoral response and increased vaccine efficacy were observed only in long period of supplementation with probiotics (Pae et al. 2012; Tsai et al. 2008). Different strains of probiotics resulted in different profiles of cytokine production in humans (Elmadfa et al. 2010; Pae et al. 2012). In addition, probiotics improve nutrient absorption and prevent colonization of pathogenic bacteria in GI tract by competition for nutrients and producing metabolic products like lactic acid and bacteriocin, a protein with antibiotic activities (Calder and Kew 2002).

20.1.1.3 Calorie Restriction and Protein Nutritional Status

CR without malnutrition can improve and delay the primary immunosenescence. This effect is believed to be due to the increased levels of antioxidant enzymes and reduction of oxidative stress, but animal studies have shown that other mechanisms like increase in IL-2 production and slow down of age-related increasing trend of TNF-α and IL-6 production may play a role (Fernandes 2008; Pae et al. 2012; Messaoudi et al. 2006; Lane et al. 2001). These studies provided evidence that CR can have effects on cellular immunity by increasing T-cell proliferation, proportion of naïve T cells, and natural killer (NK) cell activity (Lane et al. 2001). Although few studies have been done on human subjects, they confirmed that CR can improve T-cell-mediated immune response and T-cell proliferation (Ahmed et al. 2009). Some studies suggest that there might be a time window for CR initiation to benefit from its effect (Messaoudi et al. 2008; Pae et al. 2012; Meydani 2001). However, CR can be a double-edged sword as lower levels of serum albumin, as an indicator of protein intake, even in normal range, were associated with lower levels of CD3+ mature T lymphocytes and cytotoxic T lymphocytes (CTL), higher levels of immature T lymphocytes, decreased lymphocyte proliferation, and IL-2 release (Lesourd and Mazari 1999).

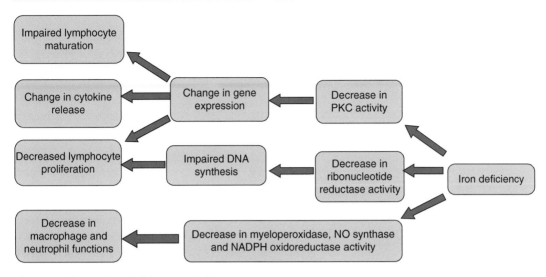

Fig. 20.3 Effects of iron deficiency on the immune system

20.1.2 Secondary Immunosenescence

In the elderly, deficiency in vitamins such as vitamin A, vitamin B12, vitamin B6, vitamin C, vitamin E, folate, niacin, and riboflavin or minerals such as iron, zinc, and selenium and subclinical macronutrient deficiency are common and may interfere with the process of primary immunosenescence. Moreover, subclinical deficiencies of macronutrients such as proteins, although may not be symptomatic, may accelerate immunosenescence (High 2001; Shepherd 2009; Lesourd 2004). We refer to these deviations as primary immunosenescence, secondary immunosenescence, or common immunosenescence (Lesourd 1997, 2006; Cunningham-Rundles et al. 2005). The extent of these deviations is determined by both host-related factors such as age, gender, and presence of infection and factors related to micronutrient like the type of micronutrient, the level of deficiency, and interaction with other micronutrients (High 2001; Shepherd 2009; Lesourd 2004; Chandra 1997).

20.1.2.1 Minerals
Iron
Iron, as a critical component of several enzymes including peroxide- and nitrous oxide-generating enzymes, plays a critical role in several metabolic pathways like electron transfer reactions and transport of oxygen radicals. It is involved in regulation of cell differentiation, cell growth, and cytokine production through regulation of different genes or activation of intracellular signaling pathway like protein kinase C (Weiss 2004). Therefore, iron plays a major role in regulation of cell-mediated immunity and functions of T lymphocytes (Fig. 20.3). Iron is involved in respiratory burst in macrophages and neutrophils, as a component of myeloperoxidase activity (Oppenheimer 2001; Maggini et al. 2007; Weiss 2002).

Iron deficiency mainly influences cell-mediated immunity. It results in low production of IL-2 and IFN which in turn result in impaired NK cell function and depressed delayed cutaneous hypersensitivity (Scrimshaw and SanGiovanni 1997; Cunningham-Rundles et al. 2005). In iron deficiency, lymphocytes and macrophages by increasing surface transferrin receptors can meet their needs for iron. Therefore, mild or even moderate iron deficiency has little effects on the immune system. But even in a mild iron deficiency state, in the presence of inflammation, macrophages sequestrate iron to limit the availability of iron to pathogens which result in limited availability of iron to other immune cells and therefore impairment of host immunity (Field et al. 2002).

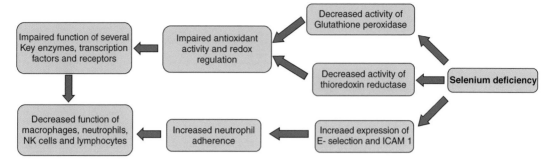

Fig. 20.4 Effects of selenium deficiency on the immune system

Zinc

Zinc deficiency is extremely frequent in the elderly and can mimic the age-related immune changes (Lesourd and Mazari 1999). Zinc is a ubiquitous player in cell division, differentiation, apoptosis, and gene transcription with its role as a cofactor for activity of more than 100 metalloenzymes associated with carbohydrate and energy metabolism, protein degradation and synthesis, nucleic acid synthesis, heme biosynthesis, and CO_2 transport (Scrimshaw and SanGiovanni 1997; Maggini et al. 2007). Zinc has an essential role in development and maintenance of the immune system particularly T cells, but its roles are so widespread that can affect both innate and adaptive immunity (Ibs and Rink 2003). Zinc is involved in maintaining of the skin and mucosal membrane integrity which is an important component of the innate immunity (Maggini et al. 2007). Zinc like iron is involved in respiratory burst, but it is also involved in cytosolic defense against oxidative stress by its role as a superoxide dismutase (Maggini et al. 2007). Zinc is an essential cofactor for the activity of thymulin, the thymic hormone responsible for thymocyte proliferation and cytokine realize modulation. Zinc, as a component of NFkB, is directly involved in the expression of different cytokines and adhesion molecules (Rink and Kirchner 2000). Zinc can prevent apoptosis by several mechanisms like interfering with interaction of glucocorticoids and its receptor and inhibiting endonuclease activity which is responsible for DNA fragmentation (Field et al. 2002).

Zinc deficiency through activation of hypothalamic–pituitary–adrenal axis results in excess release of glucocorticoids which in turn lead to reprogramming of the immune system. Decreased T-helper 1 (Th1) cytokines, TNF-α, and thymulin activity; apoptosis of lymphocytes and lymphopenia; impairment of T-helper maturation; impaired NK cell function; and reduced phagocytosis all are results of this reprogramming of the immune system which presents with impairment of cell and antibody-mediated responses and skin test anergy (Chandra 1997; Lesourd 1997; Calder and Kew 2002; Cunningham-Rundles et al. 2005; Savino et al. 2007). Severe thymic atrophy is a hallmark of zinc deficiency; however, it is associated with reduction of the number and proportion of lymphoid precursors and increase in myeloid precursors in the bone marrow (Cunningham-Rundles et al. 2005).

Selenium

Selenium, as an important component of glutathione peroxidase and thioredoxin reductase, is involved in regulation of redox state produced during inflammatory reactions and respiratory burst in immune cells and therefore plays an important role in antioxidant host defense system (Burk 2002; Arthur et al. 2003; Cunningham-Rundles et al. 2005) (Fig. 20.4). The redox regulation function of thioredoxin reductase is essential in the function of several key enzymes, transcription factors and receptors such as ribonucleotide reductase, glucocorticoid receptors, and NFkB pathway (Ryan-Harshman and Aldoori 2005; Maggini et al. 2007).

Selenium deficiency can influence both arms of the immune system. Selenium deficiency results in inefficacy of respiratory burst

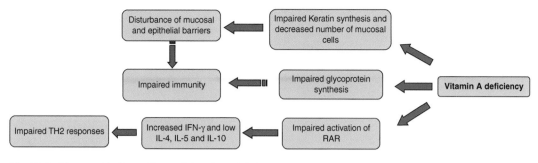

Fig. 20.5 Direct and indirect effects of vitamin A deficiency on the immune system

and impairment of macrophage and neutrophil cytotoxicity. Moreover, neutrophil adhesion is enhanced during selenium deficiency due to the increased expression of E-selectin and intercellular adhesion molecule 1 (ICAM-1) (Field et al. 2002). Selenium deficiency leads to changes in expression of cytokines and their receptors which result in decrease in T-cell proliferation and differentiation and NK cell activity.

Copper

Copper, as a component of superoxide dismutase, catalase, and glutathione peroxidase, like selenium and zinc, has an essential role in cytosolic antioxidant defense. Copper deficiency can affect several aspects of the immune response specially neutrophils, monocytes, and macrophages (Bonham et al. 2002; Maggini et al. 2007).

20.1.2.2 Vitamins

Vitamin A

Retinol, retinal, and retinoic acid, as different chemical forms of vitamin A, directly or indirectly can influence innate, cell-mediated, and humoral immunity (Fig. 20.5) (Aukrust et al. 2000). Vitamin A is needed for synthesis of a vast majority of glycoproteins such as integrins, fibronectin, and globulins which indirectly can influence the immune system (Maggini et al. 2007). Other indirect roles of vitamin A include differentiation of epithelial and mucosal barrier via regulation of Keratin synthesis and mucus-secreting cells (Maggini et al. 2007). Vitamin A can activate retinoic acid receptors (RAR) which result in regulation of cytokine release and development and differentiation of T lymphocyte specially Th-2 subsets and humoral immunity (Halevy et al. 1994; Field et al. 2002; Maggini et al. 2007).

Vitamin A deficiency results in impairment of mucosal barriers due to the impairment of basal and mucous cells proliferation, loss of gap junctions, and decrease in the proportions of preciliated and ciliated cells (Maggini et al. 2007). It also affects innate cell immunity by impairment of phagocytic and oxidative burst activity of neutrophils and macrophages (Scrimshaw and SanGiovanni 1997). Vitamin A deficiency impairs both Th1- and Th2-mediated immune responses particularly Th2 responses (Cantorna et al. 1994; Maggini et al. 2007).

Vitamin B

Vitamin B group consists of several vitamins with undeniable effects in the metabolism and therefore in the immune system. Vitamins B6, B9, and B12 constitute a triad involved in supplying one-carbon unit essential for nucleic acid and protein synthesis (Maggini et al. 2007).

Vitamin B6 deficiency like zinc deficiency can mimic the age-related immune changes (Lesourd and Mazari 1999). Vitamin B6 deficiency results in diminished cell-mediated immunity and to a less extent disturbance of humoral immunity (Rall and Meydani 1993; Chandra and Sudhakaran 1990; Scrimshaw and SanGiovanni 1997).

Vitamin B9 and vitamin B12 are both essential factors in cellular replication, and deficits in these two vitamins are associated with disturbances of both cell-mediated immunity and humoral immunity. Both of them result in thymic atrophy (Scrimshaw and SanGiovanni 1997). In addition, deficits of these vitamins result in decreased neutrophil function and phagocytosis and abnormal serum complement concentrations (Dhur et al. 1991; Scrimshaw and SanGiovanni 1997). Vitamin B9 deficiency is associated with reduced proliferation of T lymphocytes (Courtemanche et al. 2004; Maggini et al. 2007). Vitamin B12 deficiency is associated with suppressed NK cell activity, significant changes in number of lymphocytes, and T-cell subsets, i.e., CD8+ cells, CD4+ cells, and CD4+/CD8+ ratio (Dhur et al. 1991; Troen et al. 2006; Maggini et al. 2007; Courtemanche et al. 2004; Tamura et al. 1999).

Vitamin C

Vitamin C acts as a regulator of redox and scavenger of reactive oxygen species produced during respiratory burst and therefore has a deniable role in cytotoxicity of neutrophils, macrophages, and monocytes (Jacob et al. 1991; Wintergerst et al. 2006). It stimulates leukocyte functions such as neutrophil and monocyte mobility and can enhance inducible nitric oxide synthetase production in macrophages and inhibit NFκB pathway resulting in increase in macrophage function (Cunningham-Rundles et al. 2005). It enhances NK cell activity by activating PKC (Field et al. 2002). Vitamin C can enhance survival of immune cells specially T cells by regulation of metabolic checkpoints, cytokine release, and prevention of three T-cell death pathways (Hartel et al. 2004; Maggini et al. 2007). By all these effects in mind, it is completely tangible that vitamin C deficiency results in anergy in almost all components of the immune system.

Vitamin D

Vitamin D, as a lymphocyte differentiation hormone, plays an important role in modulating the immune system (Deluca and Cantorna 2001; Maggini et al. 2007; Scrimshaw and SanGiovanni 1997). Vitamin D by binding to its receptor, which exists on all immune cells except B cells, can increase bactericidal activities of neutrophils, monocytes, and macrophages by improving respiratory burst and enhance NK cell activity by

inducing the expression of antimicrobial peptides (Griffin et al. 2003; Hayes et al. 2003; Cantorna et al. 2004; Deluca and Cantorna 2001). It can also cause changes in expression of several cytokines (Cantorna et al. 2004; Deluca and Cantorna 2001; Maggini et al. 2007).

Vitamin E

Vitamin E as a potent antioxidant can support respiratory burst in neutrophils, monocytes, and macrophages (Meydani et al. 2005). Vitamin E can inhibit production of immunosuppressive factors such as PGE2 through inhibition of cyclooxygenase (COX) pathway and can modify the immune system by its effect on cytokine release (Adolfsson et al. 2001; Pae et al. 2012; Pallast et al. 1999; High 2001; Wu and Meydani 2008). Vitamin E enhances the interaction of antigen-presenting cells (APC) and immature T cells which in turn results in maturation of T cells (Pekmezci 2011; Field et al. 2002).

Vitamin E deficiency results in disturbance of humoral immunity and lymphocyte proliferation; reduced function of neutrophils, lymphocyte, NK cells, and other leukocytes; and impairment of cell-mediated immunity (Pekmezci 2011; Scrimshaw and SanGiovanni 1997; Field et al. 2002).

20.1.3 Tertiary Immunosenescence

Chen et al. defined protein–energy undernutrition or protein–calorie undernutrition as "progressive loss of both lean body mass and adipose tissue resulting from insufficient consumption of protein and energy, although one or the other may play the dominant role in the elderly" (Chen et al. 2001). Certain factors such as burns, fractures, cancer, sepsis, respiratory illness, cardiovascular disease, renal disorders, liver disease, gastrointestinal disorders, anorexia, and unrecognized dysphasia make the elderly prone to these phenomena (Price 2008). Not surprisingly, in the presence of PEM, all components of the immune system are influenced due to the high dependence on energy and amino acids for production of active protein compounds and cell division (Field et al. 2002; Scrimshaw and SanGiovanni 1997).

Fig. 20.6 Effects of PEM on the innate immunity

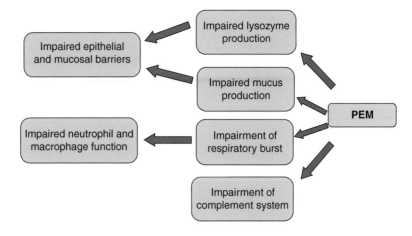

Fig. 20.7 Mechanisms of PEM-induced lymphoid atrophy

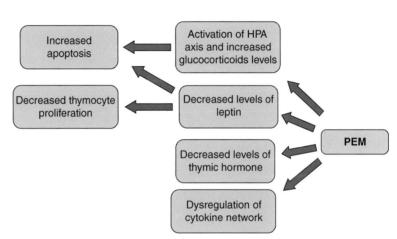

In addition, PEM is usually accompanied by micronutrient deficiencies which can result in further deterioration of the immune system (Savino and Dardenne 2010; Cunningham-Rundles et al. 2005).

20.1.3.1 Innate Immunity

PEM can cause a profound innate immunodeficiency both directly and indirectly (Fig. 20.6) (Chandra 1983). PEM results in impairment of mucosal barriers, the first defensive line of the immune system, due to decreased lysozyme concentrations and mucus production which in turn results in increase adherence of bacteria to the epithelial surfaces (Chandra 1983, 1997; Lesourd 1997). PEM also leads to impairment of respiratory burst and phagocytosis and therefore intracellular destruction of pathogens by neutrophils, monocytes, and macrophages (Redmond et al. 1991;

Savino et al. 2007; Lipschitz and Udupa 1986). There is a decrease in both concentrations and activity of most complement components particularly in C3, C5, factor B, total hemolytic activity, and opsonic activity of plasma (Chandra 1997; Lesourd 1997).

20.1.3.2 Cell-Mediated Immunity

PEM, as the main reason for tertiary immunosenescence, causes an obvious decrease in cell-mediated immune responses by a decrease in both number of T cells and their function (Chandra 1997; Lesourd 1997). PEM causes a dramatic lymphoid atrophy consisting of changes in peripheral lymphoid organs, the atrophy of the thymus, and complete loss of corticomedullary differentiation in the thymus through several mechanisms (Fig. 20.7) (Chandra 1997; Lesourd 1997; Marcos et al. 2003). This lymphoid atrophy in peripheral lymphoid organs like spleen presents with loss of lymphoid cells around small blood vessels and in lymph nodes presents with lower number of lymphocytes in paracortical areas (Chandra 1997; Lesourd 1997). There is a decrease in CD3$^+$, CD8$^+$, and specially CD4$^+$ subsets and a simultaneous increase in CD2$^+$CD3$^-$ subsets, double-negative CD2$^+$CD4$^-$CD8$^-$ subset, and CD57$^+$ NK cells. CD4$^+$/CD8$^+$ is lower compared to healthy individuals. All these changes strongly correlate with the extent of the albumin decrease and the severity of PEM (Iyer et al. 2012; Lesourd and Mazari 1999; Chandra 1997; Lesourd 1997). For example, albumin levels lower than 30 g/l have been associated with CD4$^+$ counts as low as HIV patients (<400/mm^3) (Lesourd and Mazari 1999). In the presence of PEM, lymphocyte proliferation, cytokine release, cytotoxic capacities, and as a result delayed cutaneous hypersensitivity are decreased probably due to the low serum thymic factor activity (Redmond et al. 1995; Lotfy et al. 1998; Taylor et al. 2013). In addition to major alterations in cytokine network like decreased production of IL-1, IL-2, and IFNγ, PEM impairs the responsiveness of T lymphocytes to cytokines (Lotfy et al. 1998; Chandra 1997; Lesourd 1997). The dysregulation in cytokine network results in impaired mobilization of the already low nutritional reserves which leads to low nutrition supply for leukocytes and further deterioration of the immune system (Lesourd and Mazari 1999; Chandra 1997; Lesourd 1997).

20.1.3.3 Humoral Immunity

In the presence of PEM, probably due to inhibitory factors in the plasma, there is a decrease DNA synthesis and lymphocyte proliferation. Decrease in number of antibody-producing cells results in low production of Igs (Savino et al. 2007; Chandra 1997; Lesourd 1997). Ig profiles change in PEM as there are lower concentrations of secretory IgA (sIgA) and a compensatory increase in IgM in secretions. Moreover, antibody affinity is dysregulated in these patients resulting in producing different autoantibodies (Chandra 1997; Lesourd 1997). Interestingly, antibody responses to the

T-cell-independent antigens or antigens with adjuvant are generally intact. Therefore, these changes in humoral immunity may largely be secondary to the decreased function of T helpers (Savino et al. 2007; Lesourd 1997).

20.2 Pathological Causes of Nutritional Deficiencies in the Elderly

Undernutrition in the elderly is a multifactorial phenomenon. Three main categories of physical, psychological, and social factors besides physiological anorexia of aging are responsible for susceptibility of the elderly to undernutrition (High 2001) (Fig. 20.8).

20.2.1 Physical Factors

20.2.1.1 Body Composition

Decreased muscle mass or sarcopenia, an inevitable process in aging, results from several factors including decreased motor neuron function, low levels of anabolic hormones, sedentary life and inadequate dietary protein (Roubenoff 2000; Chapman et al. 2002). These phenomena lead to a lower metabolic rate and energy requirement which in turn results in decreased dietary intake (Chapman et al. 2002; Ahmed and Haboubi 2010; Brownie 2006; Wilson and Morley 2003). In addition, skeletal muscle cells act as a strategic nutrition reserve for gluconeogenesis, synthesis of acute-phase proteins, and the immune cell proliferation during inflammatory reactions (Roubenoff 2000; Brownie 2006).

20.2.1.2 Gastrointestinal System

The GI system—from ingestion to defecation—is the target of changes in aging. Appetite physiologically decreases by aging, but factors like diminished taste, olfactory perception, and feelings of hunger which are prevalent in the elderly due to disorders, medications, and aging of the responsible organs can advance loss of appetite (Finkelstein and Schiffman 1999; Parker and Chapman 2004; Elsner 2002; Brownie 2006).

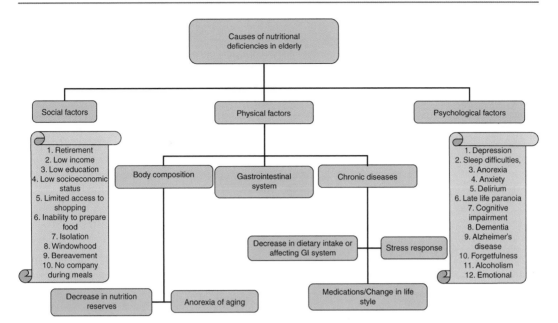

Fig. 20.8 Pathological causes of nutritional deficiencies in elderly

The diminished taste and olfactory perception result in impairment of cephalic phase of digestion. Chewing disabilities due to the loss of teeth, inappropriate dentures, dry mouth, and gingivitis limit nutritional options and make the elderly to use pureed foods with poorer nutritional quality than regular food (Finkelstein and Schiffman 1999; Elsner 2002; Omran and Morley 2000a; Brownie 2006).

In the elderly, factors such as atrophic gastritis, hypochlorhydria, decreased peristalsis and motility, low bioavailability, and impaired enzymatic capacity decrease the efficacy of GI tract for digestion, absorption, and metabolism of digested nutrients. For example, concentration of enzymes in pancreatic juice declines by aging, and small intestine loses its capacity for absorption due to decline in mucosal surface and loss of villi (Parker and Chapman 2004; Fich et al. 1989; Ahmed and Haboubi 2010; Bitar and Patil 2004; Bitar et al. 2011; Laugier et al. 1991). Impaired immune surveillance of the GI tract makes the elderly susceptible to a range of GI infections which may deteriorate the already reduced efficacy of the GI tract (Parker and Chapman 2004; Pae et al. 2012; Brownie 2006).

20.2.1.3 Chronic Diseases

Chronic diseases of the elderly impair the nutritional status by either the side effects of the disease itself or by side effects of treatment and medications.

Disease, regardless of acute or chronic, leads to a stress response and release of proinflammatory cytokines such as IL-1, TNF, and IL-6. In the presence of this stress response, already reduced nutritional reserves (due to sarcopenia) are consumed (Shatenstein 2008). In the elderly, due to decreased anabolic state, body reserves can never be fully replaced during recovery. Therefore, disease can lead to a progressive loss of body reserves and worsening nutritional status which in turn results in impaired immune system and increased susceptibility to diseases and turn on a vicious cycle (Lesourd 2006). Chronic diseases, besides increasing metabolic rate and nutrient consumption, may decrease dietary intake due to anorexia, nausea, pain, restricted mobility, and loss of coordination (Clarke et al. 1998; Shatenstein 2008). Some chronic diseases demand long-term care in nursing homes in which lack of direct attention of staff, poor positioning during meals, and forced or rapid feeding may result in undernutrition (Shatenstein 2008; Price 2008).

Chronic diseases usually require chronic use of different medications which can interfere with appetite due to impairment of taste and smell, absorption, metabolization, and excretion of the nutrients, and some like thyroxin can increase the metabolic rate and nutrient consumption (Fig. 20.9) (Clarke et al. 1998; Omran and Morley 2000a; Brownie 2006).

20.2.2 Psychological Factors

Depression, sleep difficulties, anorexia, anxiety, delirium, and more importantly late life paranoia are risk factors for decreased dietary intake (Elsner 2002; Clarke et al. 1998; Brownie 2006). Depression is the most common cause of weight loss in the elderly which is supposed to be due to enhanced levels of corticotrophin-releasing hormone, a potent anorectic neurotransmitter. In late life paranoia, the elderly decrease their food intake due to the fear of being poisoned (Cederholm and Morley 2013). In addition, cognitive impairment, dementia, Alzheimer's disease, and forgetfulness might directly or indirectly influence the nutrition both in quality and quantity. Last but not least, alcoholism which is not rare in the elderly can influence both dietary intake and nutrition absorption and metabolism (Elsner 2002; Brownie 2006). Emotional stresses play an important role in impairing the immune system due to the increased levels of oxidative stress, decreased IFN-γ release, decreased major histocompatibility complex (MHC) class II molecule expression on APCs, and activation of hypothalamic–pituitary–adrenal axis and excess release of glucocorticoids (Hays and Roberts 2006; Darnton-Hill 1992; Elsner 2002; Brownie 2006; Chapman et al. 2002).

20.2.3 Social Factors

Social factors such as retirement, low income, low education, low socioeconomic status, limited access to shopping, inability to prepare food, isolation, widowhood and bereavement, and no company during meals can strongly influence

food options and nutritional status of the elderly (Elsner 2002; Brownie 2006). Human is a social creature and is designed to eat in social groups; therefore, social isolation and eating alone can significantly decrease dietary intake (Elsner 2002; Brownie 2006; Chapman et al. 2002; Hays and Roberts 2006; Parker and Chapman 2004; Wilson and Morley 2003).

20.3 Nutritional Assessments

Undernutrition as a frequent and insidious problem in the elderly needs careful evaluation in all the elderly (Cederholm and Morley 2013; Volkert et al. 2010). The aims of nutritional assessment include evaluation of the degree of immunosenescence and risk of secondary and tertiary immunosenescence and choosing the best nutrition intervention. There is not a single biochemical marker to determine nutritional status as all biochemical markers and laboratory evaluations related to nutritional status can be biased due to the underlying diseases; therefore, assessment of nutritional status like other conditions in medicine begins with a thorough medical history and physical examination followed by necessary laboratory evaluations. The best way to minimize false-positives and false-negatives in detection of undernutrition is to follow a systematic strategy for identifying signs and symptoms of undernutrition and integration of findings from medical history, physical examination, anthropometrics, and laboratory evaluations (Vellas et al. 2001; Pepersack 2009; Brownie 2006).

20.3.1 Screening Tools

Nutritional screening can be the first line of evaluating nutritional status in the elderly. Up to now, several questionnaires have been developed to screen for undernutrition in the elderly. Of them, an inexpensive and patient-friendly screening tool is Mini Nutritional Assessment (MNA) which can classify the elderly to three categories of well nourished,

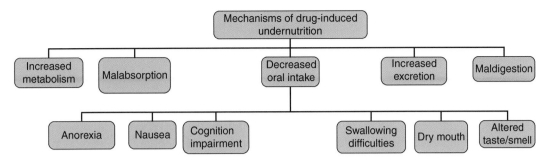

Fig. 20.9 Mechanisms of drug-induced anorexia

at risk for malnutrition, or malnourished with a high sensitivity (96 %) and specificity (98 %). It assesses nutritional status using information about general health status, dietary intake, anthropometric measurements, and subjective self-assessment (Omran and Morley 2000a; Vellas et al. 2001). Recently, a 2-stage MNA has been developed which consists of a screening stage (MNA-SF) including six items of the original MNA and the stage 2 including the remaining 12 items (Vellas et al. 2001).

20.3.2 Medical History

Obtaining a thorough medical history from an elderly is a state of the art. Several reasons make this statement true. First, cognitive decline makes history taking from the elderly very hard. Secondly, fear of losing some privileges including driver's license or even living independently makes the elderly conservative in giving information. Therefore, presence of a close family member be during history taking is recommended (Omran and Morley 2000a).

20.3.2.1 Present Illness

First of all, presentations of undernutrition should be asked from the elderly. As a key component of medical history, history of weight loss and its time period (sudden, gradual), being intentional or unintentional, should be noted. Significant weight loss is defined as loss of more than 4.5 kg or 10 % of body weight over a period of 6 months or 5 % of the body weight over a period of one month or 1–2 % of body weight per week (Martin

et al. 2007). Significant weight losses need careful evaluation as it may be a sign of insidious underlying conditions like malignancies. But insignificant weight losses even on intention, in the presence of risk factors of undernutrition, can be an alarm sign of undernutrition for a wise physician and need further assessment for micronutrient deficiencies. Poor wound healing and weakness are serious signs of undernutrition. Bone and muscle pain should be noted as well (Bates et al. 2009; Omran and Morley 2000a; High 2001; Henry et al. 2011; Swartz 2001).

Secondly, risk factors of malnutrition should be noted in history taking. Loss of appetite is an alarm sign resulting in undernutrition. Other risk factors of undernutrition can be easily remembered by the mnemonic "MEALS ON WHEELS" and "DETERMINE" (Fig. 20.10) (White 1991). Dental screening tool can be used for screening of dental problems (Martin et al. 2007; Thomson et al. 1992; Bush et al. 1996). Recurrent dieting behavior can be a sign of anorexia nervosa and require further evaluation with EAT-26 questionnaire (Miller et al. 1991). Suspicion of depression or dementia disorders requires further assessment by Geriatric Depression Scale (GDS) and Folstein Mini-Mental State Examination (MMSE), respectively (Folstein et al. 1975; Omran and Morley 2000a; Yesavage et al. 1982).

20.3.2.2 Past Medical and Surgical History

Past medical history regarding gastrointestinal, cardiovascular, pulmonary, endocrinologic, and neuromusculoskeletal disorders and chronic infections should be asked. Disorders of GI

Fig. 20.10 Mnemonic DETERMINE MEALS ON WHEELS which is used to remember risk factors of undernutrition in elderly

D E T E R M I N E   M E A L S   O N   W H E E L S

D	E	T	E	R	M	I	N	E	M	E	A	L	S	O	N	W	H	E	E	L	S
Disease	Eating poorly	Tooth loss	Economic problems	Reduced social contact	Multiple medicines	Involuntary weight loss	Needs assistance in self	Elders years above age 80	Medications	Emotional problems	**Abnormal attitudes to food**	Late life paranoia	Swallowing difficulties	Oral problems	No Money	Wandering	**Hyperthyroidism**	Entry problems	Eating problems	Low salt, low cholesterol	Shopping (food availability)

system should be evaluated with more contemplation to find previous conditions like pancreatic insufficiency, celiac disease, and Crohn's disease (Bates et al. 2009; Omran and Morley 2000a; High 2001; Henry et al. 2011; Swartz 2001).

History of past surgical procedures should be obtained as they usually have profound effects on the body reserves. Surgeries on GI system like gastrectomy or surgical resection of small intestines are of special importance. In addition, their complications like draining fistulas, abscess, open wounds, and chronic blood losses may contribute to the nutritional deficiencies (Bates et al. 2009; Omran and Morley 2000a; High 2001; Henry et al. 2011; Swartz 2001).

20.3.2.3 Drug History and Allergies

A complete drug history including not only prescribed medications but also nonprescription medications, mineral, vitamin and protein supplements, and herbal medicines should be taken (Omran and Morley 2000a). Usage of certain supplements which patients often may not consider them medications should be specifically asked during the interview (Bates et al. 2009; Omran and Morley 2000a; High 2001; Henry et al. 2011; Swartz 2001).

Allergies to certain foods like peanuts, tree nuts, shellfish, fish, eggs, soy, wheat, and milk may be present in the elderly and contribute to nutrition deficiency (Bates et al. 2009; Omran and Morley 2000a; High 2001; Henry et al. 2011; Swartz 2001).

20.3.2.4 Family History

Family history of genetic or metabolic disorder like diabetes, hypothyroidism, hyperthyroidism and history of alcoholism or psychiatric disorders

like anorexia nervosa should be directly asked (Bates et al. 2009; Omran and Morley 2000a; High 2001; Henry et al. 2011; Swartz 2001).

20.3.2.5 Personal and Social History

In the social and personal history, religions and beliefs concerning dietary restriction should be noted. Presence of certain dietary habits like vegetarianism and use of vitamin, mineral, and herbal supplements should be determined (Omran and Morley 2000a). Cigarette smoking can decrease hedonic qualities of food, and it should be noted in history. Late onset of alcoholism which is not rare in the elderly should be assessed by CAGE questionnaire or preferably by Michigan Alcoholism Screening Test (MAST) (Ewing 1984; Pokorny et al. 1972). Drug abuse like alcoholism can both endanger dietary intake and disturb nutrition absorption. Functional status is both an indicator and a reason for undernutrition and should be noted in personal history (Omran and Morley 2000a). Stress events, physical or mental, should be evaluated as they have significant negative effects on the immunity. In addition, dependency, low income, ability to shop or prepare food, having companion during meal times, and number of daily meals and snacks delicately can be asked (Bates et al. 2009; Omran and Morley 2000a; High 2001; Henry et al. 2011; Swartz 2001).

20.3.3 Physical Examination

A thorough physical examination from head to toe not only can help to diagnose underlying undernutrition but also can be helpful in determining exact type of micronutrients or

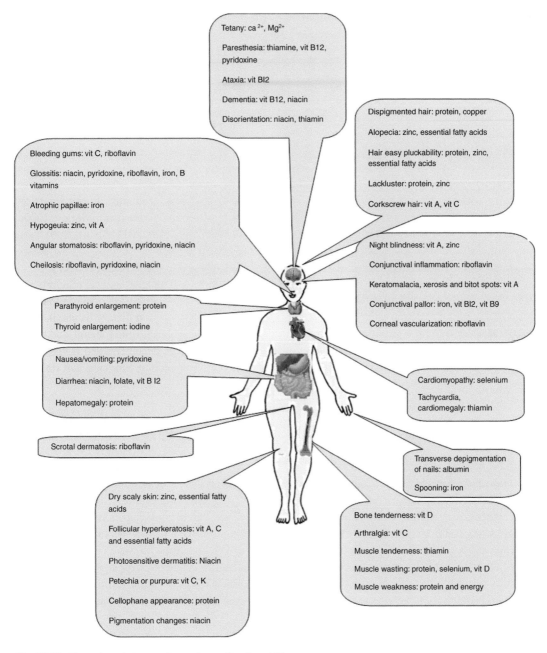

Fig. 20.11 Organ-based signs and symptoms of undernutrition

macronutrients deficiency. In addition, it prevents a false diagnosis of undernutrition by detecting signs of underlying conditions mimicking undernutrition (Fig. 20.11) (Bates et al. 2009; Omran and Morley 2000a; High 2001; Henry et al. 2011; Swartz 2001).

20.3.4 Anthropometric Assessment

Measurement of body mass index (BMI) is the first simple anthropometric assessment. Although there is controversy on the definition of normal BMI, a satisfactory BMI for the elderly with more than 65 years of age is accepted as a BMI between 24 and 27 kg/m², and a BMI between 19 and 23 kg/m² shows risk of undernutrition, and finally, based on world health organization (WHO) classification, underweight category is defined by a BMI lower than 18.5 kg/m² (38) (Omran and Morley 2000a). Compression of the intravertebral disks, osteoporosis, and other pathologies result in shortened stature in the elderly which in turn results in a pseudo increase in BMI in the elderly (Omran and Morley 2000a). So the true height should be calculated by height to arm span ratio index (Omran and Morley 2000a). In addition, ascites and edema make BMI an unreliable indicative (High 2001).

Triceps skin fold (TSF) measurement by a caliper can estimate fat stores. A TSF below the 10th percentile is indicator of undernutrition (Omran and Morley 2000a; Ahmed and Haboubi 2010). Midarm muscle circumference (MAMC) or midarm muscle area (MAMA) is an estimation of skeletal muscle mass and can be calculated using these formulas (Henry et al. 2011; Swartz 2001; Omran and Morley 2000a):

$$MAMC(cm) = MAC(cm) - \pi[TSF/10(mm)]$$

$$MAMA(cm^2) = (MAC - \pi \times TSF)^2 / 4\pi$$

Measuring electrical resistance of the body by biometric impedance analysis is a noninvasive and inexpensive method to estimate body composition (Ahmed and Haboubi 2010; Omran and Morley 2000a).

20.3.5 Dietary Intake Assessment

To assess dietary intake and estimation of the adequacy of the diet, four methods—food diaries, 24-h recall, food frequency questionnaire, and diet history—can be used (Table 20.1). Of these four methods, food diary for a period of 7 days seems more reasonable and accurate; however, recording of dietary intakes may result in change of dietary habits during the 7 days (Omran and Morley 2000a; Fernandes 2008; Grimble 2005; Henry et al. 2011; Swartz 2001).

20.3.6 Biochemical Markers

Biochemical markers of nutritional status should be assessed in order to serve several aims including:
1. Confirming the finding on medical history and physical exam regarding the nutritional status
2. Having the baseline nutritional values to evaluate efficacy of nutritional treatment
3. Planning for the essential nutritional intervention.

The most known and most commonly used marker for detection of undernutrition is the level of serum albumin. Albumin with a long half-life (18 days) can be used to show chronic nutritional status (Rothschild et al. 1972a, b). However, in addition to nutritional status, factors like hepatic synthesis, plasma distribution, and protein loss can influence albumin; so in settings like hospital admission, liver disease and congestive heart failure, nephrotic syndrome, and protein-losing enteropathies, the albumin levels cannot be relied (Courtney et al. 1982; Omran and Morley 2000b; Ahmed and Haboubi 2010).

On the other hand, transthyretin or prealbumin with the highest proportion of essential to nonessential amino acids and with a short half-life (2 days) is an indicator recent nutritional change (Nutritional Care Consensus Group 1995). End-stage liver disease, inflammation, stress, and iron deficiency can decrease prealbumin level and renal insufficiency, and steroid use can increase it (Goldberg and Brown 1987; Delpeuch et al. 1980; Smith and Goodman 1971). Total lymphocyte count (TLC) is a more useful indicator, in the presence of conditions like liver disease (Omran and Morley 2000b). In case of suspicion to micronutrient deficiencies, measuring levels of different micronutrients can be very useful (Ahmed and Haboubi 2010; Pepersack 2009; Omran and Morley 2000b).

Laboratory tests should be requested on an individual basis and based on physician judgment. However, laboratory tests like measurement of hemoglobin levels, hematocrit, transferrin saturation, levels of albumin, cholesterol, triglycerides, high-density lipoproteins (HDL) and low-density lipoproteins (LDL) in the

Table 20.1 Methods of dietary intake assessment

Method	Description	Place	Suitability for individuals or groups	Time consuming	Memory dependency	Avoidance of day-to-day variations	Dependency on the interviewer
Food diary	Information regarding the type and amount of the food and beverages is recorded by the patient	In home	Individuals	×	×	√	×
The 24-h recall	Information regarding the type and amount of food and beverages consumed during the last 24 h is recalled by the patient	During the interview	Individual	×	√	×	√
Food frequency questionnaire	Questions regarding the customary intake of key nutrients are answered by the patient	During the interview	Group	√	√	√	×
Diet history	Complete dietary history is obtained by a professional nutritionist by open-ended questions	During the interview	Individual	√	√	√	√

plasma, serum glucose, and serum folate seem reasonable tests to figure out about general nutritional status (Henry et al. 2011; Swartz 2001).

20.4 Nutritional Interventions in Immunosenescence

Nutritional intervention is one of the cost-effective approaches to delay immunosenescence. Nutritional interventions have a spectrum from changing a nutrition-related behavior, environmental condition, or aspect of health status to administration of immunonutrients via the enteral or parenteral (intravenous) routes. The latter is named immunonutrition, and every nutrient with favorable effects on the immune system is called immunonutrients (Calder 2007; Pae et al. 2012; Grimm and Calder 2002; Satyaraj 2011). Immunonutrition is becoming a popular approach

in the management of critically ill patients and surgical patients, and it can also be a feasible approach to delay immunosenescence (Barbul 2000; Koretz 2003; Calder 2007; Marik and Zaloga 2008).

The first line of any nutritional intervention is to eliminate any reversible medical, social, and physiological causes of undernutrition. Appropriate food choices should be encouraged by educational material. Dental problems and oral problems should be addressed by providing appropriate dentures, flavor enhancements, and appetite stimulants (Omran and Morley 2000a; Brownie 2006). Rehabilitation and in some cases percutaneous endoscopic gastrostomy (PEG) feeding should begin for patients with swallowing problems (Ahmed and Haboubi 2010). Treatment for chronic disease should be done, and proper modifications in diet with regard to the chronic diseases should be noted. Inappropriate medications with side effects should be changed to the ones with fewer. Factors endangering nutrition in the elderly staying at long-term care nursing home should be eliminated. Social services assistance or nursing assistance should be provided for patients with dementia and Alzheimer's or patients with functional disabilities. Treatment of depression and mood disorders by referring to a psychiatrist is recommended (Ahmed and Haboubi 2010; Pepersack 2009).

There are two types of immunonutrition in immunosenescence: (1) preventive immunonutrition or primary immunonutrition and (2) secondary immunonutrition.

Primary immunonutrition in immunosenescence aims to prevent secondary or tertiary immunosenescence and optimize the immunity in the elderly; secondary immunonutrition in immunosenescence aims to reverse secondary or tertiary immunosenescence

20.4.1 Primary Immunonutrition

Suboptimal status of nutrients predisposes body to temporary nutrient deficiency especially during the times of increased body consumption like or increased physical activities, exercise, stress, and infections. These temporary deficits may pervert the natural process of the immunosenescence in long term (Satyaraj 2011). Evidence shows that increased intake of some nutrients above the recommended levels may result in enhancement of immune function and improving immunosenescence, but increased intake of some other may not be beneficial but also have side effects on the immunity.

Three factors influence the efficacy of immunonutrition in the elderly (Field et al. 2002; Pae et al. 2012; Calder and Kew 2002):

1. Interindividual variability regarding baseline levels of immune response and genetic background
2. Nutrient–nutrient interactions
3. Variability of the different parts of the immune system in responding to micronutrients

In regard to primary nutrition, we should not have the belief that if some is good, more is better, and potential harms of oversupplementation should always be kept in mind (Volkert et al. 2010).

Overall, supplementation of the elderly with a modest physiological amount of micronutrients, especially antioxidants like vitamin E and C, and applying strategies like CR and probiotics consumption will result in improvement of the immune system; however, further studies to assess efficacy of the supplementations on resistance to infections, morbidity, and mortality are needed (Pae et al. 2012; Pepersack 2009). Future studies also should determine optimal intake of each supplement and possible side effects in oversupplementation.

20.4.2 Secondary Immunonutrition

Secondary immunonutrition is aimed at the elderly with secondary or tertiary immunosenescence due to undernutrition. Immunonutrition is a tool to improve immunosenescence and to restore decreased immune function at least partially in this group of the elderly (Lesourd 1997). It has been shown that cell-mediated immunity including both T-cell proliferation and T-cell functions can be improved by immunonutrition (Lesourd 1997). In addition, immunonutrition can enhance antibody responses to vaccines and humoral immunity (Lesourd 1997). Although several studies have pointed out that immunonutrition and refeeding therapy can reverse the process of secondary and tertiary immunosenescence, however, its efficacy in this aim probably depends on several factors like duration of undernutrition and presence of acute-phase responses (Chandra 1997). Identification of these factors, period of immunonutrition, and the essential immunonutrients for immunonutrition in secondary or tertiary immunosenescence should be determined by further studies.

References

Adolfsson O, Huber BT, Meydani SN (2001) Vitamin E-enhanced IL-2 production in old mice: naive but not memory T cells show increased cell division cycling and IL-2-producing capacity. J Immunol 167(7): 3809–3817

Ahmed T, Haboubi N (2010) Assessment and management of nutrition in older people and its importance to health. Clin Interv Aging 5:207–216

Ahmed T, Das SK, Golden JK et al (2009) Calorie restriction enhances T-cell-mediated immune response in adult overweight men and women. J Gerontol A Biol Sci Med Sci 64(11):1107–1113

Arthur JR, McKenzie RC, Beckett GJ (2003) Selenium in the immune system. J Nutr 133(5 Suppl 1): 1457S–1459S

Aukrust P, Muller F, Ueland T et al (2000) Decreased vitamin A levels in common variable immunodeficiency: vitamin A supplementation in vivo enhances immunoglobulin production and downregulates inflammatory responses. Eur J Clin Invest 30(3):252–259

Baba N, Samson S, Bourdet-Sicard R et al (2009) Selected commensal-related bacteria and Toll-like receptor 3 agonist combinatorial codes synergistically induce interleukin-12 production by dendritic cells to trigger a T helper type 1 polarizing programme. Immunology 128(1 Suppl):e523–e531

Barbul A (2000) Immunonutrition comes of age. Crit Care Med 28(3):884–885

Bates B, Bickley LS, Szilagyi PG (2009) Bates' guide to physical examination and history taking. Lippincott Williams & Wilkins, Philadelphia

Bengmark S (2006) Impact of nutrition on ageing and disease. Curr Opin Clin Nutr Metab Care 9(1):2–7

Bitar KN, Patil SB (2004) Aging and gastrointestinal smooth muscle. Mech Ageing Dev 125(12):907–910

Bitar K, Greenwood-Van Meerveld B, Saad R et al (2011) Aging and gastrointestinal neuromuscular function: insights from within and outside the gut. Neurogastroenterol Motil 23(6):490–501

BM L (ed) (2001) Handbook of Nutrition and the Aged. CRC Press, New York

Bogden JD, Louria DB (1999) Aging and the immune system: the role of micronutrient nutrition. Nutrition 15(7–8):593–595

Bonham M, O'Connor JM, Hannigan BM et al (2002) The immune system as a physiological indicator of marginal copper status? Br J Nutr 87(5):393–403

Brownie S (2006) Why are elderly individuals at risk of nutritional deficiency? Int J Nurs Pract 12(2):110–118

Burk RF (2002) Selenium, an antioxidant nutrient. Nutr Clin Care 5(2):75–79

Bush LA, Horenkamp N, Morley JE et al (1996) D-E-N-T-A-L: a rapid self-administered screening instrument to promote referrals for further evaluation in older adults. J Am Geriatr Soc 44(8):979–981

Calder PC (2007) Immunonutrition in surgical and critically ill patients. Br J Nutr 98(Suppl 1):S133–S139

Calder PC, Kew S (2002) The immune system: a target for functional foods? Br J Nutr 88(Suppl 2):S165–S177

Cantorna MT, Nashold FE, Hayes CE (1994) In vitamin A deficiency multiple mechanisms establish a regulatory T helper cell imbalance with excess Th1 and insufficient Th2 function. J Immunol 152(4):1515–1522

Cantorna MT, Zhu Y, Froicu M et al (2004) Vitamin D status, 1,25-dihydroxyvitamin D3, and the immune system. Am J Clin Nutr 80(6 Suppl):1717S–1720S

Castle SC (2000) Clinical relevance of age-related immune dysfunction. Clin Infect Dis 31(2):578–585

Cederholm T, Morley J (2013) Ageing: biology and nutrition. Curr Opin Clin Nutr Metab Care 16(1):1–2

Chandra RK (1983) Nutrition, immunity, and infection: present knowledge and future directions. Lancet 1(8326 Pt 1):688–691

Chandra RK (1997) Nutrition and the immune system: an introduction. Am J Clin Nutr 66(2):460S–463S

Chandra RK (2002) Nutrition and the immune system from birth to old age. Eur J Clin Nutr 56(Suppl 3): S73–S76

Chandra RK, Sudhakaran L (1990) Regulation of immune responses by vitamin B6. Ann N Y Acad Sci 585:404–423

Chapman IM, MacIntosh CG, Morley JE et al (2002) The anorexia of ageing. Biogerontology 3(1–2):67–71

Chen CC, Schilling LS, Lyder CH (2001) A concept analysis of malnutrition in the elderly. J Adv Nurs 36(1): 131–142

Clarke DM, Wahlqvist ML, Strauss BJ (1998) Undereating and undernutrition in old age: integrating biopsychosocial aspects. Age Ageing 27(4):527–534

Courtemanche C, Elson-Schwab I, Mashiyama ST et al (2004) Folate deficiency inhibits the proliferation of primary human CD8+ T lymphocytes in vitro. J Immunol 173(5):3186–3192

Courtney ME, Greene HL, Folk CC et al (1982) Rapidly declining serum albumin values in newly hospitalized patients: prevalence, severity, and contributory factors. JPEN J Parenter Enteral Nutr 6(2):143–145

Cunningham-Rundles S, McNeeley DF, Moon A (2005) Mechanisms of nutrient modulation of the immune response. J Allergy Clin Immunol 115(6):1119–1128; quiz 1129

Darnton-Hill I (1992) Psychosocial aspects of nutrition and aging. Nutr Rev 50(12):476–479

de Moreno de LeBlanc A, Chaves S, Carmuega E et al (2008) Effect of long-term continuous consumption of fermented milk containing probiotic bacteria on mucosal immunity and the activity of peritoneal macrophages. Immunobiology 213(2):97–108

Delcenserie V, Martel D, Lamoureux M et al (2008) Immunomodulatory effects of probiotics in the intestinal tract. Curr Issues Mol Biol 10(1–2):37–54

Delpeuch F, Cornu A, Chevalier P (1980) The effect of iron-deficiency anaemia on two indices of nutritional status, prealbumin and transferrin. Br J Nutr 43(2): 375–379

Deluca HF, Cantorna MT (2001) Vitamin D: its role and uses in immunology. FASEB J 15(14):2579–2585

Dhur A, Galan P, Hercberg S (1991) Folate status and the immune system. Prog Food Nutr Sci 15(1–2):43–60

Elmadfa I, Klein P, Meyer AL (2010) Immune-stimulating effects of lactic acid bacteria in vivo and in vitro. Proc Nutr Soc 69(3):416–420

Elsner RJ (2002) Changes in eating behavior during the aging process. Eat Behav 3(1):15–43

Ewing JA (1984) Detecting alcoholism. The CAGE questionnaire. JAMA 252(14):1905–1907

Fernandes G (2008) Progress in nutritional immunology. Immunol Res 40(3):244–261

Fich A, Camilleri M, Phillips SF (1989) Effect of age on human gastric and small bowel motility. J Clin Gastroenterol 11(4):416–420

Field CJ, Johnson IR, Schley PD (2002) Nutrients and their role in host resistance to infection. J Leukoc Biol 71(1):16–32

Finkelstein JA, Schiffman SS (1999) Workshop on taste and smell in the elderly: an overview. Physiol Behav 66(2):173–176

Folstein MF, Folstein SE, McHugh PR (1975) Mini-mental state. A practical method for grading the cognitive state of patients for the clinician. J Psychiatr Res 12(3):189–198

Galli C, Calder PC (2009) Effects of fat and fatty acid intake on inflammatory and immune responses: a critical review. Ann Nutr Metab 55(1–3):123–139

Goldberg DM, Brown D (1987) Advances in the application of biochemical tests to diseases of the liver and biliary tract: their role in diagnosis, prognosis, and the elucidation of pathogenetic mechanisms. Clin Biochem 20(2):127–148

Griffin MD, Xing N, Kumar R (2003) Vitamin D and its analogs as regulators of immune activation and antigen presentation. Annu Rev Nutr 23:117–145

Grimble RF (2005) Immunonutrition. Curr Opin Gastroenterol 21(2):216–222

Grimm H, Calder PC (2002) Immunonutrition. Br J Nutr 87(Suppl 1):S1

Guarner F, Schaafsma GJ (1998) Probiotics. Int J Food Microbiol 39(3):237–238

Halevy O, Arazi Y, Melamed D et al (1994) Retinoic acid receptor-alpha gene expression is modulated by dietary vitamin A and by retinoic acid in chicken T lymphocytes. J Nutr 124(11):2139–2146

Hartel C, Strunk T, Bucsky P et al (2004) Effects of vitamin C on intracytoplasmic cytokine production in human whole blood monocytes and lymphocytes. Cytokine 27(4–5):101–106

Hayes CE, Nashold FE, Spach KM et al (2003) The immunological functions of the vitamin D endocrine system. Cell Mol Biol (Noisy-le-grand) 49(2):277–300

Hays NP, Roberts SB (2006) The anorexia of aging in humans. Physiol Behav 88(3):257–266

Henry M, Seidel M, Jane W et al (2011) Mosby's guide to physical examination, 7th edn. Elsevier, Philadelphia

High KP (2001) Nutritional strategies to boost immunity and prevent infection in elderly individuals. Clin Infect Dis 33(11):1892–1900

Ibs KH, Rink L (2003) Zinc-altered immune function. J Nutr 133(5 Suppl 1):1452S–1456S

Iyer SS, Chatraw JH, Tan WG et al (2012) Protein energy malnutrition impairs homeostatic proliferation of memory CD8 T cells. J Immunol 188(1):77–84

Jacob RA, Kelley DS, Pianalto FS et al (1991) Immunocompetence and oxidant defense during ascorbate depletion of healthy men. Am J Clin Nutr 54(6 Suppl):1302S–1309S

Kim W, Khan NA, McMurray DN et al (2010) Regulatory activity of polyunsaturated fatty acids in T-cell signaling. Prog Lipid Res 49(3):250–261

Koretz RL (2003) Immunonutrition: can you be what you eat? Curr Opin Gastroenterol 19(2):134–139

Lane MA, Black A, Handy A et al (2001) Caloric restriction in primates. Ann N Y Acad Sci 928:287–295

Laugier R, Bernard JP, Berthezene P et al (1991) Changes in pancreatic exocrine secretion with age: pancreatic exocrine secretion does decrease in the elderly. Digestion 50(3–4):202–211

Lesourd BM (1997) Nutrition and immunity in the elderly: modification of immune responses with nutritional treatments. Am J Clin Nutr 66(2):478S–484S

Lesourd B (2004) Nutrition: a major factor influencing immunity in the elderly. J Nutr Health Aging 8(1):28–37

Lesourd B (2006) Nutritional factors and immunological ageing. Proc Nutr Soc 65(3):319–325

Lesourd B, Mazari L (1999) Nutrition and immunity in the elderly. Proc Nutr Soc 58(3):685–695

Lesourd BM, Mazari L, Ferry M (1998) The role of nutrition in immunity in the aged. Nutr Rev 56(1 Pt 2):S113–S125

Ligthart GJ, Corberand JX, Fournier C et al (1984) Admission criteria for immunogerontological studies in man: the SENIEUR protocol. Mech Ageing Dev 28(1):47–55

Lipschitz DA, Udupa KB (1986) Influence of aging and protein deficiency on neutrophil function. J Gerontol 41(6):690–694

Lotfy OA, Saleh WA, el-Barbari M (1998) A study of some changes of cell-mediated immunity in protein energy malnutrition. J Egypt Soc Parasitol 28(2):413–428

Maggini S, Wintergerst ES, Beveridge S et al (2007) Selected vitamins and trace elements support immune function by strengthening epithelial barriers and cellular and humoral immune responses. Br J Nutr 98(Suppl 1):S29–S35

Marcos A, Nova E, Montero A (2003) Changes in the immune system are conditioned by nutrition. Eur J Clin Nutr 57(Suppl 1):S66–S69

Marik PE, Zaloga GP (2008) Immunonutrition in critically ill patients: a systematic review and analysis of the literature. Intensive Care Med 34(11):1980–1990

Martin CT, Kayser-Jones J, Stotts NA et al (2007) Risk for low weight in community-dwelling, older adults. Clin Nurse Spec 21(4):203–211; quiz 212–203

Messaoudi I, Warner J, Fischer M et al (2006) Delay of T cell senescence by caloric restriction in aged long-lived nonhuman primates. Proc Natl Acad Sci U S A 103(51):19448–19453

Messaoudi I, Fischer M, Warner J et al (2008) Optimal window of caloric restriction onset limits its beneficial impact on T-cell senescence in primates. Aging Cell 7(6):908–919

Meydani M (2001) Nutrition interventions in aging and age-associated disease. Ann N Y Acad Sci 928:226–235

Meydani SN, Han SN, Wu D (2005) Vitamin E and immune response in the aged: molecular mechanisms and clinical implications. Immunol Rev 205:269–284

Miller DK, Morley JE, Rubenstein LZ et al (1991) Abnormal eating attitudes and body image in older undernourished individuals. J Am Geriatr Soc 39(5):462–466

Nutritional Care Consensus Group (1995) Measurement of visceral protein status in assessing protein and energy malnutrition: standard of care. Nutrition 11(2):169–171

Office of National Statistics (2011) Population trends. Population and Demography Division. http://www.ons.gov.uk/ons/rel/population-trends-rd/population-trends/no--145--autumn-2011/index.html. Accessed 1 Jan 2013

Omran ML, Morley JE (2000a) Assessment of protein energy malnutrition in older persons, part I: History, examination, body composition, and screening tools. Nutrition 16(1):50–63

Omran ML, Morley JE (2000b) Assessment of protein energy malnutrition in older persons, Part II: laboratory evaluation. Nutrition 16(2):131–140

Oppenheimer SJ (2001) Iron and its relation to immunity and infectious disease. J Nutr 131(2S–2):616S–633S; discussion 633S-635S

Pae M, Meydani SN, Wu D (2012) The role of nutrition in enhancing immunity in aging. Aging Dis 3(1):91–129

Pallast EG, Schouten EG, de Waart FG et al (1999) Effect of 50- and 100-mg vitamin E supplements on cellular immune function in noninstitutionalized elderly persons. Am J Clin Nutr 69(6):1273–1281

Parker BA, Chapman IM (2004) Food intake and ageing–the role of the gut. Mech Ageing Dev 125(12):859–866

Pekmezci D (2011) Vitamin E and immunity. Vitam Horm 86:179–215

Pepersack T (2009) Nutritional problems in the elderly. Acta Clin Belg 64(2):85–91

Pokorny AD, Miller BA, Kaplan HB (1972) The brief MAST: a shortened version of the Michigan Alcoholism Screening Test. Am J Psychiatry 129(3):342–345

Price DM (2008) Protein-energy malnutrition among the elderly: implications for nursing care. Holist Nurs Pract 22(6):355–360

Rall LC, Meydani SN (1993) Vitamin B6 and immune competence. Nutr Rev 51(8):217–225

Redmond HP, Leon P, Lieberman MD et al (1991) Impaired macrophage function in severe protein-energy malnutrition. Arch Surg 126(2):192–196

Redmond HP, Gallagher HJ, Shou J et al (1995) Antigen presentation in protein-energy malnutrition. Cell Immunol 163(1):80–87

Reibnegger G, Huber LA, Jurgens G et al (1988) Approach to define "normal aging" in man. Immune function, serum lipids, lipoproteins and neopterin levels. Mech Ageing Dev 46(1–3):67–82

Rink L, Kirchner H (2000) Zinc-altered immune function and cytokine production. J Nutr 130(5S Suppl):1407S–1411S

Roberts-Thomson IC, Whittingham S, Youngchaiyud U et al (1974) Ageing, immune response, and mortality. Lancet 2(7877):368–370

Rothschild MA, Oratz M, Schreiber SS (1972a) Albumin synthesis (second of two parts). N Engl J Med 286(15):816–821

Rothschild MA, Oratz M, Schreiber SS (1972b) Albumin synthesis. 1. N Engl J Med 286(14):748–757

Roubenoff R (2000) Sarcopenia and its implications for the elderly. Eur J Clin Nutr 54(Suppl 3):S40–S47

Ryan-Harshman M, Aldoori W (2005) The relevance of selenium to immunity, cancer, and infectious/inflammatory diseases. Can J Diet Pract Res 66(2):98–102

Rymkiewicz PD, Heng YX, Vasudev A et al (2012) The immune system in the aging human. Immunol Res 53(1–3):235–250

Satyaraj E (2011) Emerging paradigms in immunonutrition. Top Companion Anim Med 26(1):25–32

Savino W, Dardenne M (2010) Nutritional imbalances and infections affect the thymus: consequences on T-cell-mediated immune responses. Proc Nutr Soc 69(4):636–643

Savino W, Dardenne M, Velloso LA et al (2007) The thymus is a common target in malnutrition and infection. Br J Nutr 98(Suppl 1):S11–S16

Scrimshaw NS, SanGiovanni JP (1997) Synergism of nutrition, infection, and immunity: an overview. Am J Clin Nutr 66(2):464S–477S

Shaikh SR, Edidin M (2006) Polyunsaturated fatty acids, membrane organization, T cells, and antigen presentation. Am J Clin Nutr 84(6):1277–1289

Shatenstein B (2008) Impact of health conditions on food intakes among older adults. J Nutr Elder 27(3–4):333–361

Shepherd A (2009) Nutrition through the life span. Part 3: adults aged 65 years and over. Br J Nurs 18(5):301–302, 304–307

Sijben JW, Calder PC (2007) Differential immunomodulation with long-chain n-3 PUFA in health and chronic disease. Proc Nutr Soc 66(2):237–259

Smith FR, Goodman DS (1971) The effects of diseases of the liver, thyroid, and kidneys on the transport of vitamin A in human plasma. J Clin Invest 50(11):2426–2436

Swartz MH (2001) Textbook of physical diagnosis: history and examination, 4th edn. Saunders, Philadelphia

Tamura J, Kubota K, Murakami H et al (1999) Immunomodulation by vitamin B12: augmentation of CD8+ T lymphocytes and natural killer (NK) cell activity in vitamin B12-deficient patients by methyl-B12 treatment. Clin Exp Immunol 116(1):28–32

Taylor AK, Cao W, Vora KP et al (2013) Protein energy malnutrition decreases immunity and increases susceptibility to influenza infection in mice. J Infect Dis 207(3):501–510

Thomson WM, Brown RH, Williams SM (1992) Dentures, prosthetic treatment needs, and mucosal health in an institutionalised elderly population. N Z Dent J 88(392):51–55

Troen AM, Mitchell B, Sorensen B et al (2006) Unmetabolized folic acid in plasma is associated with reduced natural killer cell cytotoxicity among postmenopausal women. J Nutr 136(1):189–194

Tsai YT, Cheng PC, Fan CK et al (2008) Time-dependent persistence of enhanced immune response by a potential probiotic strain Lactobacillus paracasei subsp. paracasei NTU 101. Int J Food Microbiol 128(2): 219–225

Vellas B, Lauque S, Andrieu S et al (2001) Nutrition assessment in the elderly. Curr Opin Clin Nutr Metab Care 4(1):5–8

Volkert D (2002) Malnutrition in the elderly — prevalence, causes and corrective strategies. Clin Nutr 21(1):110–112

Volkert D, Saeglitz C, Gueldenzoph H et al (2010) Undiagnosed malnutrition and nutrition-related problems in geriatric patients. J Nutr Health Aging 14(5):387–392

Wahrburg U (2004) What are the health effects of fat? Eur J Nutr 43(Suppl 1):I/6–I/11

Weiss G (2002) Iron and immunity: a double-edged sword. Eur J Clin Invest 32(Suppl 1):70–78

Weiss G (2004) Chapter 11. Iron. In: Hughes DA, Darlington LG, Bendich A (eds) Diet and human immune function. Humana Press, New York

Weksler ME (1995) Immune senescence: deficiency or dysregulation. Nutr Rev 53(4 Pt 2):S3–S7

White JV (1991) Risk factors for poor nutritional status in older Americans. Am Fam Physician 44(6): 2087–2097

Wilson MM, Morley JE (2003) Invited review: aging and energy balance. J Appl Physiol 95(4):1728–1736

Wintergerst ES, Maggini S, Hornig DH (2006) Immune-enhancing role of vitamin C and zinc and effect on clinical conditions. Ann Nutr Metab 50(2):85–94

Wu D, Meydani SN (2008) Age-associated changes in immune and inflammatory responses: impact of vitamin E intervention. J Leukoc Biol 84(4):900–914

Yesavage JA, Brink TL, Rose TL et al (1982) Development and validation of a geriatric depression screening scale: a preliminary report. J Psychiatr Res 17(1):37–49

Diet and Immunosenescence

21

Giulia Accardi, Carmela Rita Balistreri,
Calogero Caruso, and Giuseppina Candore

21.1 Immunosenescence and Inflammation

The immune system, as well as the whole human body, becomes old. This leads to many changes that accumulate during the year, causing damages to the immune system and variation in the amount of different cell types.

The consequence is a lack of fidelity and efficiency during the years, hence a rise in the susceptibility of infectious, autoimmune, and inflammatory diseases in general and a reduced response to vaccines.

Immunosenescence is a cluster of modifications, actually unavoidable, that obviously constitutes a severe damage for human body and a limit for a healthy aging and longevity because of associated increase in morbidity and mortality. These changes have been described in both innate and specific immunity. A depletion of T and B cell repertoire weakens the immune system which results in an increasing chronic antigenic load that constitutes a driving force of the immunosenescence. Moreover, a saturation of immunological space with expanded clones of memory and effectors and antigen-experienced T cells and a reduction of virgin antigen-nonexperienced T cells occur. The B cell compartment is characterized with aging by a

G. Accardi, MSc • C.R. Balistreri, PhD (✉)
C. Caruso, MD • G. Candore, PhD
Department of Pathobiology and Medical
and Forensic Biotechnologies, University of Palermo,
Corso Tukory 211, Palermo 90134, Italy
e-mail: carmelarita.balistreri@unipa.it

decreased cell number as well as by improved function and quality of humoral response. This determines a loss of B clonotypic immune response to new extracellular pathogens. A switch from naïve B cells CD27⁻ to memory B cells CD27⁺ probably occurs as demonstrated by a decrease in immunoglobulin (Ig)M and IgD levels. Also a reduction in cytotoxic activity of natural killer (NK) cells correlates with the increase of infections and death in elderly. In addition, functions such as chemokine or interferon gamma (IFN-γ) secretion in response to interleukin (IL)-2 are compromised.

The development of a chronic, low-grade, inflammatory status, known as "inflammaging," is a typical aspect of immunosenescence mostly due to the increased pro-inflammatory cytokine production linked to the chronic antigenic load (Franceschi et al. 2000, 2007; Franceschi 2007). This is a critical feature in the onset of sarcopenia, frailty, and the pathogenesis of age-related chronic diseases, such as Alzheimer's disease (AD), atherosclerosis, and type 2 diabetes (Vasto et al. 2007, 2009; De Martinis et al. 2005, 2006; Ginaldi et al. 2005).

Since these pathologies share this common feature, it has been thought to include this systemic status in the concept of age-related diseasome, thus recognizing an important role for genetic and epigenetic factors involved in the regulation of inflammatory patterns in human aging. Although inflammation is a physiological event, necessary for systemic defense, its persistence over life and its possible dysregulation can be an important contributory factor in the pathogenesis of age-related

A. Massoud, N. Rezaei (eds.), *Immunology of Aging*,
DOI 10.1007/978-3-642-39495-9_21, © Springer-Verlag Berlin Heidelberg 2014

diseases. It has been allowed to focus the scientific attention on the possibility to prevent or counteract these pathologies that represent a very big problem for public health (Candore et al. 2006).

21.2 Nutrition and Immune System

21.2.1 Micronutrients

Aging is characterized by a global systemic deterioration caused by inability in homeostasis maintenance. Changes in physical and cognitive functions are evident in elderly people. Teeth loss, wrinkles, frailty, chronic inflammatory load, metabolic diseases, and increased morbidity and mortality are some of the modifications that occur during aging. It is well known that life expectancy and longevity depend on several multifactorial events determined by both genetic and environmental factors. Nutritional elements accordingly by diet have a pivotal role in these events. Nutrition can act on aging, immunity, and health in general and can also modulate gene expression with epigenetic changes.

Good and balanced nutrition is dramatically important for prevention and management of chronic age-related diseases, both directly and indirectly, and for the maintenance of healthy physical and cognitive functions. Moreover, immunomodulatory effects exerted by several nutrients such as antioxidant, fatty acid, micronutrients, specific amino acid, vitamins, and others play an important role in health status maintenance. Micronutrients are essential dietary elements for physiologic processes although in small quantities. Vitamins and trace minerals are part of micronutrients category. Their role in many physiological processes is fundamental, so their absence is deleterious for the organism and also for the immune defense.

Zinc is a trace mineral, usually present in the organism in 2.3 g, and basically bound to proteins (Vallee and Falchuk 1993). It can be disposable, thanks to its assumption from the extracellular space, but it is also contained in intracellular compartments in which it can be redistributed

and in storage protein by which it can be released (Cousins et al. 2006; Rink and Haase 2007; Truong-Tran et al. 2001). Zinc is a component of several transcription factors in which it permits the formation of zinc finger motifs; in addition, it is a component of more than 300 enzymes; it participates in cell growth and development. It has an important role in signal transduction, apoptosis, proliferation, and differentiation of immune cells (Cousins et al. 2006; Rink and Haase 2007; Truong-Tran et al. 2001; Vallee and Falchuk 1993). Although zinc plays a fundamental role in the organism, very little quantities of zinc is stored in the body. Thus, reduced intake or problems in its storage (uptake, excretion, preservation) cause severe damages, especially for the immune system. Mitogen-activated protein kinases (MAPK), protein kinase C (PKC), and nuclear factor kappa-light-chain-enhancer of activated B cells (NF-κB) are some of the related molecules and signaling pathways regulated by zinc levels. The transcriptional factor NF-κB is involved in production of proteins, such as tumor necrosis factor alpha (TNF-α). The inhibitory effect of zinc on NFκB determines a reduction on TNF-a, thus a reduction of its activity. Members of PKC family are crucially involved in both innate and adaptive immunity and zinc acts as possible mediator of this signal (Isakov and Altman 2002; Tan and Parker 2003). For example, PKC, selectively expressed in T lymphocytes, is fundamental for T cell receptor (TCR)-triggered activation of mature T cells (Csermely and Somogyi 1989). PKC can bind to plasma membrane and cytoskeleton by its N-terminal regulatory domain containing Cys_3His zinc-binding motifs. This pathway also leads to the activation of NF-κB and activator protein 1 (AP-1). Moreover, PKC promotes T cell cycle and regulates programmed T cell death (Isakov and Altman 2002; Haase and Rink 2009; Baldwin 1996). Another member, PKC has a role in T cell proliferation and interleukin (IL)-2 production. In B cells, PKC isoforms act in pre-B development, survival, and tolerance induction against self-antigen. In innate immunity, it regulates mast cell degranulation and macrophage activation (Tan and Parker 2003). However, zinc effect on B cell functions is less strong and sometimes indirect because it also leads to depletion on B cell compartment due to an increase in apoptosis for a direct regulation of apoptotic enzymes, such as caspases (Duke et al. 1983; Stennicke and Salvesen 1997).

To confirm zinc role in PKC signaling pathway activation, some studies demonstrate that zinc chelators inhibit PKC localization and action (Csermely et al. 1988; Forbes et al. 1990; Zalewski et al. 1990).

These evidences showed that the storage and the maintenance of adequate zinc level are vital for human organism. In addition to its dietary intake, the efficiency of all systems and processes related to zinc availability is essential. In elderly, zinc deficiency is prevalent due to the inadequate dietary intake resulting from physiological factors like loss of teeth, malabsorption, socioeconomic status, diseases, and medications. In fact, as many studies demonstrate, old people have less zinc intake than young individuals and elderly ill people have fewer intakes than healthy. In general, less than 50 % of old people have a good zinc intake although controversial results exist (Maret and Sandstead 2006; Briefel et al. 2000; Prasad et al. 1993). It is obvious that a lack of intracellular zinc ion bioavailability in aging could cause a status of chronic inflammation (Opipari et al. 1990; Rink and Kirchner 2000). Zinc has also a quenching activity on reactive oxygen species (ROS), so its reduction also results in an increase of these harmful molecules and ions (Frederickson et al. 2005). On the other hand, zinc itself could cause the production of ROS from mitochondrion and extramitochondrial space, as a source of oxidative stress (Frazzini et al. 2006). Moreover, a positive response about zinc importance comes from zinc supplementation studies. It has been shown that zinc supplementation in certain groups of old people increases the number of activated T helper (Th) cells and cytotoxic T lymphocytes (CTL) and percentage of T cells in total circulating lymphocytes (without a change in number). However, also in this case, controversial results exist which is probably related to different study conditions (Duchateau et al. 1981; Fortes et al. 1998; Bogden et al. 1990). Thus zinc supplementation has to be administrated carefully, taking into account the narrow range of concentration

in which this ion exerts its beneficial effect in inflammatory/immune response.

As highlighted, zinc is one of the main elements of micronutrient category individually associated with immune function in elderly. But, for the reasons mentioned before, all micronutrients could be insufficient in aged individuals and many studies report the correlation between micronutrients deficiency and changes in the immune system. Selenium, for example, is indirectly involved in cytotoxic precursor cell proliferation and clonal expansion because it upregulates IL-2 receptor expression on NK cell surface (Kiremidjian-Schumacher and Roy 1998). Vitamin E, a general term to call tocopherols and tocotrienols, is comparable to zinc in regard to its importance in the immune system. Many studies demonstrate the consequence of its deficiency both in humoral and cell-mediated immune functions (Gebremichael et al. 1984; Kowdley et al. 1992). Vitamin E is contained in immune cells, contrasting oxidative stress due to high metabolic activity in these cells. Although it is not clear the way, the supplementation of vitamin E in elderly people can selectively enhance the production of IL-2 and the activation-induced T cell proliferation in naïve but not memory T cells and can improve the delayed-type hypersensitivity reaction (Adolfsson et al. 2001; Meydani et al. 1986, 2005).

21.2.2 Gastrointestinal Immunosenescence: Cause and Effect

Aging is a systemic condition determined by a series of interaction resulting in a gradual loss of molecular and cellular fidelity. The protagonists of this interaction are, doubtlessly, environment, genetic background, immune system, and intestinal microbiota. The latter represents a real ecosystem that has to be remained in homeostatic equilibrium to guarantee human health. Intestinal microbiota are distributed from stomach to colon where they reach the peak in terms of quantity. Both Gram-positives and Gram-negatives are present. The first category, in particular *Lactobacilli and Streptococci,* mainly colonizes the stomach but is also present in the rest of the gastrointestinal system. In the distal regions, other than *Bifidobacteria* and *Enterobacteriaceae* (Gram-negative facultative aerobic), the obligatory anaerobic genera such as *Bacteroides* and *Fusobacterium* are present (Holzapfel et al. 1998). Microbiota are "friendly" component of the gastrointestinal tract, but they can become enemies, resulting in systemic dysfunctions. They are composed of more than 500 species with a distribution of 10^{10}–10^{11} colony-forming unit per gram of luminal contents in adult human (Savage 1977). Some scientists identified this microcosm as a real organ called "the microbe organ" with size similar to the liver and with a weight of about 1.5 kg (Bengmark 1998). Aging-associated dysfunctions in microbiota ecosystem certainly can contribute to age-associated pathological conditions such as metabolic syndrome, obesity, diabetes, infection, cancer inflammatory gastrointestinal diseases, constipation, cardiovascular disease, and autoimmune diseases. The main functions of these prokaryotes are digestion and nutrient absorption, complete hydrolysis of complex polysaccharides nondigestible by humans with the production of short-chain fatty acids and polyamine, synthesis of amino acids and vitamins, maintenance of systemic immune homeostasis, and its stimulation especially for the gut-associated lymphoid tissue and resistance against colonization of other pathogenic bacteria (Chung and Kasper 2010; Tiihonen et al. 2010; Turnbaugh et al. 2007; Holzapfel et al. 1998; Noack et al. 1998).

One of the most common nutritional problems among the elderly is an unbalanced diet with an insufficient intake of micronutrients, as mentioned above, such as vitamin D and B12, calcium, proteins, fruit, and vegetables; thus, fibers consequently lead to a decrease in microbial activity in the colon. Loss of teeth and reduced functionality of senses, especially taste and olfaction, lead to wrong nutritional habit. Moreover, intake of antigenic loads, microorganisms, and bacterial products, usually introduced with food, is potentially more dangerous for fragile individuals in unhealthy status. Additionally, the majority of elderly has no physical activity and is dramatically sedentary heading for a loss of muscle mass,

overweight, and impaired digestion (Tiihonen et al. 2010). The consequence is intestinal putrefaction and fermentation with an increase exposure to bacterial products, such as endotoxin, phenols, indols, and ammonia, usually in contact with the intestinal mucosa (Van Deventer et al. 1988; Cummings and Macfarlane 1997). Diet rich in protein and sulfate, present in additives, contributes to the production of more toxic products (Cummings and Macfarlane 1997). Moreover, dysbiosis, often present in aged people, causes the disruption of microflora, raising the amount of this toxin and playing a role in many chronic and degenerative diseases (Murray and Pizzorno 1998). The dysbiosis consists in qualitative and quantitative changes in the intestinal flora, their metabolic activity, and local distribution. Reasons for this condition are an incorrect diet and lifestyle, use of antibiotics and laxative, stress, and aging itself. It is important to note that change in intestinal microbiota during aging is not the same in different parts of the world because all the conditions and habits mentioned above are different. Therefore, it is possible to speculate a sort of "microbiome regionalism." For example, some studies on Irish elderly people demonstrated an increase of *Firmicutes* that remain unchanged in Italians (Biagi et al. 2010; Claesson et al. 2011).

All these changes transform the intestine in a continuous source of antigenic stimulation and new signals. These last interact with molecular pathways and determine a condition of chronic systemic and local inflammation that plays an important role in immunosenescence and consequently in frailty. Changes in enterocyte turnover may contribute into small intestine malabsorption of carbohydrate, protein, and fat. Moreover, age-related neurodegeneration that involves enteric nervous system may be a crucial element in the alteration of peristalsis (Biagi et al. 2011; Chung and Kasper 2010; Tiihonen et al. 2010).

Thus, it is possible to speculate that changes in gut microbiota have an important role in the development and maintenance of inflammaging. It was demonstrated by a study on gut microbiota that three main modifications occur in fecal microbiota of old frail people: a 26-fold reduction in the amount of *Lactobacilli* (immunostimulants and adsorption promoters), a threefold reduction in the number of *Bacteroides* (involved in polysaccharides digestion), and a sevenfold increase in the number of *Enterobacteriaceae* (potentially pathogens). It is important to note that differences exist in fecal microbiota between different countries and ages, not only between young and old, but also between aged and long-lived individuals.

21.3 Prevention: Dietary Solutions to Prevent Aging Process

21.3.1 Calorie Restriction and Modulation of Immune Response

Nowadays, the beneficiary effects of calorie restriction (CR) in extension of healthy life span are well known. Many studies exist about the role of nutrient-sensing pathways in worms, yeasts, rodents, flies, and mammals (Kaeberlein et al. 2005; Yuan et al. 2012; Anderson et al. 2009; Fontana et al. 2010). These pathways are evolutionary conserved, though with different molecular components and systemic complexity, demonstrating their importance in many species. The first evidence about beneficial effect of long-term CR in increasing life span was proposed in 1930 by McCay and colleagues (McCay et al. 1935). CR without malnutrition leads to a "standby" mode in cells and organisms and reduction in cell division and reproduction to save energy, necessary for basal metabolism (Fontana et al. 2010). The extension of life span is guaranteed by these pathways due to their capability of preserving a variety of body functions from the beginning of life. Obviously, studies in human should be the most interesting one, but they are not easily feasible. Nevertheless, in 2009 a study on humans by Ahmed et al. in 46 healthy women and men aged 20–42 years was done. The population was subjected to 10 or 30 % CR for 6 months. The results showed an increase of T cell-mediated immune response in both groups evidenced by measurement of delayed-type hypersensitivity (DTH) and T cell proliferation. Moreover, people subjected to 30 % CR showed a decrease in the production of lipopolysaccharide (LPS)-stimulated ex vivo production of T cell-suppressive eicosanoid prostaglandin E2 (PGE_2) (Ahmed et al. 2009). However, the exact mechanisms and pathway for these effects remained to be known.

Rodent and in particular mice remain the most studied model in the field of CR and immune response. Many studies have demonstrated positive roles for CR in reversing all effects of immunosenescence: the reduction in the number of naive T cells, the lower activity of NK cells and CTL production, the increase in levels of TNF-α and IL-6 in serum, the susceptibility to autoimmune diseases, the reduction in IL-2 production, and the lower response of T cell to antigens (Chen et al. 1998; Walford et al. 1973; Weindruch and Walford 1982; Weindruch et al. 1982, 1983; Spaulding et al. 1997).

21.3.2 Concluding Remarks: Mediterranean Diet and Longevity

Mediterranean diet (MD) is an eating pattern reported to contribute to better health and quality of life for those adhering to it. Given this, within Mediterranean countries, cultural and religious differences exist, resulting in a diversity in food patterns. Nowadays, the concept of "Mediterranean diets" is more commonly applied than that of merely one MD. In 1975 Ancel Keys officially introduced the MD in global scenery. This American physiologist identified saturated fat as a major factor responsible for heart diseases (Keys et al. 1986). With his studies, it was possible to establish the role of MD as the model of healthy diet useful in prevention of age-related diseases such as cancer, cardiovascular diseases, dementia, type 2 diabetes, metabolic syndrome, and inflammatory age-related diseases in general (Tyrovolas and Panagiotakos 2010; Sofi et al. 2008; Fung et al. 2010). Many studies demonstrated the beneficiary effects of MD in longevity (Berry et al. 2011; Vasto et al. 2012). The common Mediterranean dietary pattern has the following characteristics: abundance of plant foods (fruit, vegetables, legumes, breads, other forms of cereals, potatoes, beans, nuts, and seeds); fresh fruit as the typical daily dessert; olive oil as the principal source of fat; dairy products (principally cheese and yogurt), fish, and poultry consumed in low to moderate amounts; zero to four eggs consumed weekly; red meat consumed in low amounts; and wine consumed in low to moderate amounts, normally with meals. This diet is low in saturated fat, with total fat ranging from 25 to 42 % of energy throughout the Mediterranean region. This fact has conflicted with nutritional objectives in Western countries that limit total fat intake to less than 30 % of calories. «Mediterranean pyramid» describes a dietary pattern that is attractive for its famous palatability, as well as for its health benefits (Willett et al. 1995; Trichopoulou et al. 2001). The MD is known specifically for its use of olive oil, red wine, and vegetables and absence of red meat. Olive oil, in particular, plays a pivotal role in MD, taking up a central position in the pyramid. Its nutritional properties that reach the peak in the extra virgin olive oil make it a strong antioxidant. In fact olive oil contains many bioactive compounds with strong antioxidant properties. Polyphenols, including firstly oleocanthal and monounsatered fatty acids (i.e. oleic acids), are likely responsible for the inverse association with some cancers and the positive effect on the cardiovascular system (Corona et al. 2009; Pelucchi et al. 2010; Castañer et al. 2011). Moreover, olive oil should be the main source of dietary lipids. Among several kinds of oils, as seed oils, it represents the best one for cooking, thanks to its high smoke point (Casal et al. 2010).

In addition, a daily glass or two of red wine with meals has benefits for inflammation, since it contains vitamins, minerals, and anti-inflammatory agents. Wine is rich in potassium and low in sodium. Red wines have more of these elements due to the juices longer contact with the grape skins and are rich in vitamin B which comes from the grape skins as well. Protein sources for this diet are primarily fish, farm meat, and legumes. Fish, as well as nut, has anti-inflammatory effects, whereas legume carbohydrates show a low glycemic index. So, MD contains an important number of antioxidants (vitamins E and C, carotenoids, and various polyphenol compounds present in vegetables, fruits, nuts, whole grains, legumes, virgin olive oil, and wine) that are likely to play an important role in the prevention of cardiovascular diseases. MD is also rich in micronutrient, thanks to the large consumption of fruit, vegetables, and legumes. But it is important to note that not only the quality is important but also the quantity. In any case, the main point has to be the balance between all kinds of food. In fact, it was proven that a vegetarian diet with an excess of fitates results in a reduction of zinc intake. Fitates are present mostly in cereals and legumes. They cause formation of insoluble salt, resulting in low absorption of some minerals such as calcium, iron, magnesium, and zinc. Although MD contains a considerable amount of fitates, it contains the adequate provision of zinc, necessary to prevent growth and behavioral disorders in adolescent. Obviously additional studies are necessary to determine the exact amount of each food, but as many studies demonstrated, MD is the best diet to prevent many diseases and to maintain a good status of health. Another interesting study demonstrated the reduction of many circulating inflammatory biomarkers and cardiovascular disease risk factor in a study population subjected to Mediterranean diet supplemented with virgin olive oil (VOO) or mixed nuts. With respect to a third population subjected to a low-fat diet, the other two showed a decrease in soluble intercellular adhesion molecule 1 (sICAM-1) and IL-6 and a reduced immune cell activation, while C-reactive protein (CRP) decreased only in the group with VOO supplementation (Mena et al. 2009).

Finally, thanks to the high fiber content of the MD, positive effects can occur in the composition of the gut microbiota (Vrieze et al. 2010).

In literature, it has been suggested that the MD comes from regional "poverty" because some kind of foods, such as bovine meat and butter, were not very abundant due to the country climate. However, farm animals have been raised for centuries in these countries with predilection to sheep, goats, and chickens. It so happens that most cheeses made from sheep's milk are lower in cholesterol than those made from cow's milk, while olive oil, with its monounsaturated fat, is healthier than cholesterol-laden butter. In addition, the meat of sheep, goats, and even chickens contain some fat, but Mediterranean people usually eat less meat than their Northern European neighbors. Paradoxically, today, it is, instead, established that overconsumption of foods that are rich in calories, nutritionally poor, highly processed, and rapidly assimilated can lead to systemic inflammation, reduced insulin sensitivity, and several metabolic abnormalities, including obesity, hypertension, dyslipidemia, and glucose intolerance, commonly known as metabolic syndrome. These dietary patterns are common in the Western part of the world and associated with higher level of morbidity and mortality.

Dietary habits may significantly improve general health status and life quality, and MD according to international dietetic organizations might promote healthy aging. Furthermore, nutritional education from the public health practitioners could be an important way to improve health and quality of life of middle-aged and older and may be considered one of the tools to add healthy years to life. Therefore, long-term adherence to the MD can serve as an anti-inflammatory dietary pattern, which can prevent or manage diseases that are related to chronic, systemic inflammation, including cancer and cardiovascular diseases.

References

Adolfsson O, Huber BT, Meydani SN (2001) Vitamin E-enhanced IL-2 production in old mice: naive but not memory T cells show increased cell division cycling and IL-2-producing capacity. J Immunol 167: 3809–3817

Ahmed T, Das SK, Golden JK et al (2009) Calorie restriction enhances T-cell-mediated immune response in adult overweight men and women. J Gerontol A Biol Sci Med Sci 64:107–1113

Anderson RM, Shanmuganayagam D, Weindruch R (2009) Caloric restriction and aging: studies in mice and monkeys. Toxicol Pathol 37:47–51

Baldwin AS (1996) The NF-κB and IκB proteins: new discoveries and insights. Annu Rev Immunol 14: 649–681

Bengmark S (1998) Probiotics and prebiotics in prevention and treatment of gastrointestinal diseases. Gastroenterol Int 11:4–7

Berry EM, Arnoni Y, Aviram M (2011) The middle eastern and biblical origins of the Mediterranean diet. Public Health Nutr 14:2288–2295

Biagi E, Nylund L, Candela M et al (2010) Through ageing, and beyond: gut microbiota and inflammatory status in seniors and centenarians. PLoS ONE 5: e10667

Biagi E, Candela M, Franceschi C et al (2011) The aging gut microbiota: new perspectives. Ageing Res Rev 10:428–429

Bogden JD, Oleske JM, Lavenhar MA et al (1990) Effects of one year of supplementation with zinc and other micronutrients on cellular immunity in the elderly. J Am Coll Nutr 9:214–225

Briefel RR, Bialostosky K, Kennedy-Stephenson J et al (2000) Zinc intake of the U.S. population: findings from the third National Health and Nutrition Examination Survey, 1988–1994. J Nutr 130:1367–1373

Candore G, Colonna-Romano G, Balistreri CR et al (2006) Biology of longevity: role of the innate immune system. Rejuvenation Res 9:143–148

Casal S, Malheiro R, Sendas A (2010) Olive oil stability under deep-frying conditions. Food Chem Toxicol 48:2972–2979

Castañer O, Fitó M, López-Sabater MC et al (2011) The effect of olive oil polyphenols on antibodies against oxidized LDL. A randomized clinical trial. Clin Nutr 30:490–493

Chen J, Astle CM, Harrison DE (1998) Delayed immune aging in diet-restricted B6CBAT6 F1 mice is associated with preservation of naive T cells. J Gerontol A Biol Sci Med Sci 53:B330–B337

Chung H, Kasper DL (2010) Microbiota-stimulated immune mechanisms to maintain gut homeostasis. Curr Opin Immunol 22:455–460

Claesson MJ, Cusack S, O'Sullivan O et al (2011) Composition, variability, and temporal stability of the intestinal microbiota of the elderly. Proc Natl Acad Sci U S A 108:4586–4591

Corona G, Spencer JP, Dessì MA (2009) Extra virgin olive oil phenolics: absorption, metabolism, and biological activities in the GI tract: review. Toxicol Ind Health 25:285–293

Cousins RJ, Liuzzi JP, Lichten LA (2006) Mammalian zinc transport, trafficking, and signals. J Biol Chem 281:24085–24089

Csermely P, Somogyi J (1989) Zinc as a possible mediator of signal transduction in T lymphocytes. Acta Physiol Hung 74:195–199

Csermely P, Szamel M, Resch K et al (1988) Zinc can increase the activity of protein kinase C and contributes to its binding to plasma membranes in T lymphocytes. J Biol Chem 263:6487–6490

Cummings JH, Macfarlane GT (1997) Role of intestinal bacteria in nutrient metabolism. JPEN J Parenter Enteral Nutr 21:357–365

De Martinis M, Franceschi C, Monti D et al (2005) Inflamm-ageing and lifelong antigenic load as major determinants of ageing rate and longevity. FEBS Lett 579(10):2035–2039

De Martinis M, Franceschi C, Monti D et al (2006) Inflammation markers predicting frailty and mortality in the elderly. Exp Mol Pathol 80:219–227

Duchateau J, Delepesse G, Vrijens R et al (1981) Beneficial effects of oral zinc supplementation on the immune response of old people. Am J Med 70:1001–1004

Duke RC, Chervenak R, Cohen JJ (1983) Endogenous endonuclease-induced DNA fragmentation: an early event in cell-mediated cytolysis. Proc Natl Acad Sci U S A 80:6361–6365

Fontana L, Partridge L, Longo VD (2010) Extending healthy life span–from yeast to humans. Science 328: 321–326

Forbes IJ, Zalewski PD, Giannakis C et al (1990) Interaction between protein kinase C and regulatory ligand is enhanced by a chelatable pool of cellular zinc. Biochim Biophys Acta 1053:113–117

Fortes C, Forastiere F, Agabiti N et al (1998) The effect of zinc and vitamin A supplementation on immune response in an older population. J Am Geriatr Soc 46: 19–26

Franceschi C (2007) Inflammaging as a major characteristic of old people: can it be prevented or cured? Nutr Rev 65:S173–S176

Franceschi C, Bonafe M, Valensin S et al (2000) Inflammaging. An evolutionary perspective on immunosenescence. Ann N Y Acad Sci 908:244–254

Franceschi C, Capri M, Monti DI et al (2007) Inflammaging and anti-inflammaging: a systemic perspective on ageing and longevity emerged from studies in humans. Mech Ageing Dev 128:92–105

Frazzini V, Rockabrand E, Mocchegiani E et al (2006) Oxidative stress and brain aging: is zinc the link? Biogerontology 7:307–314

Frederickson CJ, Koh JY, Bush AI (2005) The neurobiology of zinc in health and disease. Nat Rev Neurosci 6:449–462

Fung TT, Hu FB, Wu K et al (2010) The Mediterranean and Dietary Approaches to Stop Hypertension (DASH) diets and colorectal cancer. Am J Clin Nutr 92: 1429–1435

Gebremichael A, Levy EM, Corwin LM (1984) Adherent cell requirement for the effect of vitamin E on in vitro antibody synthesis. J Nutr 114:1297–1305

Ginaldi L, De Martinis M, Monti D et al (2005) Chronic antigenic load and apoptosis in immunosenescence. Trends Immunol 26:79–84

Haase H, Rink L (2009) Functional significance of zinc-related signaling pathways in immune cells. Annu Rev Nutr 29:133–152

Holzapfel WH, Haberer P, Snel J et al (1998) Overview of gut flora and probiotics. Int J Food Microbiol 41: 85–101

Isakov N, Altman A (2002) Protein kinase C (theta) in T cell activation. Annu Rev Immunol 20:761–794

Kaeberlein M, Powers RW, Steffen KK et al (2005) Regulation of yeast replicative life span by TOR and Sch9 in response to nutrients. Science 310:1193–1196

Keys A, Menotti A, Karvonen MJ et al (1986) The diet and 15-year death rate in the seven countries study. Am J Epidemiol 124:903–915

Kiremidjian-Schumacher L, Roy M (1998) Selenium and immune function. Z Ernahrungswiss 37:50–56

Kowdley KV, Mason JB, Meydani SN et al (1992) Vitamin E deficiency and impaired cellular immunity related to intestinal fat malabsorption. Gastroenterology 102:2139–2142

Maret W, Sandstead HH (2006) Zinc requirements and the risks and benefits of zinc supplementation. J Trace Elem Med Biol 20:3–18

McCay CM, Crowell MF, Maynard LA (1935) The effect of retarded growth upon the length of the life span and upon the ultimate body size. J Nutr 10:63–79

Mena MP, Sacanella E, Vazquez-Agell M et al (2009) Inhibition of circulating immune cell activation: a molecular antiinflammatory effect of the Mediterranean diet. Am J Clin Nutr 89:248–256

Meydani SN, Meydani M, Verdon CP et al (1986) Vitamin E supplementation suppresses prostaglandin E1(2) synthesis and enhances the immune response of aged mice. Mech Ageing Dev 34:191–201

Meydani SN, Han SN, Wu D (2005) Vitamin E and immune response in the aged: molecular mechanisms and clinical implications. Immunol Rev 205:269–284

Murray M, Pizzorno J (1998) Encyclopedia of natural medicine. Prima Publishing, Rocklin, p 143

Noack J, Kleessen B, Proll J et al (1998) Dietary guar gum and pectin stimulate intestinal microbial polyamine synthesis in rats. J Nutr 128:1385–1391

Opipari AW Jr, Boguski MS, Dixit VM (1990) The A20 cDNA induced by tumor necrosis factor alpha encodes a novel type of zinc finger protein. J Biol Chem 265:14705–14708

Pelucchi C, Bosetti C, Negri E (2010) Olive oil and cancer risk: an update of epidemiological findings through. Curr Pharm Des 17:805–812

Prasad AS, Fitzgerald JT, Hess JW et al (1993) Zinc deficiency in elderly patients. Nutrition 9:218–224

Rink L, Haase H (2007) Zinc homeostasis and immunity. Trends Immunol 28:1–4

Rink L, Kirchner H (2000) Zinc-altered immune function and cytokine production. J Nutr 130:1407S–1411S

Savage DC (1977) Microbial ecology of the gastrointestinal tract. Annu Rev Microbiol 31:107–133

Sofi F, Cesari F, Abbate R et al (2008) Adherence to Mediterranean diet and health status: meta-analysis. BMJ 337:a1344

Spaulding CC, Walford RL, Effros RB (1997) Calorie restriction inhibits the age-related dysregulation of the cytokines TNF-alpha and IL-6 in C3B10RF1 mice. Mech Ageing Dev 93:87–94

Stennicke HR, Salvesen GS (1997) Biochemical characteristics of caspases-3, -6, -7, and −8. J Biol Chem 272:25719–25723

Tan SL, Parker PJ (2003) Emerging and diverse roles of protein kinase C in immune cell signalling. Biochem J 376:545–552

Tiihonen K, Ouwehand AC, Rautonen N (2010) Human intestinal microbiota and healthy ageing. Ageing Res Rev 9:107–116

Trichopoulou A, Naska A, Vasilopoulou E (2001) Guidelines for the intake of vegetables and fruit: the Mediterranean approach. Int J Vitam Nutr Res 71: 149–153

Truong-Tran AQ, Carter J, Ruffin RE et al (2001) The role of zinc in caspase activation and apoptotic cell death. Biometals 14:315–330

Turnbaugh PJ, Ley RE, Hamady M et al (2007) The human microbiome project. Nature 449:804–810

Tyrovolas S, Panagiotakos DB (2010) The role of Mediterranean type of diet on the development of cancer and cardiovascular disease, in the elderly: a systematic review. Maturitas 65:122–130

Vallee BL, Falchuk KH (1993) The biochemical basis of zinc physiology. Physiol Rev 73:79–118

Van Deventer SJ, Ten Cate JW, Tytgat GN (1988) Intestinal endotoxemia. Clinical significance. Gastroenterology 94: 825–831

Vasto S, Candore G, Balistreri CR et al (2007) Inflammatory networks in ageing, age-related diseases and longevity. Mech Ageing Dev 128:83–91

Vasto S, Carruba G, Lio D et al (2009) Inflammation, ageing and cancer. Mech Ageing Dev 130:40–45

Vasto S, Rizzo C, Caruso C (2012) Centenarians and diet: what they eat in the Western part of Sicily. Immun Ageing 9:10

Vrieze A, Holleman F, Zoetendal EG et al (2010) The environment within: how gut microbiota may influence metabolism and body composition. Diabetologia 53:606–613

Walford RL, Liu RK, Gerbase-Delima M et al (1973) Longterm dietary restriction and immune function in mice: response to sheep red blood cells and to mitogenic agents. Mech Ageing Dev 2:447–454

Weindruch R, Walford RL (1982) Dietary restriction in mice beginning at 1 year of age: effect on life-span and spontaneous cancer incidence. Science 215: 1415–1418

Weindruch R, Gottesman SR, Walford RL (1982) Modification of age-related immune decline in mice dietarily restricted from or after midadulthood. Proc Natl Acad Sci U S A 79:898–902

Weindruch R, Devens BH, Raff HV et al (1983) Influence of dietary restriction and aging on natural killer cell activity in mice. J Immunol 130:993–996

Willett WC, Sacks F, Trichopoulou A et al (1995) Mediterranean diet pyramid: a cultural model for healthy eating. Am J Clin Nutr 61:1402S–1406S

Yuan Y, Kadiyala CS, Ching TT et al (2012) Enhanced energy metabolism contributes to the extended life span of calorie-restricted Caenorhabditis elegans. J Biol Chem 287:31414–31426

Zalewski PD, Forbes IJ, Giannakis C et al (1990) Synergy between zinc and phorbol ester in translocation of protein kinase C to cytoskeleton. FEBS Lett 273:131–134

Dietary Intake and Impact of Zinc Supplementation on the Immune Functions in Elderly: Nutrigenomic Approach

22

Eugenio Mocchegiani, Marco Malavolta, Robertina Giacconi, and Laura Costarelli

22.1 Introduction

The elderly above the age of 60–65 years shows a higher risk of developing nutritional disorders caused by the aging process itself. Aging is accompanied with a series of physiological, biochemical, biological, and psychological changes, deteriorating the individual physical activity as well as general behavior, dietary habits, and social interactions (Meunier et al. 2005). Several clinical symptoms are linked to this situation, including dermatitis, diarrhea, and especially alterations in immunocompetence (Hambidge 2000; Cunningham-Rundles et al. 2005).

Generally, adequate nutrition plays a pivotal role in maintaining healthy status (Hambidge 2010) and immunocompetence in humans (High 1999) with possible extension of the life-span (Chernoff 2005). Among the micronutrients, zinc is essential in the elderly in terms of its impact on biological, biochemical, and immune functions (Shankar and Prasad 1998; Mocchegiani et al. 1998; Haase et al. 2006b).

Zinc deficiency affects over two billion of aged people (Prasad 2008). Nutritional zinc deficiency is widespread throughout developing countries. A lot of evidences support the belief that the main

factor associated with zinc deficiency seems to be an inadequate zinc dietary intake influenced in turn by other several intrinsic and extrinsic factors (Gibson et al. 2008). Indeed, zinc is well recognized as an essential trace element for all organisms and plays an important role in the development and integrity of the immune system affecting both innate and adaptive immune responses (Prasad 2000; Ibs et al. 2003; Bogden 2004; Haase et al. 2006b; Mocchegiani et al. 2009). Zinc is required for DNA synthesis, RNA transcription, cell division, and activation (Prasad 2007) as well as in preventing apoptosis (Fraker 2005). Zinc has also a significant role as "zinc signal" affecting the signal transduction for immune cell functions (Haase and Rink 2009a). All these effects have been identified in experimental animals and humans where an altered zinc status can affect the immunocompetence (Prasad 1998; Haase and Rink 2009b; Mocchegiani et al. 2008c). Zinc deficiency coupled with altered immune response, as occurring in aging, leads to an increased susceptibility for some age-related diseases (Vasto et al. 2006; Prasad 2009). As a consequence, several studies suggest the usefulness of a zinc supplementation in the prevention and/or treatment of diseases associated with zinc deficiency (Prasad 2009; Haase and Rink 2009b; Mocchegiani et al. 2008c). The aim of this chapter is to review some possible effects of low zinc dietary intake in aging especially at subcellular level and the main effects of zinc on immunosenescence. Moreover, we will discuss the potential role of the zinc supplementation in elderly in order to restore the immune

E. Mocchegiani, PhD (✉) • M. Malavolta, PhD
R. Giacconi, PhD • L. Costarelli, PhD
Scientific and Technologic Pole of Gerontology and Geriatrics Research of INRCA, Translational Centre of Research in Nutrition and Ageing, Italian National Research Centres on Ageing (INRCA), Ancona, Italy
e-mail: e.mocchegiani@inrca.it

A. Massoud, N. Rezaei (eds.), *Immunology of Aging*,
DOI 10.1007/978-3-642-39495-9_22, © Springer-Verlag Berlin Heidelberg 2014

response, referring to individual genetic background that is represented by metallothioneins (MT) and interleukin (IL)-6 polymorphisms (nutrigenomic approach). Such an assumption is based on the fact that the production of MT and IL-6 increases in aging leading to chronic inflammation (Mocchegiani et al. 2006), named "inflammaging" (Franceschi 2007), with subsequent altered intracellular zinc homeostasis (Mocchegiani et al. 2006).

22.2 Dietary Zinc Deficiency

Zinc deficiency is an important factor in the origin of certain common diseases that affect and cause morbidity among the elderly. Zinc is a critical trace element in human health for tissue growth, taste acuity, connective tissue growth and maintenance, immune response, prostaglandin production, bone mineralization, proper thyroid function, blood clotting, cognitive functions, fetal growth, and sperm production (Sandstead 1994). Zinc is also required for the biological activity of enzymes, for cell proliferation, and for "zinc finger" DNA motifs (Mocchegiani et al. 1998). Clinical evidences support the pathological consequences (cancer, infections, diarrhea, hypertension, cardiovascular diseases, macular degeneration, diabetes) that can occur during zinc deficiency that is a serious public health problem from young up to old age (Haase and Rink 2009b; Mocchegiani et al. 2012b) (Table 22.1). Such a deficiency in aging is typically the result of an inadequate zinc dietary intake that may occur as a response to reduced energy requirements or age-related sensory impairment (Stewart-Knox et al. 2005). It has been reported that mild zinc deficiency is a significant clinical problem in free-living elderly people: only 42.9 % have a sufficient intake of zinc (defined as >67 % of the Recommended Dietary Allowances or RDA) (Prasad et al. 1993). These data have been confirmed by other studies in different parts of the world (Andriollo-Sanchez et al. 2005; Mocchegiani et al. 2008a); German study in conjuction with phytates (Schlemmer et al. 2009) Japan study (Kogirima et al. 2007). Moreover, the

Table 22.1 Clinical consequences coupled with zinc deficiency from the young up to old age

Increased total cholesterol
Rheumatoid arthritis
Macular degeneration
Impairment of the immune response (adaptive and natural immunity)
Osteoporosis
Diarrhea
Pneumonia
Renal failure
Prostatitis
Cirrhosis
Possible development of malignant cancer (leukemia, Hodgkin disease)
Possible contributor to loss of appetite
Anorexia
Hypertension and increased risk factor of atherosclerosis
Decreased cell proliferation and increased apoptotic death (possible accelerated thymic involution)
Decreased taste acuity
Reduced concentration of transport proteins in the blood and loss in urine (albuminuria)
High susceptibility to oxidative damage from certain tissues (brain) (stroke)
Decreased absorption of dietary folate
Decreased cardiac antioxidant capacity (heart failure)
Hyperhomocysteinemia
Schizophrenia and mood disorders
Defective connective tissue
Reduced sperm production
Infertility
Sexual impotence in man and fall of libido
Irregular menstrual cycle in women
Defective sexual maturation of ovaries and testes (hypogonadism)
Weight loss and fatigue
Hair loss and alopecia
Mental lethargy
Decreased resistance to infection, causing an imbalance between Th1/ Th2 paradigm
Abnormalities in cytokine secretion and function
Neuropsychological impairment
Exacerbate hypertension (possible myocardial infarction)
Decreased functionality in monocytes, natural killer cells, granulocytes, and phagocytosis
Risk factor for the development of type 2 diabetes
Abnormalities in thyroid, sexual, pineal, pituitary, insulin, glucocorticoid hormones production
Abnormalities in the hypothalamic hormone releasing factors

Table 22.1 (continued)

Risk factor for the development of obesity
Possible development of dental caries and tooth loss
Premature aging of the skin
Dermatitis, eczema, and acne
Crohn disease and celiac disease
Slow-healing wounds
Common cold
Ulcerations

See: Evans (1986), Haase and Rink (2009b), Prasad (2009), Mocchegiani et al. (2012b)

Third National Health and Nutrition Examination Survey (NHANES) documented a decrease in zinc intake with advancing age, and only 42.5 % of old participants (age ≥ 71 years) showed an adequate zinc intake (defined as ≥ 77 % of the RDA) (Briefel et al. 2000).

Such a reduced zinc dietary intake in aging leads to low intracellular zinc ion availability, which has been well documented using specific fluorescent zinc probe (Haase et al. 2006a). The low intracellular zinc ion availability occurs despite the plasma zinc levels may be in the normal range, suggesting that the determination of plasma zinc can be misleading to detect a real zinc deficiency in elderly (Mocchegiani et al. 2006) that in turn does not reflect the reduced dietary zinc intake (Zincage project) (Mocchegiani et al. 2008a). Such a reduction may be due to many factors related to the aging process. Among them, altered intestinal absorption, alteration in zinc transporter proteins, inadequate mastication, psychosocial factors, drug interactions, and competition between zinc and other bivalent minerals (copper, iron, calcium, selenium) or vitamins may be involved. Old subjects display also a reduction in zinc cellular uptake in comparison to young adults perhaps due to the cellular senescence, which is less responsive to zinc because altered gene expressions of some zinc transporters (Zip1, Zip2, Zip3) on cellular membrane occur (Giacconi et al. 2011). Alternatively, epigenetic mechanisms might occur in the promoter region of the zinc transporters leading to an hypermethylation of the gene with subsequent decreased zinc absorption in the intestinal lumen, as supposed for the zinc transporter ZnT5

(Coneyworth et al. 2009). Anyway, regardless of the mechanism involved, the zinc dietary intake and intestinal zinc absorption are deficient in aging leading to an increased risk for the appearance of degenerative age-related diseases (Haase and Rink 2009b; Mocchegiani et al. 2012b).

Despite the amount of dietary zinc has not to exceed 40 mg/day (RDA) because it may be toxic for the functionality of various organs and systems, including the immune function (Walsh et al. 1994), the zinc absorption is strictly linked to specific saturable transport mechanisms that balance the eventual high dietary zinc intake leading to a correct intracellular zinc distribution (Sandström 1992; Menard and Cousins 1983). However, in old humans, zinc absorption, especially in the small intestine, is lower than young-adult individuals, but it is independent by zinc dietary intake (August et al. 1989). Therefore, other factors can influence zinc absorption. Among them, the amount of zinc present in the intestinal lumen, the presence of dietary promoters (e.g., human milk, animal proteins), and altered physiological states have been reported (Lonnerdal 2000). Another factor influencing the zinc absorption is the presence of phytates as well as other minerals (iron, calcium) in the diet that may act as inhibitors binding zinc or blocking its action (Lonnerdal 2000; Hambidge 2010). Studies in old animals have shown that the aging process is accompanied by alterations entailing some of the following intestinal changes: alterations in villus shape (cilia), increased collagen alteration, mitochondrial changes, crypt elongation, and prolonged replication time of cryptal cells (Thomson 2009). These changes might at least explain the altered zinc absorption in the elderly, as suggested by August et al. (August et al. 1989) and Turnlund et al. (Turnlund et al. 1982), with a reduction of 30 % in old individuals with respect to the young-adult ones. Decreased zinc absorption in elderly may also occur in large intestine owing to degenerative alterations in enterocytes and intestinal microvilli (Elmes and Jones 1980). The causes of these physiopathological alterations in large intestine are still unknown. Anyway, regardless of these factors, when the capacity of the intestinal absorption diminishes, the zinc deficiency develops with subsequent loss of appetite and impaired immune functions followed by the appearance of many clinical evidences, including hair loss, diarrhea, impotence, eye and skin lesions, weight loss, delayed wound healing, taste abnormalities, and mental lethargy (Evans 1986). Moreover other factors may affect the zinc absorption regardless by altered or deficiencies in the gut. Among them, the poor mastication and changes in oral structures, psychosocial factors, drug interactions, and the interaction of zinc with other trace elements (iron, copper) or vitamins (vit A, D, E) (Sandström 2001; Basu and Donaldson 2003; Cousins 2010; Marcellini et al. 2006). However, the more intriguing and novel aspect that can affect the zinc absorption by the diet is at subcellular level involving zinc transporters (Zip and ZnT families), MT, and the divalent metal transporter 1 (DMT1). Current evidences indicate that, within the ZnT family (involved in reducing cytosolic zinc concentrations), ZnT1, ZnT5, and ZnT6 localized to the basolateral membrane of the intestinal enterocyte may be of particular importance in intestinal zinc transport processes (Cragg et al. 2005). By contrast, the localization and functional and regulatory properties of Zip4 and Zip5 in apical enterocytes membrane indicate that they play a key role in the absorption of dietary zinc (Dufner-Beattie et al. 2004). Mutations in Zip4 are associated with the human zinc deficiency disease, such as acrodermatitis enteropathica, which displays a severe reduction in zinc uptake (Kury et al. 2002). Another zinc transporter Zip14, expressed in duodenum and jejunum and mediated by IL-6, plays also a relevant role because it is involved in zinc and iron uptake with a task in regulating compensatory mechanisms in order to avoid iron overload that can be toxic in aging (Liuzzi et al. 2006). However, it is currently unclear how aging affects the function and the gene expression of zinc transporters in enterocytes. It may be supposed that it might depend by a less efficient membrane localization of these proteins or related to impaired activity of the zinc transporters with advancing aging due to the presence of chronic inflammation. Such an assumption may be supported by the findings

in experimental models of chronic inflammation (airway inflammation) showing a positive correlation between altered mRNA zinc transporters (Zip1, Zip14, Zip4, ZnT4) and high gene expression of macrophage, monocyte, and eosinophil inflammatory-related proteins (cc16, cc18, cc19, cc111) (Lang et al. 2007). Alternatively, DNA methylation, known as an epigenetic event and modified by age, might alter the gene expressions, as supposed for CpG island in the ZnT5 and ZnT1 gene promoter regions (Coneyworth et al. 2009; Balesaria and Hogstrand 2006).

With regard to the role of MT in zinc absorption regulation, particularly in conjunction with ZnT1, MT works in maintaining free zinc concentrations within quite narrow ranges regardless by ZnT1 (Davis et al. 1998). Another transporter potentially involved in zinc uptake is DMT1: a transmembrane polypeptide found in the duodenum in the crypts and lower villi (McMahon and Cousins 1998). As these transport proteins are identified and characterized, further investigations in the whole animal as well as in humans under conditions of a range of dietary intake are however necessary in order to elucidate the amount of absorbed zinc to the amount of excreted zinc together with these subcellular processes.

22.3 Zinc Status of the Elderly

Although the upper limit of the dietary zinc intake has not to exceed 25–40 mg/day (Food and Nutritional Board 2001; Scientific Committee on Food 2002), the recommended daily allowance (RDA) for zinc in young-adult individuals and older is 11 mg/day for men and 8 mg/day for women (Maret and Sandstead 2006). An uptake below the RDA can only be seen as an indicator of potential zinc deficiency, because many other factors also play a role in decreased zinc intake. Hence, it is necessary to analyze the zinc status of each individual. The parameter of choice is often serum or plasma zinc. However, this is not the ideal parameter to determine the zinc status taking into account that many old individuals, despite increased proinflammatory cytokines known as factors for zinc depletion (Shankar and

Prasad 1998), display circulating plasma zinc levels within the normal range (about 85–90 µg/dl) (Mocchegiani et al. 2003). Other parameters may be useful to test the zinc status, such as the intracellular zinc ion bioavailability with specific zinc probes (Haase et al. 2006a) and the testing the capacity of zinc release by MT using nitric oxide (NO) donors (Mocchegiani et al. 2006). Recently, the determination of the zinc score has been validated in Zincage project (based on the determination of the zinc content in the foods and the individual quantity of the food intake). This score can represent a valid test in determining the zinc status being well correlated with the age-dependent plasma zinc levels (Kanoni et al. 2010). However, a plethora of studies report that plasma zinc levels decrease with advancing age (Haase et al. 2006b) as well as in some cell types, such as erythrocytes and lymphocytes (Prasad et al. 1993; Andriollo-Sanchez et al. 2005). Such a decrement may depend on dietary habits and life style conditions, and it varies from country to country where zinc deficiency can be more or less severe or marginal, as shown in Zincage project (Mocchegiani et al. 2008a). Also in the United States (USA), one study in a large number of elderly (age range 60–90 years.) showed that the marginal zinc deficiency appeared in more than 90 % of old subjects despite the zinc dietary intake is quite similar to RDA (11.5 mg/day) both for men and women (Ma and Betts 2000). Therefore despite of the dose recommended by RDA, old people display marginal zinc deficiency. Since the "Mediterranean diet" is variegated and contains foods (especially fish) rich of zinc (Sofi et al. 2010) usually consumed in Spain, Italy, and France and some other foods rich of zinc (read meat and legumes) are consumed in Northern European Countries and in the USA might in part justify the quite sufficient zinc dietary intake and the relative marginal zinc deficiency in elderly. But, it does not explain the reason of a remarkable subgroup in all countries of elderly subjects who achieve "successful aging" (centenarian subjects) without suffering from age-related diseases despite of the presence low zinc dietary intake and zinc deficiency (Mocchegiani et al. 2003). Taking into account

that severe zinc deficiency is strictly related to the chronic inflammation (Mocchegiani et al. 2006; Prasad 2009), the reason may be related to a lower inflammatory state in centenarians with subsequent still capacity in zinc release by MT, suggesting that the available quota of free zinc ions, despite reduced, is still sufficient in maintaining good immune performances (Mocchegiani et al. 2003), further confirming the relevance of zinc for immunosenescence and in keeping under control the inflammatory state.

22.4   Zinc and Immunosenescence

Aging is a continuous multidimensional process of physical, psychological, and social changes that compromises the normal functioning of various organs and systems, including several immunological alterations named immunosenescence, which is characterized by increased susceptibility to infections, autoimmune diseases, and cancer (Pawelec et al. 2010). The immune efficiency decreases with advancing aging, starting around 60–65 years. Alterations of the immune system during aging and zinc deprivation show many similarities, indicating the existence of a strict relationship between immunosenescence and zinc deficiency (Mocchegiani et al. 1998; Bogden 2004; Haase and Rink 2009b). The similarity is in adaptive and innate immunity as well as in neutrophil functions (chemotaxis, phagocytosis, oxidative burst). Although the total number of neutrophils is not different between old and young-adult subjects, phagocytosis, oxidative burst, and intracellular killing are impaired in aging, and neutrophils from the elderly show reduced chemotaxis and a lower resistance to apoptosis, as shown by impaired antiapoptotic effects after specific stimuli such as lipopolysaccharide (LPS), granulocyte colony-stimulating factor (G-CSF), and granulocyte-macrophage colony-stimulating factor (GM-CSF) (Schroder and Rink 2003). In this context, zinc may play a key role because a satisfactory intracellular zinc ion bioavailability preserves the oxidative burst by neutrophils, via reduction of IL-6 signalling, as observed in centenarians, who in turn display satisfactory intracellular zinc content and low grade of inflammation (Moroni et al. 2005).

22.4.1 Adaptive Immunity

With regard to adaptive immunity, the plasma concentrations of IL-6, IL-8, monocyte chemotactic protein-1 (MCP-1), macrophage inflammatory protein-1α (MIP-1α), and tumor necrosis factor alpha (TNF-α) were positively correlated with age with a progressive elevation in very old age (Mariani et al. 2006). T helper (Th)1 (interferon gamma or IFN-γ, IL-2) cytokines decrease whereas Th2 (IL-4, IL-10) cytokines increase (Cakman et al. 1996). The same trend was also observed after LPS stimulation (Gabriel et al. 2002; Cakman et al. 1997). These alterations in Th1 and Th2 cytokine productions lead to an imbalance of Th1/Th2 paradigm with a shift towards Th2 production and subsequent chronic low grade of inflammation, named "inflammaging" (Franceschi 2007). Alterations in the balance of Th1/Th2 cytokines also occur in zinc deficiency (Uciechowski et al. 2008) that is characterized by decreased IFN-γ, IL-2, and TNF-α production (Th1 cells) and increased IL-6 production by Th2 cells and macrophages (Mocchegiani et al. 1998). However, in very old age, the high levels of IL-6 are not so detrimental because of the low gene expression of IL-6 subunit receptor (gp130) that allows the presence of an inactive quota of IL-6 with subsequent reduced inflammation and good intracellular zinc content (Moroni et al. 2005).

22.4.2 T-Cell Functions

A similarity between aging and zinc deficiency exists also in T-cell pathway. The more characteristic T-cell pathway abnormalities in aging are (a) reduced T-cell proliferation in response to T-cell receptor or CD3 or mitogen stimulations (Pawelec et al. 1998); (b) altered CD4/CD8 ratio (Pawelec et al. 1998); (c) higher expression of CD95 (Fas) and lower expression of BCL-2 and p53 leading to increased apoptosis (McLeod 2000); (d) lower number of naïve (CD45RA+) and a higher number of activated memory (CD45RO+) T cells (Gregg

et al. 2005); and (e) thymic involution producing reduced number of naïve T cells and also immature because of the lack of thymic hormone activity required for T-cell maturation and differentiation (Arnold et al. 2011). The same age-related T-cell pathway alterations also occur in zinc deficiency (Mocchegiani et al. 1998; Dardenne 2002) as well as thymic involution, regardless of age, due to increased thymocyte apoptosis provoked by elevating glucocorticoid production and by the negative regulatory function by zinc in immune cell apoptosis (Taub and Longo 2005). Zinc supplementation in old mice increases the thickness of the thymic gland (especially cortical part) (Sbarbati et al. 1998) and restores the number of viable thymocytes and serum thymic hormone (thymulin) activity (Dardenne et al. 1993; Mocchegiani et al. 1995). Thus, the zinc deficiency in the elderly may also contribute to the thymic involution by augmenting apoptosis during T-cell maturation and differentiation, as observed in old (Provinciali et al. 1998) and in young zinc diet-deprived mice (King et al. 2002). On the other hand, the thymic output (measured by T-cell receptor rearrangement excision circles (TREC)) is strongly reduced during aging and in zinc deficiency leading to a reduced number of naïve mature T cells in the circulation with subsequent inability to substitute activated memory T cells, which in turn undergo to apoptosis after exposure to "foreign" antigens (Mitchell et al. 2006). By contrast, in centenarian subjects with a satisfactory zinc pool (Mocchegiani et al. 2003), the thymic output is still sufficiently maintained by IL-7 (Nasi et al. 2006), and IL-7 and its receptor act via zinc finger protein Miz-1 and SOCS1 (Saba et al. 2011), which the latter is in turn regulated by another zinc finger protein TRIM8/GERP (Toniato et al. 2002). Therefore, zinc is relevant in aging for thymic output signalling with possible new T-cell maturation and differentiation.

22.4.3 Innate Immunity

Of particular interest is the involvement of zinc in innate immunity, such as NK cells and NKT cells, and their cytotoxicity in aging. The total number of NK cells and their percentage among circulating cells increase in old people, but this effect is compensated by a reduced cytotoxic activity and reduced proliferation in response to IL-2 (Solana and Mariani 2000; Mocchegiani et al. 2009). Because the main functions of NK cells are those ones to eliminate cancer or virus-infected cells, the higher incidence of viral infections and cancer in the elderly may well be related to impairment of NK cell function. In this context, the role played by zinc may be pivotal. First of all, zinc may affect the new production of NK cells by stem cells. Zinc in vitro (10 μM) improves the development of CD34+ cell progenitors towards mature NK cells both in young (expressing CD56+ CD16– phenotype) and old age (expressing CD56– CD16+ or CD56+ CD16+ phenotypes) via increased expression of GATA-3 transcription factor (Muzzioli et al. 2009). Moreover, several studies in old animals and humans describe decreased NK cell cytotoxicity related to zinc deficiency (Mocchegiani et al. 2009) through different mechanisms involving NF-kB or Ap-1 transcriptional factors or A20 protein (Prasad 2007; Prasad et al. 2011; Bao et al. 2010). In vitro (1 μM) and in vivo zinc treatments (12 mg Zn^{++}/day) for a short period (1 month) induce complete recovery of natural killer (NK) cell cytotoxicity both in old mice and humans (Mocchegiani et al. 1995; Mariani et al. 2008). In addition, a physiological zinc treatment (15 Zn^{++}/day) for 1 month in old infected patients, other than an increased NK cell cytotoxicity, recovers the IFN-γ production leading to 50 % reduction of infection relapses (Mocchegiani et al. 2003). Findings in centenarians and in very old mice confirm the relevance of zinc in restoring NK cell function in elderly. Indeed, they have a well-preserved NK cell cytotoxicity, a good intracellular zinc ion bioavailability and satisfactory IFN-γ production (Mocchegiani et al. 2003; Miyaji et al. 2000). A very intriguing aspect is a preservation in very old age of the NKT cells bearing T-cell receptor (TCR)γδ (Mocchegiani et al. 2004), which are the first lineage of defense of the organism against virus and bacteria from early in life. NKT cells produce Th1 (IFN-γ) and Th2 (IL-4) cytokines and are functionally linked to NK cells, via IFN-γ (Biron and Brossay 2001). A dysregulation in IL-4 production by NKT cells

leads to pathology, as it occurs during a chronic inflammation and autoimmune diseases (Araujo et al. 2004). However, the main task of NKT cells is to produce IFN-γ with thus a pivotal role in antitumor cytotoxic response (Cui et al. 1997). NKT cells have been found in the thymus, liver, spleen, and bone morrow. Despite the existence of a thymus-independent differentiation pathway located in the liver for NKT cell lineage (as shown in athymic nude mice), the thymus is also a site for NKT development and the liver for NKT homing (Emoto and Kaufmann 2003). During aging, the thymus is atrophic. Therefore, the liver extrathymic function becomes prominent in order to compensate the thymic failure during aging (Abo et al. 2000). Therefore, liver NKT cell function becomes relevant in aging for host defense. Zinc also improves the liver NKT cell (mainly bearing TCRγδ) cytotoxicity in old and in very old mice, suggesting that good zinc ion bioavailability and the function of these types of NKT cells are fundamental to achieve successful aging (Mocchegiani et al. 2004).

22.4.4 Humoral Immunity

With regard to humoral immunity, changes during aging are also found with a reduction in B cell number. Such a reduction seems to be not affected by zinc deficiency but by apoptotic mechanisms (King et al. 2005). However, increased immuno-globulin productions (IgA and IgG subclasses) have been observed (Paganelli et al. 1992), and the response to vaccination with several antigens is diminished due to impaired interaction with T helper cells (Weksler and Szabo 2000). In this context, zinc might be relevant in affecting humoral immunity through its influence in cytokine production by T-cell repertoire, (IL-6, IFN-γ), suppressing the release of IL-6 (von Bulow et al. 2005) and promoting IFN-γ release by peripheral blood mononuclear cells (PBMCs) (Driessen et al. 1994). Although the role of zinc in humoral immunity is still unclear, it does not exclude the relevance of zinc for a correct inflammatory/immune response against external noxae. In particular, the zinc-gene (IL-6 and MT) interactions are pivotal in keeping under control the inflammatory/immune response with subsequent longevity, indicating these genes as "robust" for "healthy aging" (Mocchegiani et al. 2006).

22.5   Zinc-MT Gene Interaction and Inflammatory/Immune Response

MTs are essential to intracellular zinc homeostasis by sequestration and release of the metal at the occurrence and thereby controlling available free zinc ions (Palmiter 1998). The cysteine sulfur ligands in the cluster structure of MT can be reduced (zinc sequestration) or oxidized (zinc release) with thus concomitant changes in the relative amount of bound and free zinc (Maret et al. 1999). MTs are genetically polymorphic proteins with various isoforms. Humans possess genes for four isoforms located in the chromosome 16: the brain specific MT-3 isoform, the squamous epithelium-specific MT-4 isoform, and the ubiquitous MT-1 and MT-2 isoforms (West et al. 1990).

One of the first functions of MT-1 and MT-2 is to regulate intracellular zinc homeostasis and to limit oxidative damage within the cells (Palmiter 1998). Following an injurious stimulus, such as a transient inflammation, the subsequent oxidative stress induce the release of zinc from MT via NO, in order to promote the activity and expression of antioxidant enzymes, including MT itself, thus reducing the oxidative damage and the consequences of the injurious stimulus (Spahl et al. 2003). However, the increased expression of proinflammatory cytokines occurring in aging leads to increased expression of MT, which in turn sequester considerable amount of zinc making it less available for an efficient immune response (Mocchegiani et al. 2000). If, on one side, the reduced zinc ion availability in old age might indicate an excessive sequestration of zinc ions by MT, on the other side, consideration of recent findings on oxidative modification of MT leading to their loss of function suggests also a mechanism whereby these proteins can also lose their ability to buffer the intracellular

free zinc concentration (Barbato et al. 2007). In this case, MT would be unable either to bind or to consequently release zinc in response to stressors. However, it is still unclear if dysfunctional MT can be considered a typical alteration associated with specific disease/disorders or if they are a common feature of aging. However, in vitro data have shown that MT is involved in cellular senescence (Malavolta et al. 2008) with a particular role in affecting the mTOR pathway (Mocchegiani et al. 2012a). Anyway, taking into account that healthy centenarians display a low MT gene expression and satisfactory zinc ion availability despite proinflammatory cytokines (IL-6, TNF-α) increases (Mocchegiani et al. 2002), it may be suggested that this feature reflects the existence of compensatory phenomena able to counteract the effects of inflammation in these exceptional individuals. Moreover, these data suggests that a preservation of zinc homeostasis is an important feature of healthy centenarians. Therefore, the role played by the zinc-MT gene interaction is pivotal to reach successful aging and, at the same time, to escape some age-related diseases. Such a relevance of MT-zinc gene interaction fits with the "Antagonistic Pleiotropy Theory of Aging," in which one gene that is "favorable" in young-adult age may be "disadvantageous" in aging (Williams 1957). The recent discovery of novel polymorphisms of MT2A and MT1A supports this assumption. Old subjects carrying AA genotype for MT2A polymorphism display low zinc ion bioavailability, chronic inflammation by high IL-6, and altered lipid assessments, with subsequent elevated risk for atherosclerosis and diabetes type II (Giacconi et al. 2005). By contrast, polymorphism corresponding to A/C (asparagine/threonine) transition at +647 nt position in the MT1A coding region is the most involved in the women longevity (Cipriano et al. 2006).

Thus, these allelic variants may be very useful tools in order to screen old subjects at risk for zinc deficiency on genetic basis, taking into account that the actual methodological procedures to test the "zinc status" are often misleading and that laboratory investigations to assay zinc ion bioavailability are scarcely reproducible and poorly applicable to clinical practice. In this context, a novel reproducible system in testing intracellular zinc ion bioavailability has been developed using zinc fluorescent probe (Zynpir-1) associated with MT values, representing both tests valid methods to detect the intracellular zinc status (Malavolta et al. 2006).

22.6 Zinc-IL-6 Gene Interaction and Inflammatory/Immune Response

IL-6 −174G/C locus variability has been suggested: (1) to be capable of modulating on one hand the individual susceptibility to common causes of morbidity and mortality among elderly and (2) to play a crucial role in longevity (Franceschi et al. 2005). Therefore, the genetic variations of this locus of IL-6 gene are fundamental in elderly population in order to better understand the intrinsic causes of the longevity. The association of these genetic variations to the possible different immune responses is an attractive focus in elucidating the molecular mechanisms involved in immunosenescence.

The genetic variations of the IL-6 −174G/C locus have been extensively studied by different groups with, however, contradictory data. Bonafè et al. studied IL-6 promoter genetic variability at the −174C/G locus and its effect on IL-6 levels in Italian 700 people aged 60–110 years, including n. 323 centenarians. Individuals who are genetically predisposed to produce high levels of IL-6 during aging, i.e., C− men (GG genotype) at IL-6 −174C/G locus, are disadvantaged for longevity. On the other hand, the capability of C+ individuals (CC and CG genotypes) to produce low levels of IL-6 throughout life-span appears to be beneficial for longevity, at least in men. The women have, conversely, high IL-6 serum levels later in life with respect to men independently from −174C/G locus polymorphism (Bonafè et al. 2001). The inhibitory tone of estrogens on IL-6 gene expression could explain the gender difference (Bruunsgaard et al. 1999), assuming that its long-term effects last until the extreme limits of human life-span.

The major production of IL-6 in C− subjects for the whole life, including centenarians, has been also confirmed by other in vivo longitudinal studies (Rea et al. 2003). A more recent study in old and nonagenarian subjects has confirmed that IL-6 production is higher in C− carriers, and these subjects are prone to contract one of the more usual age-related inflammatory pathologies, such as atherosclerosis (Giacconi et al. 2004). Interestingly, in this last study C− old and nonagenarian subjects display also impaired innate immune response (NK cell cytotoxicity), increased MT, zinc deficiency, and low zinc ion availability in comparison to C+ carriers (Giacconi et al. 2004). These findings clearly suggest that the genetic variations of the IL-6 −174G/C locus play a key role for the longevity at immune functional level. Moreover, they suggest that the determination of the genetic variations of the IL-6 −174G/C locus associated to a comprehensive evaluation of the zinc status are an useful strategy to identify old subjects who can benefit of zinc supplementation without health risks.

22.7 Zinc Supplementation in Elderly on the Basis of MT and IL-6 Polymorphisms

One possible cause of the discrepancy existing in literature on the effect of zinc supplementation upon the immune response (see review Mocchegiani et al. 2007) in elderly may be the choice of old subjects who effectively need zinc supplementation in strict relationships with dietary habits and inflammatory status. This fact is supported by the discovery that old subjects carrying GG genotypes (named C− carriers) in IL-6 −174G/C locus display increased IL-6 production, low intracellular zinc ion availability, and impaired innate immune response coupled with enhanced MT (Mocchegiani et al. 2008b). By contrast, old subjects carrying GC and CC genotypes (named C+ carriers) in the same IL-6 -174 locus display satisfactory intracellular zinc as well as innate immune response. But, the more intriguing finding is that male carriers of C+ allele are more prone to reach centenarian age than C- carriers. Therefore, old C- subjects are more prone for zinc supplementation than old C[+] carriers. Zinc supplementation in old C- subjects restores NK cell cytotoxicity to values present in old C[+] carriers and considerably improves both zinc status, assessed by the percentage increment of granulocyte Zn (Mocchegiani et al. 2008b). When the genetic variations for IL-6 polymorphism are associated with also the genetic variations of MT1A in position +647, the plasma zinc deficiency and the altered immune response is more evident, in which innate immunity is strongly augmented, and the inflammatory status is better keep under control after zinc supplementation (Table 22.2). On the other hand, in vitro zinc (50 μM) on PBMCs from old individuals strongly reduces the gene expression of IL-1 and its receptor is (Mazzatti et al. 2008). These relevant findings suggest that the genetic variations of IL-6 and MT1A are very useful tools for the choice of old people who effectively need zinc supplementation. These results open the hypothesis that the daily requirement of zinc might be different in elderly harboring a different IL-6 and MT polymorphisms and, at the same time, they represent a valid nutrigenomic approach for zinc supplementation.

22.8 Conclusions and Perspectives

Zinc deficiency in elderly, resulting mainly from the reduced zinc dietary intake together with some age-related factors (especially intestinal absorption and subcellular processes), could compromise immune functions leading to the appearance of some degenerative diseases. Since zinc deficiency is a common event in the elderly, several researchers have documented the impact of zinc supplementation in old people in order to restore the zinc status and, as such, to prevent the disability caused by the diseases. Clinical evidences have also suggested that zinc-rich foods, as occurring in the Mediterranean diet, may be useful in the prevention of zinc deficiency in old people. However, controversial findings exist on the "real" necessity of zinc supplementation

Table 22.2 Effect of zinc supplementation on some immune parameters in elderly according to MT and IL-6 polymorphisms

	Parameter	Effects
Thymic output	T-cell receptor excision circles (TRECs)	↓↑
Immune cells senescence and apoptosis	Telomere length	–↑
	Early spontaneous apoptosis	↓
	Late Apoptosis	↓
	Oxidative stress-induced apoptosis	↓
	Mitochondrial membrane depolarization during spontaneous and dRib-induced apoptosis	↓
	Cell Cycle	–
Plasma cytokines and chemokines	IL-6, IL-8, MIP-1α	–↑
	MCP-1, RANTES	–
Immune functions	NK lytic activity	↑↑
	Basal IFN-γ, IL-8, IL-1ra, and IL-6 production	↓
	Basal IL-10 and TNFα production	↓
	Stimulated IFN-γ, IL-6, TNF-α, IL- 1ra, and IL-10 production	↑
Jak/Stat signalling and immunomodulation	IL-2 and IL-6 STAT3 and STAT5 activation	–
	Activation-induced cell death (AICD)	↑
	Cytokines and metabolic gene expression response to zinc	↑↓
T cells subsets	Activated T cells (CD3+CD25+)	↓
	CD4:CD8	–
	Frequencies of CMV-specific cells	–

Data obtained by Zincage project: Mocchegiani et al. (2008a, b, 2012b)

Legend: ↑↑ strongly increased, ↑ increased, – not modified, –↑ slightly increased, ↓↑ intervariability, ↓ decreased

because the major problem for zinc supplementation in old people is related to the choice of old subjects who effectively need zinc supplementation. The sole determination of plasma zinc is not sufficient because zinc is bound to many proteins. The testing of intracellular zinc ion bioavailability with Zinpyr-1 probe coupled with the polymorphisms of IL-6 and MT can be the added values to screen effective old subjects for zinc supplementation. Such a nutrigenomic approach is a valid tool in order to avoid zinc toxic on the immune response and, at the same time, in restoring the immune efficiency in elderly by preventing the appearance of some degenerative age-related diseases, such as cancer and infection. As a consequence, the healthy aging and longevity can be achieved. Because of the low cost of zinc supplementation, a higher consideration by the international health organizations is therefore required with specific zinc fortification programs in all countries.

Acknowledgments It has been supported by INRCA and European Commission (ZINCAGE project: FOOD-CT-2004-506850, Coordinator Dr. Eugenio Mocchegiani).

References

Abo T, Kawamura T, Watanabe H (2000) Physiological responses of extrathymic T cells in the liver. Immunol Rev 174:135–149

Andriollo-Sanchez M, Hininger-Favier I, Meunier N et al (2005) Zinc intake and status in middle-aged and older European subjects: the ZENITH study. Eur J Clin Nutr 59:S37–S41

Araujo LM, Lefort J, Nahori MA et al (2004) Exacerbated Th2-mediated airway inflammation and hyperresponsiveness in autoimmune diabetes-prone NOD mice: a critical role for CD1d-dependent NKT cells. Eur J Immunol 34:327–335

Arnold CR, Wolf J, Brunner S et al (2011) Gain and loss of T cell subsets in old age–age-related reshaping of the T cell repertoire. J Clin Immunol 31:137–146

August D, Janghorbani M, Young VR (1989) Determination of zinc and copper absorption at three dietary Zn-Cu ratios by using stable isotope methods in young adult and elderly subjects. Am J Clin Nutr 50:1457–1463

Balesaria S, Hogstrand C (2006) Identification, cloning and characterization of a plasma membrane zinc efflux transporter TrZnT-1, from fugu pufferfish (Takifugu rubripes). Biochem J 394:485–493

Bao S, Liu MJ, Lee B, Besecker B et al (2010) Zinc modulates the innate immune response in vivo to polymicrobial sepsis through regulation of NF-kappaB. Am J Physiol Lung Cell Mol Physiol 298:L744–L754

Barbato JC, Catanescu O, Murray K et al (2007) Targeting of metallothionein by L-homocysteine: a novel mechanism for disruption of Zn and redox homeostasis. Arterioscler Thromb Vasc Biol 27:49–54

Basu TK, Donaldson D (2003) Intestinal absorption in health and disease: micronutrients. Best Pract Res Clin Gastroenterol 17:957–979

Biron CA, Brossay L (2001) NK cells and NKT cells in innate defense against viral infections. Curr Opin Immunol 13:458–464

Bogden JD (2004) Influence of zinc on immunity in the elderly. J Nutr Health Aging 8:48–54

Bonafè M, Olivieri F, Cavallone L et al (2001) A gender–dependent genetic predisposition to produce high levels of IL-6 is detrimental for longevity. Eur J Immunol 31:2357–2361

Briefel RR, Bialostosky K, Kennedy-Stephenson J et al (2000) Zinc intake of the U.S. population. Findings from the third National Health and Nutrition Examination Survey 1988–1994. J Nutr 130:1367S–1373S

Bruunsgaard H, Pedersen AN, Schroll M et al (1999) Impaired production of proinflammatory cytokines in response to lipopolysaccharide (LPS) stimulation in elderly humans. Clin Exp Immunol 118:235–241

Cakman I, Rohwer J, Schutz RM et al (1996) Dysregulation between TH1 and TH2 T cell subpopulations in the elderly. Mech Ageing Dev 87:197–209

Cakman I, Kirchner H, Rink L (1997) Zinc supplementation reconstitutes the production of interferon-alpha by leukocytes from elderly persons. J Interferon Cytokine Res 17:469–472

Chernoff R (2005) Micronutrient requirements in older women. Am J Clin Nutr 81:1240S–1245S

Cipriano C, Malavolta M, Costarelli L et al (2006) Polymorphisms in MT1a gene with longevity in Italian Central female population. Biogerontology 7: 357–365

Coneyworth LJ, Mathers JC, Ford D (2009) Does promoter methylation of the SLC30A5 (ZnT5) zinc transporter gene contribute to the ageing-related decline in zinc status? Proc Nutr Soc 68:142–147

Cousins RJ (2010) Gastrointestinal factors influencing zinc absorption and homeostasis. Int J Vitam Nutr Res 80:243–248

Cragg RA, Phillips SR, Piper JM et al (2005) Regulation of zinc transporters in the human small intestine by dietary zinc supplementation. Gut 54:469–478

Cui J, Shin T, Kawano T, Sato H et al (1997) Requirement for Valpha14 NKT cells in IL-12-mediated rejection of tumors. Science 278:1623–1626

Cunningham-Rundles S, McNeeley DF, Moon A (2005) Mechanisms of nutrient modulation of the immune response. J Allergy Clin Immunol 115:1119–1128

Dardenne M (2002) Zinc and immune function. Eur J Clin Nutr 56(Suppl 3):S20–S23

Dardenne M, Boukaiba N, Gagnerault MC et al (1993) Restoration of the thymus in aging mice by in vivo zinc supplementation. Clin Immunol Immunopathol 66:127–135

Davis SR, McMahon RJ, Cousins RJ (1998) Metallothionein knockout and transgenic mice exhibit altered intestinal processing of zinc with uniform zinc-dependent zinc transporter-1 expression. J Nutr 128: 825–831

Driessen C, Hirv K, Rink L et al (1994) Induction of cyto-kines by zinc ions in human peripheral blood mono-nuclear cells and separated monocytes. Lymphokine Cytokine Res 13:15–20

Dufner-Beattie J, Kuo YM, Gitschier J et al (2004) The adaptive response to dietary zinc in mice involves the differential cellular localization and zinc regulation of the zinc transporters ZIP4 and ZIP5. J Biol Chem 279: 49082–49090

Elmes ME, Jones JG (1980) Ultrastructural changes in the small intestine of zinc deficient rats. J Pathol 130:37–43

Emoto M, Kaufmann SH (2003) Liver NKT cells: an account of heterogeneity. Trends Immunol 24:364–369

Evans GW (1986) Zinc and its deficiency diseases. Clin Physiol Biochem 4:94–98

Food and Nutrition Board, Institute of Medicine (2001) Zinc. Dietary reference intakes for vitamin A, vitamin K, boron, chromium, copper, iodine, iron, manganese, molybdenum, nickel, silicon, vanadium, and zinc. National Academy Press, Washington

Fraker PJ (2005) Roles for cell death in zinc deficiency. J Nutr 135:359–362

Franceschi C (2007) Inflammaging as a major characteris-tic of old people: can it be prevented or cured? Nutr Rev 65:S173–S176

Franceschi C, Olivieri F, Marchegiani F et al (2005) Genes involved in immune response/inflammation, IGF1/insulin pathway and response to oxidative stress play a major role in the genetics of human longevity: the les-son of centenarians. Mech Ageing Dev 126:351–361

Gabriel P, Cakman I, Rink L (2002) Overproduction of monokines by leukocytes after stimulation with lipopolysaccharide in the elderly. Exp Gerontol 37: 235–247

Giacconi R, Cipriano C, Albanese F et al (2004) The -174G/C polymorphism of IL-6 is useful to screen old subjects at risk for atherosclerosis or to reach success-ful ageing. Exp Gerontol 39:621–628

Giacconi R, Cipriano C, Muti E et al (2005) Novel -209A/G MT2A polymorphism in old patients with type 2 diabetes and atherosclerosis: relationship with inflammation (IL-6) and zinc. Biogerontology 6:407–413

Giacconi R, Malavolta M, Costarelli L et al (2011) Comparison of intracellular Zinc signals in non-adherent lymphocytes from young-adult and elderly donors: role of zinc transporters (Zip-family) and pro-inflammatory cytokines. J Nutr Biochem 23: 1256–1263

Gibson RS, Hess SY, Hotz C et al (2008) Indicators of zinc status at the population level: a review of the evi-dence. Br J Nutr 99:S14–S23

Gregg R, Smith CM, Clark FJ et al (2005) The number of human peripheral blood CD4+ CD25 high regulatory T cells increases with age. Clin Exp Immunol 140: 540–546

Haase H, Rink L (2009a) Functional significance of zinc-related signalling pathways in immune cells. Annu Rev Nutr 29:133–152

Haase H, Rink L (2009b) The immune system and the impact of zinc during aging. Immun Ageing 6:9–15

Haase H, Hebel S, Engelhardt G et al (2006a) Flow cyto-metric measurement of labile zinc in peripheral blood mononuclear cells. Anal Biochem 352:222–230

Haase H, Mocchegiani E, Rink L (2006b) Correlation between zinc status and immune function in the elderly. Biogerontology 7:421–428

Hambidge KM (2000) Human zinc deficiency. J Nutr 130(Suppl 5S):1344S–1349S

Hambidge KM (2010) Micronutrient bioavailability: dietary reference intakes and a future perspective. Am J Clin Nutr 91(Suppl 1):1430S–1432S

High KP (1999) Micronutrient supplementation and immune function in the elderly. Clin Infect Dis 28:717–722

Ibs KH, Gabriel P, Rink L (2003) Zinc and the immune sys-tem of elderly. Adv Cell Aging Gerontol 13:243–259

Kanoni S, Dedoussis GV, Herbein G et al (2010) Assessment of gene-nutrient interactions on inflam-matory status of the elderly with the use of a zinc diet score–ZINCAGE study. J Nutr Biochem 21:526–531

King LE, Osati-Ashtiani F, Fraker PJ (2002) Apoptosis plays a distinct role in the loss of precursor lym-phocytes during zinc deficiency in mice. J Nutr 132: 974–979

King LE, Frentzel JW, Mann JJ et al (2005) Chronic zinc deficiency in mice disrupted T cell lymphopoiesis and erythropoiesis while B cell lymphopoiesis and myelo-poiesis were maintained. J Am Coll Nutr 24:494–502

Kogirima M, Kurasawa R, Kubori S et al (2007) Ratio of low serum zinc levels in elderly Japanese people living in the central part of Japan. Eur J Clin Nutr 61:375–381

Kury S, Dreno B, Bezieau S et al (2002) Identification of SLC39A4, a gene involved in acrodermatitis entero-pathica. Nat Genet 31:239–240

Lang C, Murgia C, Leong M et al (2007) Anti-inflammatory effects of zinc and alterations in zinc transporter mRNA in mouse models of allergic inflammation. Am J Physiol Lung Cell Mol Physiol 292:L577–L584

Liuzzi JP, Aydemir F, Nam H et al (2006) Zip14 (Slc39a14) mediates non-transferrin-bound iron uptake into cells. Proc Natl Acad Sci U S A 103:13612–13617

Lonnerdal B (2000) Dietary factors influencing zinc absorption. J Nutr 130:1378S–1383S

Ma J, Betts NM (2000) Zinc and copper intakes and their major food sources for older adults the 1994–96 continuing survey of food intakes by individuals (CSFII). J Nutr 130:2838–2843

Malavolta M, Costarelli L, Giacconi R et al (2006) Single and three-color flow cytometry assay for intracellular zinc ion availability in human lymphocytes with Zinpyr-1 and double immunofluorescence: relationship with metallothioneins. Cytometry A 69:1043–1053

Malavolta M, Cipriano C, Costarelli L et al (2008) Metallothionein downregulation in very old age: a phenomenon associated with cellular senescence? Rejuvenation Res 11:455–459

Marcellini F, Giuli C, Papa R et al (2006) Zinc status, psy-chological and nutritional assessment in old people recruited in five European countries: ZINCAGE study. Biogerontology 7:339–345

Maret W, Sandstead HH (2006) Zinc requirements and the risks and benefits of zinc supplementation. J Trace Elem Med Biol 20:3–18

Maret W, Jacob C, Vallee BL et al (1999) Inhibitory sites in enzymes: zinc removal and reactivation by thionein. Proc Natl Acad Sci U S A 96:1936–1940

Mariani E, Cattini L, Neri S et al (2006) Simultaneous evaluation of circulating chemokine and cytokine profiles in elderly subjects by multiplex technology: relationship with zinc status. Biogerontology 7: 449–459

Mariani E, Neri S, Cattini L et al (2008) Effect of zinc supplementation on plasma IL-6 and MCP-1 production and NK cell function in healthy elderly: Interactive influence of +647 MT1a and −174 IL-6 polymorphic alleles. Exp Gerontol 43:462–471

Max Rubner-Institut (MRI) (2008) Nationale Verzehrstudie; Federal Research Institute of Nutrition and Food. Karlsruhe, Germany

Mazzatti DJ, Malavolta M, White AJ et al (2008) Effects of interleukin-6–174C/G and metallothionein 1A +647A/C single-nucleotide polymorphisms on zinc-regulated gene expression in ageing. Exp Gerontol 43:423–432

McLeod JD (2000) Apoptotic capability in ageing T cells. Mech Ageing Dev 121:151–159

McMahon RJ, Cousins RJ (1998) Mammalian zinc transporters. J Nutr 128:667–670

Menard MP, Cousins RJ (1983) Zinc transport by brush border membrane vesicles from rat intestine. J Nutr 113:1434–1442

Meunier N, Feillet-Coudray C, Rambeau M et al (2005) Impact of micronutrient dietary intake and status on intestinal zinc absorption in late middle-aged men: the ZENITH study. Eur J Clin Nutr 59:S48–S52

Mitchell WA, Meng I, Nicholson SA et al (2006) Thymic output, ageing and zinc. Biogerontology 7:461–470

Miyaji C, Watanabe H, Toma H et al (2000) Functional alteration of granulocytes, NK cells, and natural killer T cells in centenarians. Hum Immunol 61:908–916

Mocchegiani E, Santarelli L, Muzzioli M et al (1995) Reversibility of the thymic involution and of age-related peripheral immune dysfunctions by zinc supplementation in old mice. Int J Immunopharmacol 17:703–718

Mocchegiani E, Muzzioli M, Cipriano C et al (1998) Zinc, T-cell pathways, aging: role of metallothioneins. Mech Ageing Dev 106:183–204

Mocchegiani E, Muzzioli M, Giacconi R (2000) Zinc and immunoresistance to infection in aging: new biological tools. Trends Pharmacol Sci 21:205–208

Mocchegiani E, Giacconi R, Cipriano C et al (2002) MtmRNA gene expression, via IL-6 and glucocorticoids, as potential genetic marker of immunosenescence: lessons from very old mice and humans. Exp Gerontol 37:349–357

Mocchegiani E, Muzzioli M, Giacconi R et al (2003) Metallothioneins/PARP-1/IL-6 interplay on natural

killer cell activity in elderly: parallelism with nonagenarians and old infected humans. Effect of zinc supply. Mech Ageing Dev 124:459–468

Mocchegiani E, Giacconi R, Cipriano C et al (2004) The variations during the circadian cycle of liver CD1d-unrestricted NK1.1+TCR gamma/delta+cells lead to successful ageing. Role of metallothionein/IL-6/gp130/PARP-1 interplay in very old mice. Exp Gerontol 39:775–788

Mocchegiani E, Costarelli L, Giacconi R et al (2006) Nutrient-gene interaction in ageing and successful ageing. A single nutrient (zinc) and some target genes related to inflammatory/immune response. Mech Ageing Dev 127:517–525

Mocchegiani E, Giacconi R, Cipriano C et al (2007) Zinc, metallothioneins, and longevity–effect of zinc supplementation: zincage study. Ann N Y Acad Sci 1119:129–146

Mocchegiani E, Bürkle A, Fulop T (2008a) Zinc and ageing (ZINCAGE Project). Exp Gerontol 43:361–362

Mocchegiani E, Giacconi R, Costarelli L et al (2008b) Zinc deficiency and IL-6–174G/C polymorphism in old people from different European countries: effect of zinc supplementation. ZINCAGE study. Exp Gerontol 43:433–444

Mocchegiani E, Malavolta M, Muti E et al (2008c) Zinc, metallothioneins and longevity: interrelationships with niacin and selenium. Curr Pharm Des 14:2719–2732

Mocchegiani E, Giacconi R, Cipriano C et al (2009) NK and NKT cells in aging and longevity: role of zinc and metallothioneins. J Clin Immunol 29:416–425

Mocchegiani E, Costarelli L, Basso A et al (2012a) Metallothioneins, ageing and cellular senescence: a future therapeutic target. Curr Pharm Des 19:1753–1764. doi: 23061732

Mocchegiani E, Costarelli L, Giacconi R et al (2012b) Micronutrient (Zn, Cu, Fe)-gene interactions in ageing and inflammatory age-related diseases: implications for treatments. Ageing Res Rev 11:297–319

Moroni F, Di Paolo ML, Rigo A et al (2005) Interrelationship among neutrophil efficiency, inflammation, antioxidant activity and zinc pool in very old age. Biogerontology 6:271–281

Muzzioli M, Stecconi R, Moresi R et al (2009) Zinc improves the development of human CD34+ cell progenitors towards NK cells and increases the expression of GATA-3 transcription factor in young and old ages. Biogerontology 10:593–604

Nasi M, Troiano L, Lugli E et al (2006) Thymic output and functionality of the IL-7/IL-7 receptor system in centenarians: implications for the neolymphogenesis at the limit of human life. Aging Cell 5:167–175

Paganelli R, Quinti I, Fagiolo U et al (1992) Changes in circulating B cells and immunoglobulin classes and subclasses in healthy aged population. Clin Exp Immunol 90:351–354

Palmiter RD (1998) The elusive function of metallothioneins. Proc Natl Acad Sci U S A 95:8428–8430

Pawelec G, Remarque E, Barnett Y et al (1998) T cells and aging. Front Biosci 3:d59–d99

Pawelec G, Larbi A, Derhovanessian E (2010) Senescence of the human immune system. J Comp Pathol 142(Suppl 1):S39–S44

Prasad AS (1998) Zinc and immunity. Mol Cell Biochem 188:63–69

Prasad AS (2000) Effects of zinc deficiency on Th1 and Th2 cytokine shifts. J Infect Dis 182:62–68

Prasad AS (2007) Zinc: mechanisms of host defense. J Nutr 137:1345–1349

Prasad AS (2008) Zinc in human health: effect of zinc on immune cells. Mol Med 14:353–357

Prasad AS (2009) Impact of the discovery of human zinc deficiency on health. J Am Coll Nutr 28:257–265

Prasad AS, Fitzgerald JT, Hess JW et al (1993) Zinc deficiency in elderly patients. Nutrition 9:218–224

Prasad AS, Bao B, Beck FW et al (2011) Zinc-suppressed inflammatory cytokines by induction of A20-mediated inhibition of nuclear factor-κB. Nutrition 27:816–823

Provinciali M, Montenovo A, Di Stefano G et al (1998) Effect of zinc or zinc plus arginine supplementation on antibody titre and lymphocyte subsets after influenza vaccination in elderly subjects: a randomized controlled trial. Age Ageing 27:715–722

Rea IM, Ross OA, Armstrong M et al (2003) Interleukin-6-gene C/G 174 polymorphism in nonagenarian and octogenarian subjects in the BELFAST study. Reciprocal effects on IL-6, soluble IL-6 receptor and for IL-10 in serum and monocyte supernatants. Mech Ageing Dev 124:555–561

Saba I, Kosan C, Vassen L et al (2011) IL-7R-dependent survival and differentiation of early T-lineage progenitors is regulated by the BTB/POZ domain transcription factor Miz-1. Blood 117:3370–3381

Sandstead HH (1994) Understanding zinc: recent observations and interpretations. J Lab Clin Med 124:322–327

Sandström B (1992) Dose dependence of zinc and manganese absorption in man. Proc Nutr Soc 51:211–218

Sandström B (2001) Micronutrient interactions: effects on absorption and bioavailability. Br J Nutr 85(Suppl 2):S181–S185

Sbarbati A, Mocchegiani E, Marzola P et al (1998) Effect of dietary supplementation with zinc sulphate on the aging process: a study using high field intensity MRI and chemical shift imaging. Biomed Pharmacother 52:454–458

Schlemmer U, Frølich W, Prieto RM, Grases F (2009) Phytate in foods and significance for humans: food sources, intake, processing, bioavailability, protective role and analysis. Mol Nutr Food Res 53 (Suppl 2):S330–S375.

Schroder AK, Rink L (2003) Neutrophil immunity of the elderly. Mech Ageing Dev 124:419–425

Scientific Committee on Food (SCF) (2002) Opinion of the scientific committee on food on the tolerable upper intake level of Zinc. Brussels, Belgium, pp 15–25.

http://europa.eu.int/comm/food/fs/sc/scf/index_en.html

Shankar AH, Prasad AS (1998) Zn and immune function: the biological basis of altered resistance to infection. Am J Clin Nutr 68:447S–463S

Sofi F, Abbate R, Gensini GF et al (2010) Accruing evidence on benefits of adherence to the Mediterranean diet on health: an updated systematic review and meta-analysis. Am J Clin Nutr 92:1189–1196

Solana R, Mariani E (2000) NK and NK/T cells in human senescence. Vaccine 18:1613–1620

Spahl DU, Berendji-Grun D, Suschek CV et al (2003) Regulation of zinc homeostasis by inducible NO synthase-derived NO: nuclear metallothionein translocation and intranuclear Zn2+ release. Proc Natl Acad Sci U S A 100:13952–13957

Stewart-Knox BJ, Simpson EE, Parr H et al (2005) Zinc status and taste acuity in older Europeans: the ZENITH study. Eur J Clin Nutr 59:S31–S36

Taub DD, Longo DL (2005) Insights into thymic aging and regeneration. Immunol Rev 205:72–93

Thomson AB (2009) Small intestinal disorders in the elderly. Best Pract Res Clin Gastroenterol 23:861–874

Toniato E, Chen XP, Losman J et al (2002) TRIM8/GERP RING finger protein interacts with SOCS-1. J Biol Chem 277:37315–37322

Turnlund JR, Michel MC, Keyes WR et al (1982) Use of enriched stable isotopes to determine zinc and iron absorption in elderly men. Am J Clin Nutr 35:1033–1040

Uciechowski P, Kahmann L, Plumakers B et al (2008) TH1 and TH2 cell polarization increases with aging and is modulated by zinc supplementation. Exp Gerontol 43:493–498

Vasto S, Mocchegiani E, Candore G et al (2006) Inflammation, genes and zinc in ageing and age-related diseases. Biogerontology 7:315–327

von Bulow V, Rink L, Haase H (2005) Zinc-mediated inhibition of cyclic nucleotide phosphodiesterase activity and expression suppresses TNF-alpha and IL-1 beta production in monocytes by elevation of guanosine 3′,5′-cyclic monophosphate. J Immunol 175:4697–4705

Walsh CT, Sandstead HH, Prasad AS et al (1994) Zinc: health effects and research priorities for the 1990s. Environ Health Perspect 102(Suppl 2):5–46

Weksler ME, Szabo P (2000) The effect of age on the B-cell repertoire. J Clin Immunol 20:240–249

West AK, Stallings R, Hildebrand CE et al (1990) Human metallothionein genes: structure of the functional locus at 16q13. Genomics 8:513–518

Williams GC (1957) Pleiotropy, natural selection and the evolution of senescence. Evolution 11:398–411

Physiological and Pathological Role of Reactive Oxygen Species in the Immune Cells

23

Aleksandra M. Urbanska, Valerio Zolla, Paolo Verzani, and Laura Santambrogio

23.1 Introduction

Reactive oxygen, chlorine, and nitrogen species are generated under physiological conditions by different cellular organelles and molecular pathways. In most cells, reactive species are the by-product of oxidative phosphorylation, the mitochondrial molecular chain which synthesizes adenosine triphosphate (ATP); as such they are readily inactivated in order to prevent cellular oxidative damage. Reactive species are also produced in immune cells by other molecular pathways as an important innate immune mechanism against invading pathogens. Indeed, "damping" phagosome-bound pathogens with reactive species is the most effective and successful way to readily neutralize the pathogen. In this chapter, we will review the different molecular pathways involved in the production of reactive species and how reactive species play a role in innate and adaptive immune responses. Excessive or chronic production of reactive species, as observed in chronic inflammatory and degenerative conditions however, has a negative effect on immune cell function. Herein, we will also review the effects of chronic oxidative stress on dendritic cells, macrophages, granulocytes and T cells, redox homeostasis, and immune cell function.

A.M. Urbanska, PhD • V. Zolla, PhD
P. Verzani • L. Santambrogio, MD, PhD(✉)
Department of Pathology, Albert Einstein College of Medicine, New York, NY 10461, USA
e-mail: laura.santambrogio@einstein.yu.edu

23.2 Mitochondrial Respiratory Chain

The main function of mitochondria is to convert the energy found in nutrient molecules and to store it in the form of ATP in a process known as oxidative phosphorylation. The energy required to phosphorylate ADP into ATP, by the ATP synthase, is provided by the transfer of electrons through the mitochondria respiratory chain which is coupled with the pumping of protons from the matrix to the inner mitochondrial membrane (Mitchell 1961) (Fig. 23.1). Five protein complexes (I–V) form the respiratory chain. However, two complexes (complex I and III) constitute the site where electron transfer is associated with proton translocation across the mitochondrial membrane (Chance 1961). Complex I (nicotinamide adenine dinucleotide (NADH)-ubiquinone oxidoreductase) and complex III (ubiquinol-cytochrome c oxidoreductase) are the ones that generate the proton gradient required to produce the energy to synthesize ATP (Chance et al. 1979). As by-products of oxidative phosphorylation, the process of proton translocation generates reactive oxygen species (ROS) on both sides of the mitochondrial membrane. A minor source of ROS is also generated by reactions which are part of the Krebs cycle (Starkov et al. 2004).

Under physiological conditions cells are equipped with a variety of enzymes to quickly dispose of ROS including superoxide dismutase, glutathione (GSH) peroxidase, and catalase as well as some antioxidant molecules like glutathione and

A. Massoud, N. Rezaei (eds.), *Immunology of Aging*,
DOI 10.1007/978-3-642-39495-9_23, © Springer-Verlag Berlin Heidelberg 2014

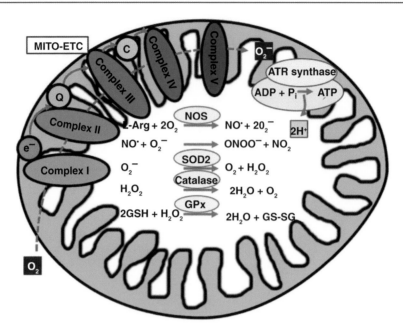

Fig. 23.1 Mitochondrial production of reactive species. The electron transport chain and oxidative phosphorylation are coupled by a proton gradient across the inner mitochondrial membrane. Electrons (e^-) from NADH and $FADH_2$ previously generated by glycolysis and citric acid cycle are transported through the five complexes (I–V) of the mitochondrial electron transport chain (MITO-ETC) to generate electrochemical gradient (proton gradient). Q – coenzyme Q (CoQ, Q or ubiquinone); C – cytochrome c; complexes I (NADH dehydrogenase), II (succinate-CoQ reductase), III (CoQ-cyt c Reductase), IV (Cytochrome Oxidase), V (ATP synthase). The oxygen from a molecule of water receives the electron forming an O_2^- superoxide anion and an H^+, which accumulate in the intermembrane space. Translocation of H^+ across the membrane through the ATP synthase provides the energy to convert ADP and a molecule of inorganic phosphate Pi into ATP. L-arginine and a molecule of oxygen generates nitric oxide radical catalyzed by the enzyme nitric oxide synthase NOS. Additionally, peroxynitrite ($ONOO^-$) formation in mitochondria is due to the constant supply of superoxide radical $O_2^{-\bullet}$ by the electron transport chain plus the facile diffusion of nitric oxide ($NO^\bullet$) to this organelle. To dispose free radicals a molecule of O_2^- is converted by the superoxide dismutases (SOD) into oxygen and hydrogen peroxide. Catalase catalyzes the decomposition of hydrogen peroxide to water and oxygen. The glutathione peroxidase (GPx) reduces hydrogen peroxide to water, where GSH represents reduced monomeric glutathione and GS–SG represents glutathione disulfide. Glutathione reductase (GSR) then reduces the oxidized glutathione to complete the cycle

vitamin E (Bai and Cederbaum 2001). However, in pathological conditions and in aging, due to an increased ROS production or decreased activity/synthesis of scavenging enzymes, cells are often unable to deal with the large amount of ROS produced. This will generate a biochemical imbalance, often referred to as "oxidative stress" where ROS molecules will quickly react with any neighboring biomolecules and oxidize them.

Mitochondria are the first target of oxidative damage cause by ROS as evidenced by extensive lipid peroxidation, protein oxidation, and mitochondrial DNA mutations (Anders et al. 2006; Lenaz 1998). Extramitochondrial ROS, on the other hand, will oxidize nuclear DNA, as well as cytosolic and organelle proteins, lipids, and carbohydrates (Turrens 2003; Pickrell et al. 2009). Aging-related oxidative stress and functional impairment of mitochondria have been linked to several chronic inflammatory and degenerative diseases as well as cancer (Pawelec et al. 2010; Muster et al. 2010).

23.3 Oxidative Burst

The importance of ROS and reactive nitrogen species (RNS) in innate immunity was first recognized in professional phagocytes undergoing a "respiratory burst" upon activation (Rada and Leto 2008; Netzer et al. 2009). This robust ROS and RNS production, in particular $O_2^{\cdot-}$ and H_2O_2, is generated by a membrane-bound, superoxide-generating enzyme, the phagocytic nicotinamide adenine dinucleotide phosphate-oxidase (NADPH). The

NADPH oxidase enzyme was discovered in 1957 when it was recognized that patients with chronic granulomatous disease (CGD) failed to generate products of the respiratory burst (Holmes et al. 1967). NADPH oxidase contains six cytochrome subunit homologs: NOX1, NOX3, NOX4, NOX5, DUOX1, and DUOX2 (Guzik and Griendling 2009; Katsuyama et al. 2012) (Fig. 23.2). The superoxide anions (O_2^-), formed by NADPH oxidase, are reduced to a more stable molecule of hydrogen peroxide (H_2O_2) and unstable radicals

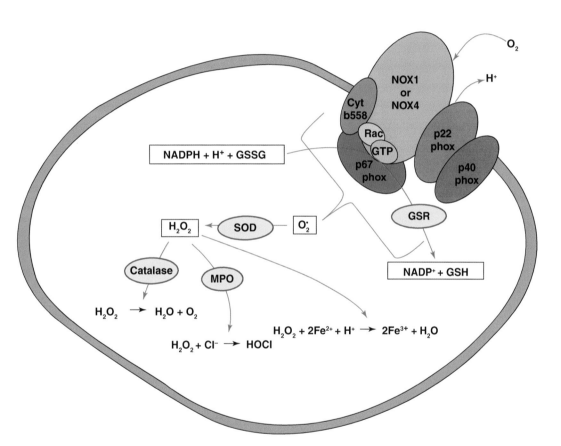

Fig. 23.2 Activation of the NADPH oxidative burst. NADPH oxidase generate free radicals ($O_2^{-\cdot}$) by transferring electrons from NADPH to molecular oxygen. This oxidase is controlled by hormones, growth factors, and other ligands which bind to receptors in the plasma membrane. NADPH oxidase consists of five subunits: gp91phox (glycoprotein-91 kDa-phagocytic-oxidase-NOX1), p22phox, p47phox-NOX4, p67phox, and p40phox and the GTPase, flavocytochrome b588 (Cyt b558), and Rac. MPO is a peroxidase enzyme which produces hypochlorous acid (HOCl) from H_2O_2. Catalase catalyzes the decomposition of hydrogen peroxide to water and oxygen. To dispose free radicals a molecule of O_2^- is converted by the superoxide dismutases (SOD) into oxygen and hydrogen peroxide. GSR reduces glutathione disulfide (GSSG) in presence of NADPH and H+ to the sulfhydryl form GSH and NADP+

of oxygen (O$^-$) and hydroxyl (OH$^\bullet$) (Bedard and Krause 2007). While not a free radical, hydrogen peroxide is also an oxidant capable of initiating lipid peroxidation chain reaction (Janero et al. 1991). In the cytosol hydrogen peroxide can be reconverted into hydroxyl radical (OH$^-$), one of the most reactive ROS, through the Fenton reaction (Korantzopoulos et al. 2007) in the presence of a catalyst such as transitional metals (manganese, copper, and iron) (Fisher 2009).

The NADPH oxidase enzyme complex serves many cellular functions requiring ROS generation, including oxygen sensing (Leto et al. 2009) redox-based cellular signaling (Fisher 2009) and biosynthetic processes (Hazen et al. 1996). However, in professional phagocytes the most important NADPH-dependent function is generation of ROS and RNS as a defense mechanism towards pathogen invasion (Winterbourn et al. 2000). ROS and RNS induce oxidative inactivation of microbial enzymes, constitutive proteins, and nucleic acids. In cells of the myelomonocytic lineage (including monocytes and polymorphonuclear leukocytes (PMN)), two additional enzymes can generate reactive species, namely, the myeloperoxidase (MPO) and bromoperoxidase (Bouayed and Bohn 2010). H_2O_2 produced by inflammatory cells oxidizes myeloperoxidase to a higher oxidation state with a redox potential in excess of 1 V. This higher oxidation state (a ferryl-oxo complex) oxidizes Cl$^-$ to HOCl, which is capable of oxidizing or chlorinating pathogen-derived macromolecules (Winterbourn et al. 2000). HOCl also reacts with amines to form chloramines or with Cl$^-$ to form Cl$_2$ gas; the latter chlorinates the nucleic acid or protein of invading pathogens (Hazen et al. 1996).

23.4 The Effect of Environment and Pollution on Cellular ROS Production

The link between production of reactive oxygen and nitrogen species and environmental factors such as chemicals, ultraviolet (UV) radiation, tobacco, alcohol, toxins, and pollutants has been established by many (Bouayed and Bohn 2010;

Bargagli 2000). Exposure to heavy metals, such as cadmium, cobalt, and lead as well as synthetic polymers like polyester terephthalate (Tang et al. 1993) and polystyrene (Liu et al. 2011) has also been shown to increase ROS production (El-Sonbaty and El-Hadedy 2012). This heterogeneous category of molecules and compounds increases reactive species production by interfering either with the mitochondrial respiratory chain, the membrane NADPH, or the metal catalyzed Fenton reaction (Poli et al. 2004).

23.5 Dendritic Cells

Dendritic cells (DCs) are sparsely but widely distributed migratory cells of bone marrow origin (Steinman 1991). They provide a critical link between the innate and adaptive immune response and they are specialized in the uptake, processing, and presentation of pathogen-derived antigens to T cells. They are the only antigen-presenting cell (APC) that can activate naive T cells (Banchereau and Steinman 1998). DCs can sense pathogen-derived products (pathogen-associated molecular patterns or PAMPs) through pattern recognition receptors (PRRs) such as Toll-like receptors (TLRs), present at their plasma membrane and in endosomal compartments (Mogensen 2009), as well as through several cytosolic sensors of the inflammasome family (Krishnaswamy et al. 2013).

Observations that ROS play an important role in innate and adaptive immune responses were first made in the 1970s when it was demonstrated that insulin along with insulin-like growth factor-II (IGF-II) receptors (Kadota et al. 1987) and insulin-like growth factor-binding protein-6 (IGFBP-6) (Xie et al. 2005) stimulated cellular H_2O_2 production (Czech et al. 1974). In a study by Rutault and co-workers, exposure of DCs to H_2O_2 was found to increase surface expression of human leukocyte antigen (HLA) class I and II (DQ and DR), as well as the co-stimulatory molecules CD40 and CD86 (Rutault et al. 1999). At the same time, H_2O_2 downregulated molecules involved in antigen capture such as CD32. The experiments also determined that H_2O_2-treated

DCs had an enhanced ability to promote T cell proliferation as compared with untreated cells. This study was among the first to demonstrate that oxygen species are a "danger" signal produced by the inflammatory microenvironment, leading to DCs activation and increased immune responses. Several additional studies confirmed the role played by ROS in activating human and rodent DCs during inflammation (Sheng et al. 2010; Zhong et al. 2013). Using UV-mediated ROS production, a strong upregulation of CD1a, HLA-DR, B7-1, and B7-2 on Langerhans cells has also been reported (Laihia and Jansen 1997).

Accumulating evidence indicates that the ability of ROS to stimulate DCs is in part due to their targeting of signaling molecules and transcription factors (Bianco et al. 2002). Major targets of

ROS include protein tyrosine phosphatases (PTP), protein tyrosine kinases (PTK), mitogen-activated protein (MAP) kinases, ion channels, and phospholipases (Droge 2002). The prototype of a redox-sensitive transcription factor is nuclear factor κB (NFκB) which is sequestered in the cytoplasm in a complex with its inhibitor IκB. ROS promote IκB degradation, initiating NFκB nuclear translocation (Mishra et al. 2008). Other redox-sensitive transcription factors include AP-1, c-Jun, and c-Fos.

An additional major pathway which generates inflammation in response to ROS occurs through the NALP3 inflammasome activation (Fig. 23.3). Inflammasomes are NOD-like receptor (NLR) and caspase-1-recruting cytoplasmic multiprotein complexes formed by a NALP protein, the

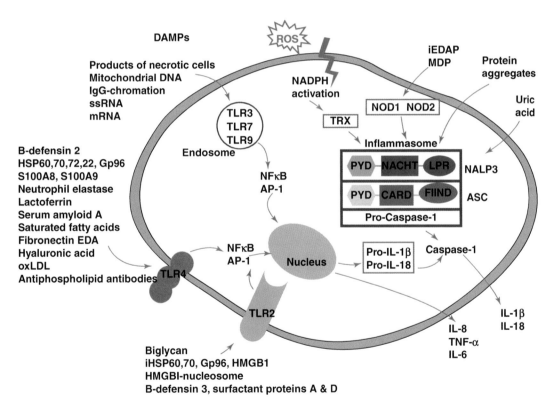

Fig. 23.3 Damage-associated molecular patterns (DAMPs). The arrays of molecular DAMPs recognized by endosomal and plasma membrane TLRs are reported for each receptor. Recognition of each ligand triggers a multitude of signaling cascades, mostly, NFκB and AP-1 mediated, leading to the secretion of pro-inflammatory cytokines including IL-1 β, IL-6, IL-8, and TNFα. Additional DAMPs (iEDAP – g-D-glutamyl-meso-diaminopimelic acid and MDP – muramyl dipeptide) trigger the Nalp3 inflammasome complex (ASC and procaspase-1) via the NOD1 and NOD2, respectively. Reactive oxygen species, uric acid crystals, and protein aggregates induce inflammasome via NADPH activation or thioredoxin reductases (TRX). IL-1 and IL-18 are released following Nalp3 inflammasome activation

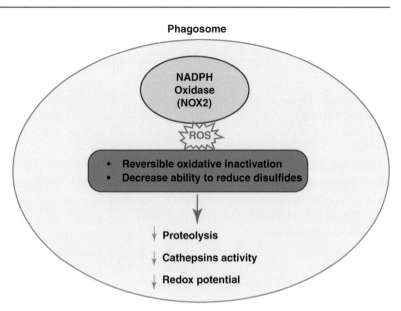

Fig. 23.4 The role of the NADPH oxidase in antigen processing. The phagosomal NADPH oxidase (NOX2) mediates the sustained production of low levels of reactive oxygen species. Low ROS levels induce reversible oxidative inactivation of local cysteine cathepsins and decreased ability to reduce disulfides. As a result, the proteolysis, cathepsins activity, and redox potential are reduced

adapter protein apoptosis-associated speck-like protein containing a CARD (ASC), which contains a caspase recruitment domain (CARD) and procaspase-1. Upon assembly they process and activate the pro-inflammatory cytokines interleukin (IL)-1β and IL-18 (Zhou et al. 2010). The NALP3 inflammasome complex is activated by a plethora of PAMPs, as well as danger-associated molecular patterns (DAMP). The NACHT, LRR, and PYD domains-containing protein 3 (NALP3) inflammasome can be activated by elevated concentrations of ROS (Chen and Nunez 2010) through activation of plasma membrane-associated nicotinamide adenine dinucleotide phosphate-oxidase (NADPH) and cytosolic thioredoxin peroxidase (TXP) and elevated concentrations of uric acid and oxidized protein aggregates.

The connection between antigen phagocytosis, phagosome formation, antigen processing, and ROS production has been explored by several laboratories (Kotsias et al. 2013). Phagosomal NADPH oxidase (NOX2) was originally shown to be recruited to the DC phagosomes to induce ROS-mediated alkalinization and to decrease antigen processing, favoring cross-presentation. It was later reported that in macrophages, NOX2 mediates the inhibition of phagosomal proteolysis through a pH-independent mechanism, by reversible oxidative inactivation of local cysteine

cathepsins (Rybicka et al. 2010) (Fig. 23.4). On the other hand, increased proteolytic activity has been reported in M2 skewed MΦ through inhibition of endosomal/lysosomal NOX2 which increases cathepsin activity (Balce et al. 2011).

Taken together these reports solidified the notion that ROS production by DCs is an important signaling mechanism that forms part of a rapid induction of innate immune responses. At the same time, however, other reports indicated that a sustained and prolonged ROS production could compromise innate immune responses (Chan et al. 2006). Indeed, chronic ROS production in DCs has been shown to negatively regulate NF-κB phosphorylation in response to lipopolysaccharide (LPS) and zymosan, although it did not compromise activation of p38 MAPK by LPS (Brown and Goldstein 1983). An additional anti-inflammatory effect by ROS production in DCs was recently reported by Jendrysik et al. (2011) who found that NOX2-dependent ROS production in DCs negatively regulated pro-inflammatory IL-12 expression by inhibiting p38-MAPK activity. It has also been proposed that perturbation of DCs function by oxidative stress induces the activation of the Nrf2-mediated pathway, which exerts negative regulatory effects on NFκB signaling, the major pathway involved in IL-12 production, co-stimulatory receptor expression, and DCs maturation. The induction of the Nrf2 pathway, in ROS-stimulated DCs, has also been linked to the induction of a Th1 toTh2 skewing and overall inhibition of Th1 immunity (Kidd 2003).

Altogether, it appears that a dichotomy between the beneficial and detrimental effects of ROS has been observed according to the length of DCs exposure to the reactive species. Indeed, in chronic inflammation, following infection or degenerative conditions, the sustained ROS production appears to be detrimental to DCs functions leading to progressive decline of their biological activities and irreversible damage.

23.6   Macrophages

Macrophages are important effectors of innate immune responses and their primary function is to phagocytose pathogens for degradation and initiate innate immune responses (VanderVen et al. 2010). Macrophages like DCs express the phagocyte NADPH oxidase, a member of NOX family, which generates reactive species to kill microbes.

As reported for other immune cells, prolonged macrophage ROS production, as observed in chronic inflammatory diseases, can be damaging to the macrophages as well as the surrounding tissue. Indeed, macrophage production of reactive carbonyls alters the extracellular matrix (ECM) network and induces tissue damage and cellular apoptosis (Cathcart 2004). Carbonyl modifications of collagens also cause increased macrophage adhesion and activation through receptors that are involved in phagocytosis (Fig. 23.5) including opsonic phagocytosis, mediated by the Fc receptor family (FcγRI, FcγRIIA, and FcγRIIA), complement receptors (CR1, CR3, and CR4), and α5β1 integrin and non-opsonic phagocytosis mediated by Dectin 1, macrophage receptor MARCO, scavenger receptor A, and αVβ5 integrin (Underhill and Goodridge 2012).

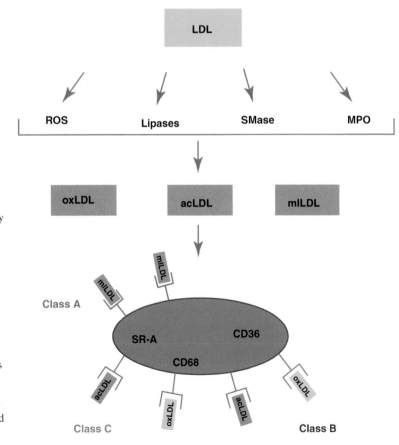

Fig. 23.5 Macrophage scavenger receptors bind oxidized lipoproteins. Highly oxidized aggregated LDLs are generated by ROS and different enzymes including SMase, lipases, and MPO. The oxidized aggregated LDLs (*acLDL* acetylated LDL, *oxLDL* oxidized LDL, *mlDL* maleylated LDL) are recognized by macrophage scavenger receptors such as SR-A (class A), CD36 (class B), and CD68 (class C). Scavenger receptor expression is upregulated by cytokines such as TNF-α and IFN-γ

TLRs are a recognition system for PAMPS. However, several oxidatively damaged biomolecules activate the TLR system such as DAMPS including heat shock protein (HSP)60, 70, 72, 22, Gp96, high mobility group box 1 (HMGB1), HMGB1-nucleosome complexes, β-defensin 3, D, eosinophil-derived neurotoxin, antiphospholipid antibodies, serum amyloid A, cardiac myosin, pancreatic adenocarcinoma upregulated factor (PAUF), carboxyethylpyrrole (CEP), monosodium urate crystals, biglycan, versican, hyaluronic acid fragments, surfactant proteins A and D, β-defensin 2, S100A8, S100A9, neutrophil elastase, antiphospholipid antibodies, lactoferrin, oxidized low-density lipoprotein (LDL), saturated fatty acids, resistin, fibronectin EDA, fibrinogen, and tenascin-C heparin sulfate fragments.

Additionally, macrophage scavenger receptors (SR), categorized into class A (SR-A1-SR-A5), class B (SR-B1-SR-B3), and class C (CD68, mucin, and lectin-like oxidized LDL receptor-1), normally function in the recognition and internalization of pathogens and apoptotic cells (Matsumoto et al. 1990) (Fig. 23.5). However, scavenger receptors also recognize altered molecular patterns present on oxidized low-density lipoprotein. For instance, SCARA1 or MSR1 multifunctional, multiligand pattern recognition receptors can bind an extraordinarily wide range of ligands, including bacterial pathogens (Dunne et al. 1994); however, it is also implicated in the pathological deposition of cholesterol during atherogenesis as a result of receptor-mediated uptake of oxidatively modified low-density lipoproteins (mLDL) (Krieger and Herz 1994; Brown and Goldstein 1983).

As a result of the action of ROS and different enzymes including sphingomyelinase (SMase), secretory phospholipase 2 (sPLA2), lipases, and MPO, the highly oxidized aggregated LDL is formed in different cells. The oxidized aggregated LDL is recognized by macrophage scavenger receptors such as SR-A, CD36, and CD68 (Brown and Goldstein 1983).

A representative receptor of class B, the plasma membrane glycoprotein receptor CD163, is a cysteine-rich receptor highly expressed on resident tissue of macrophages which acts as an innate immune sensor and inducer of local inflammation (Fabriek et al. 2009). The CD68 scavenger receptor, whose expression is restricted to mononuclear phagocytes, is a unique SR member, owing to its lysosome-associated membrane protein (LAMP)-like domain and predominant endosomal distribution (Song et al. 2011). Its function was reported to either negatively regulate antigen uptake, loading, or major histocompatibility complex class II (MHC-II) trafficking. Class C receptors recognize lipoprotein (LDL) (acLDL, acetylated LDL; and oxLDL, oxidized LDL), while CD68 recognizes primarily oxLDL.

At a more direct level, both oxidative and carbonyl stress inhibit activity of the transcriptional corepressor HDAC-2 (histone deacetylase 2), which under normoxic conditions helps to suppress pro-inflammatory gene expression (Kirkham 2007). Consequently, macrophages activated under conditions of oxidative or carbonyl stress can lead to a more enhanced inflammatory response via increased production of tumor necrosis factor alpha (TNF-α) and IL-8. Coupled with an impairment of the phagocytic response, this can lead to ineffective clearance of apoptotic cells and secondary necrosis, with the result being failure to resolve the inflammatory response and the establishment of a chronic inflammatory state (Song et al. 2011).

In conclusion, macrophages are phagocytic cells that produce and release ROS in response to phagocytosis or stimulation with various agents. The enzyme responsible for the production of superoxide and hydrogen peroxide is a multicomponent NADPH oxidase that requires assembly at the plasma membrane to function as an oxidase. In addition to participating in bacterial killing, ROS have been implicated in inflammation, in tissue injury, and in modulating cellular function.

23.7   Granulocytes

Granulocytes, discovered by Paul Ehrlich in 1879, are leukocyte subpopulations characterized by the presence of "granules," which store enzymes and other molecules important in antimicrobial functions and as mediators of inflammatory responses. Granulocytes are divided in subpopulations which include neutrophils, eosinophils, and basophils. Neutrophils, also known as PMN, are the most abundant type of granulocytes.

Neutrophils along with macrophages and dendritic cells play a key role in host defenses against invading microorganisms and have a crucial role in inflammatory processes. Neutrophils infiltrate inflamed tissues, degranulate their secretory vesicles, and release large amounts of bioactive compounds. As early as within the first minutes of stimulation, neutrophilic NADPH oxidase is activated, and cells release large quantities of superoxide anion (O_2^-) as part of the so-called respiratory burst (Ciz et al. 2012). Together with NADPH oxidase activation, several oxygen-independent events take place, such as the release of proteolytic enzymes, defensins, myeloperoxidase, and bactericidal peptides from stored intracellular granules. Neutrophils (PMNs) can exist in three different states, namely, resting, primed, and activated (Dang et al. 1999). The priming process has been demonstrated in vitro by pretreating PMNs with a sub-stimulatory concentration of pharmacological agents, which subsequently enhances the PMN response to a second stimulus. Studies show that pro-inflammatory cytokines such as granulocyte-macrophage colony-stimulating factor (GM-CSF), TNF-α, IL-1b, interferon-γ (IFN-g), and IL-8 modulate NADPH oxidase activity through a "priming" phenomenon (Gougerot-Pocidalo et al. 2002). Others reported "priming" by inducing a very weak oxidative response by neutrophils while strongly enhancing neutrophil release of ROS on exposure to a secondary applied stimulus such as bacterial N-formyl peptides (Elbim et al. 1994).

Altogether, the neutrophil oxidative burst is pivotal to pathogen defenses; however, in several chronic inflammatory conditions, it can contribute to tissue oxidative damage. Oxidative burst in rheumatoid arthritis (RA) joints is a result of the activation of innate immune system cells (Newkirk et al. 2003). Activated phagocytic cells such as neutrophils and macrophages produce free radicals in the joint area. Activated phagocytes produce reactive oxidants through the NADPH oxidase and the nitric oxide synthase (NOS). Mechanisms of free radical production differs between these cell groups. While macrophages are stimulated by the NADPH oxidase system to produce free radicals, the presence of NOS accompanied by the NADPH oxidase is necessary for neutrophils to secrete free radicals. RA neutrophils also generate enhanced amount of $ONOO^-$ by NOS (El Benna et al. 2002). A similar chronic activation of NADPH oxidase which has been linked to tissue oxidative stress has been shown in diabetes (Omori et al. 2008). It was suggested that hyperglycemia and increased advanced glycation end products prime neutrophils and increase oxidative stress inducing the translocation of p47phox to the cell membrane and preassembly with p22phox by stimulating a RAGE-ERK1/2 pathway (Erlemann et al. 2004).

Eosinophils, another subpopulation of granulocytes, are under homeostatic conditions, mostly found within the mucosal immune system (Straumann and Safroneeva 2012). They are released from hematopoietic stem cells (HSCs) into the peripheral blood in a phenotypically mature state, where they spend a short amount of time before being recruited to mucosal tissue in the lungs, gastrointestinal tract, and urogenital tract (Blanchard and Rothenberg 2009). Under inflammatory conditions, for instance, in chronic asthma or pulmonary eosinophilia, the production of type 2-associated cytokines and chemokines, particularly IL-4, IL-5, IL-13, and eotaxin-1, is increased. Eotaxin, a chemokine that selectively recruits eosinophils by inducing their chemotaxis, was found to prime the production of ROS and play a role in inducing chronic oxidative stress (Honda and Chihara 1999).

While initially similar responses of neutrophils and eosinophils to oxidative burst were reported (Petreccia et al. 1987) by Petreccia et al, a few distinctive features were found indicating substantial differences in the oxidative burst of eosinophils with respect to activation, function, and regulation (Shult et al. 1985). For example, eotaxin specifically induces significantly higher amounts of ROS in eosinophils and induces expression of the well-known eosinophil activator C5a. Eotaxin is also a GM-CSF (Peled et al. 1998).

The synthesis of a potent eosinophil chemoattractant 5-oxo-6,8,11,14-eicosatetraenoic acid (5-oxo-ETE) can be enhanced by exposure to H_2O_2 which induces dramatic increases in the levels of both GSSG and $NADP^+$ (Grant et al. 2011). Its effect on neutrophils, basophils, and monocytes is similar, promoting their infiltration into inflammatory sites (Erlemann et al. 2004). In addition, 5-oxo-ETE was able to induce infiltration of eosinophils into the skin after intradermal injection in humans (Grant et al. 2009) and to promote the survival of tumor cells by blocking the induction of apoptosis by 5-LO (Sundaram and Ghosh 2006). Because of 5-oxo-ETE chemoattractant effects on neutrophils and monocytes, this knowledge could be applied in the future in treatment of atherosclerosis, asthma, ischemia-reperfusion injury, as well as a variety of other inflammatory diseases.

Conclusions

During physiological conditions, a homeostatic balance between biosynthesis and disposal of oxygen, nitrogen, and chlorine species by immune cells is maintained. As such immune cells can take advantage of the powerful activity of ROS and RSN to kill invading pathogens or to control endosomal antigen processing and quickly dispose them to minimize unwanted oxidative reaction. However, this balance is lost in conditions associated with prolonged cellular stress, including chronic, septic, or aseptic, inflammation and degenerative conditions (Sies and Cadenas 1985); under these circumstances, the increased production/half-life of ROS and RSN will induce oxidative damage to cellular structure and contribute to decreased functionality or even cellular apoptosis (Fariss et al. 2005; Le et al. 2007).

Thus, reactive species can have beneficial effects on immune cells as well as damaging ones according to the experimental system analyzed. This can explain contradictory findings in the same cells analyzed under different experimental conditions or when experiments are performed in young or senescent cells or cells under different stressors. It can also explain why antioxidant therapy can be beneficial or detrimental under different experimental settings. Altogether, the extensive literature on reactive species in immune cells indicates that a more balanced approach is required towards the interpretation of the effects of reactive species on immune functions.

In conclusion, during the last decade several important findings and detailed molecular analysis have been reported on how reactive species are formed and their interaction with different cellular pathways. An integrative view on how the cellular redox system behaves under physiological and pathological conditions and how the same molecular players can have sometimes even opposite function under different stressors is coming to light.

References

Anders MW, Robotham JL, Sheu SS (2006) Mitochondria: new drug targets for oxidative stress-induced diseases. Expert Opin Drug Metab Toxicol 2(1):71–79

Bai J, Cederbaum AI (2001) Mitochondrial catalase and oxidative injury. Biol Signals Recept 10(3–4): 189–199

Balce DR, Li B, Allan ER et al (2011) Alternative activation of macrophages by IL-4 enhances the proteolytic capacity of their phagosomes through synergistic mechanisms. Blood 118(15):4199–4208

Banchereau J, Steinman RM (1998) Dendritic cells and the control of immunity. Nature 392(6673):245–252

Bargagli R (2000) Trace metals in Antarctica related to climate change and increasing human impact. Rev Environ Contam Toxicol 166:129–173

Bedard K, Krause KH (2007) The NOX family of ROS-generating NADPH oxidases: physiology and pathophysiology. Physiol Rev 87(1):245–313

Bianco AC, Salvatore D, Gereben B et al (2002) Biochemistry, cellular and molecular biology, and physiological roles of the iodothyronine selenodeiodinases. Endocr Rev 23(1):38–89

Blanchard C, Rothenberg ME (2009) Biology of the eosinophil. Adv Immunol 101:81–121

Bouayed J, Bohn T (2010) Exogenous antioxidants – double-edged swords in cellular redox state: health beneficial effects at physiologic doses versus deleterious effects at high doses. Oxid Med Cell Longev 3(4):228–237

Brown MS, Goldstein JL (1983) Lipoprotein metabolism in the macrophage: implications for cholesterol deposition in atherosclerosis. Annu Rev Biochem 52: 223–261

Cathcart MK (2004) Regulation of superoxide anion production by NADPH oxidase in monocytes/macrophages: contributions to atherosclerosis. Arterioscler Thromb Vasc Biol 24(1):23–28

Chan RC, Wang M, Li N et al (2006) Pro-oxidative diesel exhaust particle chemicals inhibit LPS-induced dendritic cell responses involved in T-helper differentiation. J Allergy Clin Immunol 118(2):455–465

Chance B (1961) The interaction of energy and electron transfer reactions in mitochondria. V. The energy transfer pathway. J Biol Chem 236:1569–1576

Chance B, Sies H, Boveris A (1979) Hydroperoxide metabolism in mammalian organs. Physiol Rev 59(3):527–605

Chen GY, Nunez G (2010) Sterile inflammation: sensing and reacting to damage. Nat Rev Immunol 10(12): 826–837

Ciz M, Denev P, Kratchanova M et al (2012) Flavonoids inhibit the respiratory burst of neutrophils in mammals. Oxid Med Cell Longev 2012:181295

Czech MP, Lawrence JC Jr, Lynn WS (1974) Evidence for the involvement of sulfhydryl oxidation in the regulation of fat cell hexose transport by insulin. Proc Natl Acad Sci U S A 71(10):4173–4177

Dang PM, Dewas C, Gaudry M et al (1999) Priming of human neutrophil respiratory burst by granulocyte/macrophage colony-stimulating factor (GM-CSF) involves partial phosphorylation of p47(phox). J Biol Chem 274(29):20704–20708

Droge W (2002) Free radicals in the physiological control of cell function. Physiol Rev 82(1):47–95

Dunne DW, Resnick D, Greenberg J et al (1994) The type I macrophage scavenger receptor binds to gram-positive bacteria and recognizes lipoteichoic acid. Proc Natl Acad Sci U S A 91(5):1863–1867

El Benna J, Hayem G, Dang PM et al (2002) NADPH oxidase priming and p47phox phosphorylation in neutrophils from synovial fluid of patients with rheumatoid arthritis and spondylarthropathy. Inflammation 26(6):273–278

Elbim C, Bailly S, Chollet-Martin S et al (1994) Differential priming effects of proinflammatory cytokines on human neutrophil oxidative burst in response to bacterial N-formyl peptides. Infect Immun 62(6):2195–2201

El-Sonbaty SM, El-Hadedy DE (2012) Combined effect of cadmium, lead, and UV rays on Bacillus cereus using comet assay and oxidative stress parameters. Environ Sci Pollut Res Int. Epub

Erlemann KR, Rokach J, Powell WS (2004) Oxidative stress stimulates the synthesis of the eosinophil chemoattractant 5-oxo-6,8,11,14-eicosatetraenoic acid by inflammatory cells. J Biol Chem 279(39):40376–40384

Fabriek BO, van Bruggen R, Deng DM et al (2009) The macrophage scavenger receptor CD163 functions as an innate immune sensor for bacteria. Blood 113(4):887–892

Fariss MW, Chan CB, Patel M et al (2005) Role of mitochondria in toxic oxidative stress. Mol Interv 5(2):94–111

Fisher AB (2009) Redox signaling across cell membranes. Antioxid Redox Signal 11(6):1349–1356

Gougerot-Pocidalo MA, el Benna J, Elbim C et al (2002) Regulation of human neutrophil oxidative burst by pro- and anti-inflammatory cytokines. J Soc Biol 196(1):37–46

Grant GE, Rokach J, Powell WS (2009) 5-Oxo-ETE and the OXE receptor. Prostaglandins Other Lipid Mediat 89(3–4):98–104

Grant GE, Rubino S, Gravel S et al (2011) Enhanced formation of 5-oxo-6,8,11,14-eicosatetraenoic acid by cancer cells in response to oxidative stress, docosahexaenoic acid and neutrophil-derived 5-hydroxy-6,8,11,14-eicosatetraenoic acid. Carcinogenesis 32(6):822–828

Guzik TJ, Griendling KK (2009) NADPH oxidases: molecular understanding finally reaching the clinical level? Antioxid Redox Signal 11(10):2365–2370

Hazen SL, Hsu FF, Duffin K et al (1996) Molecular chlorine generated by the myeloperoxidase-hydrogen peroxide-chloride system of phagocytes converts low density lipoprotein cholesterol into a family of chlorinated sterols. J Biol Chem 271(38):23080–23088

Holmes B, Page AR, Good RA (1967) Studies of the metabolic activity of leukocytes from patients with a genetic abnormality of phagocytic function. J Clin Invest 46(9):1422–1432

Honda K, Chihara J (1999) Eosinophil activation by eotaxin–eotaxin primes the production of reactive oxygen species from eosinophils. Allergy 54(12): 1262–1269

Janero DR, Hreniuk D, Sharif HM (1991) Hydrogen peroxide-induced oxidative stress to the mammalian heart-muscle cell (cardiomyocyte): lethal peroxidative membrane injury. J Cell Physiol 149(3):347–364

Jendrysik MA, Vasilevsky S, Yi L et al (2011) NADPH oxidase-2 derived ROS dictates murine DC cytokine-mediated cell fate decisions during CD4 T helper-cell commitment. PLoS One 6(12):e28198

Kadota S, Fantus IG, Deragon G et al (1987) Stimulation of insulin-like growth factor II receptor binding and insulin receptor kinase activity in rat adipocytes. Effects of vanadate and H2O2. J Biol Chem 262(17): 8252–8256

Katsuyama M, Matsuno K, Yabe-Nishimura C (2012) Physiological roles of NOX/NADPH oxidase, the superoxide-generating enzyme. J Clin Biochem Nutr 50(1):9–22

Kidd P (2003) Th1/Th2 balance: the hypothesis, its limitations, and implications for health and disease. Altern Med Rev 8(3):223–246

Kirkham P (2007) Oxidative stress and macrophage function: a failure to resolve the inflammatory response. Biochem Soc Trans 35(Pt 2):284–287

Korantzopoulos P, Kolettis TM, Galaris D et al (2007) The role of oxidative stress in the pathogenesis and perpetuation of atrial fibrillation. Int J Cardiol 115(2): 135–143

Kotsias F, Hoffmann E, Amigorena S et al (2013) Reactive oxygen species production in the phagosome: impact on antigen presentation in dendritic cells. Antioxid Redox Signal 18(6):714–729

Krieger M, Herz J (1994) Structures and functions of multiligand lipoprotein receptors: macrophage scavenger receptors and LDL receptor-related protein (LRP). Annu Rev Biochem 63:601–637

Krishnaswamy JK, Chu T, Eisenbarth SC (2013) Beyond pattern recognition: NOD-like receptors in dendritic cells. Trends Immunol 34:224–233

Laihia JK, Jansen CT (1997) Up-regulation of human epidermal Langerhans' cell B7-1 and B7-2 co-stimulatory molecules in vivo by solar-simulating irradiation. Eur J Immunol 27(4):984–989

Le SB, Hailer MK, Buhrow S et al (2007) Inhibition of mitochondrial respiration as a source of adaphostin-induced reactive oxygen species and cytotoxicity. J Biol Chem 282(12):8860–8872

Lenaz G (1998) Role of mitochondria in oxidative stress and ageing. Biochim Biophys Acta 1366(1–2):53–67

Leto TL, Morand S, Hurt D et al (2009) Targeting and regulation of reactive oxygen species generation by Nox family NADPH oxidases. Antioxid Redox Signal 11(10):2607–2619

Liu WF, Ma M, Bratlie KM et al (2011) Real-time in vivo detection of biomaterial-induced reactive oxygen species. Biomaterials 32(7):1796–1801

Matsumoto A, Naito M, Itakura H et al (1990) Human macrophage scavenger receptors: primary structure, expression, and localization in atherosclerotic lesions. Proc Natl Acad Sci U S A 87(23):9133–9137

Mishra D, Mehta A, Flora SJ (2008) Reversal of arsenic-induced hepatic apoptosis with combined administration of DMSA and its analogues in guinea pigs: role of glutathione and linked enzymes. Chem Res Toxicol 21(2):400–407

Mitchell P (1961) Coupling of phosphorylation to electron and hydrogen transfer by a chemi-osmotic type of mechanism. Nature 191:144–148

Mogensen TH (2009) Pathogen recognition and inflammatory signaling in innate immune defenses. Clin Microbiol Rev 22(2):240–273

Muster B, Kohl W, Wittig I et al (2010) Respiratory chain complexes in dynamic mitochondria display a patchy distribution in life cells. PLoS One 5(7):e11910

Netzer N, Goodenbour JM, David A et al (2009) Innate immune and chemically triggered oxidative stress modifies translational fidelity. Nature 462(7272):522–526

Newkirk MM, Goldbach-Mansky R, Lee J et al (2003) Advanced glycation end-product (AGE)-damaged IgG and IgM autoantibodies to IgG-AGE in patients with early synovitis. Arthritis Res Ther 5(2):R82–R90

Omori K, Ohira T, Uchida Y et al (2008) Priming of neutrophil oxidative burst in diabetes requires preassembly of the NADPH oxidase. J Leukoc Biol 84(1):292–301

Pawelec G, Derhovanessian E, Larbi A (2010) Immunosenescence and cancer. Crit Rev Oncol Hematol 75(2):165–172

Peled A, Gonzalo JA, Lloyd C et al (1998) The chemotactic cytokine eotaxin acts as a granulocyte-macrophage colony-stimulating factor during lung inflammation. Blood 91(6):1909–1916

Petreccia DC, Nauseef WM, Clark RA (1987) Respiratory burst of normal human eosinophils. J Leukoc Biol 41(4):283–288

Pickrell AM, Fukui H, Moraes CT (2009) The role of cytochrome c oxidase deficiency in ROS and amyloid plaque formation. J Bioenerg Biomembr 41(5):453–456

Poli G, Leonarduzzi G, Biasi F et al (2004) Oxidative stress and cell signalling. Curr Med Chem 11(9):1163–1182

Rada B, Leto TL (2008) Oxidative innate immune defenses by Nox/Duox family NADPH oxidases. Contrib Microbiol 15:164–187

Rutault K, Alderman C, Chain BM et al (1999) Reactive oxygen species activate human peripheral blood dendritic cells. Free Radic Biol Med 26(1–2):232–238

Rybicka JM, Balce DR, Khan MF et al (2010) NADPH oxidase activity controls phagosomal proteolysis in macrophages through modulation of the lumenal redox environment of phagosomes. Proc Natl Acad Sci U S A 107(23):10496–10501

Sheng KC, Pietersz GA, Tang CK et al (2010) Reactive oxygen species level defines two functionally distinctive stages of inflammatory dendritic cell development from mouse bone marrow. J Immunol 184(6):2863–2872

Shult PA, Graziano FM, Wallow IH et al (1985) Comparison of superoxide generation and luminol-dependent chemiluminescence with eosinophils and neutrophils from normal individuals. J Lab Clin Med 106(6):638–645

Sies H, Cadenas E (1985) Oxidative stress: damage to intact cells and organs. Philos Trans R Soc Lond B Biol Sci 311(1152):617–631

Song L, Lee C, Schindler C (2011) Deletion of the murine scavenger receptor CD68. J Lipid Res 52(8):1542–1550

Starkov AA, Fiskum G, Chinopoulos C et al (2004) Mitochondrial alpha-ketoglutarate dehydrogenase complex generates reactive oxygen species. J Neurosci 24(36):7779–7788

Steinman RM (1991) The dendritic cell system and its role in immunogenicity. Annu Rev Immunol 9:271–296

Straumann A, Safroneeva E (2012) Eosinophils in the gastrointestinal tract: friends or foes? Acta Gastroenterol Belg 75(3):310–315

Sundaram S, Ghosh J (2006) Expression of 5-oxoETE receptor in prostate cancer cells: critical role in survival. Biochem Biophys Res Commun 339(1):93–98

Tang L, Lucas AH, Eaton JW (1993) Inflammatory responses to implanted polymeric biomaterials: role of surface-adsorbed immunoglobulin G. J Lab Clin Med 122(3):292–300

Turrens JF (2003) Mitochondrial formation of reactive oxygen species. J Physiol 552(Pt 2):335–344

Underhill DM, Goodridge HS (2012) Information processing during phagocytosis. Nat Rev Immunol 12(7):492–502

VanderVen BC, Hermetter A, Huang A et al (2010) Development of a novel, cell-based chemical screen to identify inhibitors of intraphagosomal lipolysis in macrophages. Cytometry A 77(8):751–760

Winterbourn CC, Vissers MC, Kettle AJ (2000) Myeloperoxidase. Curr Opin Hematol 7(1):53–58

Xie L, Tsaprailis G, Chen QM (2005) Proteomic identification of insulin-like growth factor-binding protein-6 induced by sublethal H2O2 stress from human diploid fibroblasts. Mol Cell Proteomics 4(9): 1273–1283

Zhong J, Rao X, Deiuliis J et al (2013) A potential role for dendritic cell/macrophage-expressing DPP4 in obesity-induced visceral inflammation. Diabetes 62(1):149–157

Zhou R, Tardivel A, Thorens B et al (2010) Thioredoxin-interacting protein links oxidative stress to inflammasome activation. Nat Immunol 11(2):136–140

Oxidative Stress and Aging

24

Behjat Al-Sadat Moayedi Esfahani,
Milad Mirmoghtadaei, and Sima Balouchi Anaraki

24.1 Introduction and History

Biologists have conducted numerous empirical studies on the phenomenon of cell aging, from cells of rats to that of human beings, from fibroblasts to epithelial cells, and have concluded that in the end most cells undergo the process of aging. This is probably due to the insufficiency of physiological or cellular growth conditions and stress. Aging acts to inhibit growth and proliferation and promotes differentiation. Cells lose their potential to response to mitogens when they get old. Changes in the chromatin and gene expression of aging cells transform them to wide, chubby nonfunctional ones. As cell-to-cell communication diminishes, their adhesion to extracellular matrix increases. Such cells have lost their ability to divide and can live but a few months. Such observations show that cellular aging is a preprogrammed phenomenon which takes place in certain physiological conditions along with stress and results in cessation of cellular proliferation. In other words, aging eventually equals programmed cell death or apoptosis, a phenomenon well studied and reviewed, with

its factors already recognized; nevertheless, its physiological role in elderly prompts more studies.

In 1961, Leonard Hayflick described the aging phenomenon in this way: Aging is an inner programmed mechanism that limits cellular proliferation. This phenomenon is more apparent in fibroblast cell cultures where growth and proliferation of cells stop after several cycles. In 1998, Bodnar and his colleagues realized that the shortening of telomeres plays an important role in cell aging. Recent studies show an essential role for stress in cell deterioration. Oncoproteins such as Ras and its family can overactivate cells which will in turn lead to their inactivity and can accelerate aging. Consequently, aging takes place in two ways:

- Aging due to proliferation of cells as a result of intracellular physiological factors
- Premature aging and death of immature nonproliferative cells due to oxidative stress or other external factors

Despite the importance of this categorization, both follow the same path to ultimately result in cell death. Cells age when they are highly damaged either from external or internal factors, although in most cases both factors act synergistically to expedite the process by reducing the length of telomeres more quickly and DNA damage that causes the involvement of different cell levels to ensue premature aging. Toxins and waste products build up within cells due to different types of stress, including oxidative stress and carcinogens.

B.A.-S. Moayedi Esfahani, PharmD, SBB, MSc (✉)
S.B. Anaraki, MSc
Department of Immunology, Isfahan University
of Medical Sciences, Isfahan, Iran
e-mail: moayedi@med.mui.ac.ir

M. Mirmoghtadaei, MBBS
Department of Clinical Sciences, University of
Sharjah, Sharjah, UAE

A. Massoud, N. Rezaei (eds.), *Immunology of Aging*,
DOI 10.1007/978-3-642-39495-9_24, © Springer-Verlag Berlin Heidelberg 2014

The intricate mechanism and the relationship between each factor prompt further discussion that we will get back to later.

In the eighteenth century, Lamark divided the causes of death into two different major categories: natural death due to aging and dying because of sickness or accident. Lamark related aging to internal bodily activities. About a century later, a deeper understanding of this process was described by Weisman: Normal cell activity deteriorates gradually, either directly or indirectly (increased vulnerability to accidental death). Weisman believed somatic cells to be disposable materials for gametes. Studies on this ground have yielded different hypotheses. This variety has resulted in viewing aging from different perspectives such as in a population or an organism (either multicellular or unicellular) with different parameters that change by aging.

Nowadays, we believe senescence to consist of continuous and consecutive changes that take place in a lifetime. Free radicals including reactive oxygen species (ROS) and nitrogen reactive species (NRS) play a major role in destruction of cells, fibers, and different tissues and organs via oxidation of macromolecules such as proteins, DNA, and lipids.

In age-related diseases such as Alzheimer's and Parkinson's, there is a direct relationship between aging and increased levels of free radicals among patients. Brain is a vulnerable organ to oxidation. That is due to its high levels of oxygen consumption, unsaturated fatty acids (that can get oxidized), nonreduced metal ions, and finally the insufficiency of body's antioxidants, especially in the elderly. The presence of endogenous antioxidants in the body helps its natural defense mechanism, especially pronounced in the brain. The augmentation of oxidative damage in the elderly may be due to lack of antioxidants. Lipid peroxidation (LPO), the main cause of oxidative damage, is the result of one or all of the following factors: an extreme loss of liquid permeability, a decrease in cell membrane potential, and finally an increased permeability to metals. Increased amounts of LPO will cause a reduction in the rate of physiological reactions and consequently an increased vulnerability to different diseases.

Free radicals are involved in a wide range of diseases such as inflammatory diseases, ischemia and reperfusion, neurodegenerative diseases, diabetes, and cancer. But unfortunately we don't have any medications in the market that can act as scavengers of such wide range of oxidants. There are several reasons behind not using antioxidants in medical treatments: Oxidative stress cannot be identified as a disease. However, it can be a risk factor for different disorders. Take diabetes, for example, in which the involvement of oxidative stress is clear; however, only very few health and research centers in the United States (USA) and other parts of the world recommend the use of antioxidants. Moreover, the assessment of oxidative agents or the levels of free radicals and by the same token endogenous antioxidants is not yet a common practice in diagnostic laboratories, and physicians cannot ask for them as diagnostic tests. Furthermore, drug companies do not show much interest in antioxidants.

24.2 Molecular Mechanism of Oxidative Stress and Aging

ROS/RNS including free radicals such as superoxide (O_2^-), hydrogen peroxide (H_2O_2), and possibly hydroxyl radical (HO) are highly reactive and short-lived molecules. Due to unpaired electrons in their orbit, free radicals are unstable molecules that attack other substance within their reach and grab electron from them to stabilize themselves. ROS are the product of cellular aerobic metabolism within the mitochondria. So, any chemical or infectious agent or genetic defect that can interfere with mitochondrial function can lead to production of large amounts of ROS. In addition to mitochondria (a principal source of endogenous free radicals), peroxisomal fatty acid metabolism, cytochrome P-450 reactions, and phagocytic cells are other sites of oxidant generation. In addition, free radicals can come from external sources such as exposure to environmental pollution, radiation, cigarette smoking, carcinogenic materials, and various industrial chemicals or toxins that are found in polluted water and food (Beckman and Ames 1998).

Free radicals act as a double-edged sword based on their concentration. They are beneficial at low or moderate concentrations and play a role in many metabolic and physiological processes such as defense against infections or cellular signaling pathways. In contrast, at high concentrations, harmful effects of free radicals (oxidative stress) can cause damage to cellular components including lipids, DNA, proteins, and carbohydrates. For example, in normal conditions hydrogen peroxide is used in thyroid hormone synthesis or is involved in the myeloperoxidase reactions inside neutrophils to eliminate bacteria; at high doses however, it may participate in the oxidative destruction of macromolecules. Consequently, oxidative stress has been implicated in pathophysiology of diseases such as diabetes, heart disease, arthritis, and especially in the chronic diseases associated with the aging process such as cardiovascular and neurodegenerative diseases and cancer (Valko et al. 2007; Finkel and Holbrook 2000; Pollack and Leeuwenburgh 1999).

24.3 Antioxidants

Organisms protect themselves against harmful effects of free radicals by a complex network of antioxidant metabolites and enzymes. Antioxidants are natural free radical fighters capable of slowing or preventing oxidation of other molecules. They work by keeping ROS at an optimum level or removing them before they can damage cellular components. Antioxidants may be synthesized in the body (endogenous) or obtained from the diet (exogenous). Endogenous antioxidants are classified into two nonenzymatic (e.g., uric acid, glutathione, bilirubin, thiols, albumin, and nutritional factors, including vitamins and phenols) and enzymatic (e.g., the superoxide dismutases (SOD), the glutathione peroxidases, and catalase) groups. Antioxidants mostly obtained from diet and can protect the body from oxidative damages through different ways including (1) direct neutralizing free radicals, (2) reducing the peroxide concentrations and repairing oxidized membranes, (3) quenching iron in order to decrease the production of reactive oxygen species, and (4) using lipid metabolism as short-chain free fatty acids and cholesterol esters which are able to neutralize reactive oxygen species (Berger 2005; Fusco et al. 2007).

SODs are a set of cytosolic (copper/zinc SOD) and mitochondrial (manganese SOD) isoenzymes, depending on the trace element cofactor in their active sites. SOD converts two molecules of superoxide radical to an oxygen molecule and a hydrogen peroxide. There is a strong correlation between maximum life span of a species and its SOD activity (the first defense against ROS). For example, human SOD activity is about 16-fold greater than that of mice (Ku et al. 1993).

Glutathione peroxidase is the most abundant nonprotein endogenous hydrogen peroxide scavenger enzyme with high concentrations in both the cytosol and mitochondria. Glutathione peroxidase with its substrate glutathione (GSH) (1-g-glutamyl-1 –cysteinyl- glycine; a tripeptide found in all animal cells) forms a powerful defense against hydrogen peroxides and lipid peroxides. GSH also recycles back vitamin C and vitamin D to their native state after scavenging free radicals. Another H_2O_2 metabolizing enzyme is catalase. It metabolizes hydrogen peroxide to oxygen and water. It is found primarily in peroxisomes and less abundantly in mitochondria (Meister and Anderson 1983; Alidoost et al. 2006).

Ascorbic acid or vitamin C is a critical water-soluble free radical scavenger that humans must obtain from diet. Vitamin C interacts with GSH and vitamin E to reduce intracellular reactive oxygen species. Vitamin E is composed of a set of eight structural isomers of tocopherol and tocotrienols which are lipid-soluble antioxidant vitamins. Of these, α-tocopherol has the highest antioxidant activity and is the most important lipid-soluble antioxidant. Vitamin E is often used to attenuate oxidative stress in many pathophysiological conditions. As an antioxidant, vitamin E is important because of its ability to convert several free radicals such as superoxide, hydroxyl, and lipid peroxyl radicals into "repairable" radical forms. Moreover, when vitamin E scavenges a radical, a vitamin E radical is formed and has to be recycled back to its active form by other antioxidants (such as vitamin C) to be able to scavenge more radicals. Carotenoids are another set of lipid-soluble antioxidant vitamins. Carotenoid levels have inverse correlation with some inflammatory diseases such as atherosclerosis and cardiovascular diseases. Vitamin C, vitamin E, and carotenoids act to reduce lipid peroxidation (Herrera and Barbas 2001; Ryan et al. 2010).

Flavonoids or bioflavonoids (water-soluble pigments) are units of polyphenolic compounds that exist in most plant. Basic structure of flavonoids consists of a flavone nucleus which is connected to benzene rings. Diversity and differences in the C ring make up various flavonoids. They are concentrated in the plant seeds, skin, and core of fruits and flowering plants. Many of the plants used in medicine contain flavonoids that have antibacterial, anti-inflammatory, antiallergic, anticarcinogenic, vasodilating, and antiaging properties. For example, silymarin, a purified extract of *Silybum marianum* seeds, contains a large amount of flavonoids including silybin. Silymarin is used in liver diseases such as hepatitis and cirrhosis. It protects liver cells from membrane lipid oxidation and liver glutathione depletion (Zarban and Ziaee 2008).

Some trace elements such as selenium, copper, and zinc are sometimes considered antioxidants. But they have no antioxidant activity themselves, but are required for some antioxidant enzyme activities. Reduced metals, like iron, participate in reactions that lead to generation of reactive oxidants. With age, iron accumulates and can contribute to increased oxidative damage. So, some compounds (e.g., iron-binding proteins such as transferrin and ferritin) participate in antioxidant defense by sequestering such metal and preventing their free radical effects.

24.4 Antioxidants and Removal of Free Radicals

Nonpolar organic compounds cannot be excreted through kidneys due to their impermeability through the cell wall and need to be polarized before they can find their way into the urine. For such reactions to take place, the cytochrome P_{450} monooxygenase system must come into operation for which the body utilizes NADPH and oxygen molecules:

$$XH + O_2 + NADPH + H^+ \leftrightarrow XOH + H_2O + NADP^+$$

Iron molecules in the heme portion of the cytochrome P_{450} monooxygenase enzyme can reverse the oxidative reaction through their interaction with sulfur molecules which can be found in the enzyme's structure. During these reactions, electron is transported into cytochrome via NADPH flavoprotein and cytochrome P_{450} reductase. We can also see the application of this pathway in nutrition where cytochrome P_{450} system can play a role in oxidizing different kinds of food products. Cyclic aromatic hydrocarbons such as benzo[a]pyrene found in smoked food products can also set the cytochrome P_{450} system into action through another mechanism, and the same is true about canned foods which in turn participate in stimulating the cytochrome P_{450} pathway. This calls for a need for antioxidants to neutralize such effect.

Cytochrome P_{450} can also get activated by halogenated hydrocarbons to produce free radicals. For example, CCl_4 which was formerly used widely as a solvent in dry cleaners' shops is an important factor in producing free radicals through stimulating cytochrome P_{450} which can in turn have detrimental effects on the liver. Inhalational anesthetics like halothane can have the same impact on the liver by releasing free radicals. Despite harmful properties of such substances and numerous studies that have been conducted in this field, they are still being used in chemical and pharmaceutical industries. A compound with strong oxidizing activities that is commonly used as a chemotherapeutic agent in the treatment of wide range of cancers is Adriamycin (Doxorubicin). Since tumor cells and healthy cells compete in utilizing antioxidants, patients must have an adequate intake of antioxidants while on therapy. Same is true with regard to sun-exposed individuals and those suffering from chronic allergic diseases.

24.4.1 Removal of Free Radicals

Production of intermediate products is a necessary step to facilitate the reduction of reactive oxygen species and other toxic substances. Therefore, we can consider the action of the involved enzyme in two phases:

Phase I, Detoxification. Toxic, mutagenic, and carcinogenic substances are an indispensable part of our daily diet; examples include materials formed in the process of cooking fats, meat, protein, or other naturally occurring carcinogens present in herbal products, like certain alkaloids or the toxic substances found in fungi, just to name a few. Polycyclic aromatic hydrocarbons, benzo[a]pyrene and heterocyclic aromatic amines are other examples of materials found within processed or cooked food products. We may also consider 2-amino-1-methyl-6-phenylinidazol pyridine which can be found in concentrations 0.5–70 mg in cooked meat depending on the method and temperature it is produced.

Toxic waste products from factories, air pollution, pesticides, and other toxins that penetrate different plants and animals and eventually find their way into our bodies, and other toxins inevitably found in some pharmaceuticals are continually being ingested and can consequently harm our bodies depending on their available dosage. These in turn begin to damage our cells and tissues which may eventually result in cell death and premature aging. On the other hand, we can find substances such as isothiocyanates, dithiolethiones, allyl sulfides, and lactones in different foods which are considered antioxidants that can protect us from carcinogenic and other harmful effects of ROS and other toxins through different mechanisms.

Protecting agents can play their preventive role both at the level of initiation and proliferation of neoplastic cells. They work to stimulate and activate the endogenous antioxidant enzymes to neutralize ROS and other toxins, and therefore the effect of carcinogen. However, not all protecting agents have been discovered within our bodies, and such studies are still at their beginning. These agents can also prevent cell death and premature aging.

Phase II, Activation and neutralization of free radicals by endogenous antioxidants. As mentioned earlier, most toxic and waste products in the body are made of hydrophobic compounds, and they need to be metabolized before they can be excreted. For such reactions an oxygen molecule is required for an electron to be donated to these products (including ROS) in order for them to convert to another ion or a free radical. The intermediate products in these reactions are usually electrophilic, and their reaction with nucleophilic materials (electrons in the center of DNA) and cellular proteins requires an electron. Considering the fact that the production of these intermediate products is quintessential for removal of some waste products, the body's biologic system has to make a balance between addition and removal of electrons and consequently a balance in the intermediate products. Therefore, an imbalance in production and conversion of free radicals will result in interaction of these intermediate molecules with cellular macromolecules and will eventually result in cell injury, premature aging, or cell death (Gutteridge 1993). The enzymes that participate in the activation of free radicals are called the "phase I-activated enzymes" which include the cytochrome P_{450} superfamily, aldehyde oxidases, xanthine oxidases, and peroxides. Most oxidative reactions involving free radicals utilize the cytochrome P_{450} monooxygenase enzymatic pathway (Danielson 2002).

24.4.1.1 Response and Increased Activity in a Wide Spectrum

In phase II, neutralization takes place via endogenous enzymes to counteract free radicals that are produced in phase I enzymatic activity. Phase II enzymes will result in the reduction of intermediate products. Phase II enzymes include several families of enzymes, the most important of which include sulfurtransferases, uridine diphosphate (UDP)-glucuronosyl transferase, glutathione S-transferase, epoxide hydrolase, nicotinamide adenine dinucleotide phosphate (NAD(P)H), quinone reductase, and amine oxidases (King et al. 2000; Sheehan et al. 2001).

24.4.1.2 Activation and Neutralization of Free Radicals in Phases I and II

Despite the wide range of phase II enzymatic activity in protection against free radicals, they act only through several different mechanisms: They often neutralize the induced activation of substances due to free radicals. Such catalytic reaction however is relative and depends upon the concentration of these enzymes and their products and can also be dependent upon our diet. Liver is the main detoxification organ due to a higher concentration of these enzymes to neutralize the substances absorbed through the gut and therefore preventing their distribution into other tissues. Epithelial cells will also get activated in cases of extra free radical production, to produce more endogenous enzymes to balance out the reaction. Hence, these enzymes play a significant role in protection and prevention of cellular and tissue injuries against electrophilic substances. These agents find their way into our bodies via food and other contaminations through our lungs, guts, skin, and other organs and tissues.

24.5 The Multigenic Family of Glutathione Sulfurtransferases

Glutathione sulfurtransferases (GSTs) belong to a diverse family of isozymes that facilitate the interaction between glutathione and a wide variety of electrophilic substances, especially of lipophilic substrates. GSTs can be found in most tissues and such interactions play a major role to prevent cellular and tissue damages precipitated by free radicals. Such detoxification of endogenous compounds takes place via catalysis of the conjugation of reduced glutathione via a sulfhydryl group, thus facilitating their removal through bile or urine as mercapturic compounds. The enzymatic activity of GST family is proportional to the availability of glutathione (GSH) in the body. Therefore, those individual with a deficiency in synthesis or reduced amounts of sulfur amino acids will have a significantly less glutathione available and will consequently be much more vulnerable to oxidation-induced cellular damage. The first barrier against electrophilic compounds and lipid peroxidases is the epithelia in our small intestine, which have a relatively low synthesis of glutathione, which is in turn compensated by their uptake from bile or ingested nutrients.

Gamma-glutamylcysteine synthetase is another enzyme to help in the synthesis of glutathione which utilizes the ingested cysteine molecules. The significance of synthesis and thereby balance of glutathione has been shown to slow down the aging process and prevent certain malignancies especially lung carcinomas. This can be demonstrated when we study the higher prevalence of lung cancers in individuals with a deficiency in their GST_{MI} gene. By the same token, we can see a higher prevalence of lung cancer (besides other cancers such as larynx and gall bladder carcinomas) in chronic smokers due to a similar enzymatic synthetic defect.

24.5.1 UDP-Glucuronosyl Transferase

UDP-glucuronosyl transferases act to facilitate the excretion of electrophilic substances, including ROS via bile and urine. Formation of glucuronide compounds is considered a significant step in detoxification. Among such reactions, UDP-glucuronosyl transferases play a rather more important role when compared with glutathione conjugation and the formation of sulfur esterase, as the latter have a lower efficacy. On the other hand, the result of the former reaction is directly related to the availability of UDP-glucuronic acid as well as the activity of specific receptors for UDP-glucuronosyl transferases in the cytosol.

24.5.2 Sulfurtransferases

This group of enzymes also plays a part in catalysis of hydroxyl compounds. They function by transferring sulfur-containing groups and their binding to different harmful chemicals we take in, such as phenols that are found in food or other chemical and therapeutic compounds such as catecholamines and hydroxysteroids that are converted to ionized particles within the body. These enzymes are more efficient when there are low concentrations of free radicals to discard.

24.5.3 Epoxide Hydrolases

This enzyme functions in detoxification by converting epoxides to trans-dihydrodiols, which can be conjugated and excreted from the body. Epoxide hydrolase, either from a microsomal or cytosolic origin, operates to separate the hydraulic agent from a wide range of alkyl agents and cycloalkyl epoxides and arene oxides and balance the reaction towards trans-dihydrodiol synthesis. Epoxides and arenoxides constitute the end product of many mutagenic and carcinogenic compounds together with many other oxidant reactions such as oxidase P_{450}. Therefore, it plays an important role in regulation of carcinogens, mutagens, and other toxins and their activities and consequently has a role in the prevention of premature aging.

24.5.4 NAD(P)H: Quinone Reductase

This enzyme causes the elimination of redox cycle which takes place as a result of activation of different toxins and free radicals. This enzyme is also known by other names such as DT-diaphorase or NAD(P)H dehydrogenase. Quinone reductase (QR) is a cytosolic flavoprotein and catalyzes the following reaction:

$$NADPH + H^+ + quinone \rightleftharpoons NADP^+ + semiquinone$$

Like other enzymes that have a role in detoxification, this enzyme can also be found in all body tissues. We can notice the importance of such reaction especially when considering herbs that contain quinone, an electrophilic compound which is thus converted to phenolic compounds and will in turn attach to other glucuronides and sulfate esters with lower free radical activities.

Many herbs have been shown to contain phenolic compounds which are considered to stimulate QR activity and therefore eliminate different toxins. QR has also been shown to have a bioreductase activity against antineoplastic agents like mitomycin.

24.6 Superoxide Dismutases

Considering the role of ROS in oxidative reactions, the role of superoxide dismutases (SOD) in counteracting and outcompeting such reactions becomes evident.

There are three major families of superoxide dismutases, depending on their metal cofactor: Cu/Zn type (which binds both copper and zinc and is found in the cytoplasm outside the mitochondria), Fe and Mn types (which bind either iron or manganese that are found inside the mitochondria), and the Ni type, which binds nickel. The superoxide anion radical (O_2^-) quite rapidly and spontaneously dismutes to O_2 and hydrogen peroxide (H_2O_2). SODs are necessary because superoxide reacts with sensitive and critical cellular targets. As we age the function of ROSs deteriorates and this will result in the accumulation of oxidative agents inside the cells, especially mitochondria which are the most susceptible.

All four types of macromolecules (namely, lipids, nucleic acids, carbohydrates, and proteins) are vulnerable to damage from ROS agents. These injuries accumulate as we age and will result in a buildup of abnormal proteins and malfunctioning enzymes (Finkel and Holbrook 2000).

In 1973, Bernard Babior reported an increase in superoxide free radicals in neutrophils as a result of phagocytosis. He believed these radicals to have a bactericidal activity. He soon discovered a malicious side effect of these agents as to cause tissue injuries in the process of inflammation and that they can be protected against thereof via the action of superoxide dismutase. Other disorders such as heart attack, ischemia, shocks, and rejection of transplanted organs also seem to be affected by these free radicals' toxicity.

The role of SOD in the process of fibrosis and treatment of cholecystitis cases that lead to fibrosis has also been demonstrated. In this process fibroblasts will cause fibril collagens to arrange themselves in an order that obliterates the architecture of the involved organ or tissue, especially if it happens in lungs, kidneys, and gallbladder. While some believe such process to be irreversible, others consider it to be a dynamic reversible phenomenon. A mediator role of transforming growth factor beta 1 (TGF-β1) has recently been identified to control the antifibrotic effect of copper, zinc, and SOD and consequently reverse this process in myofibroblasts depending on their phenotype. TGF-β1 stimulates the synthesis of metalloproteases in synovial cells and fibroblasts. Thus, after the alleviation of myofibroblast injuries as a result of SOD, collagenases and metalloproteases will get activated to reverse the process. A critical role of SOD and superoxides has been demonstrated in a study on patients undergoing kidney transplantation, focusing on graft rejections and reperfusion injuries as SOD reduces first acute rejection episodes from 33 to 18.5 % and early irreversible acute rejection from 12.5 % in controls to 3.7 %. In addition there was a significant improvement of the actual 4-year graft survival rate in SOD-treated patients to 74 % compared with 52 % in controls. This study does not assess the mechanism of action of SOD; however, we can assume a reduction in immunogenicity of the allograft. The results appear significant as a hypothesis to suggest a response pattern of the immune system to some harmful signals like oxidative stress in addition to foreign antigens.

The role of superoxide radicals is thenceforth being highlighted more as molecular signals especially important in cellular division and proliferation and their mechanism of action in different disorders and such processes as metastasis, transformations, and angiogenesis. Despite the aforementioned discoveries and others on the way, there are still limitations in using SOD as medications or even in experimental labs and that is due to the weak therapeutic properties of proteins including SOD as they are easily excreted through urine and that they find their ways outside the cells very slowly. Not to mention because of their structure, they are more inclined to get

electrically charged, all of which will in turn influence their bioavailability and other pharmacodynamics and pharmacokinetic properties.

24.7 Stress-Activated Protein Kinase (SAPK) Family

This family of kinases gets activated in response to different types of stress including oxidative stress. This family includes P_{38}-MAPKα/β/γ/δ that is more vulnerable during old age. JNK1/2/3 is another member in this family (MMKs) which is an activating mediator of P_{16} in response to different age-related stresses. Studies show that fibroblasts lose their telomere length and even at a higher rate when grown inside environments with higher O_2 saturations. Despite no clear clue about the mechanism involved, we can suggest a role of oxidative stress in breaking the DNA telomeric chain (Forsyth et al. 2003; Von Zglinicki 2000).

Another possibility is DNA damage due to ROS and consequently increased activity of free radicals produced by H_2O_2 and the activation of P_{53} which will in turn accelerate the aging process.

24.8 Role of Oxidative Stress in Telomere Shortening

Telomeres are nucleoprotein structures located at the end of each chromosome as a cap in order to protect it from end-to-end fusion and degeneration. Telomere length is very heterogeneous in humans and extends for about 5–20 kb of noncoding repeats of guanine-rich tandem DNA sequences ($5'$ TTAGGG $3'$). In different individuals, telomere length is dependent not only on the kind of cell and number of cell divisions but also to age, sex, genetic, and environmental factors including ROS. At each cycle of cell division, telomeres are subjected to progressive shortening that may contribute to genomic instability, cell death, and aging. Two main reasons of telomere shortening are (1) end replication problem, which is the inability of DNA polymerase to completely replicate the $3'$ end of lagging strand during DNA replication, and (2) high sensitivity of guanine-rich telomere sequence to double-strand DNA breaks by oxidative stress (Bagherpour et al. 2009).

Telomeres are highly sensitive to damage via oxidative stress. In addition, oxidative stress can damage nucleobases or can produce single-strand breaks on genomic DNA during the life span of a cell or an organism, contributing significantly to senescence (aging). In normal conditions, the telomere structure is protected by telomerase (a telomere-repairing enzyme). Telomerase, a ribonucleoprotein complex, is involved in maintenance of chromosome ends by repairing strand DNA breaks. Oxidative damage can reduce telomerase activity in some cells. It is suggested that activation of telomerase may play an important role in the treatment of some diseases that are due to telomere shortening. Studies have shown that transferring telomerase into the cells increases both proliferation and resistant to oxidative stress. In vivo transfer of telomerase into telomerase-knockout mice improves telomere function and cirrhotic changes in mice liver cells (Tchirkov and Lansdorp 2003; Zhu et al. 2011).

24.9   Role of Apoptosis in Aging

Apoptosis is programmed cell death and is essential for eliminating infected, neoplastic, and damaged cells without inducing inflammation. Apoptosis can be induced by a wide range of stimuli such as irradiation, corticosteroids, cancer chemotherapy, chronic antigen stimulation, and oxidative stress. Oxidative stress is an important inducer of apoptosis and plays an important role in age-related diseases and immunosenescence. Immune cells like other cells are affected by oxidative stress, and this will result in lipid, protein, and DNA damages that are increased with aging (Goel and Khanduja 1998).

Immune cells undergo two different types of apoptotic processes including activation-induced cell death (AICD) and damage-induced cell death (DICD). AICD participates in the elimination of unnecessary lymphocytes derived from clonal expansion after antigenic stimulation, whereas DICD is essential for preventing neoplastic cell proliferation. In the immune system, there is a strong correlation between chronic antigenic stimulation and oxidative stress. They reduce lymphocyte sensitivity to DICD and lead to a proinflammatory stage to finally induce AICD. If clonal expansions were not controlled by apoptosis, it would rapidly result in the accumulation of senescent cells. AICD is through an extrinsic pathway that are often activated by binding of specific cell death receptors to their ligands such as cytokines. Increased AICD causes rapid lymphocytes activity and clonal expansion reduction that will lead to immune response inefficiency, whereas DICD activity reduction causes accumulation of senesces and inactivated lymphocytes, which leads to increased incidence of neoplastic lymphocytes (Ginaldi et al. 2005).

T cell receptors (TCR) interaction with their specific antigens leads to clonal expansion of specific T cells. After this stage, the number of lymphocytes increases in order to make balance in the immune system. In the elderly, high levels of proinflammatory cytokines induce AICD. In elderly people, an increased expression of tumor necrosis factor (TNF) and its receptor (CD95) and a decreased expression of CD28 facilitate apoptosis through CD95. Moreover, aging could be associated with decreased antiapoptotic protein BCL2 and increased proapoptotic protein Bax in activated lymphocytes, and reduced DICD may be related to a decreased P_{53} activity (De Martinis et al. 2007). Finally, a senescent immune system shows inadequate antigenic response due to its chronic stimulation.

24.10 Oxidative Mechanisms in Pathological Phenomena

Here, we try to point out several of the most common age-related disorders: Oxidative stress to the myocardium will result in deletion of a segment of the mitochondrial genome; lipofusion pigments which are the product of the oxidation of unsaturated fatty acids are especially found in the elderly and those suffering from neurological injuries; cataract and macular degeneration can also result from the consumption of certain chemicals or exposure to radiation.

The endogenous antioxidant system within the body, responsible for neutralizing free radicals, tends to lose its potency and functionality as we age. Aging also seems to reduce the enzymatic activity of glutathione peroxidase and SOD. Therefore, we need to assess whether this reduction of antioxidants can contribute to age-related diseases.

24.10.1 Oxidative Stress and Cataract

Age-related cataract, one of the major causes of blindness in the world, is an ocular disease caused by a wide range of etiologies including trauma, malnutrition, exposure to ultraviolet radiation, oxidative stress, and aging. In developing countries, cataract occurs in individuals older than 65 years and is mainly due to oxidative stress. H_2O_2 is the major oxidant involved in this disease. Oxidative stress can damage the eye's lens and lead to its opacification. The main function of a lens is to maintain clarity and to focus light onto the retina. Lens has high amounts of GSH and protein. The protein constitutes about 35 % of the total weight of the lens. Crystalline, lens' structural protein, contains a large amount of thiol group that needs to be in its reduced form to maintain the transparency of the lens. The solid shape of crystalline is responsible for lens transparency and provides the necessary reflective power. In an aged lens because of GSH reduction, recycling and resynthesis of this system is reduced. Therefore, lens is more susceptible to the effects of H_2O_2 and other oxidants.

24.10.2 Oxidative Stress and Asthma

Asthma is a chronic inflammatory lung disease. Several factors such as airway inflammation, bronchial hypersensitivity, and IgE-mediated immune response play important roles in the pathogenesis of asthma. Moreover, many clinical trials have suggested a role for oxidative stress in relation with the pathophysiology of asthma (Gilgun-Sherki et al. 2004). Both endogenous and exogenous ROS/RNS play a pivotal role in airway inflammation and result in the progression of this disease. Stress has an effect on airway smooth muscles and may enhance inflammation by inducing various proinflammatory mediators, enhancing mucin secretion, and stimulating bronchospasm.

ROS reduce beta-adrenergic function in lungs and render airway smooth muscles sensitive to contractions induced by acetylcholine. Inflammation and oxidative stress work together to cause permanent lung damage. During inflammation, multiple cytokines and mediators (e.g., TNF-α, fibroblast growth factor II, serotonin, and thrombin) in the lung cause oxidative activation that will eventually lead to an increase in ROS inside the cells. Two important ways to reduce oxidative stress and their effects are (i) to reduce exposure to ROS and (ii) to enhance the antioxidant defense system. Studies have shown that avoidance of exogenous oxidants such as air pollution, ozone, and nitrites can reduce the severity of asthma symptoms (Yoo Sook Cho and Moon 2010).

24.10.3 Oxidative Stress and Neurodegenerative Diseases

Age-related neurodegenerative diseases (e.g., Alzheimer's disease and Parkinson's disease) are associated with progressive dysfunction and loss of neurons and axons in the central nervous system, which is termed neurodegeneration. Neurodegeneration results from multiple factors including inflammation, infection, trauma, and oxidative stress. Central nervous system (CNS) is more sensitive to oxidative stress than other tissues and organs. Various factors in the brain lead to a higher sensitivity to reactive oxygen and nitrogen species production including (a) high oxygen uptake due to high metabolic activity, (b) high levels of polyunsaturated fatty acids which are readily oxidized by free radicals and produce toxic LPO, (c) partial defect in some enzymatic antioxidant defenses besides a low uptake of some antioxidants such as vitamin E due to the blood-brain barrier, and (d) high amounts of some reactive trace metals such as iron, released from injured cell. In addition, studies have shown that some metals such as iron and aluminum can easily pass through the blood-brain barrier by using specific or nonspecific transporters and receptors, contributing to neurotoxicity through free radical formations (Yokel 2006; Shukla et al. 2011).

The effects of oxidative stress on proteins are highly dependent on the cell type affected. For example, non-mitotic cells have more concentrations of oxidized proteins than mitotic cells. Brain contains a mixture of mitotic and non-mitotic cells. The mitotic cells in the brain including astrocytes and microglia produce cytokines and growth factors that are essential for brain homeostasis. In contrast to postmitotic cells, microglia and astrocytes are exposed to less oxidative damage. Microglia can play a dual role both as neuroprotectives and as immunological defenders. In normal conditions, microglial cells maintain CNS homeostasis by scavenging dead or damaged neuron. But immunosenescence of the CNS will lead to microglial dysfunction that enhances the production of proinflammatory cytokines, TNF-α, interleukin (IL)-1β, and free radicals including superoxide and nitric oxide. NO acts on cytochrome oxidase to stop mitochondrial respiration and finally induce apoptosis in CNS cells (Streit and Xue 2010; Gemma 2010; Van der Veen et al. 1997).

Since oxidative stress has an important role in neurodegenerative diseases, treatment with antioxidants plus using rich antioxidant foods such as fresh fruits and vegetables in order to boost endogenous antioxidant defense system can slow down the disease progression.

24.10.4 Oxidative Stress and Autoimmunity

Autoimmune diseases have a multifactorial nature in which genetic, immunological, and environmental factors are involved. Free radicals have an important role in susceptibility to a wide range of autoimmune diseases by enhancing inflammation, inducing apoptosis, and breaking down the immunological tolerances. ROS are physiological activators of some transcriptional factors of proinflammatory cytokines such as activator protein-1 (AP-1) and nuclear factor kappa-light-chain-enhancer of activated B cells (NFκB).

Many proinflammatory cytokines (TNF-α, IL-1) and inducible nitric oxide increase during the process of autoimmune rheumatic disease (ARD). Both TNF-α and IL-1 create tremendous amounts of oxidative stress. Certain cells from the cartilage of an inflamed joint (called chondrocytes) can also actively generate free radicals. In addition, endothelium, macrophages, and antigen-presenting cells show increased expression of vascular cell adhesion molecule-1 (VCAM-1) adhesion molecules and E-selectin. Activation of macrophages, polymorphonuclears, and endothelial cells during infections, surgeries, and injuries causes the release of large amounts of ROS which in turn plays an important role in inflammation and tissue damage. Higher levels of oxidative and nitrosative stress were found in systemic lupus erythematosus (SLE) patients with higher disease activity. SLE in some cases is associated with osteoporosis and atherosclerosis and ROS play a major role in its pathophysiology. In the pancreas, beta cells are highly sensitive to both reactive oxygen species and reactive nitrogen species that are involved in beta cell destruction in type 1 diabetes by inducing apoptosis.

Many autoimmune diseases such as autoimmune rheumatic disease and SLE are associated with disequilibrium between oxidant and antioxidant defense systems which is due to an overproduction of ROS or antioxidant deficiency. Hence, proper nutrition can reduce oxidative stress by boosting endogenous antioxidant defense system. For example, high doses of vitamin E administered to patients with rheumatoid arthritis reduced pain symptom in these patients. Clinical studies have shown that anti-inflammatory effects of foods rich in antioxidants are associated with downregulation of NFκB in these patients.

Studies have also shown that patients with autoimmune rheumatic diseases have reduced amounts of antioxidants such as vitamin E, vitamin C, and vitamin A which can in turn play an important role in the pathogenesis of oxidative-related diseases. In addition, serum levels of antioxidant vitamins such as alpha-tocopherol, carotene, and retinol in stored serum samples of patients diagnosed with rheumatoid arthritis or SLE for 2–15 were less than normal.

Omega-3 fatty acids reduce production of the proinflammatory cytokines such as TNF-α and IL-1 that are implicated in many autoimmune diseases (SLE, ARD). Catechin and tea polyphenols can also significantly inhibit NFκB activation. Epigallocatechin 3-gallate (EGCG), the most abundant catechin in tea, can inhibit the degeneration of IkB induced by TNF-α and can also prevent NFκB activity in normal and cancer cells. Capsiate and dihydrocapsiate are substances naturally present in chili peppers that inhibit NFκB activation in response to different factors such as TNF-α. Curcumin, an important component of turmeric, is used as an anti-inflammatory substance in eastern traditional medicine. Resveratrol, an oral polyphenol found in red grape pigments, has antioxidant properties similar to vitamin E which inhibits NFκB activation induced by IL-1β in myeloid leukemia (Sukkar and Rossi 2003).

24.10.5 Oxidative Stress and Multiple Sclerosis

Multiple sclerosis (MS) is an autoimmune disease caused by demyelination or damage to the myelin sheath around neurons. Free radicals especially peroxynitrites play a major role in the pathogenesis of MS. Production of large amounts of reactive oxygen species by activated macrophages can cause axonal damage and demyelination. ROS can induce cell death by damaging cellular lipid, protein, DNA, and especially mitochondrial structure and function. Moreover, defective antioxidant defense system in central nervous system increases the incidence of neural and axonal oxidative damage in MS patients. So, antioxidant therapy plus an appropriate diet can boost the antioxidant defense system and consequently prevent the spread of tissue damage and improve clinical symptoms of MS (Gilgun-Sherki et al. 2004).

24.10.6 Oxidative Stress and Reproduction

Many factors including genetic, physiological, and environmental may contribute to infertility. About 15–20 % of couples in the reproductive age are infertile. Numerous studies have demonstrated that oxidative stress plays an important role in pathophysiology of both male and female infertility. Free radicals, depending on their levels, have a dual role in the reproductive tract. They not only are important signaling molecules involved in the regulation of various physiological processes but also play part in pathological processes in both male and female reproductive systems. It is suggested that age-related decline in fertility is induced by oxidative damage (Agarwal et al. 2006). Different treatments are available for infertile women or men. Occasional failure of such treatments is because the mechanisms of infertility are not fully understood.

Oxidative stress disrupts the growth, development, and function of gametes. Sperm and spermatozoa are unique in their structure and function. They have specific lipid components, containing large amount of polyunsaturated fatty acid (PUFA), plasmalogens, and sphingomyelins that provide their flexibility and function. During passage through the epididymis, sperms undergo changes in their membrane lipid content. As a result of these changes, plasmalogens become the basic components of the membrane phospholipids, and molar ratio of cholesterol to phospholipids increased twofold during sperm migration in semen tubes. Docosahexaenoic acid (DHA), one of the unsaturated fatty acid in sperm membrane, has a major role in the regulation of membrane fluidity and the regulation of spermatogenesis. Sperm membrane fatty acids including DHA, phosphatidylserine, desmosterol, and arachidonic acid play important roles in regulation of directional migration of sperm surface antigens during its developmental process such as maturation, and sperm membrane fatty acids such as sulphogalactosyl-glyserolipid and lysophosphatidylcholine are involved in the interaction of sperm with ovule. They increase the fertilizing capacity of spermatozoa, induce changes in zona pellucida, and promote the fusion of sperms and ovules. In more severe cases, this lipid peroxidation could inhibit spermatogenesis completely.

In addition, oxidative stress can damage sperm DNA, genes, and proteins through DNA base oxidation (especially Guanine) or through making disulfide bonds in DNA broken chains. It can also change the morphology, structure, and function of sperms and increase their sensitivity to macrophage invasion. Low molecular weight compounds such as antioxidant vitamins (vitamin E, A, C), flavonoids, and glutathione can significantly prevent such effects.

Our understanding about the role of oxidative stress in women infertility is not complete. Oxidant/antioxidant system pervades the female reproductive tissues, which is suggestive of its role in infertility. Follicules have potent sources of ROS including macrophages, neutrophils, and activated granules cells. Jozwik et al. (1999) showed the presence of oxidative stress markers in the serum and preovulatory follicular fluid of women who underwent in vitro fertilization (IVF) with lower amounts in follicular fluid in comparison with serum which shows a higher level of antioxidants in follicular fluid protecting oocyte from oxidative damage.

24.10.7 Oxidative Stress and Hypertension

Clinical studies have shown a mutual relationship between ROS production and hypertension. In laboratory models antioxidant therapy has reduced hypertension.

Most damages caused by ROS are related to superoxide anion ($O_2^{\cdot-}$). NAD(P)H oxidase is the primary source of superoxide anion in vascular wall smooth muscle cells. Several other factors (cytokines, growth factors, vasoactive mediators, and some physiological factors) are also involved in the regulation of NAD(P)H oxidase activity. In addition, polymorphonuclears and platelets serve as important sources of $\cdot O_2^-$ in inflammatory and vascular oxidative stress. Within physiological levels, ROS act as signaling molecules that are essential for regulation of vascular contraction-relaxation, cell growth, and structural maintenance by controlling endothelial cell activity. However, at pathological levels, ROS induces vascular injury and endothelial dysfunction and will increase vascular contractions.

Renin-angiotensin II activates NAD(P)H oxidase and induces ROS generation in vascular smooth muscle cells. P_{22} phox polymorphism (one of the NAD(P)H oxidase structural units) may be involved in superoxide anion production by NAD(P)H oxidase in cardiovascular diseases.

ROS react with endothelium-derived NO and reduce its anti-arteriosclerotic effects. ROS could either increase or decrease vessel diameter depending on its level. ROS can reduce a vessel diameter through other mechanisms such as arachidonic acid oxidation via producing PGF2α (a vasoconstrictor) and inhibiting PGI2 (a vasodilator). $\cdot O_2^-$ can activate other vasoconstrictors (angiotensin II, thromboxane-A2, endothellin-1, and norepinephrine) by increasing intracellular concentrations of calcium.

24.11 Nutrition and Diet

An appropriate diet can reduce the effects of oxidative stress and prevent chronic diseases, malignancies, and premature aging. For that purpose, it is generally recommended to consume at least 5 servings of fruits and vegetable per day, especially of the Amaryllidaceae (leek) family. Fruits and vegetables generally induce the activity of endogenous antioxidants due to their vitamin, fiber, and nonnutritive photochemical contents and other trace elements and minerals (e.g., selenium, zinc, copper, manganese, and magnesium). On the other hand, the more we consume fat and meat-containing products, more carcinogens and toxins we take in. Of many studies done regarding this topic, the following few merit mentioning:

- The diversity of different cells and tissues and the availability of different enzymes with antioxidant properties
- The vital role of epithelial and endothelial cells in detection and induction of endogenous antioxidants
- Genetic diversity and the vulnerability of certain genotypes and phenotypes to carcinogens and free radicals
- Extending the capacity and functionality of these enzymes through an appropriate diet

However, what remained yet to be clarified is the effects of diet on the interaction between these enzymes and antioxidants. The activity of an antioxidant above a certain point can itself be a source of free radicals and damage different tissues. Therefore, we still need to investigate the relationship between the amount of antioxidants used and different chronic disease and the aging process. It is also not yet determined if an inappropriate diet will have an effect on the metabolism of different substrates. For instance, a diet deficient in proteins will reduce the levels of monooxygenase and subsequently cytochrome P_{450} which can play a role in cell injuries due to free radicals. Such controversy can be demonstrated in rats in a study where CCl_4 caused lower rates of hepatotoxicity compared to acetaminophen in a low-protein diet. This is probably due to decreased levels of glutathione. Diets low in certain fatty acids (e.g., linoleic acid) can also lower cytochrome P_{450}. Less correlation has been reported when investigating the influence of sugars.

Vitamin deficiencies can also reduce the level of monooxygenase. However, in some rare cases, vitamin deficiencies have been linked to an increased activity of cytochrome P_{450}.

Conclusion

Many articles have recently been published in the field of free radicals, especially investigating superoxide (O_2^-) and the enzymes that neutralize it by dismutation, and still more research is being carried out every day.

Free radicals are molecules with a missing electron. They need to receive this electron from other molecules by oxidizing them, in which process they can damage the cell membrane and the DNA which can in turn lead to a mutation and eventually malignancies. These agents can be produced within the body as a result of metabolism or be taken in through different routes such as air or water pollutions, stress, inappropriate diets (like grilled, smoked, or canned foods or fuzzy drinks and other chemicals), smoking, ionizing and nonionizing radiations (e.g., X, γ, and other electromagnetic radiations), certain saturated fats, or some chemical therapeutics. On the other hand, we can utilize oxygen more efficiently by good habits like exercise and proper breathing techniques and exposure to clean environments and an appropriate diet. Various studies have demonstrated the role of antioxidants in prevention of different diseases such as diabetes, cataract, malignancies, rheumatoid arthritis, Alzheimer's disease, Parkinson's, cardiovascular diseases, and many other age-related disorders; but unfortunately no medications have been developed to be able to scavenge such wide range of oxidant agents.

The assessment of oxidative agents or the levels of free radicals and by the same token endogenous antioxidants is not yet a common practice in diagnostic laboratories, and therefore physicians cannot ask for them as diagnostic tests. Furthermore, drug companies do not show much interest in antioxidants.

A group of scientists in the National Institute of Health were able to show a link between human aging and free radicals as they accumulate inside the cells, and that as the cells get saturated by such toxic substance, they won't be able to survive anymore and will thus be terminated. Doctor Wickenheiser, a

Canadian researcher, spent more than 10 years studying the process of aging and why some people look younger and some look older than their actual age. He concluded that this process is dependent upon oxidation of different compounds and the formation of free radicals in the body which can be reversed by using antioxidants. Nonetheless, there is involvement of genetics which is not modifiable. However, biologic age can be change by lifestyle modification. He also asserts that it is never late to start living a healthier life and to stay young as our bodies very gradually deteriorate towards death and such process can be reversed by substituting old cells with new ones.

Finally, we can recommend the following methods to prevent premature aging:

- Living a stress-free life and increasing our tolerance against downfalls
- Getting enough rest and sleep
- Incorporating exercise and a healthy diet into our lifestyle
- Proper breathing techniques
- Minimizing the intake of toxins and using appropriate amounts of antioxidants and water
- Using a recommended dose of vitamins, minerals, and supplements
- And finally, having a sense of social support and spiritual and psychological well-being

References

Agarwal A, Gupta S, Sikka S (2006) The role of free radicals and antioxidants in reproduction. Curr Opin Obstet Gynecol 18:325–332

Alidoost F, Gharagozloo M, Bagherpour B et al (2006) Effects of silymarin on the proliferation and glutathione levels of peripheral blood mononuclear cells from beta-thalassemia major patients. Int Immunopharmacol 6:1305–1310

Babior BM, Kipnes RS, Curnutte JT (1973) Biological defense mechanisms. The production by leukocytes of superoxide, a potential bactericidal agent. J Clin Invest 52:741–744

Bagherpour B, Gharagozloo M, Moayedi B (2009) The influence of iron loading and iron chelation on the proliferation and telomerase activity of human periph-eral blood mononuclear cells. Iran J Immunol 6(1):33–39

Beckman KB, Ames BN (1998) The free radical theory of aging matures. Physiol Rev 78(2):547–581

Berger MM (2005) Can oxidative damage be treated nutritionally? Clin Nutr 24(2):172–183

Cho YS, Moon HB (2010) The role of oxidative stress in the pathogenesis of asthma. Allergy Asthma Immunol Res 2(3):183–187

Danielson P (2002) The cytochrome P450 superfamily: biochemistry, evolution and drug metabolism in humans. Curr Drug Metab 3(6):561–597

De Martinis M, Franceschi C, Monti D et al (2007) Apoptosis remodeling in immunosenescence: implication for strategies to delay aging. Curr Med Chem 14(13):1389–1397

Finkel T, Holbrook NJ (2000) Oxidants, oxidative stress and the biology of ageing. Nature 408:239–247

Forsyth NR, Evans AP, Shay JW et al (2003) Developmental differences in the immortalization of lung fibroblasts by telomerase. Aging Cell 2(5):235–243

Fusco D, Colloca G, Lo Monaco MR et al (2007) Effects of antioxidant supplementation on the aging process. Clin Interv Aging 2(3):377–387

Gemma G (2010) Neuroimmunomodulation and aging. Aging Dis 1(3):169–172

Gilgun-Sherki Y, Melamed E, Offen D (2004) The role of oxidative stress in the pathogenesis of multiple sclerosis: the need for effective antioxidant therapy. J Neurol 251(3):261–268

Ginaldi L, De Martinis M, Moniti D et al (2005) Chronic antigenic load and apoptosis in immunosenescence. Trends Immunol 26(2):79–84

Goel R, Khanduja KL (1998) Oxidative stress-induced apoptosis – an overview. Curr Sci 75(12):1338

Gutteridge JMC (1993) Free radicals in disease processes – a compilation of cause and consequence. Free Radic Res Commun 19:141–158

Herrera E, Barbas C (2001) Vitamin E: action, metabolism and perspectives. J Physiol Biochem 57(2):43–56

Jozwik M, Wolczynski S, Jozwik M et al (1999) Oxidative stress markers in preovulatory follicular fluid in humans. Mol Hum Reprod 5(5):409–413

King C, Rios G, Green M et al (2000) UDP-glucuronosyltransferases. Curr Drug Metab 1(2):143–161

Ku HH, Brunk UT, Sohal RS (1993) Relationship between mitochondrial superoxide and hydrogen peroxide production and longevity of mammalian species. Free Radic Biol Med 15(6):621–627

Meister A, Anderson ME (1983) Glutathione. Annu Rev Biochem 52:711–760

Pollack M, Leeuwenburgh C (1999) Handbook of oxidants and antioxidants in exercise. Elsevier, Amsterdam

Ryan MJ, Dudash HJ, Docherty M et al (2010) Vitamin E and C supplementation reduces oxidative stress, improves antioxidant enzymes and positive muscle work in chronically loaded muscles of aged rats. Exp Gerontol 45(11):882–895

Sheehan D, Meade G, Foley V et al (2001) Structure, function and evolution of glutathione transferases: implications for classification of non-mammalian members of an ancient enzyme superfamily. Biochem J 360:1–16

Shukla V, Mishra SK, Pant HC (2011) Oxidative stress in neurodegeneration. Adv Pharmacol Sci. doi:10.1155/2011/572634

Streit WJ, Xue QS (2010) The brain's aging immune system. Aging Dis 1(3):254–261

Sukkar SG, Rossi E (2003) Oxidative stress and nutritional prevention in autoimmune rheumatic disease. Autoimmun Rev 3:199–206

Tchirkov A, Lansdorp PM (2003) Role of oxidative stress in telomere shortening in cultured fibroblasts from normal individuals and patients with ataxia–telangiectasia. Hum Mol Genet 12(3):227–232

Valko M, Leibfritz D, Moncol J et al (2007) Free radicals and antioxidants in normal physiological functions and human disease. Int J Biochem Cell Biol 39:44–84

Van der Veen RC, Hinton DR, Incardonna F et al (1997) Extensive peroxynitrite activity during progressive stages of central nervous system inflammation. J Neuroimmunol 77:1–7

von Zglinicki T (2000) Role of oxidative stress in telomere length regulation and replicative senescence. Ann N Y Acad Sci 908:99–110

Yokel RA (2006) Blood brain barrier flux of aluminum, manganese, iron and other metals suspected to contribute to metal-induced neurodegeneration. J Alzheimers Dis 10(2–3):223–253

Zarban A, Ziaee M (2008) Evaluation of antioxidant properties of silymarin and its potential to inhibit peroxyl radicals in vitro. Pak J Pharm Sci 21(3):249–254

Zhu H, Belcher M, van der Harst P (2011) Healthy aging and disease: role for telomere biology? Clin Sci 120:427–440

Skin Aging and Immune System

25

Parvin Mansouri, Reza Chalangari,
Katalin Martits Chalangari, and Zahra Saffarian

25.1 Introduction

For those of you who are reading this chapter and are 30–40 years of age, taking a look at the back of your hands is destined to be a somewhat boring experience. Yet if you look at the skin on the back of children's hands and then at the same area on your parent's hands, you cannot fail to see major differences in texture, color, and elasticity—all of which should provoke major questions. They seem to do so but, regrettably, too rarely. In both developed and developing nations, the number and proportion of older people are increasing.

By 2030, 30 % of the population will be over 65 years old. Elderly experience significantly more skin problems than do those in the younger age groups. Some of these disorders are unique to the elderly that need specialized knowledge and skill for their efficient management.

Research into skin aging is at a low ebb, and studies of skin disease in old age are similarly in short supply, this is both surprising and sad. Knowledge about the skin through the ages and its effects on the skin immune system will help us to better take care of our senior citizens. In this chapter, we have a short review on the skin structure and its immune system and immunological responses and then aging of skin and age-related changes in immune function of the skin will be discussed.

25.2 Basic Structure and Function of Skin

The skin is composed of three layers: the epidermis, dermis, and subcutaneous fat (panniculus). This organ is composed of diverse cell types of both ectodermal (e.g., keratinocytes, melanocytes, Merkel cells, neurons) and mesodermal (e.g., fibroblasts, hematopoietic, cells such as Langerhans cells, endothelial cells) lineages.

The epidermis may be divided into the following zones (starting from the innermost layer): basal layer (stratum germinativum), malpighian or prickle layer (stratum spinosum), granular layer (stratum granulosum), and horny layer (stratum corneum) that is composed of keratin and cover the viable epidermis.

25.2.1 Epidermis

The adult epidermis is composed of three basic cell types: keratinocytes, melanocyte, and Langerhans cells. In addition, Merkel cells can be found in the basal layers of the palms and soles, oral and genital mucosa, nail bed, and

P. Mansouri, MD (✉) • Z. Saffarian, MD
Dermatology Department,
Skin and Stem Cell Research Center,
Tehran University of Medical Sciences, Tehran, Iran
e-mail: mansorip@sina.tums.ac.ir

R. Chalangari, MD • K.M. Chalangari, MD
Monalisa Dermatology,
Skin and Stem Cell Research Center,
Tehran University of Medical Sciences, Tehran, Iran

A. Massoud, N. Rezaei (eds.), *Immunology of Aging*,
DOI 10.1007/978-3-642-39495-9_25, © Springer-Verlag Berlin Heidelberg 2014

follicular infundibula. Keratinocytes or squamous cells are the principal cells of the epidermis that play an active role in the immune function of the skin. Melanocytes are the pigment-producing cells derived from the neural crest and reside in the basal layer at a frequency of approximately 1 in every 10 basal keratinocytes. Langerhans cells are normally found scattered among keratinocytes of the stratum spinosum. Functionally, Langerhans cells are of the monocyte-macrophage lineage and originate in the bone marrow. They function primarily in immune response by recognition, uptake, processing, and presentation of antigens to sensitized T lymphocytes.

Epidermis is a major permeability barrier, an active member of innate immunity, has adhesion and ultraviolet protection functions.

25.2.2 Dermis

The constituents of the dermis are mesodermal in origin except for nerves. The dermis is merely a pool of acid mucopolysaccharide-containing, scattered dendritic-shaped cells, which are the precursors of fibroblasts. Dermis has three types of components-cellular: fibrous matrix, diffuse matrix, and filamentous matrix. Dermis is also the site of vascular, lymphatic, and nerve networks. Collagen, a family of fibrous proteins in human skin that represent 70 % of the dry weight of skin, is the principle component of the dermis. Elastic fibers in dermis contribute very little to resisting deformation and tearing of skin but have a role in maintaining elasticity.

Eccrine, apocrine glands, and pilosebaceous units constitute the skin adnexa. While the various adnexal structures serve specific functions, they can function as reserve epidermis after injury to the surface epidermis occurs.

Dermal mast cells play an important role in the normal immune response. Cutaneous mast cells respond to environmental changes. Dry environments result in an increase in the mast cell number and histamine production.

25.2.3 Subcutaneous Fat

Beneath the dermis lies the panniculus, lobules of fat cells, or lipocytes separated by fibrous septa composed of collagen and large blood vessels. These vessels serve to transport nutrients and immigrant cells. The tissue of the hypodermis insulates the body, serves as a reserve energy supply, cushions and protects the skin, and allows for its mobility over underlying structures. Panniculus functions as a repository of energy and an endocrine organ. The hormone leptin, secreted by adipocytes, provides a long-term feedback signal regulating fat mass.

25.3 Immune System

The human immune system is comprised of two distinct functional parts: (1) innate and (2) adaptive.

Cells of the innate immune system, including macrophages and dendritic cells (DCs), respond to biochemical structures commonly shared by a variety of different pathogens and elicit a rapid response against these pathogens. In contrast, cells of the adaptive immune system, T and B lymphocytes, bear specific antigen receptors and in comparison to the innate response, develops more slowly. A unique feature of the adaptive immune response is its ability to generate and retain memory. Although the innate and adaptive immune responses are distinct, they interact and act in synergy.

25.4 Skin and Immunity

The skin forms the body's largest interface with the environment and its principal function is that of a barrier. It protects the organism by being impermeable to a multitude of harmful exogenous substances and maintains internal homeostasis by preventing excessive water and heat loss. In addition, there is a highly specialized immune system consisting of leukocytes that are resident, recruited, or recirculated within the

Table 25.1 Cells of the adaptive and innate immune system in the skin

	Resident	Recruited	Recirculating
Innate	Keratinocytes	Monocytes	Natural killer cells
	Endothelial cells	Granulocytes	Dendritic cells
	Vascular	Basophilic	Promonocytes[a]
	Lymphatic	Eosinophilic	
	Dendritic cells	Neutrophilic	
	Mast cells	Mast cells	
	Tissue macrophages	Epitheloid cells	
Adaptive	T lymphocytes	T lymphocytes	T lymphocytes
		B lymphocytes	

[a]Indicates that there is a possibility, in this case, rather than strong evidence

tissue (Table 25.1). These cells are distributed in the epidermal and dermal layers of the skin and participate in both adaptive and innate immune responses. They are also responsible for distinguishing self from nonself which is of fundamental importance since the skin comes into daily contact with exogenous substances. Close interlinking between innate and adaptive pathways of immunity plays an important role in the initiation and amplification of immune responses in this tissue (Vukmanovic-Stejic et al. 2011).

25.5   Innate Immune Response

Immune mechanisms that are used by the host to immediately defend itself are referred to as innate immunity. These include physical barriers such as the skin and mucosal epithelium; soluble factors such as complement, antimicrobial peptides, chemokines, and cytokines; and cells, including monocytes/macrophages, DCs, natural killer cells (NK cells), and polymorphonuclear leukocytes (PMNs).

25.5.1 Physical and Chemical Barriers

Physical structures prevent most pathogens and environmental toxins from harming the host. Skin, once thought to be an inert structure, plays a vital role in protecting the individual from the external environment (Elias 2005).

25.5.2 Complement

One of the first innate defense mechanisms that await pathogens that overcome the epithelial barrier is the alternative pathway of complement. Unlike the classical complement pathway that requires antibody triggering, the lectin-dependent pathway as well as alternative pathway of complement activation can be spontaneously activated by microbial surfaces in the absence of specific antibodies (Gasque 2004).

25.5.3 Antimicrobial Peptides

The antimicrobial activity of these peptides is thought to relate to their ability to bind membranes of microbes and form pores in the membrane, leading to microbial killing. There are numerous antimicrobial peptides identified in various human tissues and secretions. Human β-defensins (HBD-1, HBD-2, HBD-3), cathelicidin (LL-37), psoriasin, and RNase 7, which have all been demonstrated to be produced by keratinocytes, and dermcidin, which is secreted in human sweat are antimicrobial peptides identified in resident skin cells (Braff et al. 2005; Schauber and Gallo 2008).

β-defensins are cysteine-rich cationic low-molecular-weight antimicrobial peptides (Harder et al. 1997). Furthermore, evidence indicating that human β-defensins attract DCs and memory T cells via CC chemokine receptor 6 (CCR6) provides a link between the innate and the adaptive immunity in skin (Yang et al. 1999).

Cathelicidins are produced by skin cells, including keratinocytes, mast cells, neutrophils, and ductal cells of eccrine glands (Nizet et al. 2001; Ong et al. 2002). Neutrophil proteases play an important role in cutaneous host defense because of its pronounced antibacterial (Nizet et al. 2001; Ong et al. 2002), antifungal (Lopez-Garcia et al. 2005), and antiviral activities (Howell et al. 2006a, b).

Dermcidin is an antimicrobial peptide expressed by human sweat glands. These peptides have broad antimicrobial activity against *S. aureus*, *E. coli*, *E. faecalis*, and *C. albicans* (Schittek et al. 2001; Senyurek et al. 2009).

25.5.4 Toll-Like Receptors

Toll-like Receptors (TLRs) recognize pathogen-associated molecular patterns (PAMPs) present in a variety of bacteria, fungi, and viruses. TLRs are expressed at sites that are exposed to microbial threats. Also activation of TLRs induces signaling pathways and TLRs directly activate host defense mechanisms that then combat the foreign invader (Akira et al. 2006).

TLR activation of a variety of cell types has been shown to trigger release of both pro-inflammatory and immunomodulatory cytokines (Hirschfeld et al. 1999; Hou et al. 2000; Medzhitov and Janeway 1997; Takeuchi et al. 1999; Yang et al. 1998).

TLRs can regulate phagocytosis either through enhancing endosomal fusion with the lysosomal compartment. In addition, activation of TLRs on immature DC leads to further maturation with enhanced T-cell stimulatory capacity (Blander and Medzhitov 2004; Doyle et al. 2004).

25.5.5 Phagocytes

Two key cells of the innate immune system are characterized by their phagocytic function: macrophages and PMNs.

PMNs are normally not present in skin; however, during inflammatory processes, these cells migrate to the site of infection and inflammation, where they are the earliest phagocytic cells to be recruited.

Activation of phagocytes by pathogens induces several important effector mechanisms, for example, triggering of cytokine production. A number of important cytokines are secreted by macrophages in response to microbes, including interleukin (IL)-l, IL-6, tumor necrosis factor alpha (TNF-α), IL-8, IL-12, and IL-10.

25.5.6 Natural Killer Cells

NK cells appear as large granular lymphocytes. Their function is to survey the body, looking for altered cells, either transformed or infected with viruses, bacteria, or parasites. These pathogens are then killed directly via perforin/granzyme- or Fas/Fas ligand (FasL)-dependent mechanisms or indirectly via the secretion of cytokines (e.g., interferon gamma or IFN-γ) (Jinquan et al. 1996).

25.5.7 Keratinocytes

Once thought to only play a role in maintaining the physical barrier of the skin, keratinocytes, the predominant cells in the epidermis, can participate in innate immunity by mounting an immune response through secretion of cytokines and chemokines, arachidonic acid metabolites, complement components, and antimicrobial peptides.

In addition to cytokines, keratinocytes secrete other factors such as neuropeptides, eicosanoids, and reactive oxygen species (Kupper and Groves 1995).

25.6   Adaptive Immune Response

25.6.1 B Lymphocytes

B cells mature in the fetal liver and adult bone marrow. They produce antibody complexes. In general, antibodies bind to microbial agents and neutralize them or facilitate uptake of the pathogen by phagocytes that destroy them. Antibodies are also responsible for mediating certain pathologic conditions in skin. In particular, antibodies against self-antigens lead to autoimmune disease (Chen et al. 2009).

25.6.2 T Lymphocytes

T cells mature in the thymus, where they are selected to live or to die. Those T cells that will have the capacity to recognize foreign antigens are positively selected and can enter the circulation. T cells release cytokines that activate NK cells and permit the growth, differentiation, and activation of B cells (Shibata et al. 2007).

25.6.3 CD4⁺ Helper T Cells

CD4$^+$ T cells are critical for helping B cells to produce antibodies by triggering their differentiation into plasma cells. To our current knowledge, CD4$^+$ T cells represent a heterogeneous cell population. Effector CD4$^+$ T cells protect against pathogens mainly by their production of T helper (Th)1, Th2, or Th17 cytokines. In contrast, regulatory CD4$^+$ T cells have the capacity to downregulate disproportionate effector responses to antigen.

25.6.4 T Helper 1/T Helper 2 Paradigm

T cells that produce IL-2, IFN-γ, and TNF are termed Th1 cells. They are the main carriers of cell-mediated immunity (CMI). Other T cells produce IL-4, IL-5, IL-6, IL-13, and IL-15. These are termed Th2 cells (Abbas et al. 1996; Mosmann et al. 1986).

Th1 cells, primarily by the release of IFN-γ, activate macrophages to kill or inhibit the growth of the pathogen and trigger cytotoxic T cells. In contrast, Th2 cells facilitate humoral responses and inhibit some cell-mediated immune responses, which results in progressive infection (Gately et al. 1998).

25.6.5 T-Regulatory Cells

An important type of immunomodulatory T cells that controls immune responses are the so-called T-regulatory cells (T-reg cells), formerly known as T-suppressor cells (Shevach et al. 2006). These cells are induced by immature antigen presenting cells (APCs)/DCs and play key roles in maintaining tolerance to self-antigens in the periphery. T-reg cells are also critical for controlling the magnitude and duration of immune responses to microbes.

25.6.6 Lymphocytes in Normal and Diseased Skin

Normal human skin contains approximately one million T cells per cm^2, 2–3 % of which reside within the epidermis, primarily in the basal and suprabasal layers. The T cells of the dermis are clustered around postcapillary venules of the superficial plexus that are situated just beneath the dermal-epidermal junction and close to adnexal appendages such as hair follicles and eccrine sweat ducts (Clark et al. 2006a).

25.6.7 Antigen-Presenting Cells

DCs, including Langerhans cells (LCs) and dermal dendritic cells (DDCs), B cells, and activated monocytes/macrophages are the major APC populations.

25.6.7.1 Langerhans Cells

In 1S6S, a medical student named Paul Langerhans, driven by his interest in the anatomy of skin nerves, identified a population of dendritically shaped cells in the suprabasal regions of the epidermis after impregnating human skin with gold salts (Langerhans 1868). These cells, which later were found in virtually all stratified squamous epithelia of mammals, are now eponymously referred to as Langerhans cells.

The expression of the Ca^{2+}-dependent lectin Langerin (CD207) is currently the single best feature discriminating LCs from other cells. Birbeck granules are cytoplasmic structures frequently displaying a tennis racket shape.

The tissue distribution of LC varies regionally in the human skin. On head, face, neck, trunk, and limb skin, the LC density ranges between 600 and 1,000/mm^2. Comparatively low densities are found in palms, soles, anogenital and sacrococcygeal skin, and the buccal mucosa. The density of human LCs decreases with age, and LC counts in skin with chronic actinic damage are significantly lower than those in skin not exposed to ultra violet (UV) light (Schuster et al. 2009).

Upon perturbation of skin homeostasis (e.g., TLR ligation, contact with chemical haptens, hypoxia), LCs gain access to antigen/allergen encountering the epidermis by distending their dendrites through epidermal tight junctions, thereby demonstrating strikingly remarkable cooperation between keratinocytes and LC (Kubo et al. 2009). After a few hours, LCs begin to enlarge, to display increased amounts of surface-bound MHC class II molecules, and to migrate downward in the dermis, where they enter afferent lymphatics and, finally, reach the lymph nodes (Larsen et al. 1990). The mechanisms governing LC migration are becoming increasingly clear. TNF-α and IL-1β are critical promoters of this process, whereas IL-10 inhibits its occurrence.

25.6.7.2 Dermal Dendritic Cells

Like LCs in the epidermis, dermal dendritic cells (DDCs) constitute another DC subpopulation in normal and inflamed skin (Meunier et al. 1993). They can be distinguished from LCs by the absence of Langerin and lack of Birbeck granules. They possess functional features of both macrophages and DCs, i.e., capacity of phagocytosis as well as antigen-presenting, migratory, and T-cell-stimulating capacities.

25.6.7.3 Inflammatory Dendritic Cells

DCs appearing in inflamed skin can be subdivided into two major subpopulations, i.e., (1) inflammatory dendritic epidermal/dermal cells (IDECs/IDDCs) and (2) plasmacytoid dendritic cells (pDCs).

25.6.7.4 Plasmacytoid Dendritic Cells

pDCs are DCs that are characterized by a highly developed endoplasmic reticulum, which results in their plasma cell-like appearance (Kohrgruber et al. 1999; Lande and Gilliet 2010). Functionally, pDCs display a unique ability to produce up to 1,000 times more natural IFNs than any other blood mononuclear cell in response to TLR

ligands and thus were also named principal type 1 IFN-producing cells (Siegal et al. 1999).

25.7 Effects of Aging

Aging is a process of progressive decreases in the maximal functioning and reserve capacity of all organs in the body, including the skin. This naturally occurring functional decline in the skin is often compounded and accelerated by chronic environmental insults, such as UV and infrared (IR) irradiation as well as environmental carcinogens present in polluted air of major urban centers.

Aging occurs at the cellular level and reflects both a genetic program and cumulative environmentally imposed damage. Mammalian cells can undergo only a limited number of cell divisions and then arrest irreversibly in a state known as replicative senescence, after which they are refractory to mitogenic stimuli. This fact has led to the perception that aging evolved in multicellular organisms as a cancer prevention mechanism.

25.8 Aging Mechanism

25.8.1 Telomeres and Aging

Telomeres, the terminal portions of eukaryotic chromosomes, consist of up to many hundreds of tandem short sequence repeats (TTAGGG in all mammals). During mitosis of somatic cells, DNA polymerase cannot replicate the final base pairs of each chromosome, resulting in progressive shortening with each round of cell division. A special reverse transcriptase, telomerase, can replicate these chromosomal cells. The enzyme is normally expressed at extremely low levels (Davis et al. 2006). Although at low levels, telomerase is expressed in epidermal cells in vivo. In skin, the relatively quiescent fibroblasts and melanocytes and keratinocytes exhibit only minor age-dependent telomere shortening of 11–25 bp (base pairs) per year. Telomeres appear to serve as a biologic clock that determines proliferative life span and functional level of the cell.

25.8.2 DNA Damage and Aging

Studies in human premature aging diseases suggest that decreased DNA repair capacity is associated with accelerated aging and that cumulative DNA damage plays a major role in the aging process. One system that is particularly susceptible to DNA damage is that of growth hormone (GH) and insulin growth factor (IGF) (Garinis et al. 2008).

Data from a study in rat showed that GH and melatonin treatment seem to have beneficial effects against age-induced damage in the central nerves system (CNS), the liver, and the skin through molecular mechanisms reducing oxidative stress and apoptosis (Tresguerres et al. 2008).

Silent information regulator proteins, sirtuins are a class of protein deacetylases implicated in slowing the aging process. It is suggested that they maintain telomere structural integrity, induce transcriptional silencing of genes that promote aging, and/or modulate mitochondrial function in response to caloric restriction (Kaeberlein 2010). Resveratrol, a phenolic substance present in red wine is thought to be sirtuin activator (Howitz et al. 2003). Several studies strongly support a role of cumulative cellular damage, particularly DNA damage, in the aging process and proficient repair of such damage in longevity.

25.8.3 Oxidative Stress

The skin, like other bodily systems, is continuously exposed to reactive oxygen species (ROS) generated during aerobic metabolism.

Although the skin contains a network of antioxidant enzymes (superoxide dismutases, catalase, and glutathione peroxidase) and non-enzymatic antioxidant molecules (vitamin E, coenzyme Q10, ascorbate, and carotenoids), this system is less than completely effective and tends to deteriorate with aging.

Oxidative stress upregulates the level of stress regulatory proteins, including hypoxia-inducible factors (HIFs) and nuclear factor kappa-light-chain-enhancer of activated B cells (NFκB). Both HIFs and NFκB induce the expression of proinflammatory cytokines like IL-1 and IL-6, vascular endothelial growth factor (VEGF), and TNF-α. These proteins are involved in immuno-regulation and cell survival (Ruland and Mak 2003), stimulate the expression of matrix-degrading metalloproteins (Kang et al. 2001), and are believed to play a central role in the aging process. Furthermore, HIFs stabilize sub-populations of malignant cells with stem cell properties (cancer stem cells). This suggests that age-associated cellular hypoxia could be involved in cancer stem cell maintenance.

Oxidative damage also affects telomeres. A recent hypothesis suggests a common cellular signaling pathway activated by DNA damage and involving the terminal portion of the telomeres (Kosmadaki and Gilchrest 2004; Li et al. 2003). The terminal portion of the 3′ telomeric strand extends beyond the complementary 5′ strand, leaving a single stranded G-rich overhang. It is suggested that during both telomere shortening and repair of telomere damage, such as that encountered by oxidative stress, the normal loop structure at the end of telomeres is disrupted, exposing the 3′ overhang that under baseline conditions is "buried" in the loop structure (Kosmadaki and Gilchrest 2004; Li et al. 2003). Exposure of the TTAGGG tandem repeat sequence then appears to activate p53 (Eller et al. 2002) and to stimulate responses known to include proliferative senescence and apoptosis (Eller et al. 2002; Li et al. 2003). Thus, the intrinsic component of skin aging involves progressive oxidative stress and telomere signaling as telomeres shorten during serial cell division and in response to oxidative DNA damage (Kosmadaki and Gilchrest 2004).

25.9 Skin Aging

Cutaneous aging includes two distinct phenomena. Intrinsic aging is a universal, presumptively inevitable change attributable to the passage of time alone; extrinsic aging is the superposition on intrinsic aging of changes attributable to chronic environmental insults, sun exposure, which are neither universal nor inevitable. Extrinsic skin aging is also commonly termed photoaging, reflecting the large and well-studied role of chronic sun exposure. The former is manifested primarily by physiologic alterations with subtle but undoubtedly important consequences for both healthy and diseased skin. The latter has major morphologic as well as physiologic manifestations and corresponds more closely to the popular notion of old skin.

Clinically, naturally aged skin is smooth, pale, and finely wrinkled. In contrast, photoaged skin is coarsely wrinkled and associated with dyspigmentation and telangiectasia. The most dramatic histological differences between intrinsic aging and photoaging occur within the dermis (Gilchrest 1989; Lavker 1979).

Alterations in collagen, the major structural component of the skin, have been suggested to be a cause of the clinical changes observed in photoaged and naturally aged skin.

25.10 Intrinsic Skin Aging

The skin changes that occur with aging (Table 25.2) lead to a gradual physiologic decline (Table 25.3). Major age-related changes in the skin's appearance include dryness (roughness), wrinkling, laxity, and a variety of benign neoplasms. Aged skin is inelastic and recovers more slowly after injury (Fig. 25.1).

The intrinsic component of skin aging involves progressive oxidative stress and telomere signaling, as telomeres shorten during serial cell division and in response to oxidative DNA damage.

Another mechanism playing a role in intrinsic aging is cellular senescence, the limited capacity of cells to divide. It is regarded by some as a cancer preventive mechanism.

Senescent cells display critically short telomeres, irreversible growth arrest, resistance to apoptosis, and altered differentiation.

Additional mechanisms include amino acid racemization, affecting protein function, and rendering them less susceptible to degradation. Finally, nonenzymatic glycosylation of extracellular matrix proteins, such as dermal collagen, leads to cross-linking with trapping and sequestration of other unaffected proteins.

25.10.1 Epidermis

The most striking and consistent histologic change is flattening of the dermal-epidermal junction with effacement of both the dermal papillae and epidermal rete pegs (Kurban and Bhawan 1990).

This results in a considerably smaller surface between the epidermis and dermis and presumably less communication and nutrient transfer. Dermal-epidermal separation occurs more readily in old skin, undoubtedly explaining the propensity of the elderly to torn skin and superficial abrasions after minor trauma.

There is an age-associated epidermal thinning of 10–50 % between the ages of 30 and 80 years (Wulf et al. 2004). Evidence suggests that epidermal keratinocytes senesce and senescent cells are more resistant to apoptosis. Therefore, such keratinocytes are more likely to accumulate mutations, increasing their risk for malignant transformation. There are controversies about the age-associated changes in the number and

Table 25.2 Histologic features of aging human skin

Epidermis	Dermis	Appendages
Flattened dermal-epidermal junction	Atrophy (loss of dermal volume)	Depigmented hair loss of hair
Variable/decreased thickness	Fewer fibroblasts	Conversion of terminal to vellus hair
Variable cell size and shape	Fewer mast cells	Abnormal nail plates
Occasional nuclear atypia	Fewer blood vessels	Fewer glands
Fewer melanocytes	Shortened capillary loops	
Fewer Langerhans cells	Abnormal nerve endings	

function of epidermal stem cells, a population of cells responsible for epidermal maintenance (Youn et al. 2004). Average thickness and degree of compaction of the stratum corneum appear constant with increasing age. There is an overall decreased lipid content in the stratum corneum of the elderly as well as decreased water content in part as a result of decrements in cholesterol synthesis. Age-associated increase in stratum corneum pH impedes lipid-processing enzyme activity (Choi et al. 2007). Age effects on

Table 25.3 Functions of human skin that decline with age

| Barrier function |
| Cell replacement |
| Chemical clearance |
| DNA repair |
| Epidermal hydration |
| Immune responsiveness |
| Mechanical protection |
| Sebum production |
| Sensory perception |
| Sweat production |
| Thermoregulation |
| Vitamin D production |
| Wound healing |

percutaneous absorption depend in part on drug structure, with hydrophilic substances such as hydrocortisone and benzoic acid being less well absorbed through the skin of old, but with hydrophobic substances such as testosterone and estradiol being equally well absorbed. Of perhaps greater clinical importance, aging markedly delays the recovery of barrier function in damaged stratum corneum.

In the elderly, the skin often appears dry and flaky, especially over the lower extremities, an area in which a remarkable age-associated decrease in the content of epidermal filaggrin has been reported. Filaggrin, required for binding of keratin filaments into macrofibrils, and its lack may cause the increased scaliness. Barrier function also may be affected by this structural change.

Epidermal turnover rate and thymidine-labeling index decrease approximately 30–50 % between the third and eighth decades, with a corresponding prolongation in stratum corneum replacement rate. Linear growth rates also decrease for hair and nails. Epidermal repair rate after wounding likewise declines with age.

A decrease in the number of enzymatically active melanocytes per unit surface area of the

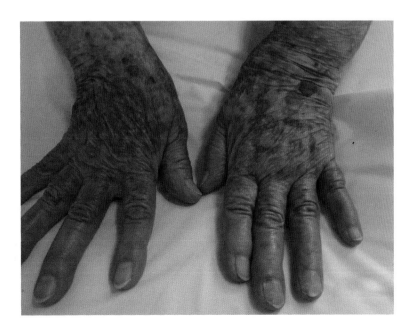

Fig. 25.1 Intrinsic skin aging, fine wrinkling, dryness, laxity, and benign neoplasms (seborrheic keratoses)

skin reduces the body's protective barrier against UV radiation. Age-associated decline in DNA repair capacity compounds the loss of protective melanin and increases the risk for skin cancer development. The number of melanocytic nevi also decrease from a peak of 15–40 in the third and fourth decade to an average of four per person after age 50 years; such nevi are rarely observed in person beyond age 80 (Plowden et al. 2004).

An endocrine function of human epidermis that declines with age is vitamin D production. Vitamin D, by binding to its nuclear receptor (1,25- dihydroxyvitamin D3 receptor or 1,25D-VDR), induces the transcription of numerous genes including those that encode proteins affecting the formation of the cornified epithelium as well as hair growth; 1,25D-VDR also activates genes that encode proteins that participate in the innate and adaptive immune responses and repress IL-17, a major inducer for autoimmune disorders such as type I diabetes mellitus, multiple sclerosis, lupus, and rheumatoid arthritis. 1,25D-VDR is also anti-inflammatory, as it decreases NFκB and cyclooxygenase (COX2) activation. Finally, 1,25D-VDR induces the activity of the tumor suppressor p53 and p21 proteins and the activity of FoxO, preventing oxidative damage and inducing DNA repair enzymes in skin. Avoidance of dairy products, insufficient sun exposure, sunscreen use, and decrease in the level of epidermal 7-dehydrocholesterol an immediate biosynthetic precursor for Vitamin D undoubtedly contribute to vitamin D deficiency in the elderly. Together, these observations suggest that age-associated decrease in Vitamin D could accelerate the aging process and argue for use of vitamin D dietary supplements in the elderly.

With regard to susceptibility to oxidative damage, there is progressive accumulation of damaged cellular proteins and lipids with aging. Furthermore, antioxidant defense systems decline with age, and, in addition, there is a decrease in DNA damage repair capacity. These changes in combination increase cellular mutability or their tendency to become senescent or both.

25.10.2 Dermis

Loss of dermal thickness approaches 20 % in elderly individuals, although in sun-protected sites significant thinning occurs only after the eighth decade. Old dermis is relatively acellular and avascular, and there is age-related loss of normal elastic fibers and dermal collagen.

Decreased inflammatory responses in the elderly are the result of decreased synthesis and secretion of keratinocyte-derived cytokines and inflammatory mediators in addition to decreased endothelial response. The striking age-associated loss of vascular bed, especially of the vertical capillary loops that occupy the dermal papillae in young skin, and increased distance from the epidermis of existing loops are thought to underlie many of the physiologic alterations in old skin, including pallor, decreased skin temperature, and the approximately 60 % reductions in basal and peak induced cutaneous blood flow.

VEGF of epidermal origin appears to play a major role in maintaining dermal vasculature, inducing the expression of antiapoptotic proteins in endothelial cells, and decreased VEGF level shown in aged mice and rabbit's skin probably contributes to endothelial cells apoptosis. Also, evidence suggests that there is an age-associated decline of both angiogenic and antiangiogenic factors, disrupting cutaneous angiogenic homeostasis. Decreased endothelial cell permeability response and decreased capacity to induce white cell adhesion contribute to the compromised immune response. Compromised thermoregulation, which predisposes the elderly to sometimes fatal heat stroke or hypothermia, may be due in part to reduced vasoactivity of dermal arterioles and, in the latter instance, to loss of heat-conserving subcutaneous fat as well. Reduction in the vascular network surrounding hair bulbs and eccrine, apocrine, and sebaceous glands may contribute to their gradual atrophy and fibrosis with age. Impaired transfer of cells as well as solutes between the extravascular and intravascular dermal compartments is suggested by several studies.

With aging, there is a decrease in the density and lumen size of lymphatic vessels accompanied by increased rigidity and decrements in lymphatic drainage, affected by decreased surrounding elastic fibers and in part because of decreased activity of enzymes that catalyze the production of nitric oxide (NO) (Gashev and Zawieja 2010).

Biochemical changes in collagen, elastin, and dermal ground substance lead to increased skin rigidity primarily due to modifications in collagen. Collagen content per unit area of skin surface decreases approximately 1 % per year throughout adult life, and the maintaining collagen fibrils appear disorganized, more compact, and granular, and they display increased collagen cross-links. Such changes almost certainly contribute to impaired wound healing in the elderly.

Beginning in early adulthood, elastic fibers decrease in number and diameter; by old age, they often appear fragmented, with small cysts and lacunae, especially near the dermal-epidermal junction most likely due to enzymatic degradation of elastin. Elastic fibers also show progressive cross-linkage and calcification with age.

At the biochemical level, there is an age-associated decrease in numerous elastic fiber components, including elastin, fibrillin, and fibulin-2. With aging, the level of fibulin-5, an extracellular matrix protein that functions as a scaffold for elastic fibers, appears to decrease before other changes are observed, suggesting that loss of fibulin-5 is a marker for skin aging (Rongioletti and Rebora 1995).

The ground substance mucopolysaccharides, glycosaminoglycans (GAGs), and proteoglycans are especially hyaluronic acid decreased. Aging also affects GAG composition and binding to elastin, impeding the drainage of molecules into lymphatic vessels. These changes may adversely influence skin turgor because proteoglycans bind 1,000 times their own weight in water and also impact collagen fiber deposition, orientation, and size.

Overall, a picture emerges of aging dermis as an increasingly rigid, inelastic, and unresponsive tissue that is less capable of undergoing modifications in response to injury or stress.

25.10.3 Subcutaneous Tissue, Muscles, and Bone

Like other striated muscles, facial muscles show accumulation of the "age pigment" lipofuscin, a marker of cellular damage.

Subcutaneous fat is depleted from distinct facial regions, but there is a prominent increase in fatty tissue in other areas. Fat in the aged face, subject to the force of gravity, contributes to sagging and drooping of the skin.

Facial bones display reduced mass with age. Bone resorption particularly in the mandible, maxilla, and frontal bones enhance the sagging of facial skin and contribute to the obliteration of the demarcation between the contour of the jaw and the neck that is so distinct in young adults.

25.10.4 Hair

By the end of the fifth decade, approximately half of the population has at least 50 % gray (white) scalp hair due to progressive and eventually total loss of melanocytes from the hair bulb (Tobin and Paus 2001). Loss of melanocytes is believed to occur more rapidly in hair than in skin because the cells proliferate and manufacture melanin at maximal rates during the anagen phase of the hair cycle, whereas epidermal melanocytes are comparatively inactive throughout their life span. More specifically, hair graying reflects loss of the melanocyte stem cell population in hair follicle bulge (Steingrimsson et al. 2005).

Scalp hair may gray more rapidly than other body hair. With aging, there is a modest decrease in the number of hair follicles due in part to atrophy and fibrosis and an increase in the proportion of telogen hair follicles. One hypothesis suggests that melanocyte loss and lack of melanosomal transfer may increase oxidative stress level in highly metabolic hair follicle keratinocytes, affecting their function and viability (Van Neste and Tobin 2004).

In postmenopausal women, hair loss and mild hirsutism are the results of decreased estrogen level and estrogen to androgen ratio.

25.10.5 Cutaneous Glands and Nerves

Eccrine glands decrease by approximately 15 % in average number during adulthood and spontaneous sweating is further reduced by more than 70 % in healthy older subjects.

There is an exponential decrease in sebum production with aging. Decreased sensory perception in old skin encompasses optimal stimulus for light touch, vibratory sensation, and corneal sensation. Cutaneous pain threshold increases up to 20 % in advancing adult age.

25.11 Effects of Menopause

Estrogens play a critical role in female development and reproduction and also influence skin and hair. Menopause typically occurs in a woman's early 50s, so that, with life expectancy in the developed world approaching 80 years (Mathers et al. 2004), women are postmenopausal for approximately one-third of their lives. Age-associated decrements in keratinocyte barrier function, immune regulation, and wound healing appear to be compounded by decreased estrogen levels and/or decreased responsiveness of cells to existing estrogens. Because both estrogen and androgen receptors are expressed by skin-derived cells, both hormones are likely to play a role in skin structure and function.

Reduction in dermal collagen content, increased cutaneous extensibility, decreased elasticity, decreased water holding capacity, increased dryness, and increased fine wrinkling are associated with decreased circulatory levels of estrogen, as are decreased sebum levels. These changes are related more to menopause than to chronologic age alone, and wrinkling is reported to be more pronounced in postmenopausal women who are not taking hormone replacement therapy than in treated women.

Estrogen and progesterone are also reported to modulate cutaneous inflammation, enhance keratinocyte proliferation and collagen synthesis, decrease the activity of MMPs, and increase the synthesis of dermal mucopolysaccharides and hyaluronic acid.

25.12 Aging and the Immune System

The immune system has two major roles: defense against external insults and internal immunologic surveillance. With advancing age, the immune system of animals and humans undergoes characteristic changes, usually resulting in decreased immune competence, termed immunosenescence. Decreased T-cell memory, loss of the naïve T-cell population, defective humoral, and cellular immunity characterize the aging immune system. Chronic inflammatory state, decreased immunity to exogenous antigens, and increased autoreactivity compromise the ability to sustain environmental insults. With aging, increased ROS within cells leads to oxidative stress and contributes to low-grade inflammation. Additionally, mitochondrial electron transfer during oxidative phosphorylation is compromised with aging and results in leakage of proinflammatory ROS into the cytoplasm. This ROS imbalance contributes to immune senescence beginning with decline in the innate immune response and culminating with impaired adaptive immune responses. These changes contribute to the increased incidence of infections and malignancies in the elderly (De la Fuente et al. 2005; Grolleau-Julius et al. 2010; Peters et al. 2009).

25.13 Skin Immune System in Aging

Immunosenescence also affect the skin, the largest immunologically active organ of the body (Sunderkotter et al. 1997). There is a decrease in cutaneous immune function in older humans that leads to increased bacterial (such as Streptococcus- and Staphylococcus-induced cellulitis) and fungal infections (often candidiasis) (Laube 2004) and contributes to the increase in cutaneous malignancies. This indicates that defective cutaneous immunity develops during aging (Desai et al. 2006; Lasithiotakis et al. 2008).

On the other hand, qualities of the skin are age-related changes but are not primarily linked to the immune system can exert an influence on the immune response. For example, the increased fragility of aged skin and decreased excretory function of skin glands favors infection with bacteria, reduction in cutaneous vasculature (Johnson 1994), and increased permeability of older vessels (Bilato and Crow 1996) are likely to influence recruitment of an inflammatory infiltrate.

25.13.1 T Lymphocytes

Normal, healthy human skin contains large numbers of antigen-experienced CD4[+] and CD8[+] T cells (Clark et al. 2006b; Schaerli et al. 2004). According to some calculations, there are approximately 20 billion skin-resident T cells in healthy human skin, nearly twice the number present in circulation (Clark et al. 2006b).

There is evidence that certain immunological reactions involving T cells deteriorate with growing age (Farthing and Walton 1994). Sensitization to substances, such as 2.4-dinitrochloro benzene, is markedly reduced in the elderly population (Waldorf et al. 1968). Cutaneous cell-mediated immunity to so-called recall antigens may be reduced in elderly (Johnson 1994; Maxwell and McCluskey 1986). Aging mice also reveal diminished cell-mediated immunity (Snyder and Hogenesch 1996). Such an age-associated decrease in immunological functions involving T cells could be caused by a decline in the number of T cells or by a deterioration of T-cell functions.

In contrast to the controversies about the total number of T cells or CD4-CD8 subtypes, there is a wide agreement that during aging there is an intriguing shift among T lymphocytes from native T cells to memory T cells (Schwab et al. 1997; Stulnig et al. 1995).

T-reg cells play a crucial role in regulating the magnitude of an immune response. 5–10 % of T-cells resident in normal human skin express forkhead box P3 (Foxp3) and have other characteristics of T regulative (Agius et al. 2009; Clark et al. 2006a; Vukmanovic-Stejic et al. 2008). T regs circulate between the skin and lymph nodes, in the steady state and immune response (Tomura et al. 2010). These cells can directly inhibit both T cells and antigen presenting cells such as dendritic cells and macrophages (Schwarz and Schwarz 2010; Tiemessen et al. 2007).

T-reg cells also can inhibit TNF-α secretion by macrophages (Taams et al. 2005). There is a significant increase in the T reg in the skin of old subjects. Overrepresentation of T-reg cells in old skin may explain the decreased TNF-α secretion by cutaneous macrophages in old humans (Agius et al. 2009).

25.13.2 B Lymphocytes

A diminution in antibody responsiveness in aged humans or mice has long been known (Sunderkotter et al. 1997). Qualitative alterations are more important for the altered antibody response (Sansoni et al. 1993).

Clinically, these abnormalities include reduced neutralization of invading microbes, increased occurrence of monoclonal gammopathies, and increased levels of autoantibodies (Sunderkotter et al. 1997). In elderly humans, an impaired humoral immune response in vaccinations against influenza virus is caused by differences in IgG1 antibody production (Sunderkotter et al. 1997). Well known to the dermatologist is the increased occurrence of usually benign monoclonal gammopathies in elderly individuals since they are frequently associated with dermatoses such as scleromyxedema, necrobiotic xanthogranuloma, subcorneal pustulosis, or erythema elevatum diutinum (Sunderkotter et al. 1997).

Bullous pemphigoid is an autoimmune disease of elderly people, for example, while the classic autoantibody-mediated systemic lupus erythematosus is not.

25.13.3 Skin APC and Aging

Main components of the innate immune system in the skin are Langerhans cells, dermal dendritic cells, and skin resident macrophages.

In general, the number and phenotype of cutaneous DCs are comparable in young and old subjects during aging however migration, phagocytosis and, capacity to stimulate T cells may be decreased (Kovacs et al. 2009; Mahbub et al. 2011; Shaw et al. 2010).

25.13.3.1 Langerhans Cells

Epidermal LCs act as sentinels of the adaptive immune system and are adept at processing antigen. Following an external challenge, a proportion of epidermal LCs is mobilized and migrates to local skin-draining lymph nodes. In order to migrate, LCs require independent signals from both interleukin IL-1β and tumor necrosis factor TNF-α (Ogden et al. 2011). Investigations demonstrated a reduction in the number of epidermal LCs in elderly subjects (Gilchrest et al. 1982).

According to *Ogden S.* et al., the ability of peripheral blood monocytes to differentiate into LCs was not impaired in aged subjects, but ability of LC to migrate to draining lymph nodes has been shown to decline with age (Ogden et al. 2011).

25.13.3.2 Plasmacytoid Dendritic Cells

PDCs are a unique dendritic cell subset, which is present in the normal skin in very small numbers. However, they play an important role in viral infection (for example, Varicella zoster virus or VZV) and inflammatory skin disorders (such as psoriasis, lupus erythematosus, and lichen planus), also in skin tumors (melanoma, BCC, SCC, CTCL) (Conrad et al. 2009). There is clear evidence that PDC cytokine secretion is reduced with age (Panda et al. 2010; Shodell and Siegal 2002). The evidence that older people often have problems with VZV reactivation, causing shingles, supports the possibility of the impaired function of PDC in the skin, through decreased migration, activation, or cytokine secretion (Vukmanovic-Stejic et al. 2011).

25.13.4 Monocytes and Macrophages

Macrophages and monocytes play an important role in the immune response by fulfilling three major tasks: phagocytosis and elimination of microbes or foreign bodies, presentation of antigen, and production of an unsurpassed amount of cytokines. During aging, monocyte counts are not significantly decreased but a number of macrophage functions decline with aging, including diminished TLR expression, reduced phagocytic capacity, and a decline in secretion of chemokines and cytokines (Shaw et al. 2010).

25.14 Photoaging

25.14.1 Spectrum of UV Light

The sun emits UV radiation as part of an electromagnetic spectrum. It is usually subdivided, rather arbitrarily, into UVA (400–315 nm), UVB (315–290 nm), and UVC (290–200 nm). More than 95 % of the sun's UV radiation that reaches the earth's surface is UVA. UV radiation can be absorbed by biologic molecules (DNA, protein, lipids) and it can damage and kill unprotected cells.

To survive in our environment, all living organisms had to develop protective mechanisms in order to prevent UV-induced killing and to maintain the stability of their genome. Such defenses include the development of UV-absorbing surface layers, enzymatic and nonenzymatic antioxidative defenses, repair processes, and removal of damaged cells. Through evolution, humans have lost most of the UV-protective fur, which remains an effective UV-protector only on the scalp (of most individuals). Nevertheless, the human skin is quite effective in protecting the rest of the organism from the harmful effects of solar UV irradiation, since UV radiation does not penetrate any deeper than the skin.

Some of the UV light reaching the skin is absorbed by biomolecules, thus eliciting photochemical and photobiological responses. A light absorbing molecule is called a chromophore.

Both short-term and long-term effects of exposure to UV light are wavelength-dependent (Yarosh et al. 2008).

25.14.2 UV Light and the Skin

Visible, short-term, cutaneous effects of UV radiation include sunburn that is beyond this chapter.

Fig. 25.2 Photoaged versus intrinsically aged skin of an elderly man. Habitually sun-exposed skin above the collar line is prominently wrinkled and lax, in contrast with the equally chronologically aged but sun-protected skin of the lower neck and shoulder. Despite the striking difference in appearance, both areas manifest age-associated functional decrements

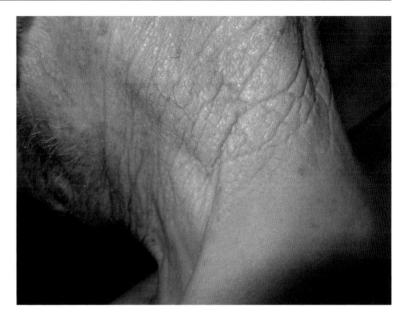

Long-term effects of chronic sun exposure include photoaging and photocarcinogenesis. Sun exposure and its effects on cutaneous immunity integrate a complex network of biologic processes. Sun damage alters many of the key pathways involved in generating an appropriate immune response to an antigen (Hanneman et al. 2006).

25.14.3 Mechanism and Clinical Findings

In contrast to photocarcinogenesis, where the anti-inflammatory effects of UV light play a pivotal role, photoaging is characterized by a chronic inflammatory response to UV light.

UV-induced erythema is characterized by infiltrating neutrophils. Neutrophils are potent cells packed with proteolytic enzymes, including neutrophil elastase and metalloproteinases. Furthermore, activated neutrophils generate and release ROS. Infiltrating neutrophils can thus damage collagen fibers and particularly elastic fibers (Rijken and Bruijnzeel-Koomen 2011).

Results of a study showed that neutrophil infiltration and neutrophil elastase (NE) activity are elevated in the chronic UVB-irradiation skin of hairless mouse and confirmed the involvement of NE in matrix metalloproteinase (MMP) activation. These data suggest that NE indirectly plays a role in skin photoaging through MMP activation. Drugs that interfere with neutrophil influx are potential antiphotoaging agents (Takeuchi et al. 2010).

A prominent feature of photoaged skin is elastosis, a process characterized clinically by yellow discoloration and a sometimes pebbly surface (Fig. 25.2) and histologically by tangled masses of degraded elastic fibers that form an amorphous mass composed of disorganized tropoelastin and fibrillin (Fig. 25.3). At dermo-epidermal junction, fibrillin is reduced (Halder 1998). In addition, the amount of ground substance increases in photodamaged skin, whereas the amount of collagen decreases, in part because of increased metalloproteinase activity. This MMP-mediated collagen destruction accounts, in a large part, for the connective tissue damage that occurs due to photoaging. These investigators also claimed that collagen synthesis is reduced more in photoaged human skin than in naturally aged skin in vivo (Fisher et al. 1996, 1997; Talwar et al. 1995). Photodamaged skin frequently displays an increased number of hyperplastic fibroblasts as well as increased inflammatory cells (Fig. 25.4), including mast cells, histiocytes, and other

Fig. 25.3 Photodamaged facial skin and large masses of deranged elastic fibers characterize solar elastosis

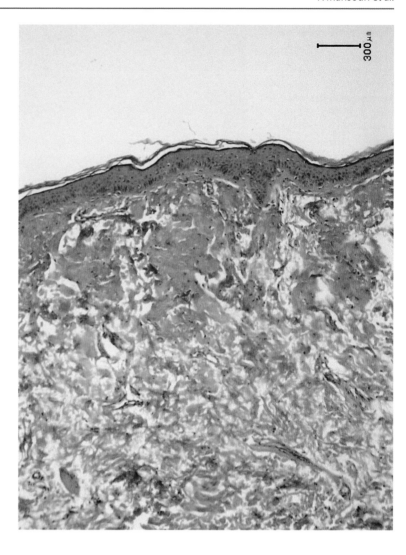

mononuclear cells, giving rise to the term helio-dermatitis [literally, "cutaneous inflammation due to sun" (Fig. 25.5)]. It has been reported that signals resulting from UVA exposure in the eye pass through the contrast nervous system, thus leading to the secretion of alpha-melanocyte stimulating hormone (α-MSH) and adrenocorticotropic hormone (ACTH) from the hypothalamus, which results in the immunosuppression (Hiramoto et al. 2009). In addition, the same group previously reported that UVA exposure in the eye induces the activation of mast cells through the autonomic nervous system (Yamate et al. 2011).

In a recent study, the effects of long-term UVA irradiation of the eye on photoaging of the skin in mice were evaluated. The plasma level of α-melanocyte stimulating hormone (α-MSH),

nitrogen oxides (NO$_2$/NO$_3$), TNF-α, and prostaglandin (PG)E$_2$ content all increased after UVA irradiation. However, the level of α-MSH increased more by eye irradiation than skin irradiation. In addition, UVA irradiation of the eye and dorsal skin increased the number of mast cells and fibroblasts. Furthermore, the expression of the melanocortin-1 receptor (MC1R) was increased on the fibroblast surface by UVA irradiation of the eye. These results indicate that the signal evoked by UVA irradiation of the eye, through the hypothalamo-pituitary proopiomelanocortin system, upregulated the production of α-MSH and increased expression of MC1R in fibroblast. This hormone controls the collagen generation from fibroblasts, thus suggesting that photoaging was induced by UVA irradiation of the eye (Hiramoto et al. 2012).

Fig. 25.4 Marked dermal inflammatory infiltrate associated with the heliodermatitis that is characteristic of ongoing and chronic actinic exposure

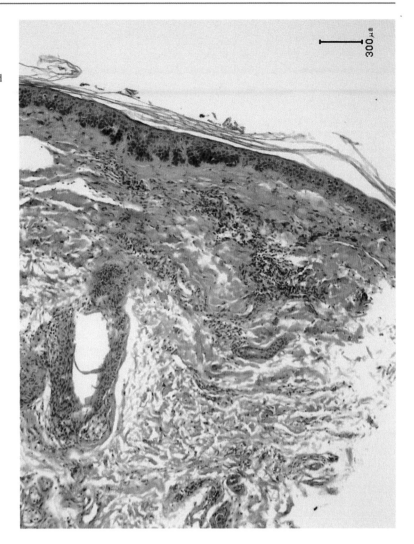

The role of α-MSH as a regulator of the extracellular matrix of the skin was supported by the recent studies demonstrating that α-MSH suppressed the collagen synthesis induced by transforming growth factor beta (TGF-β_1), a key profibrotic cytokine implicated in the pathogenesis of fibrotic disorders, including systemic sclerosis (Bohm et al. 2004). Therefore, there appears to be a mechanism wherein the α-MSH/MC1R system controls the generation of collagen. The elucidation of this mechanism may, therefore, lead to the development of new measures for preventing photoaging. Moreover, the cytoprotective and DNA damage-reducing effects of α-MSH may be of special interest for patients with diseases associated with increased UV susceptibility

(Hiramoto et al. 2012). Dermal vasculature in mildly photodamaged skin displays venule wall thickening; in severely photodamaged skin, thin vessel walls with compromised perivascular veil cells display dilations (telangiectases).

In contrast with chronologically aged skin, photodamaged epidermis is frequently acanthotic, although severe atrophy, loss of polarity, and cellular atypia also can be seen. Initial pigmentary changes of photoaging can sometimes be seen just weeks or months after sunburn "sunburn freckles." Additional changes are described in Table 25.4.

Since natural sunlight is polychromatic, other wavelengths may have some effects on the human skin. Recent work demonstrates that IR and heat

Fig. 25.5 Photoaging: heliodermatitis. Pronounced furrowing, yellow discoloration, and pebbly surface (solar elastosis)

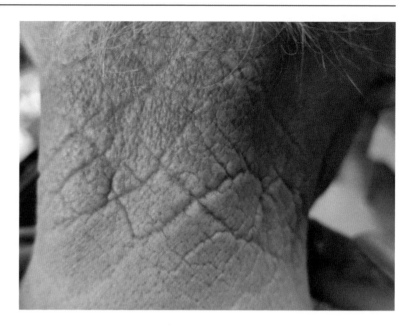

Table 25.4 Features of photoaged skin

Clinical	Histologic
Dryness (roughness)	Increased compaction of stratum corneum, increased thickness of granular cell layer, reduced epidermal thickness, reduced epidermal mucin content
Actinic keratosis	Nuclear atypia, loss of orderly, progressive keratinocyte maturation; irregular epidermal hyperplasia and/or hypoplasia; occasional dermal inflammation
Irregular Pigmentation	
Freckling	Reduced or increased number of hypertrophic, strongly DOPA-positive melanocytes
Lentigines	Elongation of epidermal rete ridges; increase in number and melanization of melanocytes
Guttate hypomelanosis	Reduced number of atypical melanocytes
Diffuse irreversible hyperpigmentation (bronzing)	Increased number of DOPA-positive melanocytes and increased melanin content per unit area and increased number of dermal melanophages
Wrinkling	
Fine surface lines	None detected
Deep furrows	Contraction of septae in the subcutaneous fat
Stellate pseudoscars	Absence of epidermal pigmentation, altered fragmented dermal collagen
Elastosis (fine nodularity and/or coarseness)	Nodular aggregations of fibrous to amorphous material in the papillary dermis
Inelasticity	Elastotic dermis
Telangiectasia	Ectatic vessels often with atrophic walls
Venous lakes	Ectatic vessels often with atrophic walls
Purpura (easy bruising)	Extravasated erythrocytes and increased perivascular inflammation
Comedones (maladie de Favre et Racouchot)	Ectasia of the pilosebaceous follicular orifice
Sebaceous hyperplasia	Concentric hyperplasia of sebaceous glands

Basal cell carcinoma and squamous cell carcinoma also occur in photoaged skin but, unlike the table entries, affect only a minority of individuals exposure each induces cutaneous angiogenesis and inflammatory cellular infiltration, disrupts the dermal extracellular matrix by inducing MMP, and alters dermal structural proteins, thereby adding to premature skin aging (Cho et al. 2009). Data from a study demonstrate that human skin mast cells are activated and recruited by UV, as well as by IR and heat, all of which are components of sunlight. Mast cells might modulate the skin aging processes by influencing the function of many different surrounding cells in skin, including keratinocytes (KCs) and fibroblasts (FBs) by their mediator (Kim et al. 2009).

Photoaging is most apparent in Whites but also occurs in Asians, Hispanics, and Africans. Individuals with skin phototypes I and II (white) generally show atrophic and dysplastic skin changes with actinic keratoses and epidermal malignancies, whereas the individuals with darker skin phototypes III and IV manifest hypertrophic responses such as furrowing, lentigines, and coarseness. It usually involves the face, neck, or extensor surfaces of the upper extremities most severely (Munavalli et al. 2005). The differences in clinical appearance of photoaged skin between Whites and other groups are primarily due to differences in their UV defense systems. In the latter three groups, melanin is a major form of protection, whereas in Whites, melanin plays a lesser role, and stratum corneum thickening is relatively more important. One study reported a sun protection factor for black epidermis of 13.4 compared to 3.4 for white epidermis (Kaidbey et al. 1979).

Major clinical features of photoaging in Asian skin are solar lentigines and mottled pigmentation. Moderate-to-severe wrinkling occurs in Asians but only in the sixth decade (Chung et al. 2001; Halder and Richards 2004).

Due to its ability to penetrate deeper into the dermis, UVA in particular is thought to play an important role in the dermal changes of photoaging, but it is thought to be as important in photocarcinogenesis, since all UV-induced skin cancers (basal and squamous cell carcinomas (SCCs and BCCs) and melanomas) arise from cells that reside within the epidermis, not from dermal cells.

25.14.4 UV Effects on the Cutaneous Immune System

Sunburn exemplifies the profound effect that UV light has on the skin's immune function, in this case a proinflammatory effect. Several clinical observations Table 25.5 provide evidence for the proinflammatory/immune-stimulating effects of UV light on the skin. On the other hand, UV light clearly has anti-inflammatory/immunosuppressive properties as well, exemplified by the efficacy of UV phototherapy in the treatment of inflammatory skin disorders. Proinflammatory, anti-inflammatory, and immunomodulatory changes occur side-by-side within different arms of cellular and humoral immune reaction cascade.

UV light-induced effects on the immune system involve not only the areas of skin directly exposed to UV light but also non-irradiated sites. An example of systemic immunostimulating effects is the UV-induced exacerbation of systemic disease in patients with systemic lupus erythematosus. Recently, it has been suggested that the immunosuppressive effects of UV light affect primarily the adaptive, antigen-specific immune system, while immunostimulatory effects target the innate immune systems (Schwarz 2010).

Cellular photoreceptors that mediate the signaling that leads to UV-induced immune responses are as follows: DNA (via formation of DNA damage or DNA photoproducts), urocanic acid in the stratum corneum (via UV-induced isomerization from the trans- to the cis-isoform), and membrane lipids (via UV-induced alteration of the membrane redox potential). The immunosuppressive effects of UVB are well established, but evidence is accumulating that UVA also has prominent effects.

25.15 Photocarcinogenesis

UVR from the sun is the most prevalent carcinogen in human, particularly among Caucasians. In the case of photocarcinogenesis, UV exposure provides a one-two punch—not only does it generate DNA damage that leads to mutation formation and malignant transformation, but its immunosuppressive properties, including the

Table 25.5 Effects of ultraviolet light on the immune system

Clinical observations
Suggestive of proinflammatory/immune-stimulating effects:
Sunburn
Dermatoheliosis
Photodermatoses (phototoxic and photoallergic)
Photoaggravation of inflammatory skin diseases (e.g., psoriasis, atopic dermatitis, pityriasis rubra pilaris)
Induction of autoimmune connective tissue diseases (e.g., cutaneous lupus erythematosus (LE), flares of systemic LE)
Efficacy of UV phototherapy for the treatment of skin infections (e.g., lupus vulgaris)
Suggestive of anti-inflammatory/immunosuppressive effects:
Activation of recurrent orolabial herpes simplex
Increased risk of photocarcinogenesis in the setting of immunosuppression (e.g., solid organ transplant recipients)
Efficacy of UV phototherapy for the treatment of inflammatory skin diseases
Cellular and molecular events in UV-irradiated skin
Mediating proinflammatory/immune-stimulating effects:
Release of proinflammatory mediators by resident and nonresident skin cells (e.g., serotonin, prostaglandins, IL-l, IL-6, IL-B, TNF-α)
Induction of antimicrobial peptides (hypothesized to explain why UV-irradiated skin is not prone to bacterial infections)
Mediating anti-inflammatory/immunosuppressive effects:
Depletion of Langerhans cells or modulation of their antigen-presenting function
Release of anti-inflammatory mediators by resident and nonresident skin cells (e.g., IL-l 0, a-MSH)
Induction of regulatory T cells (antigen-specific)

induction of specific tolerance to antigens from UV-induced skin tumors, reduce the ability of the host immune-defense system to recognize and remove malignant cells. UV irradiation also impairs immune surveillance against cells infected with oncogenic viruses (e.g., certain human papillomavirus (HPV) types) and may thereby further promote skin cancer formation. This may explain why cutaneous SCCs develop more frequently than BCCs in immunosuppressed patients (e.g., solid organ transplant recipients), in contrast to immunocompetent individuals, in whom BCCs occur more commonly than SCCs. Patients infected with human immunodeficiency virus (HIV) do have a moderately increased incidence of SCC, but these tumors at sun-exposed sites are associated with HPV.

The advantage of reduced immune reactivity following exposure to UV light is the prevention of illicit (auto) immune reactions to transiently UV-altered cells. Any shift in the balance between pro- and anti-inflammatory responses toward a more immunosuppressed state increases the risk of UV-induced tumor formation, as occurs in chronically immunosuppressed patients. However, tilting this balance toward proinflammatory responses and autoimmunity increases the risk of developing photodermatoses or photoaggravated skin diseases such as lupus erythematosus. The critical nature of this balance is also exemplified by the observation that effective photoprotection commonly leads to spontaneous resolution of actinic keratoses.

As photocarcinogenesis commonly occurs in photoaged skin, this further demonstrates the simultaneous occurrence of pro- and anti-inflammatory responses to UV light. Both processes, photoaging and photocarcinogenesis, usually require several years of sun exposure before clinical manifestations are apparent.

Novel, pathway-based approaches to prevent or treat skin cancer are being developed. Educational and behavioral approaches are keys to minimizing skin cancer rates in future.

25.16 Ultraviolet Immunosuppression

Sun exposure and its effects on cutaneous immunity integrate a complex network of biologic processes. Sun damage alters many of the key pathways involved in generating an appropriate immune response to an antigen (Hanneman et al. 2006).

25.16.1 Antigen-Presenting Cells

Epidermal LCs are the principal APCs in the skin. They have an extensive network of dendrites reaching up to the stratum corneum to detect and recognize foreign antigens that contact the epidermal surface. They comprise the major immune-surveillance network of the skin. Cutaneous immunity depends on proper functioning of LCs. Exposure to UVB radiation (280–320 nm) has been shown to alter LC number, morphology, and antigen-presenting function. Within hours of UV exposure, LCs begin migrating from the irradiated epidermis, without the functional maturity to mount an immune response. In response to foreign antigen, UV-irradiated LCs fail to stimulate Th1 cells but preferentially activate Th2 cells, resulting in increased generation of suppressor T cells. Thus, migration of LCs coupled with differential activation of Th subsets after antigen exposure translates to a decreased or absent ability to mount an appropriate immune response. Consequently, microbial antigens may be tolerated and tumor growth rather than rejection occurs. Similar to UVB, UVA radiation (320–400 nm) also causes a reduction in LC number and disruption of their functional capacity (Dumay et al. 2001). These effects of UVA may partially explain its suppressive effects on in vivo contact sensitivity that have been observed in both animal and human studies (Fourtanier et al. 2000).

25.16.2 Cytokines

UV-induced immune suppression is modulated through the participation of a number of cytokines including but not limited to IL-1β, TNF-α, IL-10, and IL-12. After UV exposure, immunosuppressive cytokines TNF-α and IL-10 are released from damaged keratinocytes. TNF-α is a proinflammatory cytokine that causes the upregulation of intercellular adhesion molecule (ICAM) and major histocompatibility complex (MHC) class I and class II. TNF-α and IL-1β have been implicated in directing LC migration after UV radiation.

Several studies indicate that the IL-10 released by UV-irradiated keratinocytes modulates antigen presentation by LCs such that there is preferential activation of Th2 cells that then secrete additional immune-suppressive cytokines (IL-4 and IL-10) and suppress cell-mediated immune responses (Ullrich 1994). The release of cytokines by UV comes not only from damaged keratinocytes but also from additional sources as well. UVB-induced damage to cutaneous nerves induces the release of neuropeptides such as calcitonin gene-related peptide and substance P from nerve endings, which causes dermal mast cell degranulation and thus the release of additional IL-10 and TNF-α (Granstein and Matsui 2004). CD11b⁺ macrophages after UVB exposure are yet another large source of IL-10 (Kodali et al. 2005; Schmitt et al. 2000).

IL-12 is a cytokine produced by polymorphonuclear cells, keratinocytes, and APCs. It is one of the crucial cytokines involved in activation of Th1 lymphocytes and blockade of Th2 activity. Because of this capacity, it has been speculated that IL-12 could neutralize the effects of IL-10 and thus overcome UV-induced immune suppression. A study demonstrated that the ability of IL-12 to prevent UV immune suppression depends on DNA repair (Schwarz et al. 2005). After UV exposure, IL-12 is downregulated, likely due in part to increased levels of prostaglandin E2. Decreased IL-12 further contributes to UV-induced immune suppression (Kodali et al. 2005; Murphy 1998; Stevens and Bergstresser 1998). Based on data demonstrating that IL-12 can interfere with UV-induced T-suppressor cells and counteract the effects of IL-10, it may have significant therapeutic potential to block UV-induced immune suppression (Hanneman et al. 2006).

25.16.3 T Lymphocytes

T-suppressor cells play a critical role in UV immune suppression and induction of tolerance, thereby preventing rejection of UV radiation-induced tumors. They have been shown to originate from the draining lymph nodes of UV-irradiated mice and have been associated with increased production of IL-10, TGF-β, and inhibition of IL-12 (Shreedhar et al. 1998). They are commonly referred to as CD4$^+$ CD25$^+$ T cells. A study have demonstrated that after in vitro expansion of these T cells, they secreted a Tr-1 like cytokine pattern, characterized by high levels of IL-10, TGF-β, IFN-γ, low levels of IL-2, and no IL-4. It was also demonstrated that the T cells responsible for transferring tolerance express the cytotoxic T-lymphocyte antigen 4 (CTLA-4) cell surface marker (Schwarz et al. 2005). CTLA-4 (CD152) is a surface marker expressed on activated T lymphocytes that cross-links the B7-2 molecule on APCs (Oosterwegel et al. 1999). This leads to downregulation of IL-2 and inhibition of a variety of immune responses. Another group of immune-effector cells, known as NK T cells, has also been reported to mediate UV-immune suppression and skin tumor development (Moodycliffe et al. 2000). NK T cells express intermediate amounts of T-cell receptor molecules on their surface and coexpress surface antigens normally found on NK cells. These cells compose only 2–3 % of the splenic T-cell population and are believed to exert their suppressive function via secretion of high levels of IL-4, similar to Th2 cells, within hours of primary CD3 stimulation (Hanneman et al. 2006).

25.16.4 Chromophores: DNA and Urocanic Acid

For immune suppression to occur, UV energy must be converted into a biologic signal. Photoreceptors in the skin, such as DNA, urocanic acid, membrane lipids, and proteins, are believed to perform this function (Ullrich 2002). As mentioned previously, there is a strong correlation between DNA damage and certain cytokines involved in modifying immune responses. DNA repair enzymes in the form of bacterial T4 endonuclease V liposomes prevent UV-induced upregulation of the immunosuppressive cytokines IL-10

andTNF-α in vivo (Wolf et al. 2000). Investigators have shown that topical application of DNA repair enzymes from Micrococcus luteus partially prevented simulated solar radiation (SSR)-induced suppression of contact hypersensitivity (CHS) to dinitrochlorobenzene in human subjects, indicating that damage to DNA by SSR contributes to UV-immune suppression (Ke MS et al. 2004).

Trans-urocanic acid (Trans-UCA) is a natural substance formed from deamination of histidine during keratinization, which leads to its accumulation in the stratum corneum. Exposure to UV causes photoisomerization of trans-UCA to cis-UCA, which exerts immune-suppressive properties. In the early 1980s, the first suggestion that UCA might be involved in UV-immune suppression came with the discovery that trans-UCA has a maximal absorption spectra of 270 nm and thus could be a natural sunscreen. It was later discovered, using a mouse model, that inhibition of contact hypersensitivity (CHS) has a similar absorption peak at 270 nm. These identical absorption spectra then strongly implicated UCA as a chromophore for UV-immune suppression. Furthermore, when tape stripping was performed to remove stratum corneum, UV-immune suppression was prevented (Hanneman et al. 2006). Both in vitro and in vivo studies have suggested that the immune-suppressive properties of cis-UCA may be due to modulation of cytokines such as TNF-α, IL-10, and IL-12, as well as LC depletion (Beissert and Schwarz 1999; Holan et al. 1998). In vivo studies have shown that UV-irradiated mice treated topically with cis-UCA have enhanced tumor growth, whereas those treated with anti-cis-UCA antibodies had a decreased incidence of tumor formation (Reeve et al. 1989).

25.16.5 Other Possible Contributory Molecules

Another possible mediator involved especially in UVA-induced immune suppression is nitric oxide (NO). Studies using topical NO inhibitor suggest that NO production may be a particularly important oxidative event causing epidermal LC depletion in response to UVA irradiation (Yuen et al. 2002).

One of the supposed beneficial effects of UVB radiation is the production of vitamin D in the skin, as well as conversion of provitamin D_3 (7-dehydrocholestereol) to the active vitamin D_3 metabolite (1,25 dihydroxyvitamin D_3) (Reichrath and Rappl 2003). Current data suggest that vitamin D and its related analogues inhibit differentiation and induce a persistent state of immaturity in DCs via alterations in surface ligands and production and release of cytokines. VDR ligands also induce generation of $CD4^+$, $CD25^+$ T-reg cells that secrete inhibitory cytokines and inhibit Ag-specific T-cell activation. As mentioned previously, all of these effects depend on the presence of the vitamin D receptor (Griffin and Kumar 2003; Reichrath and Rappl 2003).

UV radiation also alters cellular redox equilibrium and causes reactive oxygen species formation and membrane lipid peroxidation. Oxidative damage to cellular components may likewise contribute to immune suppression. Using a murine epidermal DC line, hydrogen peroxide was shown to mediate UVB impairment of antigen presentation (Caceres-Dittmar et al. 1995). The ability of various antioxidants to interfere with UV-induced immune suppression and tolerance induction suggests further that UV-induced oxidative stress contributes to immune suppression (Nakamura et al. 1997; van den Broeke and Beijersbergen van Henegouwen 1995).

25.17 Skin Disease in the Elderly

There is an increased susceptibility to cutaneous disease and injury by aging. Such disorders often appear to be the consequence of age-associated intrinsic losses of cutaneous cellular function. However, many dermatoses observed more commonly in the elderly reflect the higher prevalence of systemic diseases, such as diabetes, vascular insufficiency, and various neurologic syndromes. The increased prevalence of some disorders also may reflect reduced local skin care due to immobility or neurologic impairment. As well, subtle age-associated changes in immune status may contribute.

Reduced tolerance to systemically administered drugs is well documented in the elderly due to decrements in lean body mass, metabolism, and renal excretion (Vestal and Cusack 1990).

Selected common cutaneous disorders in the elderly are discussed briefly in the following (Table 25.6).

25.17.1 Tumors

Benign proliferative growths are especially characteristic of aging skin. Acrochordons, cherry angiomas, seborrheic keratoses, and lentigines begin to appear in middle age and are numerous in nearly every adult beyond age 65 years.

25.17.1.1 Seborrheic Keratoses

Seborrheic keratoses are benign papules or plaques that are highly variable in size and color. Because their number increases with aging, independent of sun exposure, they are considered by some as a biomarker of intrinsic aging (Yaar and Gilchrest 2001). Seborrheic keratoses represent clonal proliferations of both keratinocytes and melanocytes (Nakamura et al. 2001). They have no malignant potential. Although the pathogenesis of these keratoses is not completely understood, lesional keratinocytes express high levels of endothelin-1 and lesional melanocytes have increased tyrosinase expression (Teraki et al. 1996).

25.17.2 Skin Cancer

The age-specific incidence of skin cancer, including melanoma, increases with age (Berneburg et al. 1999), presumably due in part to cumulative exposure to carcinogens over a lifetime interspersed with cell division, with the attendant risk of mutation. There are also well-documented age-associated decreases in DNA repair capacity (Goukassian et al. 2000; Moriwaki et al. 1996) and immunosurveillance

Table 25.6 Presumptive pathophysiology of common cutaneous disorders in the elderly

Disorder	Pathophysiology
Benign neoplasia	
Seborrheic keratosis	Focal epidermal homeostatic loss leading to increased endothelin-1
Malignant neoplasia	
Squamous cell carcinoma and actinic keratosis	Ultraviolet-induced DNA damage
Basal cell carcinoma	Decreased DNA damage repair capacity
Malignant melanoma	Cumulative age-associated DNA damage
Merkel cell carcinoma	Decreased DNA damage repair capacity; polyoma virus
Angiosarcoma	
Papulosquamous disorders	
Psoriasis	Changes in patient's environment leading to Koebnerization
	Systemic medications
Xerosis/asteatotic dermatitis	Disturbance of epidermal maturation (decreased filaggrin production and/or altered lipid profile)
	Decreased water content in outer layers of stratum corneum slower corneocyte transit
Pruritus	Penetration of irritants through damaged stratum corneum (?)
	Altered sensory threshold (neuropathy) (?)
	Metabolic disorder
	Endocrine disorder
	Malignant neoplasm
	Adverse drug reaction
	Parasitic infestation
Infections	Compromised local cutaneous health predisposing to growth of infective organism
	Age-associated decreased immune function
	Underlying systemic disorder associated with decreased immune function
Ulcers	Impaired wound healing capacity (decreased levels of growth factors, decreased cellular proliferative capacity, increased perivascular fibrin deposition)
	Decreased mobility
	Underlying systemic disorder
	Compromised local cutaneous health (venous stasis, arteriosclerosis, hypertension)
Bullous pemphigoid	Flattening of the dermal-epidermal junction
	Increased circulating autoantibodies
Photosensitivity reactions	Medications with unsaturated ring structures

(Kessler 1993), as well as subtle loss of proliferative homeostasis.

The major etiologic factor for skin cancer is UV irradiation. The importance of exposure timing, dose rate, and total UVR exposure differ between the types of skin cancer. Habitual sun exposure of fair-skinned individuals induces SCC as well as actinic keratoses.

In contrast, the risk of BCCs and particularly malignant melanoma is related not only to total sun exposure but also to intense intermittent sun exposure (Kricker et al. 1995).

Although all types of melanoma have increased age-specific incidences (Sachs et al. 2001), lentigo malignant melanoma overwhelmingly develops in the 1960s or later in habitually sun-exposed skin (Morris and Sober 1989).

Merkel cell carcinoma is a rare cutaneous tumor thought to arise from a pluripotential cell that displays neuroendocrine differentiation. More than 90 % of patients diagnosed with this tumor are older than age 50 (Gupta et al. 2006; Moll et al. 1994).

Also the most common form of angiosarcoma occurs on the head and neck of the elderly.

25.17.3 Papulosquamous Disorders

25.17.3.1 Xerosis and Asteatotic Dermatitis

Xerosis is a dry, rough quality of skin that is almost universal in the elderly and may be attributed to a subtle disturbance of epidermal maturation, such as inadequate filaggrin production (Tezuka et al. 1994) or altered lipid profile (Ghadially et al. 1995). Water content of the viable epidermis is normal, but there is some reduction in the outermost layers of the stratum corneum (Elias and Ghadially 2002). There is no explanation for pruritus that often accompanies xerosis (Gilchrest 1995).

Asteatotic eczema, a condition frequently found in the elderly during the wintertime, is dermatitis superimposed on xerosis. It is often caused by low humidity in a heated environment. It manifests by dry, fissured skin with fine scale and is usually localized to the pretibial region.

25.17.3.2 Pruritus

Pruritus is perhaps the most common skin-related complaint of the elderly. In a majority of cases, pruritus is attributable only to xerosis, often exacerbated by low humidity, frequent bathing, or application of irritants to the skin. However, in up to 10–50 % of patients, pruritus may have other etiologies. These include metabolic or endocrine disorders, such as diabetes mellitus, renal failure, thyroid disease, or hepatic disease, in particular the obstructive type. Pruritus can be a manifestation of a malignant neoplasm, in particular lymphoma or leukemia or polycythemia vera. Adverse drug reactions can manifest as pruritus. Finally, infestations such as scabies lead to intense pruritus (Frances et al. 1991).

25.17.4 Infectious Processes

25.17.4.1 Bacterial

Impetigo and folliculitis in the elderly are usually caused by Staphylococci, in contrast to the pediatric, usually caused by Streptococci. Cellulitis is an infectious inflammatory disease involving the subcutaneous tissue. In elderly may present with only subtle rubor, tumor, calor, and dolor.

Erysipelas, a β-hemolytic streptococcal infection of skin, is more common in elderly.

Also, necrotizing fasciitis is a rare cutaneous infection, but it is more frequent in the elderly (Elgart 2002).

25.17.4.2 Parasitic

Scabies can occur in any age, but nursing homes provide a fertile ground for rapid spread of the infestation. In the elderly, because of their decreased immunity, lesions may be atypical and display less inflammation and pruritus (Uitto and Pulkkinen 1996).

25.17.4.3 Dermatophytes and Yeasts

Onychomycosis is present in approximately 40 % of patients after age 60 years, and tinea pedis is present in approximately 80 % of this population. Indeed, in elderly diabetic patients, interdigital tinea pedis may ulcerate and predispose to bacterial cellulitis.

Also cutaneous infections due to Candida albicans are common in the elderly (Martin and Elewski 2002).

25.17.4.4 Viral

The incidence of herpes zoster peaks at age 75 years. Postherpetic neuralgia, uncommon in patients younger than 40 years old, occurs in more than 40 % of patients aged 60–69 years and 50 % of 70-year-old patients or older (Mathers et al. 2004). Decreased cellular immunity and impaired wound healing in the elderly may account for slower resolution of the acute eruption (Weitz et al. 1987).

25.17.5 Ulcers

Chronic ulcers of all etiologies are more common in the elderly. The most common are leg ulcers, usually in the setting of chronic venous insufficiency. Exudation of macromolecules such as fibrinogen into the dermis may block the passage of oxygen and nutrients and growth factors required for tissue homeostasis.

Decubitus ulcers are proportionately far more common in elderly hospitalized patients than in younger (Paquette and Falanga 2002).

25.17.5.1 Bullous Pemphigoid

Bullous pemphigoid is far more common after age 60 years than in younger persons, a predilection that may be explained in part by the age-associated increases in circulating autoantibodies and ease of dermal-epidermal separation (Yaar and Gilchrest 1987). Bullous pemphigoid is a self-limited condition that frequently resolves within 6–12 months, but elderly patients may experience increased morbidity and mortality because of debilitated general health or as a side effect of treatment.

25.17.6 Drug Eruptions

Adverse drug reactions of all kinds increase with age, in part because the elderly consume more medications than younger age groups and because of medical conditions, including impaired renal, cardiac, or hepatic function, which compromise drug metabolism or excretion. The most frequently observed adverse cutaneous drug reactions are pruritus, exanthems, and urticaria, but drug-induced autoimmune reactions, including pemphigus, bullous pemphigoid, and lupus, also occur in the elderly.

References

Abbas AK, Murphy KM, Sher A (1996) Functional diversity of helper T lymphocytes. Nature 383(6603): 787–793

Agius E, Lacy KE, Vukmanovic-Stejic M et al (2009) Decreased TNF-alpha synthesis by macrophages restricts cutaneous immunosurveillance by memory CD4+ T cells during ageing. J Exp Med 206(9): 1929–1940

Akira S, Uematsu S, Takeuchi O (2006) Pathogen recognition and innate immunity. Cell 124(4):783–801

Beissert S, Schwarz T (1999) Mechanisms involved in ultraviolet light-induced immunosuppression. J Investig Dermatol Symp Proc 4(1):61–64

Berneburg M, Grether-Beck S, Kurten V et al (1999) Singlet oxygen mediates the UVA-induced generation of the photoageing-associated mitochondrial common deletion. J Biol Chem 274(22):15345–15349

Bilato C, Crow MT (1996) Atherosclerosis and the vascular biology of ageing. Aging (Milano) 8(4):221–234

Blander JM, Medzhitov R (2004) Regulation of phagosome maturation by signals from toll-like receptors. Science 304(5673):1014–1018

Bohm M, Raghunath M, Sunderkotter C et al (2004) Collagen metabolism is a novel target of the neuropeptide alpha-melanocyte-stimulating hormone. J Biol Chem 279(8):6959–6966

Braff MH, Bardan A, Nizet V et al (2005) Cutaneous defense mechanisms by antimicrobial peptides. J Invest Dermatol 125(1):9–13

Caceres-Dittmar G, Ariizumi K, Xu S et al (1995) Hydrogen peroxide mediates UV-induced impairment of antigen presentation in a murine epidermal-derived dendritic cell line. Photochem Photobiol 62(1):176–183

Chen K, Xu W, Wilson M et al (2009) Immunoglobulin D enhances immune surveillance by activating antimicrobial, proinflammatory and B cell-stimulating programs in basophils. Nat Immunol 10(8):889–898

Cho S, Shin MH, Kim YK et al (2009) Effects of infrared radiation and heat on human skin ageing in vivo. J Investig Dermatol Symp Proc 14(1):15–19

Choi EH, Man MQ, Xu P et al (2007) Stratum corneum acidification is impaired in moderately aged human and murine skin. J Invest Dermatol 127(12): 2847–2856

Chung JH, Lee SH, Youn CS et al (2001) Cutaneous photodamage in Koreans: influence of sex, sun exposure, smoking, and skin color. Arch Dermatol 137(8): 1043–1051

Clark RA, Chong B, Mirchandani N et al (2006a) The vast majority of CLA+ T cells are resident in normal skin. J Immunol 176(7):4431–4439

Clark RA, Chong BF, Mirchandani N et al (2006b) A novel method for the isolation of skin resident T cells from normal and diseased human skin. J Invest Dermatol 126(5):1059–1070

Conrad C, Meller S, Gilliet M (2009) Plasmacytoid dendritic cells in the skin: to sense or not to sense nucleic acids. Semin Immunol 21(3):101–109

Davis T, Haughton MF, Jones CJ et al (2006) Prevention of accelerated cell ageing in the Werner syndrome. Ann N Y Acad Sci 1067:243–247

De la Fuente M, Hernanz A, Vallejo MC (2005) The immune system in the oxidative stress conditions of ageing and hypertension: favorable effects of antioxidants and physical exercise. Antioxid Redox Signal 7(9–10):1356–1366

Desai A, Krathen R, Orengo I et al (2006) The age of skin cancers. Sci Aging Knowledge Environ 2006(9):pe13

Doyle SE, O'Connell RM, Miranda GA et al (2004) Toll-like receptors induce a phagocytic gene program through p38. J Exp Med 199(1):81–90

Dumay O, Karam A, Vian L et al (2001) Ultraviolet AI exposure of human skin results in Langerhans cell depletion and reduction of epidermal antigen-presenting cell function: partial protection by a broad-spectrum sunscreen. Br J Dermatol 144(6): 1161–1168

Elgart ML (2002) Skin infections and infestations in geriatric patients. In: Gilchrest BA (ed) Geriatric dermatology. W. B. Saunders, Philadelphia, p 89

Elias PM (2005) Stratum corneum defensive functions: an integrated view. J Invest Dermatol 125(2):183–200

Elias PM, Ghadially R (2002) The aged epidermal permeability barrier: basis for functional abnormalities. Clin Geriatr Med 18(1):103–120, vii

Eller MS, Puri N, Hadshiew IM et al (2002) Induction of apoptosis by telomere 3′ overhang-specific DNA. Exp Cell Res 276(2):185–193

Farthing PM, Walton LJ (1994) Changes in immune function with age. In: Squier CA, Hill MW (eds) The effects of ageing in oral mucosa and skin. CRC Press, Boca Raton, pp 113–120

Fisher GJ, Datta SC, Talwar HS et al (1996) Molecular basis of sun-induced premature skin ageing and retinoid antagonism. Nature 379(6563):335–339

Fisher GJ, Wang ZQ, Datta SC et al (1997) Pathophysiology of premature skin ageing induced by ultraviolet light. N Engl J Med 337(20):1419–1428

Fourtanier A, Gueniche A, Compan D et al (2000) Improved protection against solar-simulated radiation-induced immunosuppression by a sunscreen with enhanced ultraviolet A protection. J Invest Dermatol 114(4):620–627

Frances C, Boisnic S, Hartmann DJ et al (1991) Changes in the elastic tissue of the non-sun-exposed skin of cigarette smokers. Br J Dermatol 125(1):43–47

Garinis GA, van der Horst GT, Vijg J et al (2008) DNA damage and ageing: new-age ideas for an age-old problem. Nat Cell Biol 10(11):1241–1247

Gashev AA, Zawieja DC (2010) Hydrodynamic regulation of lymphatic transport and the impact of ageing. Pathophysiology 17(4):277–287

Gasque P (2004) Complement: a unique innate immune sensor for danger signals. Mol Immunol 41(11):1089–1098

Gately MK, Renzetti LM, Magram J et al (1998) The interleukin-12/interleukin-12-receptor system: role in normal and pathologic immune responses. Annu Rev Immunol 16:495–521

Ghadially R, Brown BE, Sequeira-Martin SM et al (1995) The aged epidermal permeability barrier. Structural, functional, and lipid biochemical abnormalities in humans and a senescent murine model. J Clin Invest 95(5):2281–2290

Gilchrest BA (1989) Skin ageing and photoageing: an overview. J Am Acad Dermatol 21(3 Pt 2):610–613

Gilchrest BA (1995) Pruritus in the elderly. Semin Dermatol 14(4):317–319

Gilchrest BA, Murphy GF, Soter NA (1982) Effect of chronologic ageing and ultraviolet irradiation on Langerhans cells in human epidermis. J Invest Dermatol 79(2):85–88

Goukassian D, Gad F, Yaar M et al (2000) Mechanisms and implications of the age-associated decrease in DNA repair capacity. FASEB J 14(10):1325–1334

Granstein RD, Matsui MS (2004) UV radiation-induced immunosuppression and skin cancer. Cutis 74(5 Suppl):4–9

Griffin MD, Kumar R (2003) Effects of 1alpha,25(OH)2D3 and its analogs on dendritic cell function. J Cell Biochem 88(2):323–326

Grolleau-Julius A, Ray D, Yung RL (2010) The role of epigenetics in ageing and autoimmunity. Clin Rev Allergy Immunol 39(1):42–50

Gupta SG, Wang LC, Penas PF et al (2006) Sentinel lymph node biopsy for evaluation and treatment of patients with Merkel cell carcinoma: The Dana-Farber experience and meta-analysis of the literature. Arch Dermatol 142(6):685–690

Halder RM (1998) The role of retinoids in the management of cutaneous conditions in blacks. J Am Acad Dermatol 39(2 Pt 3):S98–S103

Halder RM, Richards GM (2004) Photoageing in patients of skin of color. In: Rigel DS, Weiss RA, Lim HW, Dover JS (eds) Photoageing. Marcel Dekker, Inc, New York, p 55

Hanneman KK, Cooper KD, Baron ED (2006) Ultraviolet immunosuppression: mechanisms and consequences. Dermatol Clin 24(1):19–25

Harder J, Bartels J, Christophers E et al (1997) A peptide antibiotic from human skin. Nature 387(6636):861

Hiramoto K, Jikumaru M, Yamate Y et al (2009) Ultraviolet A irradiation of the eye induces immunomodulation of skin and intestine in mice via hypothalomo-pituitary-adrenal pathways. Arch Dermatol Res 301(3):239–244

Hiramoto K, Yamate Y, Kobayashi H et al (2012) Long-term ultraviolet A irradiation of the eye induces photoageing of the skin in mice. Arch Dermatol Res 304(1):39–45

Hirschfeld M, Kirschning CJ, Schwandner R et al (1999) Cutting edge: inflammatory signaling by Borrelia burgdorferi lipoproteins is mediated by toll-like receptor 2. J Immunol 163(5):2382–2386

Holan V, Kuffova L, Zajicova A et al (1998) Urocanic acid enhances IL-10 production in activated CD4+ T cells. J Immunol 161(7):3237–3241

Hou L, Sasaki H, Stashenko P (2000) Toll-like receptor 4-deficient mice have reduced bone destruction following mixed anaerobic infection. Infect Immun 68(8):4681–4687

Howell MD, Gallo RL, Boguniewicz M et al (2006a) Cytokine milieu of atopic dermatitis skin subverts the innate immune response to vaccinia virus. Immunity 24(3):341–348

Howell MD, Wollenberg A, Gallo RL et al (2006b) Cathelicidin deficiency predisposes to eczema herpeticum. J Allergy Clin Immunol 117(4):836–841

Howitz KT, Bitterman KJ, Cohen HY et al (2003) Small molecule activators of sirtuins extend Saccharomyces cerevisiae lifespan. Nature 425(6954):191–196

Jinquan T, Vorum H, Larsen CG et al (1996) Psoriasin: a novel chemotactic protein. J Invest Dermatol 107(1):5–10

Johnson GK (1994) Effects of ageing on the microvasculature and microcirculation in skin and oral mucosa. In: Squier CA, Hill MW (eds) The effects of ageing in oral mucosa and skin. CRC Press, Boca Raton, pp 99–105

Kaeberlein M (2010) Lessons on longevity from budding yeast. Nature 464(7288):513–519

Kaidbey KH, Agin PP, Sayre RM et al (1979) Photoprotection by melanin–a comparison of black and Caucasian skin. J Am Acad Dermatol 1(3):249–260

Kang S, Fisher GJ, Voorhees JJ (2001) Photoageing: pathogenesis, prevention and treatment. In: Gilchrest BA (ed) Geriatric dermatology. W. B. Saunders, Philadelphia, p 643

Ke MS et al (2004) Effects of T4 endonuclease liposomes and RNA fragments on UV-induced DNA damage. J Invest Dermatol 122(3):A146

Kessler I (1993) Epidemiological considerations in the role of dendritic/Langerhans cells in human cancer. In Vivo 7(3):305–312

Kim MS, Kim YK, Lee DH et al (2009) Acute exposure of human skin to ultraviolet or infrared radiation or heat stimuli increases mast cell numbers and tryptase expression in human skin in vivo. Br J Dermatol 160(2):393–402

Kodali S, Beissert S, Granstein RD (2005) Physiology and pathology of skin photoimmunology. In: Cutaneous Immunology and clinical immunodermatology. CRC Press, Boca Raton, pp 457–474

Kohrgruber N, Halanek N, Groger M et al (1999) Survival, maturation, and function of CD11c- and CD11c+ peripheral blood dendritic cells are differentially regulated by cytokines. J Immunol 163(6):3250–3259

Kosmadaki MG, Gilchrest BA (2004) The role of telomeres in skin ageing/photoageing. Micron 35(3):155–159

Kovacs EJ, Palmer JL, Fortin CF et al (2009) Ageing and innate immunity in the mouse: impact of intrinsic and extrinsic factors. Trends Immunol 30(7):319–324

Kricker A, Armstrong BK, English DR et al (1995) Does intermittent sun exposure cause basal cell carcinoma? a case-control study in Western Australia. Int J Cancer 60(4):489–494

Kubo A, Nagao K, Yokouchi M et al (2009) External antigen uptake by Langerhans cells with reorganization of epidermal tight junction barriers. J Exp Med 206(13): 2937–2946

Kupper TS, Groves RW (1995) The interleukin-1 axis and cutaneous inflammation. J Invest Dermatol 105(1 Suppl):62S–66S

Kurban RS, Bhawan J (1990) Histologic changes in skin associated with ageing. J Dermatol Surg Oncol 16(10): 908–914

Lande R, Gilliet M (2010) Plasmacytoid dendritic cells: key players in the initiation and regulation of immune responses. Ann N Y Acad Sci 1183:89–103

Langerhans P (1868) Ueber die Nerven der menschlichen Haut. Archiv für pathologische Anatomie und Physiologie und für klinische Medicin 44(2–3):325–337

Larsen CP, Steinman RM, Witmer-Pack M et al (1990) Migration and maturation of Langerhans cells in skin transplants and explants. J Exp Med 172(5):1483–1493

Lasithiotakis K, Leiter U, Meier F et al (2008) Age and gender are significant independent predictors of survival in primary cutaneous melanoma. Cancer 112(8): 1795–1804

Laube S (2004) Skin infections and ageing. Ageing Res Rev 3(1):69–89

Lavker RM (1979) Structural alterations in exposed and unexposed aged skin. J Invest Dermatol 73(1):59–66

Li GZ, Eller MS, Firoozabadi R et al (2003) Evidence that exposure of the telomere 3′ overhang sequence induces senescence. Proc Natl Acad Sci U S A 100(2):527–531

Lopez-Garcia B, Lee PH, Yamasaki K et al (2005) Antifungal activity of cathelicidins and their potential role in Candida albicans skin infection. J Invest Dermatol 125(1):108–115

Mahbub S, Brubaker AL, Kovacs EJ (2011) Ageing of the innate immune system: an update. Curr Immunol Rev 7(1):104–115

Martin ES, Elewski BE (2002) Cutaneous fungal infections in the elderly. In: Gilchrest BA (ed) Geriatric dermatology. W. B. Saunders, Philadelphia, p 59

Mathers CD, Iburg KM, Salomon JA et al (2004) Global patterns of healthy life expectancy in the year 2002. BMC Public Health 4:66

Maxwell AP, McCluskey DR (1986) Assessment of cell-mediated immunity in a British population using multiple skin test antigens. Clin Allergy 16(4):365–369

Medzhitov R, Janeway CA Jr (1997) Innate immunity: impact on the adaptive immune response. Curr Opin Immunol 9(1):4–9

Meunier L, Gonzalez-Ramos A, Cooper KD (1993) Heterogeneous populations of class II MHC+ cells in human dermal cell suspensions. Identification of a small subset responsible for potent dermal antigen-presenting cell activity with features analogous to Langerhans cells. J Immunol 151(8):4067–4080

Moll I, Bohnert E, Herbst C et al (1994) Establishment and characterization of two Merkel cell tumor cultures. J Invest Dermatol 102(3):346–353

Moodycliffe AM, Nghiem D, Clydesdale G et al (2000) Immune suppression and skin cancer development: regulation by NKT cells. Nat Immunol 1(6):521–525

Moriwaki S, Ray S, Tarone RE et al (1996) The effect of donor age on the processing of UV-damaged DNA by cultured human cells: reduced DNA repair capacity and increased DNA mutability. Mutat Res 364(2): 117–123

Morris BT, Sober AJ (1989) Cutaneous malignant melanoma in the older patient. In: Gilchrest BA (ed) Clinics in geriatric medicine, vol 5. W. B. Saunders, Philadelphia, p 171

Mosmann TR, Cherwinski H, Bond MW et al (1986) Two types of murine helper T cell clone. I. Definition according to profiles of lymphokine activities and secreted proteins. J Immunol 136(7):2348–2357

Munavalli GS, Weiss RA, Halder RM (2005) Photoageing and nonablative photorejuvenation in ethnic skin. Dermatol Surg 31(9 Pt 2):1250–1260; discussion 1261

Murphy G (1998) The acute effects of ultraviolet radiation on the skin. In: JLM H (ed) Photoimmunology. Chapman & Hall, London, pp 43–52

Nakamura T, Pinnell SR, Darr D et al (1997) Vitamin C abrogates the deleterious effects of UVB radiation on cutaneous immunity by a mechanism that does not depend on TNF-alpha. J Invest Dermatol 109(1): 20–24

Nakamura H, Hirota S, Adachi S et al (2001) Clonal nature of seborrheic keratosis demonstrated by using the polymorphism of the human androgen receptor locus as a marker. J Invest Dermatol 116(4):506–510

Nizet V, Ohtake T, Lauth X et al (2001) Innate antimicrobial peptide protects the skin from invasive bacterial infection. Nature 414(6862):454–457

Ogden S, Dearman RJ, Kimber I et al (2011) The effect of ageing on phenotype and function of monocyte-derived Langerhans cells. Br J Dermatol 165(1):184–188

Ong PY, Ohtake T, Brandt C et al (2002) Endogenous antimicrobial peptides and skin infections in atopic dermatitis. N Engl J Med 347(15):1151–1160

Oosterwegel MA, Greenwald RJ, Mandelbrot DA et al (1999) CTLA-4 and T cell activation. Curr Opin Immunol 11(3):294–300

Panda A, Qian F, Mohanty S et al (2010) Age-associated decrease in TLR function in primary human dendritic cells predicts influenza vaccine response. J Immunol 184(5):2518–2527

Paquette D, Falanga V (2002) Leg ulcers. In: Gilchrest BA (ed) Geriatric dermatology. W. B. Saunders, Philadelphia, p 77

Peters T, Weiss JM, Sindrilaru A et al (2009) Reactive oxygen intermediate-induced pathomechanisms contribute to immunosenescence, chronic inflammation and autoimmunity. Mech Ageing Dev 130(9):564–587

Plowden J, Renshaw-Hoelscher M, Engleman C et al (2004) Innate immunity in ageing: impact on macrophage function. Aging Cell 3(4):161–167

Reeve VE, Greenoak GE, Canfield PJ et al (1989) Topical urocanic acid enhances UV-induced tumour yield and malignancy in the hairless mouse. Photochem Photobiol 49(4):459–464

Reichrath J, Rappl G (2003) Ultraviolet light (UV)-induced immunosuppression: is vitamin D the missing link? J Cell Biochem 89(1):6–8

Rijken F, Bruijnzeel-Koomen CA (2011) Photoaged skin: the role of neutrophils, preventive measures, and potential pharmacological targets. Clin Pharmacol Ther 89(1):120–124

Rongioletti F, Rebora A (1995) Fibroelastolytic patterns of intrinsic skin ageing: pseudoxanthoma-elasticum-like papillary dermal elastolysis and white fibrous papulosis of the neck. Dermatology 191(1):19–24

Ruland J, Mak TW (2003) Transducing signals from antigen receptors to nuclear factor kappaB. Immunol Rev 193:93–100

Sachs DL, Marghoob AA, Halpern A (2001) Skin cancer in the elderly. In: Gilchrest BA (ed) Geriatric dermatology. W. B. Saunders, Philadelphia, p 715

Sansoni P, Cossarizza A, Brianti V et al (1993) Lymphocyte subsets and natural killer cell activity in healthy old people and centenarians. Blood 82(9):2767–2773

Schaerli P, Ebert L, Willimann K et al (2004) A skin-selective homing mechanism for human immune surveillance T cells. J Exp Med 199(9):1265–1275

Schauber J, Gallo RL (2008) Antimicrobial peptides and the skin immune defense system. J Allergy Clin Immunol 122(2):261–266

Schittek B, Hipfel R, Sauer B et al (2001) Dermcidin: a novel human antibiotic peptide secreted by sweat glands. Nat Immunol 2(12):1133–1137

Schmitt DA, Walterscheid JP, Ullrich SE (2000) Reversal of ultraviolet radiation-induced immune suppression by recombinant interleukin-12: suppression of cytokine production. Immunology 101(1):90–96

Schuster C, Vaculik C, Fiala C et al (2009) HLA-DR+ leukocytes acquire CD1 antigens in embryonic and fetal human skin and contain functional antigen-presenting cells. J Exp Med 206(1):169–181

Schwab R, Szabo P, Manavalan JS et al (1997) Expanded CD4+ and CD8+ T cell clones in elderly humans. J Immunol 158(9):4493–4499

Schwarz T (2010) The dark and the sunny sides of UVR-induced immunosuppression: photoimmunology revisited. J Invest Dermatol 130(1):49–54

Schwarz A, Schwarz T (2010) UVR-induced regulatory T cells switch antigen-presenting cells from a stimulatory to a regulatory phenotype. J Invest Dermatol 130(7):1914–1921

Schwarz A, Maeda A, Kernebeck K et al (2005) Prevention of UV radiation-induced immunosuppression by IL-12 is dependent on DNA repair. J Exp Med 201(2):173–179

Senyurek I, Paulmann M, Sinnberg T et al (2009) Dermcidin-derived peptides show a different mode of action than the cathelicidin LL-37 against Staphylococcus aureus. Antimicrob Agents Chemother 53(6):2499–2509

Shaw AC, Joshi S, Greenwood H et al (2010) Ageing of the innate immune system. Curr Opin Immunol 22(4):507–513

Shevach EM, DiPaolo RA, Andersson J et al (2006) The lifestyle of naturally occurring CD4+ CD25+ Foxp3+ regulatory T cells. Immunol Rev 212:60–73

Shibata K, Yamada H, Hara H et al (2007) Resident Vdelta1+ gammadelta T cells control early infiltration of neutrophils after Escherichia coli infection via IL-17 production. J Immunol 178(7):4466–4472

Shodell M, Siegal FP (2002) Circulating, interferon-producing plasmacytoid dendritic cells decline during human ageing. Scand J Immunol 56(5):518–521

Shreedhar VK, Pride MW, Sun Y et al (1998) Origin and characteristics of ultraviolet-B radiation-induced suppressor T lymphocytes. J Immunol 161(3):1327–1335

Siegal FP, Kadowaki N, Shodell M et al (1999) The nature of the principal type 1 interferon-producing cells in human blood. Science 284(5421):1835–1837

Snyder PW, Hogenesch H (1996) Immune system. In: Mohr U, Dungworth DL, Capen CC, Carlton WW, Sundberg JP, Ward JM (eds) Pathobiology of the ageing mouse, vol 1. International Life Sciences Institute Press, Washington, DC, pp 189–203

Steingrimsson E, Copeland NG, Jenkins NA (2005) Melanocyte stem cell maintenance and hair graying. Cell 121(1):9–12

Stevens GL, Bergstresser PR (1998) Photodermatology. In: Hawk JLM (ed) Photoimmunology. Chapman & Hall, London, pp 54–67

Stulnig T, Maczek C, Bock G et al (1995) Reference intervals for human peripheral blood lymphocyte subpopulations from 'healthy' young and aged subjects. Int Arch Allergy Immunol 108(3):205–210

Sunderkotter C, Kalden H, Luger TA (1997) Ageing and the skin immune system. Arch Dermatol 133(10): 1256–1262

Taams LS, van Amelsfort JM, Tiemessen MM et al (2005) Modulation of monocyte/macrophage function by human CD4+CD25+ regulatory T cells. Hum Immunol 66(3):222–230

Takeuchi O, Hoshino K, Kawai T et al (1999) Differential roles of TLR2 and TLR4 in recognition of gram-negative and gram-positive bacterial cell wall components. Immunity 11(4):443–451

Takeuchi H, Gomi T, Shishido M et al (2010) Neutrophil elastase contributes to extracellular matrix damage induced by chronic low-dose UV irradiation in a hairless mouse photoageing model. J Dermatol Sci 60(3):151–158

Talwar HS, Griffiths CE, Fisher GJ et al (1995) Reduced type I and type III procollagens in photodamaged adult human skin. J Invest Dermatol 105(2):285–290

Teraki E, Tajima S, Manaka I et al (1996) Role of endothelin-1 in hyperpigmentation in seborrhoeic keratosis. Br J Dermatol 135(6):918–923

Tezuka T, Qing J, Saheki M et al (1994) Terminal differentiation of facial epidermis of the aged: immunohistochemical studies. Dermatology 188(1):21–24

Tiemessen MM, Jagger AL, Evans HG et al (2007) CD4+CD25+Foxp3+ regulatory T cells induce alternative activation of human monocytes/macrophages. Proc Natl Acad Sci U S A 104(49):19446–19451

Tobin DJ, Paus R (2001) Graying: gerontobiology of the hair follicle pigmentary unit. Exp Gerontol 36(1): 29–54

Tomura M, Honda T, Tanizaki H et al (2010) Activated regulatory T cells are the major T cell type emigrating from the skin during a cutaneous immune response in mice. J Clin Invest 120(3):883–893

Tresguerres JA, Kireev R, Tresguerres AF et al (2008) Molecular mechanisms involved in the hormonal prevention of ageing in the rat. J Steroid Biochem Mol Biol 108(3–5):318–326

Uitto J, Pulkkinen L (1996) Molecular complexity of the cutaneous basement membrane zone. Mol Biol Rep 23(1):35–46

Ullrich SE (1994) Mechanism involved in the systemic suppression of antigen-presenting cell function by UV irradiation. Keratinocyte-derived IL-10 modulates antigen-presenting cell function of splenic adherent cells. J Immunol 152(7):3410–3416

Ullrich SE (2002) Photoimmune suppression and photocarcinogenesis. Front Biosci 7:d684–d703

van den Broeke LT, Beijersbergen van Henegouwen GM (1995) Topically applied N-acetylcysteine as a protector against UVB-induced systemic immunosuppression. J Photochem Photobiol B 27(1):61–65

Van Neste D, Tobin DJ (2004) Hair cycle and hair pigmentation: dynamic interactions and changes associated with ageing. Micron 35(3):193–200

Vestal RE, Cusack BJ (1990) Pharmacology and ageing. In: Schneider EL, Rowe JW (eds) Handbook of the biology of ageing. Academic Press, San Diego, p 349

Vukmanovic-Stejic M, Agius E, Booth N et al (2008) The kinetics of CD4+Foxp3+ T cell accumulation during a human cutaneous antigen-specific memory response in vivo. J Clin Invest 118(11):3639–3650

Vukmanovic-Stejic M, Rustin MH, Nikolich-Zugich J et al (2011) Immune responses in the skin in old age. Curr Opin Immunol 23(4):525–531

Waldorf DS, Willkens RF, Decker JL (1968) Impaired delayed hypersensitivity in an ageing population. Association with antinuclear reactivity and rheumatoid factor. JAMA 203(10):831–834

Weitz JI, Crowley KA, Landman SL et al (1987) Increased neutrophil elastase activity in cigarette smokers. Ann Intern Med 107(5):680–682

Wolf P, Maier H, Mullegger RR et al (2000) Topical treatment with liposomes containing T4 endonuclease V protects human skin in vivo from ultraviolet-induced upregulation of interleukin-10 and tumor necrosis factor-alpha. J Invest Dermatol 114(1): 149–156

Wulf HC, Sandby-Moller J, Kobayasi T et al (2004) Skin ageing and natural photoprotection. Micron 35(3): 185–191

Yaar M, Gilchrest BA (1987) Bullous pemphigoid: disease of the ageing immune system. In: Ahmed AR (ed) Clinics in Dermatology. Lippincott, Philadelphia, p 135

Yaar M, Gilchrest BA (2001) Ageing and photoageing of keratinocytes and melanocytes. Clin Exp Dermatol 26(7):583–591

Yamate Y, Hiramoto K, Kasahara E et al (2011) Ultraviolet-A irradiation to the eye modulates intestinal mucosal functions and properties of mast cells in the mouse. Photochem Photobiol 87(1): 191–198

Yang RB, Mark MR, Gray A et al (1998) Toll-like receptor-2 mediates lipopolysaccharide-induced cellular signalling. Nature 395(6699):284–288

Yang RB, Mark MR, Gurney AL et al (1999) Signaling events induced by lipopolysaccharide-activated toll-like receptor 2. J Immunol 163(2):639–643

Yarosh D, Dong K, Smiles K (2008) UV-induced degradation of collagen I is mediated by soluble factors released from keratinocytes. Photochem Photobiol 84(1):67–68

Youn SW, Kim DS, Cho HJ et al (2004) Cellular senescence induced loss of stem cell proportion in the skin in vitro. J Dermatol Sci 35(2):113–123

Yuen KS, Nearn MR, Halliday GM (2002) Nitric oxide-mediated depletion of Langerhans cells from the epidermis may be involved in UVA radiation-induced immunosuppression. Nitric Oxide 6(3):313–318

Aging Immunity and the Impact of Physical Exercise

26

Guillaume Spielmann, Austin B. Bigley, Emily C. LaVoy, and Richard J. Simpson

26.1 Introduction

Regular physical exercise is associated with increased longevity and a lower risk of developing cardiovascular disease (CVD), diabetes, metabolic syndrome, hypertension, infectious illnesses, and cancer (Lynch et al. 1996; Kodama et al. 2009; Evenson et al. 2003; Blair et al. 1996; Barlow et al. 2006). Over the last quarter century, there has been considerable interest in the effects of exercise on the aging immune system. Immunosenescence, the canopy term used to describe the progressive decline in normal immune function with age, has been attributed to the etiology of many age-related diseases. This includes cancer, pneumonia/influenza, septicemia, and nephritis, which are among the ten leading causes of death in persons aged 65 years or older in the United States (US) (Heron and Tejada-Vera 2009). Regular exercise has been purported as a simple lifestyle factor that could help negate the onset of immunosenescence and reduce the burden of immune-related health problems in the elderly population. The methods used to study the effects of exercise on the aging immune system are highly varied. Cross-sectional experimental designs are oftentimes used to discriminate between exercise trained and untrained older adults, whereas more and more studies are now incorporating longitudinal randomized controlled trials to examine the effects of an exercise training intervention on various aspects of immunity. Exercise training interventions usually incorporate aerobic- and/or resistance-based exercise lasting from 8 weeks to 12 months, and the subjects enrolled in these studies range from healthy middle-aged adults to frail elderly nursing home residents. Among the most common outcome measures used to assess the effects of exercise on the aging immune system are T-cell proliferative responses to mitogens, serum antibody titers following vaccination, cytotoxic activity of natural killer (NK) cells, the function of phagocytic cells, the numbers and composition of leukocyte subtypes, and circulating levels of inflammatory mediators (Haaland et al. 2008). Although vast inconsistencies in experimental design can often complicate the interpretation of the available literature, more and more evidence is emerging to indicate that exercise is in fact capable of negating immunosenescence. In this chapter, we address the effects of regular exercise on immunosenescence and the associated immune risk profile (IRP) in older humans. We have defined older humans as aged 60 years or more and, although we have focused mostly on studies involving human subjects, data from animal models are referred to when appropriate human data are lacking.

G. Spielmann, PhD • A.B. Bigley • E.C. LaVoy
R.J. Simpson, PhD (✉)
Laboratory of Integrated Physiology,
Department of Health and Human Performance,
University of Houston,
Houston, TX 77204, USA
e-mail: rjsimpson@uh.edu

A. Massoud, N. Rezaei (eds.), *Immunology of Aging*,
DOI 10.1007/978-3-642-39495-9_26, © Springer-Verlag Berlin Heidelberg 2014

26.2 Aging, Immunosenescence, and the Immune Risk Profile

Longitudinal aging studies that have been ongoing since the mid-1990s identified a cluster of immunological biomarkers referred to as IRP that predict mortality at 2-, 4-, and 6-year follow-up in a very old Swedish population (Pawelec et al. 2009; Ferguson et al. 1995). The IRP includes an inverted CD4+:CD8+ T-cell ratio, poor T-cell proliferative responses to mitogens, low levels of interleukin (IL)-2 production, high ratio of late (i.e., CD27-/CD28-) to early (i.e., CD27+/CD28+) stage differentiated CD8+ T cells, increased proportion of T cells expressing markers associated with senescence (i.e., killer cell lectin-like receptor subfamily G member 1 or KLRG1, CD57), and seropositivity to cytomegalovirus (CMV). CMV is a ubiquitous β-herpesvirus that establishes lifelong infection in over 50 % of the US population (Bate et al. 2010). As CMV is capable of frequent and intermittent reactivation, it is believed to drive immunosenescence of the T-cell compartment due to a sustained antigenic load that may lead to T-cell exhaustion and proliferative arrest. CMV reactivation causes an insidious inflation of the memory T-cell pool and, in conjunction with a lowering output of naïve T cells from the atrophying thymus in aging humans, the repertoire of naïve T cells capable of recognizing and responding to novel infectious agents is substantially lowered (Brunner et al. 2010). This is referred to as a lowering of the "immune space" and is hypothesized to allow rapidly evolving pathogens (i.e., influenza, rhinovirus, respiratory syncytial virus, or RCV) to disseminate more readily in the aging host (Saurwein-Teissl et al. 2002).

A common criticism of the IRP is that it is too focused on adaptive immunity. It has now become apparent that the innate arm of the immune system is not impervious to the effects of immunosenescence. For instance, the proliferation and natural cytotoxicity of NK cells has been shown to decrease with age (Gayoso et al. 2011), while defects in neutrophil phagocytosis and chemotaxis is also evident with increasing age (Shaw et al. 2010). Moreover, monocyte expression of co-stimulatory molecules (i.e., CD80/CD86) and production of cytokines also show age-related impairments, particularly in the context of toll-like receptor (TLR) signaling (van Duin and Shaw 2007; Shaw et al. 2011). A marked association with aging is increased levels of circulatory inflammatory mediators. This has been coined "inflamm-aging" and describes a chronic, mostly asymptomatic, low-grade inflammatory state that can eventually lead to chronic illnesses in the elderly such as cardiovascular disease, type 2 diabetes mellitus, Alzheimer's disease, osteoporosis, and certain cancers. Indeed, circulating levels of inflammatory mediators such as IL-6, interleukin-1 receptor antagonist (IL-1RA), and C-reactive protein (CRP) are considered useful prognostic markers in very old people (Jylha et al. 2007). Here we describe the impact of aging and exercise on innate immunity and those aspects of adaptive immunity that have been associated with the IRP.

26.3 Exercise, Aging, and Innate Immunity

26.3.1 Neutrophils

Neutrophils are the initial responders at sites of tissue injury and infection where they play a critical role in the initiation of inflammation (Kumar and Sharma 2010). They are the most abundant phagocytes in circulating blood and they help the host combat rapidly proliferating bacteria, yeast, and fungal infections through the generation of free radicals and the release of proteolytic enzymes and microbicidal peptides from cytoplasmic granules (Shaw et al. 2010, 2011). Neutrophils are attracted to the site of immunological insult by a process known as chemotaxis that is driven by the release of pro-inflammatory cytokines, such as tumor necrosis factor alpha (TNF-α), IL-1, and IL-8 by tissue-resident macrophages (Hume et al. 2002). The available data concerning the effect of aging on the number of circulating neutrophils is highly ambiguous. Most studies report no change in the number of neutrophils with healthy aging (Chatta and Dale 1996; Born et al. 1995; Fulop et al. 1985); however, it has also been reported that the number of circulating neutrophils decreases (De Martinis et al. 2004) and increases with age (Bruunsgaard and Pedersen 2000). Interestingly, elevated neutrophil counts are associated with chronic, low-grade inflammation and increased 2-year mortality in the elderly (Ferrando-Martinez et al. 2013). Collectively, these data suggest that neutrophil count does not change with healthy aging, but can become elevated as part of so-called inflamm-aging.

The functional capabilities of neutrophils appear to be impaired by aging as most studies report decreased chemotaxis, phagocytosis, and free radical production with advancing age (Peters et al. 2009; Butcher et al. 2001; Fulop et al. 1997). These changes are associated with decreased surface expression of CD16, a marker of neutrophil functional capability and viability that is required for phagocytosis of opsonized target cells (Butcher et al. 2001). It is important to note, however, that not all studies support an age-related impairment of neutrophil phagocytosis and migratory functions (Plackett et al. 2004). In experimental models of human skin abrasion and gingivitis, older adults appear to have similar neutrophil migration, adhesion, and infiltration properties as the young; however, there is some evidence for reduced and/or impaired neutrophil chemotaxis in response to infection with age (Plackett et al. 2004). This could potentially allow bacteria to persist in the host and also extend inflammation beyond the site of infection (Shaw et al. 2010). The idea that impaired neutrophil function contributes to impaired bacterial immunity in the aged is further supported by an age-dependent decrease in phagocytosis of *Escherichia coli* and *Staphylococcus aureus* by neutrophils (Wenisch et al. 2000). Additionally, neutrophil susceptibility to spontaneous and cytokine-induced apoptosis is greater in aged individuals (Fulop et al. 1997). This impaired apoptosis resistance may interfere with the normal process of inflammation whereby activated macrophages prolong the lifespan of neutrophils at the site of inflammation through the release of pro-survival cytokines (Solana et al. 2012). Further, neutrophil-driven recruitment of dendritic cells to loci of infection may also be impaired as evidenced by decreased plasma levels of the human neutrophil-derived alarmin cathelicidin (LL37) with age (Alvarez-Rodriguez et al. 2012). Collectively, these data suggest a broad decrease in neutrophil function with age that affects both their direct effector functions and their interactions with other cells of the innate immune system.

The age-related functional decrements that have been observed in neutrophil function have been corroborated by observations of impaired cell signaling. There is a marked age-dependent decline in intracellular signaling through the mitogen-activated protein kinases (MAPK), janus kinase/signal transducer and activator of transcription (JAK/STAT), and phosphatidylinositol-3-kinase and protein kinase B (PI3K-Akt) pathways in neutrophils (Larbi et al. 2005). This decline in signaling is not due to loss of receptors, but rather inadequate signaling through receptors due to loss of lipid raft integrity (Fortin et al. 2008; Guichard et al. 2005). Inadequate lipid raft integrity prevents proper assembly of the nicotinamide adenine dinucleotide phosphate (NADPH) oxidase complex with subsequent loss of free radical generation (Guichard et al. 2005). Similarly, signaling through pattern recognition receptors (PRR) that allow neutrophils to discriminate between self and "nonself" is also disrupted due to altered trafficking of signaling molecules in and out of lipid rafts (Shaw et al. 2011). Ca^{2+} flux during cell signaling is also impaired in the aged, which results in reduced microbicidal capacity and free radical generation by neutrophils (Plackett et al. 2004). Further, anti-apoptotic signaling downstream of inflammatory mediators (i.e., IL-2, lipopolysaccharides (LPS), granulocyte-macrophage colony-stimulating factor (GM-CSF), and granulocyte colony-stimulating factor (G-CSF)) is decreased in the elderly (Plackett et al. 2004). Thus, an age-dependent impairment in cell signaling through a variety of pathways results in neutrophils that have fewer effector functions and are present for a shorter period of time during infection.

Despite marked age-related changes in neutrophil function, relatively little is known about the impact of exercise training. Cross-sectional studies have reported a decline in neutrophil number in elderly men that exercise regularly (de Gonzalo-Calvo et al. 2012; Michishita et al. 2008); however, most longitudinal studies have reported no change in neutrophil number following exercise training interventions in healthy elderly (Walsh et al. 2011; Woods et al. 1999). However, exercise training has been shown to reduce blood neutrophil counts in overweight women with concomitant reductions in insulin resistance and BMI (Michishita et al. 2008), suggesting that chronic exercise may reduce neutrophils and other pro-inflammatory mediators in those showing symptoms of chronic low-grade inflammation. With regard to neutrophil function, a moderate intensity exercise training regimen has been reported to increase neutrophil chemotaxis and phagocytosis (Syu et al. 2012), and regular exercise is associated with a lower age-related decline in neutrophil phagocytosis (Yan et al. 2001). Strenuous exercise has also been reported to delay apoptosis (Mooren et al. 2012) and modulate pro-inflammatory gene expression in neutrophils (Radom-Aizik et al. 2008). Unfortunately, the effect of exercise training on the decline in neutrophil function with age has been understudied. One study investigating the effect of a 15-week exercise training intervention on postmenopausal women found that exercise had no effect on neutrophil granulation or oxidative burst (Fairey et al. 2005). In addition, Takahashi et al. (2013) reported that a 12-week training intervention consisting of low-volume walking exercises resulted in decreased neutrophil activation and basal oxidative stress in the elderly. Future studies should investigate the effects of chronic exercise on the most discernable age-related decrements in neutrophil function, such as impaired Microbidical capacity and chemotaxis to infectious agents (Shaw et al. 2010).

26.3.2 Monocytes/Macrophages

Monocytes and macrophages are important intermediaries between the innate and adaptive immune systems. They have strong effector capabilities against viruses, bacteria, and tumors, while also being potent antigen presenting cells (APCs) (Cros et al. 2010; Geissmann et al. 2010). Circulating monocytes can typically be classified into two main categories: classical (CD14^{high}/CD16$^-$) and pro-inflammatory (CD14^{low}/CD16$^+$) (Passlick et al. 1989). Pro-inflammatory monocytes are characterized by their high production of TNF-α in response to ligation of TLR2 and TLR4 (Belge et al. 2002). Classical monocytes represent a less mature phenotype with weaker effector functions and lower tissue-migratory potential as evidenced by their expression of CD62L, CD64, and C-C chemokine receptor type 2 (CCR2) coupled to low expression of chemokine (C-X-C motif) receptor 1 (CXCR1) (Solana et al. 2012). A portion of circulating monocytes will differentiate into tissue-resident macrophages. Macrophages are frontline phagocytes and antigen-presenting cells that contribute to wound healing and priming of adaptive immune responses (Mege et al. 2011). Macrophages can be classified as M1-type (classically activated or "pro-inflammatory") or M2-type (alternatively activated or "anti-inflammatory") based on the nature of their interactions with lymphocytes. M1 macrophages are activated by the T-helper (Th)1 cytokine interferon gamma (IFN-γ) and secrete high levels of the pro-inflammatory cytokine IL-12, while M2 macrophages are activated by the Th2 cytokine IL-4 and secrete high levels of the anti-inflammatory cytokine IL-10 (Biswas and Mantovani 2010).

The absolute number of monocytes in blood increases with aging, which is mostly attributable to pro-inflammatory, "nonclassical" CD14^{dim}/CD16^{bright} cells (Merino et al. 2011). This preferential expansion of the pro-inflammatory monocyte subset with aging leads to an increased proportion of CD16$^+$ cells relative to younger individuals (Nyugen et al. 2010). An increased number of pro-inflammatory monocytes are associated with elevated atherosclerotic activity and increased incidence of inflammation-dependent diseases (Dopheide et al. 2012). Thus, it is likely that an increase in the size of the pro-inflammatory monocyte pool contributes to "inflamm-aging" and the increased incidence of cardiovascular disease in the elderly.

The age-dependent shift of monocytes toward a pro-inflammatory phenotype is associated with marked functional decrements (Panda et al. 2010; Cretel et al. 2010). Phagocytosis and free radical production by monocytes and macrophages is decreased with healthy aging (Gomez et al. 2008). Antigen presentation by macrophages is also impaired with aging due largely to a decreased expression of major histocompatibility complex (MHC) class II molecules (Solana et al. 1991; Villanueva et al. 1990), and decreased production of IL-12 following activation (Plowden et al. 2004; Wu et al. 2008). In aged individuals, baseline production of pro-inflammatory cytokines (IL-6 and IL-8) by monocytes is elevated (Franceschi et al. 2007); however, LPS-stimulated pro-inflammatory cytokine production has been reported to be decreased in most studies (Renshaw et al. 2002; van Duin and Shaw 2007). Similarly, macrophage production of pro-inflammatory cytokines (TNF-α, IFN-γ, and IL-6) is decreased in response to antigen challenge in the elderly (Agius et al. 2009). Thus, it appears that monocytes/macrophages contribute to the chronic low-grade inflammation of aging and that this permanent state of semi-activation renders the cells less responsive to antigenic stimulation.

The functional changes observed in monocytes and macrophages with aging are associated with dysregulated signaling through TLRs. TLR1-/TLR2-induced IL-6 and TNF-α production is lost in the elderly due in part to reduced expression of TLR1 and TLR4 (van Duin and Shaw 2007). Induction of co-stimulatory proteins CD80 and CD86 following TLR stimulation is reduced as well (van Duin et al. 2007), which suggests that monocytes have a reduced capacity to prime T cells during antigen presentation. Defective TLR signaling has also been implicated in the defective chemotaxis of macrophages toward sites of tissue injury in the elderly (Plowden et al. 2004; Ashcroft et al. 1998).

The effects of exercise on monocyte surface expression of TLRs have received a considerable amount of research attention in the past decade. Particular emphasis has been placed on TLR4 due to its increased expression on monocytes in chronic inflammatory conditions such as sepsis (Armstrong et al. 2004) and type 2 diabetes (Reyna et al. 2008). Early cross-sectional studies reported reduced monocyte TLR4 expression in trained versus untrained elderly (McFarlin et al. 2004, 2006); however, these studies failed to account for potential changes in the composition of monocyte subsets that have different preexisting expression levels of TLRs (i.e., pro-inflammatory vs. classical monocytes) (Simpson et al. 2009). While acute exercise has been shown to downregulate expression of TLRs 1, 2, and 4 on circulating monocytes and dampen their downstream functional responses (Lancaster et al. 2005), longitudinal exercise studies have yet to uncover any significant effect of training on monocyte TLR4 expression in the elderly (Timmerman et al. 2008; Shimizu et al. 2011). Exercise training, however, has been reported to have significant effects on monocyte subset composition and function. For example, Timmerman et al. reported that a 12-week training program consisting of aerobic and resistance exercise resulted in a decreased proportion of CD14[+]/CD16[+] monocytes in blood and reduced LPS-stimulated production of the pro-inflammatory cytokine TNF-α (Timmerman et al. 2008). Not all monocyte functions appear to be positively modulated by exercise, however, as another 12-week program of concurrent aerobic and resistance exercise training was reported to have no effect on the phagocytic activity of monocytes (Schaun et al. 2011). Overall, the current literature, while brief, suggests that chronic exercise may reduce the contribution of monocytes to inflamm-aging, while enhancing their antigen presenting capabilities in the aged.

The literature concerning the effects of exercise on age-related decrements in macrophage function is extremely sparse. Acute exercise has been reported to increase the effector functions of macrophages (i.e., phagocytosis, microbiocidal activity, and chemotaxis), while decreasing accessory functions, such as MHC class II molecule expression and antigen presentation (Woods et al. 2000). Aging is associated with an impairment of this acute exercise response as evidenced by decreased exercise-induced cytokine production by macrophages (Przybyla et al. 2006). While studies investigating the effects of exercise on macrophage function, especially in the aged, are quite rare, there is promising data coming from murine models. For example, Kawanishi et al. reported that exercise training induces phenotypic switching from pro-inflammatory M1 type to anti-inflammatory M2 type in adipose tissue-resident macrophages and inhibits infiltration of adipose tissue by M1-type macrophages (Kawanishi et al. 2010). This finding suggests that exercise may inhibit the age-associated increase in the production of pro-inflammatory mediators by adipose tissue, which is strongly linked to chronic diseases such as coronary artery disease and type 2 diabetes (Shimizu et al. 2013). These results, however, remain to be confirmed in humans.

26.3.3 Dendritic Cells

Dendritic cells (DCs) are the most potent APCs of the innate immune system, and they are required for the initiation of cell-mediated immunity (Romagnani et al. 2005). DCs can be separated into two major categories: myeloid DCs (mDCs) and plasmacytoid DCs (pDCs). mDCs are critical to the induction of the Th1 immune response (Kawai and Akira 2007). Through their production of IL-12 and surface expression of co-stimulatory molecules, mDCs are able to send naive CD4$^+$ T cells in the direction of a Th1 phenotype, prime antigen-specific CD8$^+$ T cells, and activate NK cells (Reis e Sousa et al. 1997; Lanzavecchia et al. 2001). pDCs are essential to the immune response to viruses through production of type I and type III interferons (IFN-I/IFN-III) (Siegal et al. 1999) and antigen presentation to CD4$^+$ and CD8$^+$ T cells (Romagnani et al. 2005; Ferlazzo et al. 2004; Lande et al. 2010).

The data concerning the effect of age on dendritic cell number is highly equivocal. The numbers of mDCs and pDCs have been reported to decline with age or be unaltered by age (Agrawal et al. 2012; Della Bella et al. 2007; Shodell and Siegal 2002). While there is no consensus regarding dendritic cell number changes with aging, there are clear age-dependent decrements in DC function. Aging is associated with impaired PI3K

signaling (Agrawal et al. 2007) and amplified baseline nuclear factor kappa-light-chain-enhancer of activated B cells (NFκB), activation in mDCs (Agrawal et al. 2009). This age-dependent decline in PI3K signaling has been linked to decreased IL-12 production, antigen presentation, and migratory capacity (Della Bella et al. 2007; Agrawal and Gupta 2011). On the other hand, the higher basal levels of NFκB are associated with elevated unstimulated production of pro-inflammatory cytokines (TNF-α and IL-6) and increased reactivity to self-antigens (Agrawal et al. 2009). Thus, it appears that mDCs contribute directly to nonspecific inflammation and decreased immune self-tolerance, two hallmarks of immunosenescence.

The function of pDCs is impaired with aging as well. The responsiveness of TLR7 and TLR9 to viral antigens is lower in the pDCs of the elderly (Jing et al. 2009; Agrawal and Gupta 2011), which results in decreased TLR7/TLR9-dependent production of IFN-I/IFN-III and impaired antigen presentation (Sridharan et al. 2011). As with mDCs, the ability of pDCs to produce pro-inflammatory cytokines is maintained even in the absence of stimulation (Agrawal et al. 2008). Thus, it appears that both categories of DCs contribute to inflamm-aging and the age-related decline in adaptive immunity.

In spite of the likely role that altered DC function plays in immunosenescence and impaired immune self-tolerance, few studies have investigated the impact of exercise on DC frequency or function (Walsh et al. 2011). A recent study showed that both mDCs and pDCs are mobilized into the peripheral blood compartment in response to acute aerobic exercise, while Nicket et al. found that mDC numbers increased but pDC numbers decreased after marathon running (Nickel et al. 2012). In addition, treadmill running has been reported to mobilize DCs without altering their activation status or allostimulatory function (Ho et al. 2001). The literature concerning longitudinal effects of exercise training on DC number and function is even sparser. Liu et al. report a marked increase in the frequency of both mDCs (CD11c$^+$) and pDCs (CD123$^+$) following 6 months of Tai Chi exercises in middle aged and elderly women (Liu et al. 2012). While these changes were correlated with concomitant increases in the frequency of IL-4- and IFN-γ-expressing T cells, no direct measures of DC function were determined (Liu et al. 2012). Thus, no studies have yet investigated the effect of chronic exercise on DC function. However, some longitudinal exercise studies have investigated changes in DC function using rat models. For example, 5 weeks of endurance training in Sprague–Dawley rats was found to enhance DC-induced leukocyte activation through increased IL-12 production and MHC Class II expression in bone marrow-derived DCs, suggesting that exercise training may enhance the ability of DCs to present antigens and prime T-cell responses (Chiang et al. 2007). Given the importance of DCs to self-tolerance and their possible involvement in immunosenescence, the effects of exercise training on DC differentiation and function in the elderly requires further investigation.

26.3.4 NK Cells

NK cells are cytotoxic effectors of the innate immune system that are able to distinguish between healthy autologous cells and target cells (i.e., malignant or virally infected cells) to prevent dysregulated NK-cell killing. NK cells can be separated into major categories: $CD56^{dim}$ and $CD56^{bright}$. $CD56^{dim}$ NK cells make up 90 % of the total NK-cell pool in blood and are characterized by high cytotoxic functions (De Maria and Moretta 2011). $CD56^{bright}$ NK cells are considered immunoregulatory due to their high capacity to secrete cytokines (such as IFN-γ) and chemokine when stimulated (Wendt et al. 2006; Farag et al. 2003). Though categorized as part of the innate immune system, NK cells possess several properties associated with adaptive immunity. Evidence taken from mouse models and acute viral infections in humans suggests that NK cells express antigen-specific receptors, proliferate in response to infection, and generate long-lived memory cells (Sun and Lanier 2011). What separates NK cells from cytotoxic $CD8^+$ T cells is

their ability to kill target cells spontaneously in the absence of activation or prior antigen exposure (Vivier et al. 2011).

NK-cell cytotoxicity declines with age on a per cell basis; however, overall cytotoxicity is maintained in healthy aging due to an increased percentage and absolute number of NK cells (Le Garff-Tavernier et al. 2010; Solana and Mariani 2000; Mariani et al. 1994). The decreased per cell killing, observed with aging, is associated with a decline in NK-cell expression of activating receptors, such as NKp30 (Sanchez-Correa et al. 2011; Tarazona et al. 2009) and NKp46 (Almeida-Oliveira et al. 2011). Studies of the effects of aging on inhibitory human leukocyte antigen (HLA)-specific killer immunoglobulin-like receptors (KIR) are inconsistent. Multiple studies have reported no effect of aging on inhibitory KIR expression (Le Garff-Tavernier et al. 2010; Almeida-Oliveira et al. 2011; Gayoso et al. 2011); however Lutz et al. (2005) reported an increase in inhibitory KIR expression with aging that was accompanied by a reciprocal decrease in expression of the inhibitory receptor complex CD94/NKG2A. The shifting of NK cells towards a KIR+/NKG2A phenotype with aging suggests a proportional shift toward a more differentiated phenotype (Beziat et al. 2010). Lending further support to the notion that NK-cell differentiation accelerates with age, there is an age-dependent decline in the percentage and absolute number of $CD56^{bright}$ NK cells that occurs in tandem with an expansion of the $CD56^{dim}$ subset (Borrego et al. 1999; Chidrawar et al. 2006).

The phenotypic changes observed in NK cells with advancing age are accompanied by functional decrements. For example, a drop in IL-2 driven production of chemokines has been observed in the elderly and attributed to the loss of $CD56^{bright}$ NK cells (Mariani et al. 2002). The capacity of NK cells to express IFN-γ when stimulated by cytokines, however, is maintained in spite of the increased $CD56^{dim}:CD56^{bright}$ ratio due to increased per-cell production of IFN-γ by $CD56^{bright}$ NK cells (Le Garff-Tavernier et al. 2010). The ability of NK cells to expand as part of the Th1 immune response also appears to be impaired as IL-2-driven proliferation of NK cells is decreased in older donors (Borrego et al. 1999) due in part to an increased proportion of NK cells expressing the putative terminal differentiation marker CD57 (Simpson et al. 2008). These CD57[+] NK cells have lower replicative potential than their CD57[−] counterparts; however, their ability to kill target cells and secrete IFN-γ when stimulated is maintained (Lopez-Verges et al. 2010). Interestingly, some of the aging effects on NK-cell phenotype may be more accurately attributed to CMV infection, which is more common in the elderly (Bate et al. 2010). For example, aging is associated with a downregulation of KLRG1 expression (Hayhoe et al. 2010) in combination with upregulation of CD57 (Simpson et al. 2008), phenotypic alterations which have been observed in young adults infected with CMV (Bigley et al. 2012).

The effect of exercise training on NK-cell function has been investigated using multiple cross-sectional and longitudinal designs, which have often yielded contradictory results. For example, it has been reported that elderly women with relatively high aerobic capacity have higher NK-cell cytotoxic activity (NKCA) than their less-fit counterparts (Nieman et al. 1993); however, other studies have reported no difference in NKCA between active and inactive elderly (Shinkai et al. 1995; Yan et al. 2001). Studies employing resistance and aerobic training interventions in the elderly have yielded similarly equivocal results. Woods et al. showed that elderly individuals who completed a 6-month aerobic training intervention had increased NKCA per cell relative to control subjects who performed stretching and flexibility exercises over the same time interval (Woods et al. 1999). However, Campbell et al. reported no change in NKCA in postmenopausal women following a 12-month aerobic training program, despite a significant increase in maximal oxygen uptake (Campbell et al. 2008). Additionally, Nieman et al. (1990, 1993) reported no effect of aerobic exercise training on NKCA in older women, despite previously documenting that exercise training increased NKCA in obese, young women. This data suggests that perhaps exercise training only increases NKCA in "unhealthy"

people regardless of age. Studies investigating the effect of resistance training on NK-cell function in the elderly are also highly inconsistent. McFarlin et al. reported that NKCA increased 136 % in elderly women who completed a 10-week resistance training intervention (McFarlin et al. 2005); however, a previous study reported no increase in NKCA in elderly women who participated in a 10-week resistance training intervention, despite documenting a 148 % increase in strength (Flynn et al. 1999). Future research should take a broader view of NK-cell function as all of the studies described above measured NKCA against only one cell line, K562. Future studies should investigate the effect of exercise training on NK-cell killing of other cell lines and measure other aspects of NK-cell function, such as IFN-γ production and cytokine-driven proliferation.

Changes in NK-cell function due to exercise training could be the result of altered composition of NK-cell subsets. The surface expression of inhibitory receptors (i.e., KLRG1 and CD158a) and the terminal differentiation marker CD57 are known to be altered with age and latent CMV infection (Bigley et al. 2013; Hayhoe et al. 2010; Simpson et al. 2008). The increased expression of CD57 on NK cells with advancing age is likely to have a significant impact on NK cell-function as CD57[+] NK cells show enhanced production of IFN-γ and increased cytotoxicity when activated through CD16; however, their proliferative capacity is reduced and they display decreased cytotoxicity when stimulated with the cytokines IL-12 and IL-18 (Lopez-Verges et al. 2010). Thus, it is important to investigate the effect of exercise training on NK-cell surface receptors and a broader range of NK-cell functions. To this point, only one study has investigated the effects of exercise training on the frequency of NK-cell subsets and it used a young fit population. Suzui et al. reported an increased CD56[bright] to CD56[dim] ratio with a concomitant reduction in NKCA in young female volleyball players who had just completed a period of intensified training (Suzui et al. 2004). Future studies should examine the effects of exercise training on the composition of NK-cell subsets in the elderly and how said changes impact on the functional capabilities of NK cells.

26.4 Exercise, Aging, and Adaptive Immunity

26.4.1 T-Cell Phenotype

Advancing age is associated with many changes in T-cell phenotype and function. Throughout the lifespan, naïve T cells are gradually replaced with expanded clones of antigen-experienced effector and memory cells. These late-differentiated cells occupy immune space, reducing the number of antigen-virgin cells able to respond to novel pathogens. Furthermore, after many rounds of cell division the late-differentiated cells undergo cell cycle arrest. While unable to proliferate, these senescent cells are frequently apoptosis resistant and tend to accumulate, further reducing immune space (Brunner et al. 2010). Several therapies have been proposed to remove senescent T cells, including therapeutic vaccination, monoclonal antibody therapy, and cytokine therapy. There is also interest in exercise as an inexpensive alternative to these treatments. An acute bout of aerobic exercise leads to a transitory increase in the number of highly differentiated and senescent T cells in the peripheral blood followed by a decrease below resting values during recovery from exercise. The fate of the mobilized senescent cells is not known, but it has been suggested that they undergo apoptosis in tissues such as the intestines (Hoffman-Goetz and Quadrilatero 2003; Kruger et al. 2008) from an exercise-induced increase in pro-apoptotic factors including reactive oxygen species and glucocorticoids as well as increased expression of CD95 (Mooren et al. 2002; Simpson et al. 2007; Simpson 2011). Regular exercise could therefore be a means to clear senescent cells from the blood (Simpson 2011). In support of this, cross-sectional comparisons between the physically active and sedentary elderly find that those who regularly exercise have lower proportions of KLRG1$^+$CD28$^-$ and KLRG1$^+$CD57$^+$ senescent T cells (Table 26.1). Spielmann et al. recently demonstrated that, independently of age, high aerobic capacity is inversely associated with the accumulation of senescent T cells and that the association of increasing age with a decreased proportion of naïve T cells is abrogated in individuals with an above-average maximal oxygen uptake score (VO$_{2max}$). These findings hold even after adjusting for potential confounders, including percentage body fat and latent herpesvirus infections (Spielmann et al. 2011).

These cross-sectional observations lead to the question of whether or not some of the deleterious effects of aging on T cells can be reversed through an exercise-training program. Unfortunately, most longitudinal studies conducted to date have not been promising, as exercise interventions in the previously sedentary elderly have generally not found alteration in T-cell phenotypes (Table 26.2). Woods et al. found that a 6-month supervised aerobic exercise program consisting of brisk walking 3 days each week did not alter numbers of naïve and memory CD4$^+$ and CD8$^+$ T cells (Woods et al. 1999). However, this study used CD45RA and CD45RO as naïve and memory T-cell markers, which are now considered to be imperfect markers as CD45RA can be reexpressed by later differentiated effector memory T cells (Dunne et al. 2002). A more recent study examined the expression of surface markers associated with T-cell activation and co-stimulation, but found that 32 weeks of a functionally oriented training program including both endurance and resistance exercise among frail nursing home residents (mean age: 88 years) did not alter the proportion of CD4$^+$ or CD8$^+$ T cells expressing CD25, CD28, and HLA-DR (Kapasi et al. 2003). Similar results were found following a 12-month moderate-intensity resistance training program among clinically healthy, sedentary elderly women (60–77 years) as no changes in CD25, CD28, CD45RA, CD45RO, CD69, CD95, or HLA-DR were reported among CD4 and CD8 T cells (Raso et al. 2007). In contrast, 6 months of supervised aerobic and resistance training 5 days a week led to an increase in CD28 expression on CD4 T cells among the healthy, previously sedentary men and women (61–76 years) who participated (Shimizu et al.

Table 26.1 Findings from cross-sectional studies that have examined associations between exercise training status and specific aspects of immunosenescence in older humans

Reference	Subjects	Training status definition	Findings (compared to untrained status)
Nieman et al. (1993)	Untrained women 73.5 ± 1.2 years ($n=30$); trained women aged 72.5 ± 1.8 years ($n=12$)	*Trained*: regularly competing in endurance races and participated in >1 h of exercise daily for at least 5 years previous, VO_{2max}, 31.3 ± 0.9 $ml \cdot kg^{-1} \cdot min^{-1}$ *Untrained*: less than three moderate-vigorous endurance exercise sessions of 20-min duration per week for previous 6 months, VO_{2max}, 18.7 ± 0.9 $ml \cdot kg^{-1} \cdot min^{-1}$	↑ NK-cell cytotoxicity; ↑ T-cell proliferation; ↑ lymphocyte counts; ↓ frequency of URTI symptoms
Shinkai et al. (1995)	Untrained men 65.8 ± 3.5 years ($n=19$); trained men 63.8 ± 3.3 years ($n=17$)	*Trained*: members of local senior running club, VO_{2max}, 38.8 ± 1.3 $ml \cdot kg^{-1} \cdot min^{-1}$ *Untrained*: local sedentary participants not engaged in structured exercise training, VO_{2max}, 29.2 ± 0.9 $ml \cdot kg^{-1} \cdot min^{-1}$	↑ IL-2, IL-4, and IFN-γ production; ↑ T-cell proliferation; → NK-cell cytotoxicity; → lymphocyte counts
Yan et al. (2001)	Untrained middle-aged men 51.6 ± 4.3 years ($n=22$); untrained elderly men 66.3 ± 3.2 years ($n=20$); trained middle-aged men 50.7 ± 8.2 years ($n=18$); trained elderly men 65.1 ± 4.5 years ($n=28$)	*Trained*: daily exercise activity of 4–6 MET *Untrained*: daily exercise activity of 1–3 MET	↓ CD4:CD8 ratio in elderly group; ↓ proportion of NK cells in elderly group; → NK-cell activity; ↑ neutrophil phagocytosis in elderly group
Ogawa et al. (2003)	Untrained women 63 ± 1 years ($n=12$; trained women 63 ± 1 years ($n=9$)	*Trained*: members of a walking group, VO_{2peak}, 32.3 ± 1 $ml \cdot kg^{-1} \cdot min^{-1}$ *Untrained*: sedentary, VO_{2peak}, 27.8 ± 0.9 $ml \cdot kg^{-1} \cdot min^{-1}$	↑ IL-2⁺/CD8⁺, IL-4⁺/CD8⁺, and IL-4⁺/CD4⁺ T cell numbers; → IFN-γ:IL-4 ratio
Colbert et al. (2004)	Men and women aged 70–79 years ($n=3,075$)	Exercise duration and energy expenditure estimated from subject self reports	↓ Plasma CRP, IL-6 and TNF-α concentrations
Ludlow et al. (2008)	Men and women 60.3 ± 4.9 years ($n=69$)	Subjects grouped into quartiles according to self-reported daily energy expenditure	↑ Leukocyte telomere length in moderate exercisers (991–2,340 Kcal/week) compared to low (<990 Kcal/week) and high (>3,541 Kcal/week) exercisers. → Leukocyte telomerase activity
Spielmann et al. (2011)	Healthy men aged 18–61 years ($n=102$)	Subjects grouped into tertiles according to age-adjusted VO_{2max} scores	↑ Proportion of naïve CD8⁺ T cells; ↓ proportions of senescent/exhausted CD4⁺ and CD8⁺ T cells
Beshgetoor et al. (2004)	Female master's athletes 41 ± 4.3 years ($n=20$) and female nonathletes 42 ± 3.6 years ($n=19$)	*Trained*: regularly competing in endurance races, had been training and competing for 11.7 ± 8.3 years, participated in >8 h of exercise weekly *Untrained*: do not participate in regular exercise	↑ Proportion of PMA-stimulated T cells expressing IL-2; → T cell, CD4⁺ T cell, CD8⁺ T-cell numbers
Gueldner et al. (1997)	Healthy women aged 60–98 years ($n=46$)	*Active* ($n=25$): self-reported as lifetime "exercisers" and currently enrolled in formal exercise classes *Inactive* ($n=21$): self-reported as sedentary	↑ CD25 expression among lymphocytes following anti-CD3 stimulation

→ No difference due to exercise training status, ↑ greater response, ↓ lower response

CD cluster of differentiation, *URTI* upper respiratory tract infection, *MET* metabolic equivalent, *CRP* C-reactive protein, *IL* interleukin, *TNF* tumor necrosis factor, *IFN* interferon, VO_{2max} maximal oxygen uptake, *NK* natural killer

Table 26.2 Findings from randomized control trials that have examined the effects of exercise training on specific aspects of immunosenescence in older humans

Reference	Subjects	Exercise training protocol	Findings (compared to control group)
Nieman et al. (1993)	Sedentary healthy women 73.5 ± 1.2 years ($n=30$)	*Experimental group* ($n=14$): 12 weeks of walking exercise at 60 % heart rate reserve, 30–40-min sessions, five times per week	$\rightarrow$ NK-cell cytotoxicity; $\rightarrow$ T-cell proliferation; $\rightarrow$ lymphocyte, T cell, CD4$^+$ T cell, CD8$^+$ T cell, NK-cell counts; $\downarrow$ frequency of URTI symptoms
		Control group ($n=16$): 12 weeks of range of movement and flexibility exercise with heart rate values close to resting values, 30–40-min sessions, five times per week	
Woods et al. (1999)	Sedentary healthy men and women 65.3 ± 0.8 years ($n=29$)	*Experimental group* ($n=14$): 6 months of progressive supervised aerobic exercise (duration, 10–40-min sessions; intensity, 50–65 % VO_{2max}), three times per week	$\uparrow$ T-cell proliferation; $\uparrow$ NK-cell cytotoxicity; $\rightarrow$ neutrophil, lymphocyte, CD4$^+$ T cell, CD8$^+$ T cell, monocyte counts; $\rightarrow$ memory (CD45RO$^+$) CD4$^+$ T-cell counts; $\rightarrow$ CD4:CD8 T-cell ratio
		Control group ($n=15$): 6 months of range of movement and flexibility exercise at the same frequency as the experimental group	
Kapasi et al. (2003)	Frail elderly nursing home residents ($n=190$)	*Experimental group* ($n=94$): 8 months of functionally orientated endurance and resistance exercise, four times per day, 5 days per week	$\rightarrow$ T-cell proliferation; $\rightarrow$ lymphocyte subpopulations or activation markers (CD28, CD25, HLA-DR); $\rightarrow$ infection incidence
		Control group ($n=96$): no structured exercise training	
Fairey et al. (2005)	Sedentary postmenopausal female breast cancer survivors aged 59 ± 6 years ($n=52$)	*Experimental group* ($n=24$): 15 weeks of progressive aerobic exercise training, 70–75 % VO_{2peak}, 15–35-min sessions, three times per week	$\uparrow$ Unstimulated T-cell proliferation; $\uparrow$ NK-cell cytotoxicity; $\rightarrow$ neutrophil oxidative burst; $\rightarrow$ T cell-stimulated cytokine (IL-1α, TNFα, IL-6, IL-4, IL-10, TGF-β_1) production; $\rightarrow$ T cell, B cell, CD14$^+$ monocyte, NK-cell numbers; $\rightarrow$ T-cell CD28, CD45RO, or CD25 expression
		Control group ($n=28$): no structured exercise training	
Kohut et al. (2004)	Healthy sedentary adults aged 73.07 ± 5.6 years ($n=27$)	*Experimental group* ($n=14$): 10 months of aerobic exercise training, 65–75 % heart rate reserve, 25–30-min sessions, three times per week	$\uparrow$ Mean fold increase in antibody titer to influenza A vaccine; $\uparrow$mononuclear cell granzyme B expression in response to live influenza virus stimulation
		Control group ($n=13$): no structured exercise training	
Campbell et al. (2008)	Healthy sedentary postmenopausal women ($n=108$) aged 50–75 years	*Experimental group* ($n=14$): 12 months of progressive aerobic and resistance exercise training, 40–75 % maximal heart rate, 16–45-min sessions, two times per week	$\rightarrow$ CD4:CD8 T-cell ratio; $\rightarrow$ NK-cell cytotoxicity; $\rightarrow$ T-cell proliferation; $\rightarrow$ lymphocyte, T cell, CD4$^+$ T cell, CD8$^+$ T cell, NK-cell, B-cell counts
		Control group ($n=13$): 12 months of 60-min stretching and relaxation sessions, one time per week	

(continued)

Table 26.2 (continued)

Reference	Subjects	Exercise training protocol	Findings (compared to control group)
Shin et al. (2008)	Obese women aged 46.8 ± 6.4 years ($n=16$)	*Experimental group* ($n=8$): 6 months of supervised treadmill walking/running at 60 % VO_{2peaks}, 45-min sessions, three times per week. *Control group* ($n=8$): no structured exercise training	→ Leukocyte telomere length; ↑ antioxidant activity in response to acute exercise; ↓ oxidative stress in response to acute exercise
Woods et al. (2009)	Healthy men and women aged 69.9±0.4 years ($n=144$)	*Experimental group* ($n=74$): 10 months of progressive cardiovascular exercise (45–70 % VO_{2max}) 10–60-min sessions, three times per week. *Control group* ($n=70$): flexibility and stretching exercise, 75-min sessions, two times per week	↑ Duration of seroprotective response to trivalent influenza vaccine; ↓ illness severity and sleep disturbances
Shimizu et al. (2011)	Healthy men and women aged 61–79 years ($n=24$)	*Experimental group* ($n=12$): 12 weeks of progressive endurance and resistance training, two times per week. *Control group* ($n=12$): no structured exercise training	↑ CD8+/CD28+ T-cell numbers; → lymphocyte, T cell, CD4+ T cell, CD8+ T-cell numbers; ↑ CD14+/CD80+ monocyte numbers; → CD14+/TLR-4+ monocyte numbers
Shimizu et al. (2008)	Healthy men and women aged 61–79 years ($n=48$)	*Experimental group* ($n=28$): 6 months of supervised endurance and resistance training, five times per week. *Control group* ($n=20$): no structured exercise training	↑CD4+ T cell, CD4+/CD28+ T cell, and CD4+/IFN-γ+ T-cell numbers; → CD4+/IL-4+ T-cell numbers; →lymphocyte, T-cell numbers
Raso et al. (2007)	Healthy women aged 60–77 years ($n=42$)	*Experimental group* ($n=21$): 12 months of progressive, moderate-intensity resistance training (55 % 1 RM) 3 sets of 12 repetitions for five exercises, three times per week. *Control group* ($n=21$): no structured exercise training	→NK-cell cytotoxicity; → T-cell proliferation; → lymphocyte, T cell, B cell, NK cell, CD4+ T cell, CD8+ T-cell numbers; → T-cell CD45RA, CD45RO, CD28, CD95, CD25, CD69, or HLA-DR expression
Fahlman et al. (2000)	Healthy women aged 70–87 years ($n=29$)	*Experimental group* ($n=15$): 10 weeks of progressive endurance training, 20–50-min sessions, three times per week. *Control group* ($n=14$): no structured exercise training	→ T cell, CD4+ T cell, CD8+ T cell, NK-cell numbers;→ T-cell proliferation; →NK-cell cytotoxicity; →CD4:CD8 ratio
Flynn et al. (1999)	Healthy women aged 67–84 years ($n=30$)	*Experimental group* ($n=15$): 10 weeks of progressive resistance training, three times per week. *Control group* ($n=15$): no structured exercise training	↓B-cell numbers; → T cell, CD4+ T cell, CD8+ T cell, NK-cell numbers; → T-cell proliferation; →CD4:CD8 ratio
Okutsu et al. (2008)	Healthy men and women aged 60–81 years ($n=65$)	*Experimental group* ($n=32$): 25 weeks of endurance and resistance exercise, 2-h sessions, two times per week. *Control group* ($n=33$): no structured exercise training	↑DTH response to tuberculin PPD; → T cell, CD4+ T cell, CD8+ T cell, NK-cell numbers; →CD4:CD8 ratio

Drela et al. (2004)	Healthy women aged 62–86 years (n=42)	*Experimental group (n=30):* 24 months of progressive moderate aerobic exercise *Control group (n=12):* no structured exercise training	↑Proportion of lymphocyte-stimulated IL-2 expression; → proportion of lymphocyte-stimulated IL-4, IFN-γ expression; →lymphocyte, T cell, NK-cell, B-cell numbers; →CD4:CD8 ratio
Rall et al. (1996)	Healthy men and women 65–80 years (n=14)	*Experimental group (n=8):* 12 weeks of progressive resistance training with "warm-up" water exercises, 60-min sessions, two times per week *Control group (n=6):* 15 min of "warm-up" water exercises, two times per week	→T-cell-stimulated IL-1β, IL-2, TNF-α, IL-6, PGE-2 production; → T-cell proliferation; →CD4:CD8 ratio

→ No difference between experimental and control groups, ↑ greater than control group, ↓ less than control group

CD cluster of differentiation, *URTI* upper respiratory tract infection, *TGF* transforming growth factor, *IL* interleukin, *TNF* tumor necrosis factor, *TLR* toll-like receptor, VO_{2max} maximal oxygen uptake, *NK* natural killer

2008). The same researchers also found that a 12-week program of twice weekly aerobic and resistance training exercises in healthy elderly men and women (mean age: 67 years) increased the number of CD28 expressing CD8 T cells (Shimizu et al. 2011).

26.4.2 CD4:CD8 Ratio

Aging is associated with changes in the number of CD4$^+$ T cells relative to CD8$^+$ T cells. Persistent antigen stimulation and the apoptosis-resistant nature of late-differentiated CD8$^+$ T cells lead to an accumulation of CD8$^+$ T cells relative to CD4$^+$ T cells; a CD4:CD8 ratio less than 1 usually indicates a lowered naïve T-cell repertoire. Indeed, a CD4:CD8 ratio less than 1.0 is one parameter of the IRP. Unfortunately, the literature generally indicates that exercise does not impact the CD4:CD8 T-cell ratio in resting blood samples. Six weeks of supervised aerobic exercise did not change the CD4:CD8 ratio in elderly subjects (mean age: 70 years) (Woods et al. 1999), nor did 10 weeks of aerobic (Fahlman et al. 2000) or resistance (Flynn et al. 1999) exercise training. Longer interventions have also failed to find an effect on the CD4:CD8 ratio among the elderly, although aerobic and resistance exercise training programs ranging from 25 weeks (Okutsu et al. 2008), 12 months (Campbell et al. 2008), and 24 months (Drela et al. 2004) have been tried. While it seems that exercise does not impact the CD4:CD8 ratio in clinically healthy older adults, none of these studies have included subjects that entered the experiment with ratios <1, leaving open the possibility that exercise training may improve some aspects of immunity among individuals already in the IRP. One promising study found that 9 months of resistance training increased the CD4:CD8 ratio in human immunodeficiency virus (HIV)-infected elderly patients from 0.63 to 0.81 (Souza et al. 2008). Unfortunately, however, this experiment lacked a control group and so the CD4:CD8 ratio may have increased due to something other than the exercise intervention. Conversely, aging may also lead to elevated CD4:CD8 ratios. Several studies have found that sedentary elderly have greater CD4:CD8 ratios than sedentary individuals in a younger age cohort. Habitual exercise may alter these ratios where the active elderly have ratios closer to that of the younger groups. Yan et al. found an age-related elevation in the CD4:CD8 ratio among older sedentary men compared to middle-aged controls, but none in trained elderly men (Yan et al. 2001). The cross-sectional study by Shinkai et al. also found that the sedentary elderly (mean age: 65 years) had a significantly greater CD4:CD8 ratio compared to the younger (mean age: 24 years) controls, but the active elderly did not (Shinkai et al. 1995).

26.4.3 T-Cell Proliferation

The effect of physical fitness on various measures of T cell in the elderly has also been studied. Aging is generally associated with a loss of in vitro-stimulated T-cell proliferation and alterations in cytokine secretion and signaling processes, such as loss of IL-2 synthesis and expression of IL-2 receptors (DelaRosa et al. 2006; Xu et al. 1993). Cross-sectional studies typically demonstrate that the physically fit have a greater T-cell proliferative response to mitogens in vitro, indicating an enhanced ability of the T cells to be activated. For example, 65–85-year-old women with high aerobic fitness levels have greater T-cell proliferation in response to phytohemagglutinin (PHA) compared to untrained elderly women (Nieman et al. 1993). Similarly, Shinkai et al. (1995) found that recreational-level male runners aged 60 years and older have a 44 % greater T-cell proliferation in response to PHA and a 51 % improvement in response to pokeweed mitogen relative to non-running men of a similar age (Shinkai et al. 1995). While the absolute number of T cells did not differ between the physically fit and sedentary in both these studies, it remains possible that the differences in proliferative ability reflect differences in the proportions of naïve or late-differentiated T cells between the two groups. The effect of training interventions on T-cell proliferation has also been studied and has yielded mixed results. The cross-sectional study conducted by Nieman et al. discussed above also contained an exercise intervention, where sedentary elderly women participated in either a 12-week aerobic (30–40 min walking, 5 days per week) or flexibility training program. While the participants of the aerobic program did have a significant increase in VO_{2max} compared to those who underwent the flexibility intervention, no measurable change in T-cell proliferation was found (Nieman et al. 1993). Neither did 32 weeks of a functionally oriented training program with frail nursing home residents (Kapasi et al. 2003), 12 months of moderate intensity resistance training (Raso et al. 2007), nor 12 months of progressive aerobic and resistance exercises with postmenopausal women (Campbell et al. 2008) find an improvement in T-cell proliferative responses to PHA. In contrast, Woods et al. found a nominally beneficial effect among previously sedentary men and women (mean age: 65 years) who engaged in 6 months of supervised progressive aerobic exercise three times a week, with a greater T-cell response to concanavalin A (Woods et al. 1999). However, significant increases in T-cell proliferation among the control group (12 weeks of movement and flexibility exercises) were also reported. It may be that some researchers failed to notice changes in T-cell proliferation because their experimental protocol only employed one type of mitogen or did not measure unstimulated T-cell proliferation. Fairey et al. did not find any changes in the response to PHA, but did find that 15 weeks of progressive aerobic exercise training increased unstimulated T-cell proliferation among postmenopausal breast cancer survivors (Fairey et al. 2005).

26.4.4 T-Cell Cytokine Signaling

Another way to assess T-cell function is to measure their ability to send and receive signals through cytokines. IL-2 signaling has been of special interest, as the activation and proliferation of T cells depends on the secretion of IL-2 and the expression of IL-2 receptors. The secretion and expression of high-affinity IL-2 receptors decreases with age and is associated with the IRP (DelaRosa et al. 2006; Xu et al. 1993). Both cross-sectional (Table 26.1) and longitudinal (Table 26.2) studies have found that regular exercise is associated with improved IL-2 signaling in the elderly. Elderly women who had participated in a walking program for 4 years had a greater number of CD8[+] T cells expressing IL-2 compared to sedentary controls (Ogawa et al. 2003). Similarly, female masters athletes (>40 years) had a greater percent of CD4[+] T cells that expressed IL-2 compared to nonathletes following phorbol myristate acetate (PMA) stimulation (Beshgetoor et al. 2004). Shinkai et al. also found that stimulated peripheral blood mononuclear cells (PBMCs) from elderly athletes secreted greater amounts of IL-2 compared to age-matched sedentary controls, perhaps explaining their observation of greater T-cell proliferation among the athletes (Shinkai et al. 1995). One longitudinal study found that 24 months of aerobic exercise training in elderly women (aged 62–86 years) led to an increased percent of lymphocytes expressing IL-2 following in vitro stimulation compared to controls (Drela et al. 2004). Unfortunately, this study did not identify the lymphocyte subsets responsible for the increased expression. Another study that used a 12-week progressive resistance training intervention in previously sedentary elderly did not find any differences in IL-2 production by PBMCs (Rall et al. 1996). There has been less research in IL-2 receptor expression, although Gueldner et al. reported greater surface expression of the IL-2 L chain receptor CD25 following CD3 simulation among elderly women that self-identified as "active," compared to inactive controls (Gueldner et al. 1997). In contrast, an exercise intervention among frail nursing home residents did not find a change in unstimulated CD25 expression on CD4[+] or CD8[+] T cells following the 32-week intervention (Kapasi et al. 2003). Another IL-2 receptor, the IL-2 J chain receptor (CD122), may be more important in cell signaling than CD25, but the effect of habitual exercise on this receptor has yet to be studied.

The balance between Th1 and Th2 responses may be comprised in the elderly, as aging leads to Th2-type dominance (Shearer 1997) that may result in T cell-mediated dysfunction. It has been proposed that exercise can shift the balance back toward Th1-type responses (Malm 2004). Many groups have reported that moderate exercise tends to lead to a shift toward Th1-type cytokine responses, whereas strenuous or exhaustive exercise causes Th2-type dominance (Ostrowski et al. 1999; Pedersen and Bruunsgaard 2003). Exercise-induced changes in glucocorticoids can alter Th-mediated responses, but likely inhibit the Th1-cell production of IL-12 and IFN-γ while upregulating IL-4, IL-10, and IL-13 secretion by Th2 cells, resulting in an increased Th2 response (Elenkov 2004). This shift towards Th2 cytokine responses has been observed in animal models, even after relatively short training periods (Lowder et al. 2006; Ru and Peijie 2009). Using older mice, Kohut et al. found that moderate exercise training increased antigen-specific cell production of Th1 cytokines but not Th2 cytokines (Kohut et al. 2001). This effect was not found in younger mice, indicating that age may interact with exercise in Th1/Th2 shifts. Regardless, data from studies with elderly humans have not found an effect of exercise on Th1 or Th2 cytokines. Ogawa et al. found no difference in the ratio of IFN-γ to IL-4 between elderly females who participated in a walking program and those who did not. Twelve weeks of resistance training did not alter PBMC production of any cytokines examined, including IL-1β, TNF-α, IL-6, or prostaglandin E2 (PGE2) (Rall et al. 1996). Despite finding changes in IL-2 expression, 24 months of aerobic exercise did not alter stimulated expression of IFN-γ or IL-4 (Drela et al. 2004).

26.4.5 Regulatory, Th17, and Gamma-Delta T cells

CD4$^+$CD25$^+$ T cells expressing forkhead box 3 (FOXP3) are classified as T regulatory cells (Tregs). Tregs play an important role in the maintenance and regulation of the immune system, as they suppress excessive immune responses to both self and innocuous antigens through curbing the activation, proliferation, and functions of a variety of cells. The dysfunction of Tregs may result in autoimmune diseases, allergies, and asthma (Sakaguchi et al. 2010), and a role for Tregs in immunosenescence has been proposed (Wang et al. 2010). For example, Hwang et al. found that CD4$^+$CD25$^+$FOXP3$^+$ T cells from elderly individuals were more potent suppressors of IL-10 production in target cells, indicating that the capacity of Tregs in regulating IL-10 production may be affected during aging (Hwang et al. 2009). Murine models suggest that Tregs are also altered by exercise training. Lowder et al. found that repeated bouts of moderate intensity exercise increased the number and suppressive function of CD4$^+$CD25$^+$FOXP3$^+$ Tregs in the lungs and lymph nodes in the mouse model of asthma (Lowder et al. 2010). In contrast, Wang et al. did not find an affect of moderate-intensity training in healthy mice, but did find an increase in Tregs following 6 weeks of high intensity, prolonged exercise (Wang et al. 2012). The authors suggest that an increase in Tregs following high-intensity training may suppress the immune system and lead to the increased risk of infections associated with high levels of training. A few researchers have examined the responses of Tregs to exercise in humans. Wilson et al. found a significant increase in CD4$^+$CD25$^+$FOXP3$^+$ cells following a single bout of acute exercise in elite adolescent swimmers (Wilson et al. 2009). Twelve weeks of Tai Chi Chuan exercise training in middle-aged volunteers was also found to increase the levels of CD4$^+$CD25$^+$ T cells (Yeh et al. 2006); however CD25$^+$ expression on CD4$^+$ T cells is not considered a reliable marker for indentifying Tregs. A follow-up study found that FoxP3 expression did not increase with Tai Chi Chuan exercise in healthy volunteers, but was increased in patients with type 2 diabetes mellitus (Yeh et al. 2009). The increases in Tregs following exercise in the murine asthma model and with individuals with type 2 diabetes suggest that the exercise responses of Tregs differ between healthy individuals and those with altered immune systems. Unfortunately, changes in Treg function and number following exercise in the elderly have not yet been examined.

Th17 are a subset of CD4[+] helper T cells that develop independently from the Th1 and Th2 lineage. They are distinguished by their production of IL-17 and play a role in host defense against extracellular pathogens through mediation of neutrophil and macrophage recruitment to infection sites. A role for these cells in the pathogenesis of multiple inflammatory conditions and autoimmune disorders has also been found. Naïve and memory Th17 cells in humans have been shown to be affected by aging, with the elderly producing more IL-17 from naïve CD4[+] T cells, but less IL-17 from memory CD4 T cells compared to the young (Walsh et al. 2011). Little is known about the response of Th17 cells or IL-17 to either acute or chronic exercise. An increase in serum levels of IL-17 has been observed in rats following a strenuous bout of treadmill running (Duzova et al. 2009), and Lowder et al. has shown a significant decrease in IL-17 in vitro production in exercise-trained asthmatic mice (Lowder et al. 2010). The effect of exercise on Th17 cells in humans or in aging is not yet known. Another subset of T cells is the γδ T cells, which have a tissue-migrating phenotype and infiltrate epithelial-rich tissue such as the skin, intestines, and the reproductive tract. γδ T cells recognize non-peptide antigens such as lipids and aid in bacterial elimination, wound repair, and delayed-type hypersensitivity (DTH) reactions. They also display cytolytic activity against a wide range of tumor cell lines in vitro in a TCR-dependent manner and so have been widely studied in anticancer immunotherapy (Chiplunkar et al. 2009). However the impact of aging on γδ T cells has so far received little attention (Pawelec et al. 2010), although it appears that the number of γδ T cells increases with age (Mazzoccoli et al. 2011). γδ T cells have been observed to be mobilized into the blood compartment following acute stress and exercise (Anane et al. 2009; Bigley et al. 2012), but the effect of chronic exercise training on these cells is not yet known.

Differing results between longitudinal studies likely arise from differences in the exercise protocol used, and the different ways the out-come measures were examined. The initial health status of the participants may also influence results of a longitudinal study, where subjects with weakened immune systems may respond better to exercise than the already healthy subjects typically recruited. Although Kapasi et al. did not find an effect of exercise in frail nursing home residents, the exercise intervention consisted of basic mobility exercises such as standing, walking, and bathroom visits, whereas Fairey et al. used progressive cycling exercise adjusted to 70–75 % of the participants' peak oxygen consumption (Fairey et al. 2005; Kapasi et al. 2003). Another possibility is the length of the intervention and intensity of the exercise program. Many of the elder athletes used in the cross-sectional studies had been maintaining a high level of activity for at least 5 years, and some of the inclusion criteria have been quite strict (>1 h/day for the last 5 years) (Nieman et al. 1993; Shinkai et al. 1995). Clearly, more research using different populations is required for future studies.

26.5 Exercise and Inflamm-Aging

The cellular changes that occur with age are not the only factors accountable for the state of relative immunosuppression observed in the elderly. Aging is also associated with an impairment of the localized and transient inflammatory response, necessary to control pathogen incursion and dissemination. This state of subclinical, low-grade chronic inflammation, termed inflamm-aging (Franceschi et al. 2000), is associated with increased concentrations of circulating cytokines and inflammatory mediators such as C-reactive protein, IL-1β, IL-6, IL-15, and TNF-α (Bruunsgaard et al. 1999; Ershler et al. 1993; Forsey et al. 2003; Bartlett et al. 2012) accompanied by a decrease in anti-inflammatory cytokines such as IL-10 (Lio et al. 2002). In addition to predicting frailty in the elderly (Baylis et al. 2013), inflamm-aging is believed to play a central role in the development of many chronic diseases, such as cardiovascular disease (Libby 2006), type 2 diabetes mellitus (Pedersen et al. 2003), neurodegenerative disease (Giunta et al. 2008), and certain cancers (Allavena et al. 2008; Mantovani and Pierotti 2008). Some markers of inflamm-aging, such as the increased plasma levels of circulating IL-1ra, IL-6, and CRP, have also been shown to predict mortality in nonagenarians (Jylha et al. 2007). While inflamm-aging has been proposed to augment CMV reactivation (Pawelec et al. 2010) and further contribute to the IRP in the elderly, a recent longitudinal study has shown that the level of chronic low inflammation in the elderly is independent of CMV infection (Bartlett et al. 2012).

Regular physical activity moderates the levels of circulating pro-inflammatory cytokines (Petersen and Pedersen 2005), helps to prevent the development of many diseases, improves the inflamm-aging-associated insulin resistance seen in the elderly (Nieto-Vazquez et al. 2008; Kodama et al. 2007), and is also associated with a reduction in all-cause mortality (Blair and Jackson 2001). Using exercise to reduce inflamm-aging could therefore be an efficient therapeutic approach to delay the onset of chronic diseases associated with low-grade inflammation. This is further supported by cross-sectional studies highlighting the deleterious impact of physical inactivity on low-grade systemic inflammation in otherwise healthy subjects (Colbert et al. 2004; Kullo et al. 2007; Pedersen and Bruunsgaard 2003; Taaffe et al. 2000). Moreover, other measures of poor physical fitness, such as low muscular strength, have shown that elderly with low handgrip strength presented a higher level of inflammation than their stronger counterparts (Tiainen et al. 2010; Cesari et al. 2004). On the contrary, physical activity has been associated with reduction in circulating levels of the pro-inflammatory cytokines IL-6 and TNF-α in the elderly (Phillips et al. 2010; Nicklas et al. 2008) and a lower LPS-stimulated in vitro secretion of IL-6, TNF-α, and IL-1β (Phillips et al. 2010). In a large cross-sectional population-based study, Elosua et al. assessed the association between self-reported physical activity along with physical performances of over a thousand 65 years and older individuals (Elosua et al. 2005). They found that men and women elderly practicing regular

moderate physical activity had significantly lower levels of CRP and IL-6, compared to age-matched sedentary individuals. Interestingly, even subjects that reportedly practiced low-physical activity were found to have reduced CRP in men and IL-6 in women (Elosua et al. 2005). Similarly, levels of circulating IL-6 and CRP are positively associated with the time required to walk 400 m or 6 miles (Elosua et al. 2005; Taaffe et al. 2000). However, conflicting results show that this association disappears when more accurate techniques are used to determine physical fitness, such as maximal oxygen consumption treadmill tests (Valentine et al. 2009).

The use of moderate intensity aerobic exercise has also shown to be an effective therapeutic method to reduce the production of TNF-α and IFN-γ by mitogen-stimulated PBMCs in sedentary subjects at risk for ischemic heart disease (Smith et al. 1999). In addition to producing less pro-inflammatory cytokines, those mitogen-stimulated PBMCs secreted more anti-inflammatory cytokines IL-4, IL-10, and transforming growth factor beta 1 (TGF-β1) than the controls at the end of the 6-month training period (Smith et al. 1999). Using sedentary elderly (>64 years old) with low initial physical fitness, Kohut et al. (2006) showed that a 10-month training program (65–80 % HR reserve, three times a week for 30–45 min a day) elicited a reduction in circulating CRP, IL-6, and IL-18 when compared to the non-exerciser control group (Kohut et al. 2006). Shorter exercise training interventions of 2 months also elicit reduction in the circulating pro-inflammatory monocyte chemotactic protein-1 (MCP-1) and in nitric oxide synthase mRNA levels in PBMCs isolated from older adults (Gano et al. 2011). This effect was also seen in vivo when Kadoglou et al. showed that exercise training helped to reduce the levels of circulating CRP and TNF-α in patients with type 2 diabetes (Kadoglou et al. 2007a, b).

Aging is associated with many confounding factors that could influence the process of inflamm-aging. For instance, adiposity is associated with inflamm-aging independently of age; therefore, weight management interventions could exert positive effects on the age-related low-grade inflammation (Church et al. 2010). However, several studies have shown that the anti-inflammatory effects of exercise are independent from reductions in body fat (Balducci et al. 2010; Fischer et al. 2007).

26.6 Exercise and Viral Infections

The chronic state of low-grade inflammation observed in the elderly is thought to potentially aggravate the incidence of viral infections (Stout-Delgado et al. 2009). Viral infections hold major clinical implications in the elderly, and certain viruses, such as influenza virus, are responsible for up to 36,000 fatalities and over 200,000 hospitalizations in the United States each year (CDC 2011). In addition to newly acquired viruses, excessive reactivation of latent viruses in immunosupressed elderly can pose threat to their health and survival. Herpes viruses such as herpes simplex virus (HSV-1 and HSV-2), varicella zoster virus (VZV), Epstein-Barr virus (EBV), and CMV are highly prevalent in the general population. Herpes viruses are often clinically asymptomatic in the immunocompetent host, but they persist in a lifelong latency and will be periodically reactivated in response to physical or psychological stress (Almanzar et al. 2005; Padgett et al. 1998; Uchakin et al. 2011). While the rate at which those reactivations occur is unknown, the stress-reducing properties of regular physical activity (Salmon 2001) may reduce the frequency of viral reactivation, and thus help delay persistent virus-induced immunosenescence.

Exercise may also reduce local inflammation by shifting from a type I to a type II immune response and consequently help to prevent viral infection and/or increase viral clearance (Martin et al. 2009). Indeed, studies have shown that moderate exercise training would induce a shift from the pro-inflammatory cytokine profile (type I) to an anti-inflammatory cytokine profile (type II) in influenza-infected mice (Lowder et al. 2006) and protecting them from death (Lowder et al. 2005). While acute bouts of exercise also

appear to transiently reduce influenza-induced symptoms in mice (Sim et al. 2009), regular moderate exercise training helps to lower local inflammatory markers, such as IL-6, TNF-α, MCP-1, macrophage inflammatory protein-1β (MIP-1β), KC, and regulated upon activation normal T cell expressed and presumably secreted (RANTES) (Sim et al. 2009). In addition to these local changes, both acute and chronic moderate exercise helped to reduce viral load and to improve morbidity (Sim et al. 2009). The differences in the effect of exercise dose on the immune system have been well documented, and while exhaustive exercise is considered immunosuppressive and highly stressful in young individuals and animals (Davis et al. 1997; Nieman et al. 1995; Peters and Bateman 1983), it does not appear to reduce antibody responses (Kapasi et al. 2000) or viral-specific T-cell responses in old mice (Kapasi et al. 2005). However, contradicting studies have reported that mice exercised to exhaustion had increased morbidity and mortality in response to high doses of HSV-1, when compared to moderate and non-exercisers (Davis et al. 2004). In addition, viral replication, inflammation, necrosis in the myocardium, and mortality in response to Coxsackie B virus are also increased in animals after strenuous exercise (Gatmaitan et al. 1970; Ilback et al. 1989).

Most studies on the effect of exercise on experimentally induced viral infections have been performed on animals for obvious ethical reasons. However, a few longitudinal studies have assessed the impact of regular physical activity on the response to preexisting viral infections in humans. Dependent on exercise dose, both immuno-protective and suppressant effects have been observed. A study conducted on adults in Hong Kong reported that, while low to moderate frequency of exercise led to a decrease in the risk of influenza-associated mortality in adults, a high frequency of exercise did not (Wong et al. 2008). In addition, bouts of high-intensity exercise are known to increase the risk for upper respiratory tract infections (URTI) (Nieman 1997a, b; Nieman et al. 2003), while moderate-intensity physical activity prevents the apparition of URTI symptoms (Nieman et al. 1990).

Similarly, postmenopausal obese women following moderate-intensity exercise training also report fewer cold symptoms than their non-exercising counterparts (Chubak et al. 2006). The exact mechanisms that underpin the protective effects of exercise against infections are not fully understood, but may involve the transient postexercise rise in salivary antimicrobial proteins, such as LL-37 and human neutrophil peptides 1, 2, and 3 (HNP 1–3) (Usui et al. 2011; Davison et al. 2009), bolstering the first line of defense against primary viral infection.

26.7 Exercise and Vaccination

The progressive decline in the function of the immune system associated with human aging is associated with poor vaccine efficacy (Grubeck-Loebenstein et al. 2009; Koch et al. 2007), leaving the elderly vulnerable to viral infections. It is notoriously difficult to seroconvert those aged 70 years and older against viruses like influenza, which is perhaps why the elderly account for >90 % of the deaths from influenza infection (Hannoun et al. 2004). While the efficacy of current vaccines in generating protective antibody titers is evaluated to 70–90 % in young adults, only 17–53 % of vaccination will have a similar effect in the elderly (Goodwin et al. 2006). The disrupted cell-mediated and humoral responses to influenza vaccination seen in healthy elderly are also associated with impaired cytokine secretion (Bernstein et al. 1998).

Physical exercise has been proposed as a cheap, safe, and efficient way to improve vaccine responses in the elderly. It was shown that when older adults (aged >64 years) were immunized with a trivalent influenza virus before and after a 10-month aerobic training intervention, vaccine efficacy, measured as the mean fold increase in antibody titer to two strains of influenza A virus (H1N1 and H3N2), was greatly improved in comparison to non-exerciser controls (Kohut et al. 2004). In addition, cross-sectional studies have shown that elderly men and women with higher cardiovascular fitness had greater antibody responses to influenza vaccines (Keylock et al.

2007). Seroprotection also appears to be increased in community-dwelling elderly (average age 70 years) who followed a 10-month cardiovascular training program up to 24 weeks after receiving the influenza vaccine (Woods et al. 2009). In addition, elderly men and women with higher cardiovascular fitness have greater antibody responses to influenza vaccine. Indirect beneficial effects of physical activity on vaccine efficacy in the elderly have also been proposed. Shimizu et al. (2011) showed that 12 weeks of exercise training elicited an increase in $CD28^+/CD8^+$ T cells and $CD80^+$ monocytes in the elderly, which in turn were positively associated with the antibody response to the influenza vaccine (Sambhara et al. 1998; van Duin et al. 2007). It is, however, interesting to note that the beneficial effect of exercise on vaccination appears to be dose dependent, and while studies using moderate-intensity exercise trainings observed improvements in vaccination efficacy, those using low-intensity exercise training did not (Keylock et al. 2007).

The effects of exercise training on in vivo immune response such as DTH skin reactions have also been examined. Physically active elderly have higher anti-keyhole limpet hemocyanin (KLH) immunoglobulin (Ig)M, IgG, IgG1, and DTH responses than their sedentary counterparts (Smith et al. 2004), and when participating in a 25-week training intervention, healthy elderly exhibited enhanced DTH skin reaction to tuberculin-purified protein derivative (Okutsu et al. 2008). Greater serum IgG1 and IgM concentrations against KLH were also observed in elderly who completed a 10-month aerobic exercise training intervention (Grant et al. 2008).

Eccentrically biased muscle-damaging bouts of exercise prior to influenza vaccination have also shown to increase serum antibody responses and IFN-γ production compared to control trials (Edwards et al. 2006, 2007). While this seems to be limited to individuals who had relatively poor immune responses to the vaccine (Campbell et al. 2010), it indicates that the improved vaccine efficacy in response to exercise seen in previously sedentary elderly may be due to transient immune perturbations as opposed to a permanent restoration of the immune system caused by long-term exercise training.

Conclusion

It is clear that the etiology of immunosenescence is multifaceted and can impact on both arms of the immune system. Poorer vaccine responses and increased rates of infection and malignancy seen in the elderly are likely due to defects in the normal functioning of the immune system. Regular physical exercise has been associated with increased immunity and may serve as a simple lifestyle intervention to counteract the deleterious effects of immunosenescence. Some of the positive effects of exercise for older adults include increased responses to vaccines (Kohut et al. 2004; Woods et al. 2009), greater NK-cell function (McFarlin et al. 2005; Nieman et al. 1993; Woods et al. 1999) reductions in circulatory inflammatory mediators (Pedersen and Bruunsgaard 2003), increased neutrophil phagocytic activity (Yan et al. 2001), lowered inflammatory response to bacterial challenge (Phillips et al. 2010), reduced frequencies of exhausted/senescent T cells in the periphery (Spielmann et al. 2011), increased T-cell proliferation (Nieman et al. 1993; Shinkai et al. 1995), and longer leukocyte telomere lengths (Ludlow et al. 2008; Cherkas et al. 2008). Moreover, immune responses and outcomes of viral infections and malignancies due to exercise training have also been reported to be improved in animal studies (Lowder et al. 2005, 2006; Hojman et al. 2011). These findings provide a strong indication that habitual exercise has immune regulatory properties and may help delay the onset of immunosenescence.

Although many of the immune biomarkers that are positively displayed in exercising elderly are key components of the IRP, which, in turn, has been shown to predict morbidity and mortality in older humans (Ferguson et al. 1995; Pawelec et al. 2009), it is not known if exercise training can reverse, as well as prevent, those impaired immune responses

that have been associated with immunosenescence. This is because most longitudinal exercise training studies (Table 26.2) have failed to document the positive effects of exercise on immunity that have been consistently reported in studies with a cross-sectional design (Table 26.1). A problem with the randomized control trials, however, is that the exercise training intervention is mostly applied to otherwise healthy untrained people. Vast differences in the mode, duration, and intensity of the exercise training intervention also cloud interpretation of the available data. In contrast, exercise training intervention studies in "unhealthy" people such as cancer survivors (Fairey et al. 2005), obese individuals (Nieman et al. 1990), and those living with HIV (Perna et al. 1999) mostly report positive effects on immunity. Exercise may therefore contribute to the reversal of immunosenescence in those individuals considered to be "at risk." Future studies that examine the effects of exercise training in diseased cohorts, frail elderly, or people assigned to the IRP category may indeed reveal immune restorative properties of regular exercise.

References

Agius E, Lacy KE, Vukmanovic-Stejic M, Jagger AL, Papageorgiou AP, Hall S, Reed JR, Curnow SJ, Fuentes-Duculan J, Buckley CD et al (2009) Decreased TNF-alpha synthesis by macrophages restricts cutaneous immunosurveillance by memory CD4+ T cells during aging. J Exp Med 206:1929–1940

Agrawal A, Gupta S (2011) Impact of aging on dendritic cell functions in humans. Ageing Res Rev 10:336–345

Agrawal A, Agrawal S, Cao JN, Su H, Osann K, Gupta S (2007) Altered innate immune functioning of dendritic cells in elderly humans: a role of phosphoinositide 3-kinase-signaling pathway. J Immunol 178:6912–6922

Agrawal A, Agrawal S, Tay J, Gupta S (2008) Biology of dendritic cells in aging. J Clin Immunol 28:14–20

Agrawal A, Tay J, Ton S, Agrawal S, Gupta S (2009) Increased reactivity of dendritic cells from aged subjects to self-antigen, the human DNA. J Immunol 182:1138–1145

Agrawal A, Sridharan A, Prakash S, Agrawal H (2012) Dendritic cells and aging: consequences for autoimmunity. Expert Rev Clin Immunol 8:73–80

Allavena P, Garlanda C, Borrello MG et al (2008) Pathways connecting inflammation and cancer. Curr Opin Genet Dev 18(1):3–10

Almanzar G, Schwaiger S, Jenewein B et al (2005) Long-term cytomegalovirus infection leads to significant changes in the composition of the CD8+ T cell repertoire, which may be the basis for an imbalance in the cytokine production profile in elderly persons. J Virol 79(6):3675–3683

Almeida-Oliveira A, Smith-Carvalho M, Porto LC, Cardoso-Oliveira J, Ribeiro Ados S, Falcao RR, Abdelhay E, Bouzas LF, Thuler LC, Ornellas MH et al (2011) Age-related changes in natural killer cell receptors from childhood through old age. Hum Immunol 72:319–329

Alvarez-Rodriguez L, Lopez-Hoyos M, Garcia-Unzueta M, Amado JA, Cacho PM, Martinez-Taboada VM (2012) Age and low levels of circulating vitamin D are associated with impaired innate immune function. J Leukoc Biol 91:829–838

Anane LH, Edwards KM, Burns VE et al (2009) Mobilization of gammadelta T lymphocytes in response to psychological stress, exercise, and beta-agonist infusion. Brain Behav Immun 23(6):823–829

Armstrong L, Medford AR, Hunter KJ, Uppington KM, Millar AB (2004) Differential expression of Toll-like receptor (TLR)-2 and TLR-4 on monocytes in human sepsis. Clin Exp Immunol 136:312–319

Ashcroft GS, Horan MA, Ferguson MW (1998) Aging alters the inflammatory and endothelial cell adhesion molecule profiles during human cutaneous wound healing. Lab Invest 78:47–58

Balducci S, Zanuso S, Nicolucci A et al (2010) Anti-inflammatory effect of exercise training in subjects with type 2 diabetes and the metabolic syndrome is dependent on exercise modalities and independent of weight loss. Nutr Metab Cardiovasc Dis 20(8):608–617

Barlow CE, LaMonte MJ, Fitzgerald SJ et al (2006) Cardiorespiratory fitness is an independent predictor of hypertension incidence among initially normotensive healthy women. Am J Epidemiol 163(2):142–150

Bartlett DB, Firth CM, Phillips AC et al (2012) The age-related increase in low-grade systemic inflammation (Inflammageing) is not driven by cytomegalovirus infection. Aging Cell 11(5):912–915

Bate SL, Dollard SC, Cannon MJ (2010) Cytomegalovirus seroprevalence in the United States: the national health and nutrition examination surveys, 1988–2004. Clin Infect Dis 50(11):1439–1447

Baylis D, Bartlett DB, Syddall HE et al (2013) Immune-endocrine biomarkers as predictors of frailty and mortality: a 10-year longitudinal study in community-dwelling older people. Age (Dordr) 35:963–971

Belge KU, Dayyani F, Horelt A, Siedlar M, Frankenberger M, Frankenberger B, Espevik T, Ziegler-Heitbrock L (2002) The proinflammatory CD14+CD16+DR++ monocytes are a major source of TNF. J Immunol 168:3536–3542

Bernstein ED, Gardner EM, Abrutyn E et al (1998) Cytokine production after influenza vaccination in a healthy elderly population. Vaccine 16(18):1722–1731

Beshgetoor D, Arrues S, McGuire K (2004) Effect of competitive training on T cell mediated immune function in Master's female athletes. Int J Sports Med 25(7):553–558

Beziat V, Descours B, Parizot C, Debre P, Vieillard V (2010) NK cell terminal differentiation: correlated stepwise decrease of NKG2A and acquisition of KIRs. PLoS One 5:e11966

Bigley AB, Lowder TW, Spielmann G et al (2012) NK cells have an impaired response to acute exercise and a lower expression of the inhibitory receptors KLRG1 and CD158a in humans with latent cytomegalovirus infection. Brain Behav Immun 26(1):177–186

Bigley AB, Spielmann G, LaVoy ECP, Simpson RJ (2013) Can exercise-related improvements in immunity influence cancer prevention and prognosis in the elderly? Maturitas 76:51–56

Biswas SK, Mantovani A (2010) Macrophage plasticity and interaction with lymphocyte subsets: cancer as a paradigm. Nat Immunol 11:889–896

Blair SN, Jackson AS (2001) Physical fitness and activity as separate heart disease risk factors: a meta-analysis. Med Sci Sports Exerc 33(5):762–764

Blair SN, Kampert JB, Kohl HW 3rd et al (1996) Influences of cardiorespiratory fitness and other precursors on cardiovascular disease and all-cause mortality in men and women. JAMA 276(3):205–210

Born J, Uthgenannt D, Dodt C, Nunninghoff D, Ringvolt E, Wagner T, Fehm HL (1995) Cytokine production and lymphocyte subpopulations in aged humans. An assessment during nocturnal sleep. Mech Ageing Dev 84:113–126

Borrego F, Alonso MC, Galiani MD, Carracedo J, Ramirez R, Ostos B, Pena J, Solana R (1999) NK phenotypic markers and IL2 response in NK cells from elderly people. Exp Gerontol 34:253–265

Brunner S, Herndler-Brandstetter D, Weinberger B et al (2010) Persistent viral infections and immune ageing. Ageing Res Rev 10(3):362–369

Bruunsgaard H, Pedersen BK (2000) Special feature for the Olympics: effects of exercise on the immune system: effects of exercise on the immune system in the elderly population. Immunol Cell Biol 78:523–531

Bruunsgaard H, Andersen-Ranberg K, Jeune B et al (1999) A high plasma concentration of TNF-alpha is associated with dementia in centenarians. J Gerontol A Biol Sci Med Sci 54(7):M357–M364

Butcher SK, Chahal H, Nayak L, Sinclair A, Henriquez NV, Sapey E, O'Mahony D, Lord JM (2001) Senescence in innate immune responses: reduced neutrophil phagocytic capacity and CD16 expression in elderly humans. J Leukoc Biol 70:881–886

Campbell PT, Wener MH, Sorensen B et al (2008) Effect of exercise on in vitro immune function: a 12-month randomized, controlled trial among postmenopausal women. J Appl Physiol 104(6):1648–1655

Campbell JP, Edwards KM, Ring C et al (2010) The effects of vaccine timing on the efficacy of an acute eccentric exercise intervention on the immune response to an influenza vaccine in young adults. Brain Behav Immun 24(2):236–242

CDC (2011) Update: influenza activity—United States, 2010–11 season, and composition of the 2011–12 influenza vaccine. MMWR Morb Mortal Wkly Rep 60:7

Cesari M, Penninx BW, Pahor M et al (2004) Inflammatory markers and physical performance in older persons: the InCHIANTI study. J Gerontol A Biol Sci Med Sci 59(3):242–248

Chatta GS, Dale DC (1996) Aging and haemopoiesis. Implications for treatment with haemopoietic growth factors. Drugs Aging 9:37–47

Cherkas LF, Hunkin JL, Kato BS et al (2008) The association between physical activity in leisure time and leukocyte telomere length. Arch Intern Med 168(2): 154–158

Chiang LM, Chen YJ, Chiang J, Lai LY, Chen YY, Liao HF (2007) Modulation of dendritic cells by endurance training. Int J Sports Med 28:798–803

Chidrawar SM, Khan N, Chan YL, Nayak L, Moss PA (2006) Ageing is associated with a decline in peripheral blood CD56bright NK cells. Immun Ageing 3:10

Chiplunkar S, Dhar S, Wesch D et al (2009) Gammadelta T cells in cancer immunotherapy: current status and future prospects. Immunotherapy 1(4):663–678

Chubak J, McTiernan A, Sorensen B et al (2006) Moderate-intensity exercise reduces the incidence of colds among postmenopausal women. Am J Med 119(11):937–942

Church TS, Earnest CP, Thompson AM et al (2010) Exercise without weight loss does not reduce C-reactive protein: the INFLAME study. Med Sci Sports Exerc 42(4):708–716

Colbert LH, Visser M, Simonsick EM et al (2004) Physical activity, exercise, and inflammatory markers in older adults: findings from the Health, Ageing and Body Composition Study. J Am Geriatr Soc 52(7): 1098–1104

Cretel E, Veen I, Pierres A, Bongrand P, Gavazzi G (2010) Immunosenescence and infections, myth or reality? Med Mal Infect 40:307–318

Cros J, Cagnard N, Woollard K, Patey N, Zhang SY, Senechal B, Puel A, Biswas SK, Moshous D, Picard C et al (2010) Human CD14dim monocytes patrol and sense nucleic acids and viruses via TLR7 and TLR8 receptors. Immunity 33:375–386

Davis JM, Kohut ML, Colbert LH et al (1997) Exercise, alveolar macrophage function, and susceptibility to respiratory infection. J Appl Physiol 83(5):1461–1466

Davis JM, Murphy EA, Brown AS et al (2004) Effects of moderate exercise and oat beta-glucan on innate immune function and susceptibility to respiratory infection. Am J Physiol Regul Integr Comp Physiol 286(2):R366–R372

Davison G, Allgrove J, Gleeson M (2009) Salivary antimicrobial peptides (LL-37 and alpha-defensins HNP1-3), antimicrobial and IgA responses to prolonged exercise. Eur J Appl Physiol 106(2):277–284

de Gonzalo-Calvo D, Fernandez-Garcia B, de Luxan-Delgado B, Rodriguez-Gonzalez S, Garcia-Macia M, Suarez FM, Solano JJ, Rodriguez-Colunga MJ, Coto-Montes A (2012) Long-term training induces a healthy inflammatory and endocrine emergent biomarker profile in elderly men. Age (Dordr) 34:761–771

De Maria A, Moretta L (2011) Revisited function of human NK cell subsets. Cell Cycle 10:1178–1179

De Martinis M, Modesti M, Ginaldi L (2004) Phenotypic and functional changes of circulating monocytes and polymorphonuclear leucocytes from elderly persons. Immunol Cell Biol 82:415–420

DelaRosa O, Pawelec G, Peralbo E et al (2006) Immunological biomarkers of ageing in man: changes in both innate and adaptive immunity are associated with health and longevity. Biogerontology 7(5–6): 471–481

Della Bella S, Bierti L, Presicce P, Arienti R, Valenti M, Saresella M, Vergani C, Villa ML (2007) Peripheral blood dendritic cells and monocytes are differently regulated in the elderly. Clin Immunol 122:220–228

Dopheide JF, Obst V, Doppler C, Radmacher MC, Scheer M, Radsak MP, Gori T, Warnholtz A, Fottner C, Daiber A et al (2012) Phenotypic characterisation of proinflammatory monocytes and dendritic cells in peripheral arterial disease. Thromb Haemost 108:1198–1207

Drela N, Kozdron E, Szczypiorski P (2004) Moderate exercise may attenuate some aspects of immunosenescence. BMC Geriatr 4:8

Dunne PJ, Faint JM, Gudgeon NH et al (2002) Epstein-Barr virus-specific CD8(+) T cells that re-express CD45RA are apoptosis-resistant memory cells that retain replicative potential. Blood 100(3):933–940

Duzova H, Karakoc Y, Emre MH et al (2009) Effects of acute moderate and strenuous exercise bouts on IL-17 production and inflammatory response in trained rats. J Sports Sci Med 8(2):219–224

Edwards KM, Burns VE, Reynolds T et al (2006) Acute stress exposure prior to influenza vaccination enhances antibody response in women. Brain Behav Immun 20(2):159–168

Edwards KM, Burns VE, Allen LM et al (2007) Eccentric exercise as an adjuvant to influenza vaccination in humans. Brain Behav Immun 21(2):209–217

Elenkov IJ (2004) Glucocorticoids and the Th1/Th2 balance. Ann N Y Acad Sci 1024:138–146

Elosua R, Bartali B, Ordovas JM et al (2005) Association between physical activity, physical performance, and inflammatory biomarkers in an elderly population: the InCHIANTI study. J Gerontol A Biol Sci Med Sci 60(6):760–767

Ershler WB, Sun WH, Binkley N et al (1993) Interleukin-6 and ageing: blood levels and mononuclear cell production increase with advancing age and in vitro production is modifiable by dietary restriction. Lymphokine Cytokine Res 12(4):225–230

Evenson KR, Stevens J, Cai J et al (2003) The effect of cardiorespiratory fitness and obesity on cancer mortality in women and men. Med Sci Sports Exerc 35(2):270–277

Fahlman M, Boardley D, Flynn MG et al (2000) Effects of endurance training on selected parameters of immune function in elderly women. Gerontology 46(2):97–104

Fairey AS, Courneya KS, Field CJ et al (2005) Randomized controlled trial of exercise and blood immune function in postmenopausal breast cancer survivors. J Appl Physiol 98(4):1534–1540

Farag SS, VanDeusen JB, Fehniger TA, Caligiuri MA (2003) Biology and clinical impact of human natural killer cells. Int J Hematol 78:7–17

Ferguson FG, Wikby A, Maxson P et al (1995) Immune parameters in a longitudinal study of a very old population of Swedish people: a comparison between survivors and nonsurvivors. J Gerontol A Biol Sci Med Sci 50(6):B378–B382

Ferlazzo G, Pack M, Thomas D, Paludan C, Schmid D, Strowig T, Bougras G, Muller WA, Moretta L, Munz C (2004) Distinct roles of IL-12 and IL-15 in human natural killer cell activation by dendritic cells from secondary lymphoid organs. Proc Natl Acad Sci U S A 101:16606–16611

Ferrando-Martinez S, Romero-Sanchez MC, Solana R, Delgado J, de la Rosa R, Munoz-Fernandez MA, Ruiz-Mateos E, Leal M (2013) Thymic function failure and C-reactive protein levels are independent predictors of all-cause mortality in healthy elderly humans. Age (Dordr) 35:251–259

Fischer CP, Berntsen A, Perstrup LB et al (2007) Plasma levels of interleukin-6 and C-reactive protein are associated with physical inactivity independent of obesity. Scand J Med Sci Sports 17(5):580–587

Flynn MG, Fahlman M, Braun WA et al (1999) Effects of resistance training on selected indexes of immune function in elderly women. J Appl Physiol 86(6):1905–1913

Forsey RJ, Thompson JM, Ernerudh J et al (2003) Plasma cytokine profiles in elderly humans. Mech Ageing Dev 124(4):487–493

Fortin CF, McDonald PP, Lesur O, Fulop T Jr (2008) Aging and neutrophils: there is still much to do. Rejuvenation Res 11:873–882

Franceschi C, Bonafe M, Valensin S et al (2000) Inflammageing. An evolutionary perspective on immunosenescence. Ann N Y Acad Sci 908:244–254

Franceschi C, Capri M, Monti D, Giunta S, Olivieri F, Sevini F, Panourgia MP, Invidia L, Celani L, Scurti M et al (2007) Inflammaging and anti-inflammaging: a systemic perspective on aging and longevity emerged from studies in humans. Mech Ageing Dev 128:92–105

Fulop T Jr, Foris G, Worum I, Leovey A (1985) Age-dependent alterations of Fc gamma receptor-mediated effector functions of human polymorphonuclear leucocytes. Clin Exp Immunol 61:425–432

Fulop T Jr, Fouquet C, Allaire P, Perrin N, Lacombe G, Stankova J, Rola-Pleszczynski M, Gagne D, Wagner JR, Khalil A et al (1997) Changes in apoptosis of human polymorphonuclear granulocytes with aging. Mech Ageing Dev 96:15–34

Gano LB, Donato AJ, Pierce GL et al (2011) Increased proinflammatory and oxidant gene expression in circulating mononuclear cells in older adults: amelioration by habitual exercise. Physiol Genomics 43(14):895–902

Gatmaitan BG, Chason JL, Lerner AM (1970) Augmentation of the virulence of murine coxsackievirus B-3 myocardiopathy by exercise. J Exp Med 131(6):1121–1136

Gayoso I, Sanchez-Correa B, Campos C et al (2011) Immunosenescence of human natural killer cells. J Innate Immun 3(4):337–343

Geissmann F, Gordon S, Hume DA, Mowat AM, Randolph GJ (2010) Unravelling mononuclear phagocyte heterogeneity. Nat Rev Immunol 10:453–460

Giunta B, Fernandez F, Nikolic WV et al (2008) Inflammageing as a prodrome to Alzheimer's disease. J Neuroinflammation 5:51

Gomez CR, Nomellini V, Faunce DE, Kovacs EJ (2008) Innate immunity and aging. Exp Gerontol 43:718–728

Goodwin K, Viboud C, Simonsen L (2006) Antibody response to influenza vaccination in the elderly: a quantitative review. Vaccine 24(8):1159–1169

Grant RW, Mariani RA, Vieira VJ et al (2008) Cardiovascular exercise intervention improves the primary antibody response to keyhole limpet hemocyanin (KLH) in previously sedentary older adults. Brain Behav Immun 22(6):923–932

Grubeck-Loebenstein B, Della Bella S, Iorio AM et al (2009) Immunosenescence and vaccine failure in the elderly. Aging Clin Exp Res 21(3):201–209

Gueldner SH, Poon LW, La Via M et al (1997) Long-term exercise patterns and immune function in healthy older women. A report of preliminary findings. Mech Ageing Dev 93(1–3):215–222

Guichard C, Pedruzzi E, Dewas C, Fay M, Pouzet C, Bens M, Vandewalle A, Ogier-Denis E, Gougerot-Pocidalo MA, Elbim C (2005) Interleukin-8-induced priming of neutrophil oxidative burst requires sequential recruitment of NADPH oxidase components into lipid rafts. J Biol Chem 280:37021–37032

Haaland DA, Sabljic TF, Baribeau DA et al (2008) Is regular exercise a friend or foe of the ageing immune system? A systematic review. Clin J Sport Med 18(6):539–548

Hannoun C, Megas F, Piercy J (2004) Immunogenicity and protective efficacy of influenza vaccination. Virus Res 103(1–2):133–138

Hayhoe RP, Henson SM, Akbar AN, Palmer DB (2010) Variation of human natural killer cell phenotypes with age: identification of a unique KLRG1-negative subset. Hum Immunol 71:676–681

Heron M, Tejada-Vera B (2009) Deaths: leading causes for 2005. Natl Vital Stat Rep 58(8):1–97

Ho CS, Lopez JA, Vuckovic S, Pyke CM, Hockey RL, Hart DN (2001) Surgical and physical stress increases circulating blood dendritic cell counts independently of monocyte counts. Blood 98:140–145

Hoffman-Goetz L, Quadrilatero J (2003) Treadmill exercise in mice increases intestinal lymphocyte loss via apoptosis. Acta Physiol Scand 179(3):289–297

Hojman P, Dethlefsen C, Brandt C et al (2011) Exercise-induced muscle-derived cytokines inhibit mammary cancer cell growth. Am J Physiol Endocrinol Metab 301(3):E504–E510

Hume DA, Ross IL, Himes SR, Sasmono RT, Wells CA, Ravasi T (2002) The mononuclear phagocyte system revisited. J Leukoc Biol 72:621–627

Hwang KA, Kim HR, Kang I (2009) Ageing and human CD4(+) regulatory T cells. Mech Ageing Dev 130(8): 509–517

Ilback NG, Fohlman J, Friman G (1989) Exercise in cox-sackie B3 myocarditis: effects on heart lymphocyte subpopulations and the inflammatory reaction. Am Heart J 117(6):1298–1302

Jing Y, Shaheen E, Drake RR, Chen N, Gravenstein S, Deng Y (2009) Aging is associated with a numerical and functional decline in plasmacytoid dendritic cells, whereas myeloid dendritic cells are relatively unaltered in human peripheral blood. Hum Immunol 70: 777–784

Jylha M, Paavilainen P, Lehtimaki T et al (2007) Interleukin-1 receptor antagonist, interleukin-6, and C-reactive protein as predictors of mortality in nonagenarians: the vitality 90+ study. J Gerontol A Biol Sci Med Sci 62(9):1016–1021

Kadoglou NP, Iliadis F, Angelopoulou N et al (2007a) The anti-inflammatory effects of exercise training in patients with type 2 diabetes mellitus. Eur J Cardiovasc Prev Rehabil 14(6):837–843

Kadoglou NP, Perrea D, Iliadis F et al (2007b) Exercise reduces resistin and inflammatory cytokines in patients with type 2 diabetes. Diabetes Care 30(3):719–721

Kapasi ZF, Catlin PA, Joyner DR et al (2000) The effects of intense physical exercise on secondary antibody response in young and old mice. Phys Ther 80(11): 1076–1086

Kapasi ZF, Ouslander JG, Schnelle JF et al (2003) Effects of an exercise intervention on immunologic parameters in frail elderly nursing home residents. J Gerontol A Biol Sci Med Sci 58(7):636–643

Kapasi ZF, McRae ML, Ahmed R (2005) Suppression of viral specific primary T cell response following intense physical exercise in young but not old mice. J Appl Physiol 98(2):663–671

Kawai T, Akira S (2007) Signaling to NF-kappaB by Toll-like receptors. Trends Mol Med 13:460–469

Kawanishi N, Yano H, Yokogawa Y, Suzuki K (2010) Exercise training inhibits inflammation in adipose tissue via both suppression of macrophage infiltration and acceleration of phenotypic switching from M1 to M2 macrophages in high-fat-diet-induced obese mice. Exerc Immunol Rev 16:105–118

Keylock KT, Lowder T, Leifheit KA et al (2007) Higher antibody, but not cell-mediated, responses to vaccination in high physically fit elderly. J Appl Physiol 102(3):1090–1098

Koch S, Larbi A, Ozcelik D et al (2007) Cytomegalovirus infection: a driving force in human T cell immunosenescence. Ann N Y Acad Sci 1114:23–35

Kodama S, Shu M, Saito K et al (2007) Even low-intensity and low-volume exercise training may improve insulin resistance in the elderly. Intern Med 46(14): 1071–1077

Kodama S, Saito K, Tanaka S et al (2009) Cardiorespiratory fitness as a quantitative predictor of all-cause mortality and cardiovascular events in healthy men and women: a meta-analysis. JAMA 301(19):2024–2035

Kohut ML, Boehm GW, Moynihan JA (2001) Moderate exercise is associated with enhanced antigen-specific cytokine, but not IgM antibody production in aged mice. Mech Ageing Dev 122(11):1135–1150

Kohut ML, Arntson BA, Lee W et al (2004) Moderate exercise improves antibody response to influenza immunization in older adults. Vaccine 22(17–18): 2298–2306

Kohut ML, McCann DA, Russell DW et al (2006) Aerobic exercise, but not flexibility/resistance exercise, reduces serum IL-18, CRP, and IL-6 independent of beta-blockers, BMI, and psychosocial factors in older adults. Brain Behav Immun 20(3):201–209

Kruger K, Lechtermann A, Fobker M et al (2008) Exercise-induced redistribution of T lymphocytes is regulated by adrenergic mechanisms. Brain Behav Immun 22(3):324–338

Kullo IJ, Khaleghi M, Hensrud DD (2007) Markers of inflammation are inversely associated with VO2 max in asymptomatic men. J Appl Physiol 102(4):1374–1379

Kumar V, Sharma A (2010) Neutrophils: Cinderella of innate immune system. Int Immunopharmacol 10: 1325–1334

Lancaster GI, Khan Q, Drysdale P, Wallace F, Jeukendrup AE, Drayson MT, Gleeson M (2005) The physiological regulation of toll-like receptor expression and function in humans. J Physiol 563:945–955

Lande R, Gilliet M (2010) Plasmacytoid dendritic cells: key players in the initiation and regulation of immune responses. Ann N Y Acad Sci 1183:89–103

Lanzavecchia A, Sallusto F (2001) Regulation of T cell immunity by dendritic cells. Cell 106:263–266

Larbi A, Douziech N, Fortin C, Linteau A, Dupuis G, Fulop T Jr (2005) The role of the MAPK pathway alterations in GM-CSF modulated human neutrophil apoptosis with aging. Immun Ageing 2:6

Le Garff-Tavernier M, Beziat V, Decocq J, Siguret V, Gandjbakhch F, Pautas E, Debre P, Merle-Beral H, Vieillard V (2010) Human NK cells display major phenotypic and functional changes over the life span. Aging Cell 9:527–535

Libby P (2006) Inflammation and cardiovascular disease mechanisms. Am J Clin Nutr 83(2):456S–460S

Lio D, Scola L, Crivello A et al (2002) Gender-specific association between −1082 IL-10 promoter polymorphism and longevity. Genes Immun 3(1):30–33

Liu J, Chen P, Wang R, Yuan Y, Li C (2012) Effect of Tai Chi exercise on immune function in middle-aged and elderly women. J Sports Med Doping Stud 2(119): 1–7

Lopez-Verges S, Milush JM, Pandey S, York VA, Arakawa-Hoyt J, Pircher H, Norris PJ, Nixon DF, Lanier LL (2010) CD57 defines a functionally distinct population of mature NK cells in the human CD56dimCD16+ NK-cell subset. Blood 116:3865–3874

Lowder T, Padgett DA, Woods JA (2005) Moderate exercise protects mice from death due to influenza virus. Brain Behav Immun 19(5):377–380

Lowder T, Padgett DA, Woods JA (2006) Moderate exercise early after influenza virus infection reduces the Th1 inflammatory response in lungs of mice. Exerc Immunol Rev 12:97–111

Lowder T, Dugger K, Deshane J et al (2010) Repeated bouts of aerobic exercise enhance regulatory T cell responses in a murine asthma model. Brain Behav Immun 24(1):153–159

Ludlow AT, Zimmerman JB, Witkowski S et al (2008) Relationship between physical activity level, telomere length, and telomerase activity. Med Sci Sports Exerc 40(10):1764–1771

Lutz CT, Moore MB, Bradley S, Shelton BJ, Lutgendorf SK (2005) Reciprocal age related change in natural killer cell receptors for MHC class I. Mech Ageing Dev 126:722–731

Lynch J, Helmrich SP, Lakka TA et al (1996) Moderately intense physical activities and high levels of cardiorespiratory fitness reduce the risk of non-insulin-dependent diabetes mellitus in middle-aged men. Arch Intern Med 156(12):1307–1314

Malm C (2004) Exercise immunology: the current state of man and mouse. Sports Med 34(9):555–566

Mantovani A, Pierotti MA (2008) Cancer and inflammation: a complex relationship. Cancer Lett 267(2):180–181

Mariani E, Monaco MC, Cattini L, Sinoppi M, Facchini A (1994) Distribution and lytic activity of NK cell subsets in the elderly. Mech Ageing Dev 76:177–187

Mariani E, Meneghetti A, Neri S, Ravaglia G, Forti P, Cattini L, Facchini A (2002) Chemokine production by natural killer cells from nonagenarians. Eur J Immunol 32:1524–1529

Martin SA, Pence BD, Woods JA (2009) Exercise and respiratory tract viral infections. Exerc Sport Sci Rev 37(4):157–164

Mazzoccoli G, Vendemiale G, De Cata A et al (2011) Change of gammadeltaTCR-expressing T cells in healthy ageing. Int J Immunopathol Pharmacol 24(1):201–209

McFarlin BK, Flynn MG, Campbell WW, Stewart LK, Timmerman KL (2004) TLR4 is lower in resistance-trained older women and related to inflammatory cytokines. Med Sci Sports Exerc 36:1876–1883

McFarlin BK, Flynn MG, Phillips MD et al (2005) Chronic resistance exercise training improves natural killer cell activity in older women. J Gerontol A Biol Sci Med Sci 60(10):1315–1318

McFarlin BK, Flynn MG, Campbell WW, Craig BA, Robinson JP, Stewart LK, Timmerman KL, Coen PM (2006) Physical activity status, but not age, influences inflammatory biomarkers and toll-like receptor 4. J Gerontol A Biol Sci Med Sci 61:388–393

Mege JL, Mehraj V, Capo C (2011) Macrophage polarization and bacterial infections. Curr Opin Infect Dis 24:230–234

Merino A, Buendia P, Martin-Malo A, Aljama P, Ramirez R, Carracedo J (2011) Senescent CD14+CD16+ monocytes exhibit proinflammatory and proatherosclerotic activity. J Immunol 186:1809–1815

Michishita R, Shono N, Inoue T, Tsuruta T, Node K (2008) Associations of monocytes, neutrophil count, and C-reactive protein with maximal oxygen uptake in overweight women. J Cardiol 52:247–253

Mooren FC, Bloming D, Lechtermann A et al (2002) Lymphocyte apoptosis after exhaustive and moderate exercise. J Appl Physiol 93(1):147–153

Mooren FC, Volker K, Klocke R, Nikol S, Waltenberger J, Kruger K (2012) Exercise delays neutrophil apoptosis by a G-CSF-dependent mechanism. J Appl Physiol 113:1082–1090

Nickel T, Emslander I, Sisic Z, David R, Schmaderer C, Marx N, Schmidt-Trucksass A, Hoster E, Halle M, Weis M et al (2012) Modulation of dendritic cells and toll-like receptors by marathon running. Eur J Appl Physiol 112:1699–1708

Nicklas BJ, Hsu FC, Brinkley TJ et al (2008) Exercise training and plasma C-reactive protein and interleukin-6 in elderly people. J Am Geriatr Soc 56(11):2045–2052

Nieman DC (1997a) Immune response to heavy exertion. J Appl Physiol 82(5):1385–1394

Nieman DC (1997b) Risk of upper respiratory tract infection in athletes: an epidemiologic and immunologic perspective. J Athl Train 32(4):344–349

Nieman DC, Nehlsen-Cannarella SL, Markoff PA et al (1990) The effects of moderate exercise training on natural killer cells and acute upper respiratory tract infections. Int J Sports Med 11(6):467–473

Nieman DC, Henson DA, Gusewitch G et al (1993) Physical activity and immune function in elderly women. Med Sci Sports Exerc 25(7):823–831

Nieman DC, Henson DA, Sampson CS et al (1995) The acute immune response to exhaustive resistance exercise. Int J Sports Med 16(5):322–328

Nieman DC, Dumke CI, Henson DA et al (2003) Immune and oxidative changes during and following the Western States Endurance Run. Int J Sports Med 24(7):541–547

Nieto-Vazquez I, Fernandez-Veledo S, Kramer DK et al (2008) Insulin resistance associated to obesity: the link TNF-alpha. Arch Physiol Biochem 114(3):183–194

Nyugen J, Agrawal S, Gollapudi S, Gupta S (2010) Impaired functions of peripheral blood monocyte subpopulations in aged humans. J Clin Immunol 30:806–813

Ogawa K, Oka J, Yamakawa J et al (2003) Habitual exercise did not affect the balance of type 1 and type 2 cytokines in elderly people. Mech Ageing Dev 124(8–9):951–956

Okutsu M, Yoshida Y, Zhang X et al (2008) Exercise training enhances in vivo tuberculosis purified protein derivative response in the elderly. J Appl Physiol 104(6):1690–1696

Ostrowski K, Rohde T, Asp S et al (1999) Pro- and anti-inflammatory cytokine balance in strenuous exercise in humans. J Physiol 515(Pt 1):287–291

Padgett DA, Sheridan JF, Dorne J et al (1998) Social stress and the reactivation of latent herpes simplex virus type 1. Proc Natl Acad Sci U S A 95(12):7231–7235

Panda A, Qian F, Mohanty S, van Duin D, Newman FK, Zhang L, Chen S, Towle V, Belshe RB, Fikrig E et al (2010) Age-associated decrease in TLR function in primary human dendritic cells predicts influenza vaccine response. J Immunol 184:2518–2527

Passlick B, Flieger D, Ziegler-Heitbrock HW (1989) Identification and characterization of a novel monocyte subpopulation in human peripheral blood. Blood 74:2527–2534

Pawelec G, Derhovanessian E, Larbi A et al (2009) Cytomegalovirus and human immunosenescence. Rev Med Virol 19(1):47–56

Pawelec G, Akbar A, Beverley P et al (2010) Immunosenescence and Cytomegalovirus: where do we stand after a decade? Immun Ageing 7:13

Pedersen BK, Bruunsgaard H (2003) Possible beneficial role of exercise in modulating low-grade inflammation in the elderly. Scand J Med Sci Sports 13(1):56–62

Pedersen M, Bruunsgaard H, Weis N et al (2003) Circulating levels of TNF-alpha and IL-6-relation to truncal fat mass and muscle mass in healthy elderly individuals and in patients with type-2 diabetes. Mech Ageing Dev 124(4):495–502

Perna FM, LaPerriere A, Klimas N et al (1999) Cardiopulmonary and CD4 cell changes in response to exercise training in early symptomatic HIV infection. Med Sci Sports Exerc 31(7):973–979

Peters EM, Bateman ED (1983) Ultramarathon running and upper respiratory tract infections. An epidemiological survey. S Afr Med J 64(15):582–584

Peters T, Weiss JM, Sindrilaru A, Wang H, Oreshkova T, Wlaschek M, Maity P, Reimann J, Scharffetter-Kochanek K (2009) Reactive oxygen intermediate-induced pathomechanisms contribute to immunosenescence, chronic inflammation and autoimmunity. Mech Ageing Dev 130:564–587

Petersen AM, Pedersen BK (2005) The anti-inflammatory effect of exercise. J Appl Physiol 98(4):1154–1162

Phillips MD, Flynn MG, McFarlin BK et al (2010) Resistance training at eight-repetition maximum reduces the inflammatory milieu in elderly women. Med Sci Sports Exerc 42(2):314–325

Plackett TP, Boehmer ED, Faunce DE, Kovacs EJ (2004) Aging and innate immune cells. J Leukoc Biol 76:291–299

Plowden J, Renshaw-Hoelscher M, Gangappa S, Engleman C, Katz JM, Sambhara S (2004) Impaired antigen-induced CD8+ T cell clonal expansion in aging is due to defects in antigen presenting cell function. Cell Immunol 229:86–92

Przybyla B, Gurley C, Harvey JF, Bearden E, Kortebein P, Evans WJ, Sullivan DH, Peterson CA, Dennis RA (2006) Aging alters macrophage properties in human skeletal muscle both at rest and in response to acute resistance exercise. Exp Gerontol 41:320–327

Radom-Aizik S, Zaldivar F Jr, Leu SY, Galassetti P, Cooper DM (2008) Effects of 30 min of aerobic exercise on gene expression in human neutrophils. J Appl Physiol 104:236–243

Rall LC, Roubenoff R, Cannon JG et al (1996) Effects of progressive resistance training on immune response in ageing and chronic inflammation. Med Sci Sports Exerc 28(11):1356–1365

Raso V, Benard G, DA Silva Duarte AJ et al (2007) Effect of resistance training on immunological parameters of healthy elderly women. Med Sci Sports Exerc 39(12):2152–2159

Reis e Sousa C, Hieny S, Scharton-Kersten T, Jankovic D, Charest H, Germain RN, Sher A (1997) In vivo microbial stimulation induces rapid CD40 ligand-independent production of interleukin 12 by dendritic cells and their redistribution to T cell areas. J Exp Med 186:1819–1829

Renshaw M, Rockwell J, Engleman C, Gewirtz A, Katz J, Sambhara S (2002) Cutting edge: impaired Toll-like receptor expression and function in aging. J Immunol 169:4697–4701

Reyna SM, Ghosh S, Tantiwong P, Meka CS, Eagan P, Jenkinson CP, Cersosimo E, Defronzo RA, Coletta DK, Sriwijitkamol A et al (2008) Elevated toll-like receptor 4 expression and signaling in muscle from insulin-resistant subjects. Diabetes 57:2595–2602

Romagnani C, Della Chiesa M, Kohler S, Moewes B, Radbruch A, Moretta L, Moretta A, Thiel A (2005) Activation of human NK cells by plasmacytoid dendritic cells and its modulation by CD4+ T helper cells and CD4+ CD25hi T regulatory cells. Eur J Immunol 35:2452–2458

Ru W, Peijie C (2009) Modulation of NKT cells and Th1/Th2 imbalance after alpha-GalCer treatment in progressive load-trained rats. Int J Biol Sci 5(4):338–343

Sakaguchi S, Miyara M, Costantino CM et al (2010) FOXP3+ regulatory T cells in the human immune system. Nat Rev Immunol 10(7):490–500

Salmon P (2001) Effects of physical exercise on anxiety, depression, and sensitivity to stress: a unifying theory. Clin Psychol Rev 21(1):33–61

Sambhara S, Switzer I, Kurichh A et al (1998) Enhanced antibody and cytokine responses to influenza viral antigens in perforin-deficient mice. Cell Immunol 187(1):13–18

Sanchez-Correa B, Morgado S, Gayoso I, Bergua JM, Casado JG, Arcos MJ, Bengochea ML, Duran E, Solana R, Tarazona R (2011) Human NK cells in acute myeloid leukaemia patients: analysis of NK cell-activating receptors and their ligands. Cancer Immunol Immunother 60:1195–1205

Saurwein-Teissl M, Lung TL, Marx F et al (2002) Lack of antibody production following immunization in old age: association with CD8(+)CD28(−) T cell clonal expansions and an imbalance in the production of Th1 and Th2 cytokines. J Immunol 168(11):5893–5899

Schaun MI, Dipp T, Rossato Jda S, Wilhelm EN, Pinto R, Rech A, Plentz RD, Homem de Bittencourt PI, Reischak-Oliveira A (2011) The effects of periodized concurrent and aerobic training on oxidative stress parameters, endothelial function and immune response in sedentary male individuals of middle age. Cell Biochem Funct 29:534–542

Shaw AC, Joshi S, Greenwood H et al (2010) Ageing of the innate immune system. Curr Opin Immunol 22(4):507–513

Shaw AC, Panda A, Joshi SR et al (2011) Dysregulation of human Toll-like receptor function in ageing. Ageing Res Rev 10(3):346–353

Shearer GM (1997) Th1/Th2 changes in ageing. Mech Ageing Dev 94(1–3):1–5

Shimizu K, Kimura F, Akimoto T et al (2008) Effect of moderate exercise training on T-helper cell subpopulations in elderly people. Exerc Immunol Rev 14:24–37

Shimizu K, Suzuki N, Imai T et al (2011) Monocyte and T cell responses to exercise training in elderly subjects. J Strength Cond Res 25(9):2565–2572

Shimizu I, Yoshida Y, Katsuno T, Minamino T (2013) Adipose tissue inflammation in diabetes and heart failure. Microbes Infect 15:11–17

Shin YA, Lee JH, Song W et al (2008) Exercise training improves the antioxidant enzyme activity with no changes of telomere length. Mech Ageing Dev 129(5):254–260

Shinkai S, Kohno H, Kimura K et al (1995) Physical activity and immune senescence in men. Med Sci Sports Exerc 27(11):1516–1526

Shodell M, Siegal FP (2002) Circulating, interferon-producing plasmacytoid dendritic cells decline during human ageing. Scand J Immunol 56:518–521

Siegal FP, Kadowaki N, Shodell M, Fitzgerald-Bocarsly PA, Shah K, Ho S, Antonenko S, Liu YJ (1999) The nature of the principal type 1 interferon-producing cells in human blood. Science 284:1835–1837

Sim YJ, Yu S, Yoon KJ et al (2009) Chronic exercise reduces illness severity, decreases viral load, and results in greater anti-inflammatory effects than acute exercise during influenza infection. J Infect Dis 200(9):1434–1442

Simpson RJ (2011) Ageing, persistent viral infections, and immunosenescence: can exercise "make space"? Exerc Sport Sci Rev 39(1):23–33

Simpson RJ, Florida-James GD, Cosgrove C et al (2007) High-intensity exercise elicits the mobilization of senescent T lymphocytes into the peripheral blood compartment in human subjects. J Appl Physiol 103(1):396–401

Simpson RJ, Cosgrove C, Ingram LA, Florida-James GD, Whyte GP, Pircher H, Guy K (2008) Senescent T-lymphocytes are mobilised into the peripheral blood compartment in young and older humans after exhaustive exercise. Brain Behav Immun 22:544–551

Simpson RJ, McFarlin BK, McSporran C, Spielmann G, o Hartaigh B, Guy K (2009) Toll-like receptor expression on classic and pro-inflammatory blood monocytes

after acute exercise in humans. Brain Behav Immun 23:232–239

Smith JK, Dykes R, Douglas JE et al (1999) Long-term exercise and atherogenic activity of blood mononuclear cells in persons at risk of developing ischemic heart disease. JAMA 281(18):1722–1727

Smith TP, Kennedy SL, Fleshner M (2004) Influence of age and physical activity on the primary in vivo antibody and T cell-mediated responses in men. J Appl Physiol 97(2):491–498

Solana R, Mariani E (2000) NK and NK/T cells in human senescence. Vaccine 18:1613–1620

Solana R, Villanueva JL, Pena J, De la Fuente M (1991) Cell mediated immunity in ageing. Comp Biochem Physiol A Comp Physiol 99:1–4

Solana R, Tarazona R, Gayoso I, Lesur O, Dupuis G, Fulop T (2012) Innate immunosenescence: effect of aging on cells and receptors of the innate immune system in humans. Semin Immunol 24:331–341

Souza PM, Jacob-Filho W, Santarem JM et al (2008) Progressive resistance training in elderly HIV-positive patients: does it work? Clinics (Sao Paulo) 63(5):619–624

Spielmann G, McFarlin BK, O'Connor DP et al (2011) Aerobic fitness is associated with lower proportions of senescent blood T cells in man. Brain Behav Immun 25(8):1521–1529

Sridharan A, Esposo M, Kaushal K, Tay J, Osann K, Agrawal S, Gupta S, Agrawal A (2011) Age-associated impaired plasmacytoid dendritic cell functions lead to decreased CD4 and CD8 T cell immunity. Age (Dordr) 33:363–376

Stout-Delgado HW, Du W, Shirali AC et al (2009) Ageing promotes neutrophil-induced mortality by augmenting IL-17 production during viral infection. Cell Host Microbe 6(5):446–456

Sun JC, Lanier LL (2011) NK cell development, homeostasis and function: parallels with CD8(+) T cells. Nat Rev Immunol 11:645–657

Suzui M, Kawai T, Kimura H, Takeda K, Yagita H, Okumura K, Shek PN, Shephard RJ (2004) Natural killer cell lytic activity and CD56(dim) and CD56(bright) cell distributions during and after intensive training. J Appl Physiol 96:2167–2173

Syu GD, Chen HI, Jen CJ (2012) Differential effects of acute and chronic exercise on human neutrophil functions. Med Sci Sports Exerc 44:1021–1027

Taaffe DR, Harris TB, Ferrucci L et al (2000) Cross-sectional and prospective relationships of interleukin-6 and C-reactive protein with physical performance in elderly persons: MacArthur studies of successful ageing. J Gerontol A Biol Sci Med Sci 55(12):M709–M715

Takahashi M, Miyashita M, Kawanishi N, Park JH, Hayashida H, Kim HS, Nakamura Y, Sakamoto S, Suzuki K (2013) Low-volume exercise training attenuates oxidative stress and neutrophils activation in older adults. Eur J Appl Physiol 113(5):1117–1126

Tarazona R, Gayoso I, Alonso C, Peralbo E, Casado J, Sanchez-Correa B, Morgado S, Solana R (2009) NK cells in human ageing. In: Handbook on Immunosenescence. Springer, Netherlands, pp 531–544

Tiainen K, Hurme M, Hervonen A et al (2010) Inflammatory markers and physical performance among nonagenarians. J Gerontol A Biol Sci Med Sci 65(6):658–663

Timmerman KL, Flynn MG, Coen PM, Markofski MM, Pence BD (2008) Exercise training-induced lowering of inflammatory (CD14+CD16+) monocytes: a role in the anti-inflammatory influence of exercise? J Leukoc Biol 84:1271–1278

Uchakin PN, Parish DC, Dane FC et al (2011) Fatigue in medical residents leads to reactivation of herpes virus latency. Interdiscip Perspect Infect Dis 2011: 571340

Usui T, Yoshikawa T, Orita K et al (2011) Changes in salivary antimicrobial peptides, immunoglobulin A and cortisol after prolonged strenuous exercise. Eur J Appl Physiol 111(9):2005–2014

Valentine RJ, Misic MM, Rosengren KS et al (2009) Sex impacts the relation between body composition and physical function in older adults. Menopause 16(3): 518–523

van Duin D, Shaw AC (2007) Toll-like receptors in older adults. J Am Geriatr Soc 55(9):1438–1444

van Duin D, Allore HG, Mohanty S et al (2007) Prevaccine determination of the expression of costimulatory B7 molecules in activated monocytes predicts influenza vaccine responses in young and older adults. J Infect Dis 195(11):1590–1597

Villanueva JL, Solana R, Alonso MC, Pena J (1990) Changes in the expression of HLA-class II antigens on peripheral blood monocytes from aged humans. Dis Markers 8:85–91

Vivier E, Raulet DH, Moretta A, Caligiuri MA, Zitvogel L, Lanier LL, Yokoyama WM, Ugolini S (2011) Innate or adaptive immunity? The example of natural killer cells. Science 331:44–49

Walsh NP, Gleeson M, Pyne DB et al (2011) Position statement. Part two: maintaining immune health. Exerc Immunol Rev 17:64–103

Wang L, Xie Y, Zhu LJ et al (2010) An association between immunosenescence and CD4(+)CD25(+) regulatory T cells: a systematic review. Biomed Environ Sci 23(4):327–332

Wang J, Song H, Tang X et al (2012) Effect of exercise training intensity on murine T-regulatory cells and

vaccination response. Scand J Med Sci Sports 22(5): 643–652

Wendt K, Wilk E, Buyny S, Buer J, Schmidt RE, Jacobs R (2006) Gene and protein characteristics reflect functional diversity of CD56dim and CD56bright NK cells. J Leukoc Biol 80:1529–1541

Wenisch C, Patruta S, Daxbock F, Krause R, Horl W (2000) Effect of age on human neutrophil function. J Leukoc Biol 67:40–45

Wilson LD, Zaldivar FP, Schwindt CD et al (2009) Circulating T-regulatory cells, exercise and the elite adolescent swimmer. Pediatr Exerc Sci 21(3): 305–317

Wong CM, Lai HK, Ou CQ et al (2008) Is exercise protective against influenza-associated mortality? PLoS One 3(5):e2108

Woods JA, Ceddia MA, Wolters BW et al (1999) Effects of 6 months of moderate aerobic exercise training on immune function in the elderly. Mech Ageing Dev 109(1):1–19

Woods J, Lu Q, Ceddia MA, Lowder T (2000) Special feature for the Olympics: effects of exercise on the immune system: exercise-induced modulation of macrophage function. Immunol Cell Biol 78:545–553

Woods JA, Keylock KT, Lowder T et al (2009) Cardiovascular exercise training extends influenza vaccine seroprotection in sedentary older adults: the immune function intervention trial. J Am Geriatr Soc 57(12):2183–2191

Wu D, Meydani SN (2008) Age-associated changes in immune and inflammatory responses: impact of vitamin E intervention. J Leukoc Biol 84:900–914

Xu X, Beckman I, Bradley J (1993) Age-related changes in the expression of IL-2 and high-affinity IL-2 binding sites. Int Arch Allergy Immunol 102(3):224–231

Yan H, Kuroiwa A, Tanaka H et al (2001) Effect of moderate exercise on immune senescence in men. Eur J Appl Physiol 86(2):105–111

Yeh SH, Chuang H, Lin LW et al (2006) Regular tai chi chuan exercise enhances functional mobility and CD4CD25 regulatory T cells. Br J Sports Med 40(3): 239–243

Yeh SH, Chuang H, Lin LW et al (2009) Regular Tai Chi Chuan exercise improves T cell helper function of patients with type 2 diabetes mellitus with an increase in T-bet transcription factor and IL-12 production. Br J Sports Med 43(11):845–850

Index